FUNDAMENTAL NURSING SKILLS

8 - ob
· peds
@ Fri. night

Aug 24 - Clinical?
before lecture
maybe @

So Bend
Dr. maybe
on Sat.

2 problem
areas
writting
ND +
goals

meds
Pull meds before
melissa gets there
med sheet out
& ready to go

focus on
DV —

78 %
81
———
165
82
21165

Springhouse Corporation
Springhouse, Pennsylvania

STAFF

Executive Director, Editorial
Stanley Loeb

Senior Publisher
Matthew Cahill

Art Director
John Hubbard

Clinical Project Director
Patricia Dwyer Schull, RN, MSN

Editors
Stephen Daly, Edith McMahon, June Norris

Clinical Editors
Sandra Ludwig Nettina, RN,C, MSN; Linda Roy, RN, MSN, CCRN; Julie N. Tackenberg, RN, MA, CNRN; Beverly Ann Tscheschlog, RN; Nina Poorman Welsh, RN

Drug Information Editor
George J. Blake, RPh, MS

Copy Editors
Cynthia Breuninger (supervisor), Priscilla DeWitt, Terri Goshko, Nancy Papsin

Designers
Stephanie Peters (associate art director), Kristina Gabage

Illustrators
John Carlance, Jacalyn Facciolo, Jean Gardner, Bob Jackson, Nancy Lou Makris, Bob Neumann, Judy Newhouse, Mary Stangl, Larry Ward

Cover
Kevin Curry, Maria Errico (designers), John Gallagher (photographer)

Art Production
Robert Perry (manager), Heather Bernhardt, Donald Knauss, Robert Wieder

Typography
David Kosten (director), Diane E. Paluba (manager), Elizabeth Bergman, Joyce Rossi Biletz, Phyllis Marron, Robin Mayer, Valerie Rosenberger

Manufacturing
Deborah Meiris (director), T.A. Landis, Anna Brindisi

Production Coordination
Patricia McCloskey

Editorial Assistants
Maree DeRosa, Beverly Lane, Mary Madden

Material in this book was adapted from *Nursing Procedures*, ©1992 by Springhouse Corporation.

Library of Congress Cataloging-in-Publication Data

Fundamental nursing skills.
    p.   cm.
    Includes bibliographical references and index.
    1. Nursing   I. Springhouse Corporation.
    [DNLM: 1. Nursing Process. WY 100 F978 1993]
RT41.F875   1993
610.73—dc20
DNLM/DLC   93-17823
ISBN 0-87434-596-0   CIP

Printed in the United States of America.

FNS-010793

CONTENTS

CONTRIBUTORS AND CONSULTANTS

Ruth E. Blauer, RN, MS, CNA
Director, Education Department
Rutland (Vt.) Regional Medical Center

Vicki L. Buchda, RN, MS
Director, Special Care
Maryvale Samaritan Medical Center
Phoenix, Ariz.

Sherry Buffington, RN, CCRN, CLA (ASCP)
Staff nurse, ICCU
Doylestown (Pa.) Hospital

Dorothy A. Calabrese, RN, MSN, CURN
Clinical nurse specialist, urology and oncology
Cleveland Clinic Foundation

Carla M. Clark, RN, MS
Nurse research clinician
Good Samaritan Regional Medical Center
Phoenix, Ariz.

Bonita Gail Largent Cloyd, RN, BSN, CETN
Enterostomal therapist
Western Baptist Hospital
Paducah, Ky.

Shirley J. Edwards, RN, MSN, OCN
Clinical nurse specialist, oncology
Saint John's Hospital and Health Center
Santa Monica, Calif.

Marsha L. England, RN, CRNI, AA
Charge nurse, I.V. therapy
Saint John's Hospital and Health Center
Santa Monica, Calif.

Diane Broadbent Friedman, RN, MSN, CS
Research nurse coordinator
Milton S. Hershey Medical Center
Hershey, Pa.

Jan Fuchs, RN, MS, CNN
Head nurse
Peritoneal Dialysis Unit
Cleveland Clinic Foundation

Jean B. Gordon, RN, OCN
Oncology clinical instructor
Saint Barnabas Medical Center
Livingston, N.J.

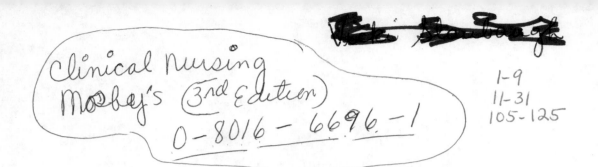

FUNDAMENTAL NURSING SKILLS

Susan J. Hart, RN,C, MSN, CCRN
Clinical nurse specialist, critical care
Saint Barnabas Medical Center
Livingston, N.J.

Charles Krozek, RN, BA, MN
Nursing education coordinator
Saint John's Hospital and Health Center
Santa Monica, Calif.

Kathleen M. Malloch, RN, BS, MBA, CNA
Clinical nursing administrator
Maryvale Samaritan Medical Center
Phoenix, Ariz.

Clara Martin, RN
Infection control assistant
Texas Children's Hospital
Houston

Rebecca M. McCaskey, RN, BA, MEd
Clinical nurse educator
Warren Grant Magnuson Clinical Center
National Institutes of Health
Bethesda, Md.

Karen M.J. McCleave, RN, MS, CFNP, CIC
Supervisor, employee health and infection control
Maryvale Samaritan Medical Center
Phoenix, Ariz.

Cheryl Milford, RN, MS, CCRN
Nursing staff development specialist
Ohio State University, Columbus

Mary Beth Modic, RN, MSN
Quality monitor, nursing quality management
Cleveland Clinic Foundation

Carolyn J. Montgomery, MDiv, ThM
Chaplain
Doylestown (Pa.) Hospital

Deirdre P. Mountjoy, RN, MS
Staff development instructor
Maryvale Samaritan Medical Center
Phoenix, Ariz.

Jody Pelusi, RN, MSN, OCN, RT
Clinical nurse specialist, oncology
Maryvale Samaritan Medical Center
Phoenix, Ariz.

Anna Pignanelli, BSN
Clinical instructor, surgical and oncology nursing
Cleveland Clinic Foundation

Marla J. Prizant-Weston, RN, MS, CCRN
Clinical nurse specialist, critical care
Desert Samaritan Medical Center
Phoenix, Ariz.

Frances W. Quinless, RN, PhD
Chair, Department of Nursing Education and Services
University of Medicine and Dentistry of New Jersey
Newark, N.J.

Susan F. Rudy, RN, BSN
Clinical coordinator, oral surgery and otolaryngology
Warren Grant Magnuson Clinical Center
National Institutes of Health
Bethesda, Md.

Ann Schneidman, RN, MS, NS
Pulmonary nurse consultant
Phoenix, Ariz.

Daniele Shollenberger, RN, MSN
Clinical nurse specialist
Allentown Hospital-Lehigh Valley Hospital Center
Allentown, Pa.

Marylou Nesbitt Snow, RN, MS, OCN
Clinical nurse specialist, oncology
Desert Samaritan Medical Center
Mesa, Ariz.

Dori Taylor, RN, PhD, CNA
Director, nursing education and research
Assistant clinical professor
John Dempsey Hospital
University of Connecticut, Farmington

Kathryn I. Weber, RN
Staff nurse, I.V. Therapy
Saint John's Hospital and Health Center
Santa Monica, Calif.

FOREWORD

Whether you're a nursing student or a practicing nurse, *Fundamental Nursing Skills* will help you master essential clinical techniques. This definitive one-volume resource explains and shows how to perform virtually every fundamental nursing procedure—nearly 200 in all. What's more, the volume uses the nursing process to provide you with the concepts and skills necessary for today's nursing practice.

Fundamental Nursing Skills opens with six chapters devoted to broad nursing topics: fundamental procedures (including comprehensive guidelines for a systematic head-to-toe patient assessment), infection control, specimen collection for diagnostic testing, physical treatments, drug administration, and intravascular therapy. The following seven chapters cover procedures related to specific body systems. Throughout all of the chapters, more than 500 illustrations, photographs, and charts enhance the text. In fact, several common procedures, such as nasogastric tube insertion and cardiopulmonary resuscitation, contain step-by-step photographic or illustrated directions.

To help you use this book, each nursing skill is covered in the same easy-to-follow format. Each starts with an introduction that defines and briefly describes the procedure, explains its purpose, and points out any contraindications.

Next, *Equipment* lists all the items you'll need to perform the procedure and, where appropriate, identifies the items available as kits. *Preparation of equipment,* which follows, explains all the steps that must be taken to ensure the procedure's effectiveness.

Implementation takes you step by step through the procedure in clear, concise style. Rationales, highlighted by *italicized type,* explain why each major step is performed. Where necessary, you'll also find suggestions for patient teaching and discharge planning. Next, *Special considerations* lists additional concerns related to the procedure, such as ways to avoid common problems, variations in performing the procedure, warnings and, where appropriate, insights from the latest medical and nursing research.

When appropriate, the *Complications* section alerts you to possible patient problems resulting from the procedure. Finally, *Documentation* tells you about procedure-specific items that should be included in your notes or on the patient's medical record. Besides fostering professional responsibility and accountability, accurate and complete documentation is essential for meeting regulatory standards and determining accurate reimbursement. And it helps you avoid potential legal problems.

Throughout the book, special graphic devices called logos draw your attention to important recurring topics. For example, all emergency procedures in the book, such as cardiopulmonary resuscitation, are identified by a special symbol at their start. Another logo identifies the topic of home care. Still another logo, *Equipment,* explains and sometimes shows devices, such as those for intermittent infusion. *Troubleshooting* alerts you to equipment problems that may arise and explains how to prevent or correct them.

Fundamental Nursing Skills is an essential addition to your clinical library, whether you're a nursing student, a practicing nurse, a nurse educator, or an administrator. It's also indispensable for any nurse returning to practice. Designed to save you time and improve your skills and confidence, this book will help you give quality patient care in any setting.

Marguerite K. Schlag, RN, MSN, EdD
　Director, Nursing Education and Development
　Robert Wood Johnson University Hospital
　New Brunswick, N.J.

FUNDAMENTAL NURSING SKILLS

CHAPTER 1

FUNDAMENTAL PROCEDURES

FRANCES W. QUINLESS, RN, PhD
RUTH E. BLAUER, RN, MS, CNA

Introduction

Patients come to hospitals because they need skilled clinical observation and treatment. According to the American Hospital Association, about 37 million people undergo hospitalization each year, and for most, it's a trying experience. After all, hospitalization challenges the patient's sense of privacy and control of his life. He must relinquish at least part of his normal routine. He must rely on you and your co-workers to meet his fundamental needs. Depending on the complexity of his health problem, he and his family may also require teaching, counseling, coordination of services, development of community support systems, and help in coping with health-related changes in his life.

In many hospitals, staff nurses, primary nurses, and clinical nurse specialists deliver all these vital services. This chapter serves as a starting point to help you understand and perform many of these tasks confidently and effectively. It thoroughly covers all the fundamentals: admission, transfer and discharge procedures; assessment (including a section on writing a nursing care plan); ensuring patient safety and mobility (including proper use of restraints and assistive devices); practicing correct body mechanics and patient transfer techniques; and using special orthopedic beds. The chapter also includes a comprehensive review of personal hygiene and comfort measures, nutrition, elimination, surgical care, spiritual care, and postmortem care.

Before turning to these nursing care specifics, however, review the broader aims of your care, such as helping the patient cope with restricted mobility; giving him a comfortable, stimulating environment; making sure his hospital stay is free of hazards; promoting an uneventful recovery; and helping him return to his normal life.

Dealing with restricted mobility

Whenever a patient's condition impairs or prevents mobility, your nursing goals are to promote his independence by motivating him and helping him set goals, to prevent injury and the complications of immobility, to teach him needed skills, and to foster a positive body image, especially if he faces long-term or permanent immobility.

Promoting a comfortable environment

By manipulating physical factors in the patient's environment—temperature, humidity, lighting—you can affect his comfort, condition, and at times, his response to treatment. For example, a room temperature of 68° to 72° F (20° to 22° C) and a relative humidity of 30% to 60%, although comfortable for most patients, may be too cold for elderly patients. Also, proper artificial or natural lighting helps duplicate the day-night cycle.

Providing sensory stimulation

Sensory stimulation (such as therapeutic touch) contributes to patient well-being. Although the amount and type of required stimulation varies with each patient, you can prevent sensory overload or deprivation by accurately assessing his needs. When evaluating stimuli in the patient's environment, remember that illness is a stressor that may intensify the patient's responses, especially to noise and odors.

Promoting safety

Besides weakening the patient, illness and any accompanying treatment may impair his judgment and contribute to accidents. Be alert to hazards in the patient's environment and teach him and his family to recognize them. When caring for a patient with restricted mobility, you must help him as he is moved, lifted, and transported. By using proper body mechanics and appropriate assistive devices, you can prevent injury, fatigue, and discomfort for your patient and yourself.

Preventing complications

For the bedridden patient, immobility poses special hazards, such as pressure on bony prominences; venous, pulmonary, and urinary stasis; and disuse of muscles and joints. These can lead to such complications as pressure ulcers, thrombi, phlebitis, pneumonia, urinary calculi, and contractures. To prevent complications, be sure to use correct positioning, meticulous skin care, assistive devices, and regular turning and range-of-motion exercises.

Promoting rehabilitation

The first step toward rehabilitation typically is progressive ambulation, which should begin as soon as possible—if necessary, using such assistive devices as a cane, crutches, or a walker. Effective rehabilitation also may require you to teach positioning, transfer, and mobilization techniques to the patient and his family. Demonstrating a technique—such as transfer from bed to wheelchair—during hospitalization helps the patient and his family to understand it. Allowing them to practice it under your supervision gives them the confidence to perform it at home. Encourage them to provide positive reinforcement to motivate the patient to work toward his goals.

ADMISSION, TRANSFER, AND DISCHARGE PROCEDURES
Admission

Admission to the nursing unit prepares the patient for his hospital stay. Whether the admission is scheduled or follows emergency treatment, effective admission procedures should accomplish the following goals: verify the patient's identity and assess his clinical status, make him as comfortable as possible in his new and potentially threatening environment, introduce him to roommates and staff, orient him to the physical environment and routine activities, and provide supplies and special equipment needed for daily care.

Because admission procedures can color the patient's perception of the hospital environment, they have a significant impact on subsequent treatment. Admission routines that are efficient and show appropriate concern for the patient ease his anxiety and promote cooperation and receptivity to treatment. Conversely, admission routines that the patient perceives as careless or excessively impersonal can heighten anxiety, reduce cooperation, impair his response to treatment, and perhaps aggravate symptoms.

Equipment
Hospital gown ■ personal property form ■ valuables envelope ■ admission form ■ nursing assessment form, if appropriate ■ thermometer ■ emesis basin ■ bedpan or urinal ■ bath basin ■ water pitcher, cup, and tray ■ urine specimen container, if needed.

An admission pack usually contains soap, comb, toothbrush, toothpaste, mouthwash, water pitcher, cup, tray, lotion, facial tissues, and thermometer (if you won't be using an electronic thermometer). Because the patient's pack is included in his hospital bill, he can take it home at the end of his stay. An admission pack helps prevent cross-contamination and increases nursing efficiency by providing basic items at each patient's bedside.

Implementation
• Obtain a gown and an admission pack for the patient.
• Position the bed as the patient's condition requires. If the patient is ambulatory, place the bed in the low position; if he is arriving on a stretcher, place the bed in the high position. Fold down the top linens.
• Adjust the lights, temperature, and ventilation in the room. If the patient requires emergency or special equipment, such as oxygen or suction, prepare it for use.

Admitting the adult patient
• When the patient arrives on the unit, greet him by his proper name and introduce yourself and any staff present. Be sure to speak slowly and clearly.
• Compare the name and hospital number on the patient's identification bracelet with that listed on the admission form. Verify the name and its spelling with the patient. Notify the admission office of any corrections.
• Quickly review the admission form and the doctor's orders. Note the reason for admission, any restrictions on activity or diet, and any orders for diagnostic tests requiring specimen collection.
• Escort the patient to his room and, if he's not in great distress, introduce him to his roommate. Then wash your hands and help him change into a hospital gown or pajamas; if the patient is sharing a room, provide privacy. Itemize all valuables, clothing, and prostheses on the nursing assessment form; if your hospital doesn't use such a form, itemize the patient's belongings in your notes. Encourage the patient to store valuables or money in the hospital safe or, preferably, to send them home along with any medications he may have brought. Show the ambulatory patient where the bathroom and closets are located.
• Take and record the patient's vital signs, and collect specimens if ordered. Measure the patient's height and weight if his condition allows it. If the patient can't stand, use a chair or bed scale and ask him his height. *Knowing the patient's height and weight is important for planning treatment and diet and for calculating medication and anesthetic dosages.*
• Show the patient how to use the equipment in his room. Be sure to include the call system, bed controls, TV controls, telephone, and lights.
• Explain the hospital routine. Tell the patient when to expect meals, vital sign checks, and medications. Inform him of the visiting hours and of any restrictions on visiting.
• Take a complete patient history. Include all previous hospitalizations, illnesses, and surgeries; current drug therapy; and food or drug allergies. Ask the patient to tell you why he came to the hospital. Record the answers (in the patient's own words) as the chief complaint. Follow up with a physical assessment, emphasizing complaints. If you discover any marks, bruises, or discolorations, record them on the nursing assessment form.
• After assessing the patient, inform him of any tests that have been ordered and when they're scheduled. Describe what he should expect.
• Before leaving the patient's room, make sure he's comfortable and safe. Adjust his bed, and place the call button and other equipment (such as water pitcher and cup,

emesis basin, and facial tissues) within easy reach. Raise the side rails.
• Post patient care reminders (concerning such topics as allergies or special needs) at the patient's bedside *to notify co-workers*. (See *Using patient care reminders* for examples.)

Admitting the pediatric patient
• Your initial goal will be to establish a friendly, trusting relationship with the child and his parents *to help relieve fears and anxiety, which can hinder treatment*. Remember that a child under age 3 may fear separation from his parents; an older child may worry about what will happen to him in the hospital.
• Speak directly to the child, and allow him to answer questions before obtaining more information from his parents.
• While orienting the parents and child to the unit, describe the layout of the room and bathroom, and tell them the location of the playroom, television room, and snack room, if available.
• Teach the child how to call the nurse. Stress that she will be available at all times to take care of all his needs, such as getting him a drink or helping him to the bathroom.
• Explain the institution's rooming-in and visiting policies *so the parents can take every opportunity to be with their child*.
• Inquire about the child's usual routine *so that favorite foods, bedtime rituals, toileting, and adequate rest can be incorporated into the hospital routine*.
• Encourage the parents to bring some of their child's favorite toys, blankets, or other items to the hospital *to make the child feel more at home amid unfamiliar surroundings*.

Special considerations
If the patient doesn't speak English and isn't accompanied by a bilingual family member, contact the appropriate resource (usually the social services department) to secure an interpreter.

Keep in mind that the patient admitted to the emergency department (ED) requires different procedures than the patient admitted to other departments. (See *Managing emergency admissions,* page 6.)

If the patient brings medication from home, take an inventory and record this information on the nursing assessment form. Instruct the patient not to take any medication unless authorized by the doctor. Send authorized medication to the hospital pharmacy for identification and relabeling. Send other medication home with a responsible family member, or store it in the designated area outside the patient's room until he's discharged. *Use*

Using patient care reminders

When placed at the head of the patient's bed, care reminders call attention to the patient's special needs and help ensure consistent care by communicating these needs to the hospital staff, the patient's family, and other visitors.

You can use a specially designed card or a plain piece of paper to post *important information* about the patient, such as the following:
• Allergies
• Dietary restrictions
• Fluid restrictions
• Specimen collection
• Patient deaf or hearing-impaired in right or left ear
• Foreign-language speaker

You can also use care reminders to post *special instructions,* such as the following:
• Complete bed rest
• No BP on right arm
• Turn q 1 hour
• NPO
• I & O

Never violate the patient's privacy by posting his diagnosis, details about surgery, or any information he might find embarrassing.

---

of unauthorized medication may interfere with treatment or cause an overdose.

Find out the patient's normal routine, and ask him if he would like to make any adjustments to the hospital regimen; for instance, he may prefer to shower at night instead of in the morning. *By accommodating the patient with such adjustments whenever possible, you can ease his anxiety and help him feel more in control of his potentially threatening situation.*

Documentation
After leaving the patient's room, complete the nursing assessment form or your notes, as specified by your institution. The completed form should include the patient's vital signs, height, weight, allergies, and drug and health history; a list of his belongings and those that he sent home with family members; the results of your physical assessment (see "Physical assessment" elsewhere in this chapter); and a record of specimens collected for diagnostic tests.

Managing emergency admissions

For the patient admitted through the emergency department (ED), treating his immediate needs overshadows routine admission procedures. After ED treatment, the patient arrives on the nursing unit with a temporary identification bracelet, a doctor's order sheet, and a record of treatment. Read this record and talk to the nurse who cared for the patient in the ED to ensure continuity of care and to gain insight into the patient's condition and behavior.

Next, record any ongoing treatment, such as an I.V. infusion, in your notes. Take and record the patient's vital signs, and follow the doctor's orders for treatment. If the patient is conscious and not in great distress, explain any treatment orders. Otherwise, delay your explanation. If family members accompany the patient, ask them to wait in the lounge while you assess the patient and begin treatment. Permit them to visit the patient after he's settled in his room. When the patient's condition allows, proceed with routine admission procedures.

Transfer

Patient transfer—either within the hospital or to another care facility—requires thorough preparation and careful documentation. Preparation includes an explanation of the transfer to the patient and his family, discussion of the patient's condition and care plan with the staff at the receiving unit or facility, and arrangements for transportation if necessary. Documentation of the patient's condition before and during transfer and adequate communication between nursing staffs ensure continuity of nursing care and provide legal protection for the transferring hospital and its staff.

Equipment
Admission inventory of belongings ■ patient's chart, medication record, and nursing Kardex ■ medications ■ bag or suitcase.

Implementation
• Explain the transfer to the patient and his family. Assess his physical condition *to determine the means of transfer,* such as a wheelchair or a stretcher.

• Using the admissions inventory of belongings as a checklist, collect the patient's property. Be sure to check the entire room, including the closet, bedside stand, overbed table, and bathroom. If the patient is being transferred to another facility, don't forget valuables or personal medications that have been stored.
• Gather the patient's medications from the cart and the refrigerator. If the patient is being transferred to another unit, send them to the receiving unit; if he's being transferred to another facility, return them to the hospital pharmacy.
• Notify the hospital's business office and other appropriate departments of the transfer.
• Have a staff person notify the dietary department, the pharmacy, and the hospital telephone operator of the transfer (if within the hospital).
• Contact the nursing staff on the receiving unit, and review the patient's condition, drug regimen, and nursing care plan with them *to ensure continuity of care.*

Transfer within the hospital
• If the patient is being transferred from or to an intensive care unit, your hospital may require new care orders from the patient's doctor. If so, review the new orders with the nursing staff at the receiving unit.
• Send the patient's chart, laboratory request slips, Kardex, special equipment, and other required materials to the receiving unit.
• Use a wheelchair to transport the ambulatory patient to the newly assigned room unless it's on the same unit as his present one, in which case he may be allowed to walk. Use a stretcher to transport the bedridden patient.
• Introduce the patient to the nursing staff at the receiving unit. Then take the patient to his room and, depending on his condition, place him in the bed or seat him in a chair. Introduce him to his new roommate, if appropriate, and tell him about any unfamiliar equipment in the room.

Transfer to an extended care facility
• Make sure the patient's doctor has written the transfer order on his chart and has completed the special transfer form. This form should include the patient's diagnosis, care summary, drug regimen, and special care instructions, such as diet and physical therapy.
• Complete the nursing summary, including the patient's assessment, progress, required nursing treatments, and special needs, *to ensure continuity of care.*
• Keep one copy of the transfer form and the nursing summary with the patient's chart, and forward the other copies to the receiving facility. However, don't send the patient's medications, Kardex, or chart.

Transfer to an acute care facility

• Make sure the doctor has written the transfer order on the patient's chart and has completed the transfer form as discussed above. Then complete the nursing summary.

• Depending on the doctor's instructions, send one copy of the transfer form and the nursing summary and photocopies of the pertinent excerpts from the patient's chart — such as laboratory test and X-ray results, patient history and physical progress notes, and vital sign records — to the receiving facility with the patient. Or, following your facility's policy, substitute a written summary of the patient's condition and hospital history for the excerpts from the patient's chart. *This information legally protects the transferring hospital and its staff and completes the patient's chart.*

Special considerations

If the patient requires an ambulance to take him to another facility, arrange transportation with the hospital's social services department. Ensure that the necessary equipment is assembled to provide care during transport.

Documentation

Record the time and date of transfer, the patient's condition during transfer, the name of the receiving unit or facility, and the means of transportation.

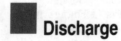

Discharge

Although discharge from the hospital is usually considered routine, effective discharge requires careful planning and continuing assessment of the patient's needs during his hospitalization. Ideally, discharge planning begins shortly after admission. Discharge planning aims to teach the patient and his family about his illness and its effect on his life-style; to provide instructions for home care; to communicate dietary or activity instructions; and to explain the purpose, adverse effects, and scheduling of drug treatment. It can also include arranging for transportation, follow-up care if necessary, and coordination of outpatient or home health care services.

Equipment

Wheelchair, unless the patient leaves by ambulance ■ patient's chart ■ patient instruction sheet ■ discharge summary sheet ■ plastic bag or patient's suitcase for personal belongings.

Dealing with a discharge against medical advice

Occasionally, the patient or his family may demand discharge against medical advice (AMA). If this occurs, notify the doctor immediately. If the doctor fails to convince the patient to remain in the hospital, he'll ask the patient to sign an AMA form releasing the hospital from legal responsibility for any medical problems the patient may experience after discharge.

If the doctor isn't available, discuss the discharge form with the patient and obtain his signature. If the patient refuses to sign the AMA form, don't detain him. *This violates his legal rights.* After the patient leaves, document the incident thoroughly in your notes and notify the doctor.

Implementation

• Before the day of discharge, inform the patient's family of the time and date of discharge. If his family can't arrange transportation, notify the social services department. (Always confirm arranged transportation on the day of discharge.)

• Obtain a written discharge order from the doctor. If the patient discharges himself against medical advice, obtain the appropriate hospital form. (See *Dealing with a discharge against medical advice.*)

• If the patient requires home medical care, confirm arrangements with the appropriate community agency or hospital department.

• On the day of discharge, review the patient's discharge care plan, initiated on admission and modified during his hospitalization, with the patient and his family. List prescribed drugs on the patient instruction sheet along with the dosage, prescribed time schedule, and adverse reactions that he should report to the doctor. Ensure that the drug schedule is consistent with the patient's life-style *to prevent improper administration and to promote patient compliance.* (See *Discharge teaching goals,* page 8.)

• Review procedures the patient or his family will perform at home. If necessary, demonstrate these procedures, provide written instructions, and check performance with a return demonstration.

• List dietary and activity instructions, if applicable, on the patient instruction sheet, and review the reasons for them. If the doctor orders bed rest, make sure the patient's family can provide daily care and will obtain necessary equipment.

Discharge teaching goals

Your discharge teaching should aim to ensure that the patient:
□ understands his illness
□ complies with his drug therapy
□ carefully follows his diet
□ manages his activity level
□ understands his treatments
□ recognizes his need for rest
□ knows about possible complications
□ knows when to seek follow-up care.
  Remember that your discharge teaching must include the patient's family or other caregivers to ensure that the patient receives proper home care.

• Check with the doctor about the patient's next office appointment; if the doctor hasn't yet done so, inform the patient of the date, time, and location. If scheduling is your responsibility, make an appointment with the doctor, outpatient clinic, physical therapy, X-ray department, or other health services, as needed. If the patient can't arrange transportation, notify the social services department.
• Retrieve the patient's valuables from the hospital safe and review each item with him. Then obtain the patient's signature *to verify receipt of his valuables.*
• Obtain from the pharmacy any drugs the patient brought to the hospital. Return these to the patient if drug therapy is unchanged. If giving a new prescription, provide an explanation of the dosage, schedule, and adverse effects.
• If appropriate, take and record the patient's vital signs on the discharge summary form. Notify the doctor if any signs are abnormal, such as an elevated temperature. *If necessary, the doctor may alter the patient's discharge plan.*
• Help the patient get dressed if necessary.
• Collect the patient's personal belongings from his room, compare them with the admission inventory of belongings, and help place them in his suitcase or a plastic bag.
• After checking the room for misplaced belongings, help the patient into the wheelchair, and escort him to the hospital's exit; if the patient is leaving by ambulance, help him onto the litter. If the patient's family hasn't already made arrangements for payment, contact the business office.
• After the patient has left the area, strip the bed linens and notify the housekeeping staff that the room is ready for terminal cleaning.

Special considerations
Whenever possible, involve the patient's family in discharge planning *so they can better understand and perform patient care procedures.* Before the patient is discharged, perform a physical assessment. If you detect abnormal signs or the patient develops new symptoms, notify the doctor and delay discharge until he has seen the patient.

Documentation
Although hospital policy determines the extent and form of discharge documentation, you'll usually record the time and date of discharge, the patient's physical condition, special dietary or activity instructions, the type and frequency of home care procedures, the patient's drug regimen, the dates of follow-up appointments, the mode of departure and name of the patient's escort, and a summary of the patient's hospitalization if necessary.

ASSESSMENT
Temperature

Body temperature represents the balance between heat produced by metabolism, muscular activity, and other factors and heat lost through the skin, lungs, and body wastes. A stable temperature pattern promotes proper function of cells, tissues, and organs; a change in this pattern usually signals the onset of illness.

Temperature can be measured with a mercury, a digital electronic, or a chemical-dot thermometer. Oral temperature in adults normally ranges from 97° to 99.5° F (36.1° to 37.5° C); rectal temperature, the most accurate reading, is usually 1° F higher; axillary temperature, the least accurate, reads 1° to 2° F (0.6° to 1.1° C) lower.

Temperature normally fluctuates with rest and activity. Lowest readings typically occur between 4 and 5 a.m.; the highest readings occur between 4 and 8 p.m. Other factors also influence temperature, including sex, age, emotional condition, and environment. Keep the following principles in mind. Women normally have higher temperatures than men, especially during ovulation. Normal temperature is highest in neonates and lowest in elderly persons. Heightened emotions raise temperature; depressed emotions lower it. A hot external environment can raise temperature; a cold environment lowers it.

Equipment
Mercury or electronic thermometer for oral or rectal use, or chemical-dot thermometer ■ water-soluble lubricant or petroleum jelly (for rectal temperature) ■ facial tissue ■

Types of thermometers

TYPE	OPERATING PRINCIPLE	ADVANTAGES	DISADVANTAGES
Mercury			
Oral	Heat expands mercury.	• Easy to store • Inexpensive • Readily available • Eliminates risk of cross-contamination if used by one patient	• Accuracy varies despite manufacturers' efforts to standardize. • Breakage and cross-contamination may occur if the thermometer is used by multiple patients. • Temperature is recorded more slowly than with other types of thermometers. • The mercury column is difficult to read.
Rectal			
Electronic digital			
Institutional	Heat alters the amount of current running through a resistor.	• Rapid recording and easy-to-read temperature • Extremely accurate (institutional unit must be properly charged and calibrated) • Eliminates risk of glass breakage • Easy to store	• Institutional unit is expensive, but the nursing time saved may offset the cost. • Institutional unit requires periodic recharging and recalibration. • Cross-contamination may occur.
Individual			
Chemical-dot	Heat initiates a chemical reaction.	• Eliminates risk of cross-contamination and breakage • Records temperature faster than mercury thermometer	• Improper storage may cause an inaccurate reading. • An adapter is needed for rectal use. • The plastic strip in the patient's mouth may cause discomfort.

disposable thermometer sheath or probe cover (except for chemical-dot thermometer) ■ alcohol sponge.

Preparation of equipment
A thermometer may be included as part of the admission pack. If it is, keep it at the patient's bedside and, on discharge, allow him to take it home. Otherwise, obtain a thermometer from the nurse's station or central supply department, and bring it to the patient's bedside. If you use an electronic thermometer, make sure it has been recharged. (See *Types of thermometers.*)

Implementation
• Explain the procedure to the patient, and wash your hands.

Using a mercury thermometer

• Hold the thermometer between your thumb and index finger at the end opposite the bulb.

• If the thermometer has been soaking in a disinfectant, rinse it in cold water. *Rinsing removes chemicals that may irritate oral or rectal mucous membranes or axillary skin.* Avoid using hot water *because it expands the mercury, which could break the thermometer.* Using a twisting motion, wipe the thermometer from the bulb upward.

• Then quickly snap your wrist several times while holding the thermometer to shake it down. *Shaking causes the mercury to descend into the bulb.* The mercury will then expand in response to the patient's body temperature and be forced upward.

• To use a disposable sheath over the mercury thermometer, disinfect the thermometer with an alcohol sponge. Insert it into the disposable sheath opening, then twist to tear the seal at the dotted line. Pull it apart. *Using a sheath decreases contamination and reduces cleaning time.*

Using an electronic thermometer

• Insert the probe into a disposable probe cover. If taking a rectal temperature, lubricate the probe cover *to reduce friction and ease insertion.* Leave the probe in place until the maximum temperature appears on the digital display.

Using a chemical-dot thermometer

• Remove the thermometer from its protective dispenser case by grasping the handle end with your thumb and forefinger, moving the handle up and down to break the seal, and pulling the handle straight out. Be sure to keep the thermometer sealed until use *because opening it activates the dye dots.*

Taking an oral temperature

• Position the tip of the thermometer under the patient's tongue, as far back as possible, on either side of the frenulum linguae. *Placing the tip in this area promotes contact with abundant superficial blood vessels and contributes to an accurate reading.*

• Instruct the patient to close his lips but to avoid biting down with his teeth. *Biting can break a mercury thermometer, cutting the mouth or lips or causing ingestion of broken glass or mercury.*

• Leave a mercury thermometer in place for at least 2 minutes or a chemical-dot thermometer for 45 seconds *to register temperature,* or wait until the maximum temperature is displayed on the electronic thermometer. (With some electronic units, a buzzer sounds when the maximum temperature is reached; with others, a light appears.)

• For a mercury thermometer, remove and discard the disposable sheath, then read the temperature at eye level, noting it before shaking down the thermometer. For an electronic thermometer, note the temperature, then remove and discard the probe cover. For the chemical-dot thermometer, read the temperature as the last dye dot that has changed color, or fired, then discard the thermometer and its dispenser case.

Taking a rectal temperature

• Position the patient on his side with his top leg flexed, and drape him to provide privacy. Then fold back the bed linens to expose the anus.

• Squeeze the lubricant onto a facial tissue *to prevent contamination of the lubricant supply.*

• Lubricate about ½" (1.3 cm) of the thermometer tip for an infant or about 1½" (3.8 cm) for an adult. *Lubrication reduces friction and thus eases insertion.* This step may be unnecessary when using disposable rectal sheaths *because they're prelubricated.*

• Lift the patient's upper buttock, and insert the thermometer about ½" for an infant or 1½" for an adult. Gently direct the thermometer along the rectal wall toward the umbilicus. *This will avoid perforating the anus or rectum or breaking the thermometer. It also will help ensure an accurate reading because the thermometer will register hemorrhoidal artery temperature instead of fecal temperature.* Feces may increase the patient's apparent temperature *because of the heat given off during decomposition.*

• Hold the mercury thermometer in place for 2 to 3 minutes or the electronic thermometer until the maximum temperature is displayed. *Holding it prevents damage to rectal tissues caused by displacement or loss of the thermometer into the rectum. Note:* Electronic thermometers usually provide a separate rectal probe that may be color coded to distinguish it more easily from the oral probe.

• Carefully remove the thermometer, wiping it as necessary.

• Wipe the patient's anal area *to remove any lubricant or feces.*

Taking an axillary temperature

• Position the patient comfortably with the axilla exposed.

• Gently pat the axilla dry with a facial tissue *because moisture conducts heat.* Avoid harsh rubbing, *which generates heat.*

• Ask the patient to place his hand over his chest and to grasp his opposite shoulder, lifting his elbow.

• Position the thermometer in the axilla, with the tip pointing toward the patient's head.

• Tell the patient to continue grasping his shoulder and to lower his elbow and hold it against his chest. *This promotes skin contact with the thermometer.*

Contraindication — Any symptom or circumstance indic-
(Indicare: to point ating the inappropriateness of a
out) form of treatment otherwise advisable.

Pulse • **11**

• Leave a mercury thermometer in place for 10 minutes; leave an electronic thermometer in place until it displays the maximum temperature. Axillary temperature takes longer to register than oral or rectal temperature *because the thermometer isn't enclosed in a body cavity.*

• Grasp the end of the thermometer and remove it from the axilla.

Special considerations

Oral measurement is contraindicated in patients who are unconscious, disoriented, or seizure-prone; in young children and infants; and in patients with oral or nasal impairment that necessitates mouth breathing. Rectal measurement is contraindicated in patients with diarrhea, recent rectal or prostatic surgery or injury *because it may injure inflamed tissue,* or recent myocardial infarction *because anal manipulation may stimulate the vagus nerve, causing bradycardia or another rhythm disturbance.*

Drinking hot or cold liquids, chewing gum, or smoking may alter oral temperature readings. Wait 15 minutes after these activities before taking a temperature. Bathing may alter axillary temperature.

Use the same thermometer for repeated temperature taking *to avoid spurious variations caused by equipment differences.* Store chemical-dot thermometers in a cool area *because exposure to heat activates the dye dots.*

Don't avoid taking an oral temperature when the patient is receiving nasal oxygen *because oxygen administration raises oral temperature by only about 0.3° F (0.17° C).*

Documentation

Record the time, route, and temperature on the patient's chart.

Pulse

Blood pumped by the heart into an already-full aorta during ventricular contraction creates a fluid wave that travels from the heart to the peripheral arteries. This recurring wave—called a pulse—can be palpated at locations on the body where an artery crosses over bone or firm tissue. (See *Pulse points.*) In adults and children over age 3, the radial artery in the wrist is the most common palpation site because it's easily accessible and the artery can be compressed readily against the radius. In infants and children under age 3, a stethoscope is used to listen to the heart itself rather than palpating a pulse. Because auscultation is done at the heart's apex, this is called the apical pulse.

Pulse points

Shown below are anatomic locations where an artery crosses bone or firm tissue and can be palpated for a pulse.

An apical-radial pulse is taken by simultaneously counting apical and radial beats—the first by auscultation at the apex of the heart, the second by palpation at the radial artery. Some heartbeats detected at the apex aren't strong enough to be detected at peripheral sites. When this occurs, the apical pulse rate is higher than the radial; the difference between the two rates is the pulse deficit.

Pulse taking involves determining the rate (number of beats per minute), rhythm (pattern or regularity of the beats), and volume (amount of blood pumped with each beat). If the pulse is faint or weak, use a Doppler ultrasound blood flow detector if available. (See *Detecting blood flow with Doppler ultrasound,* page 12.)

Detecting blood flow with Doppler ultrasound

More sensitive than palpation for determining pulse rate, the Doppler ultrasound blood flow detector is especially useful when a pulse is faint or weak. Unlike palpation, which detects arterial wall expansion and retraction, this instrument detects the motion of red blood cells.

Doppler probe with amplifier

To use the Doppler device
• Apply a small amount of coupling gel or transmission gel (not water-soluble lubricant) to the ultrasound probe.
• Position the probe on the skin directly over the selected artery. In the top illustration, the probe is over the posterior tibial artery.
• When using a Doppler model like the one in the top illustration, turn the instrument on and, moving counterclockwise, set the volume control to the lowest setting. If your model doesn't have a speaker, plug in the earphones and slowly raise the volume. The Doppler ultrasound stethoscope shown at lower right is basically a stethoscope fitted with an audio unit, volume control, and transducer, which amplifies the movement of red blood cells.
• To obtain the best signals with either device, tilt the probe 45 degrees from the artery, making sure to put gel between the skin and the probe. Slowly move the probe in a circular motion to locate the center of the artery and the Doppler signal—a hissing noise at the heartbeat. Avoid moving the probe rapidly because this distorts the signal.
• Count the signals for 60 seconds to determine the pulse rate.
• After you've measured the pulse rate, clean the probe with a soft cloth soaked in antiseptic solution or soapy water. Don't immerse the probe or bump it against a hard surface.

Doppler ultrasound stethoscope

Equipment
Watch with second hand ▪ stethoscope (for auscultating apical pulse) ▪ Doppler ultrasound blood flow detector if necessary.

Preparation of equipment
If you're not using your own stethoscope, disinfect the earpieces with an alcohol sponge before and after use *to prevent cross-contamination.*

Implementation
• Wash your hands, and tell the patient that you intend to take his pulse.

• Make sure the patient is comfortable and relaxed *because an awkward, uncomfortable position may affect the heart rate.*

Taking a radial pulse
• Place the patient in a sitting or supine position, with his arm at his side or across his chest.
• Gently press your index, middle, and ring fingers on the radial artery, inside the patient's wrist. You should feel a pulse with only moderate pressure; *excessive pressure may obstruct blood flow distal to the pulse site.* Don't use your thumb to take the patient's pulse *because its own strong pulse may be confused with the patient's.*

Identifying pulse patterns

TYPE	RATE	RHYTHM (PER 3 SECONDS)	CAUSES AND INCIDENCE
Normal	60 to 80 beats/minute; in neonates, 120 to 140 beats/minute	● ● ● ●	• Varies with such factors as age, physical activity, and sex (men usually have lower pulse rates than women)
Tachycardia	Above 100 beats/minute	●●●●●●●	• Accompanies stimulation of the sympathetic nervous system by emotional stress—anger, fear, anxiety—or certain drugs, such as caffeine • May result from exercise and from certain health conditions, such as congestive heart failure, anemia, and fever (which increases oxygen requirements and therefore pulse rate)
Bradycardia	Below 60 beats/minute	● ● ●	• Accompanies stimulation of the parasympathetic nervous system by drugs—especially digitalis—and such conditions as cerebral hemorrhage and heart block • May also be present in fit athletes
Irregular	Uneven time intervals between beats (for example, periods of regular rhythm interrupted by pauses or premature beats)	●●●● ●●●	• May indicate cardiac irritability, hypoxia, digitalis overdose, potassium imbalance, or sometimes more serious arrhythmias if frequent premature beats • Occasional premature beats normal

• After you've located the pulse, count the beats for 60 seconds, or, if it's more convenient, count for 30 seconds and multiply by 2. *Counting for a full minute provides a more accurate picture of irregularities.* While counting the rate, assess pulse rhythm and volume by noting the pattern and strength of the beats. If you detect an irregularity, repeat the count, *because pulse irregularities are important signs.* Note if the irregularity occurs in a pattern or randomly. If doubt remains, take an apical pulse. (See *Identifying pulse patterns.*)

Taking an apical pulse
• Help the patient to a supine position and drape him if necessary.
• Warm the diaphragm or bell of the stethoscope in your hand before applying it to the patient's chest. *Placing a cold stethoscope against the skin may startle the patient and momentarily increase the heart rate.* Keep in mind that the bell transmits low-pitched sounds more effectively than the diaphragm.
• Place the diaphragm or bell of the stethoscope over the apex of the heart, which normally is located at the fifth intercostal space left of the midclavicular line. Then insert the earpieces into your ears. Count the beats for 60 seconds (or count for 30 seconds and multiply by 2) and note their rhythm and volume. Also evaluate the intensity (loudness) of heart sounds.
• Remove the stethoscope and make the patient comfortable.

Taking an apical-radial pulse
• Two nurses work together to obtain the apical-radial pulse; one palpates the radial pulse while the other auscultates the apical pulse with a stethoscope. Both must use the same watch when counting beats.

• Help the patient to a supine position and drape him if necessary.
• Locate the apical and radial pulses.
• Determine a time to begin counting. Then each nurse should count beats for 60 seconds.

Special considerations
When the peripheral pulse is irregular, take an apical pulse to measure the heartbeat more directly. If the pulse is faint or weak, use a Doppler ultrasound blood flow detector if available.

If a second nurse is not available to help take an apical-radial pulse, you can hold the stethoscope in place with the hand that holds the watch while palpating the radial pulse with the other hand. You can then feel any discrepancies between the apical and radial pulses.

Documentation
Record pulse rate, rhythm, and volume and the time of measurement. "Full" or "bounding" describes a pulse of increased volume; "weak" or "thready," decreased volume. When recording apical pulse, include intensity of heart sounds. When recording apical-radial pulse, chart the rate according to the pulse site—for example, A/R pulse of 80/76.

Respiration

Controlled by the respiratory center in the lateral medulla oblongata, respiration is the exchange of oxygen and carbon dioxide between the atmosphere and body cells. External respiration, or breathing, is accomplished by the diaphragm and chest muscles and delivers oxygen to the lower respiratory tract and alveoli.

Four measures of respiration—rate, rhythm, depth, and sound—reflect the body's metabolic state, diaphragm and chest-muscle condition, and airway patency. Respiratory rate is recorded as the number of cycles (with inspiration and expiration comprising one cycle) per minute; rhythm, as the regularity of these cycles; depth, as the volume of air inhaled and exhaled with each respiration; and sound, as the audible digression from normal, effortless breathing.

Equipment
Watch with second hand.

Implementation
• The best time to assess your patient's respirations is immediately after taking the pulse rate. Keep your fingertips over the radial artery, and don't tell the patient you're counting respirations. If you tell him, *he'll become conscious of his respirations and the rate may change.*
• Count respirations by observing the rise and fall of the patient's chest as he breathes. Or position the patient's opposite arm across his chest and count respirations by feeling its rise and fall. Consider one rise and one fall as one respiration.
• Count respirations for 30 seconds and multiply by 2 or count for 60 seconds if respirations are irregular *to account for variations in respiratory rate and pattern.* As you count respirations, be alert for and record such breath sounds as stertor, stridor, wheezing, and an expiratory grunt. *Stertor* is a snoring sound resulting from secretions in the trachea and large bronchi. Listen for it in patients with neurologic disorders and in those who are comatose. *Stridor* is an inspiratory crowing sound that occurs with upper airway obstruction in laryngitis, croup, or the presence of a foreign body. When listening for stridor in infants and children with croup, also observe for sternal, substernal, or intercostal retractions. *Wheezing* is caused by partial obstruction in the smaller bronchi and bronchioles. This high-pitched, musical sound is common in patients with emphysema or asthma. In infants, an *expiratory grunt* indicates imminent respiratory distress. In older patients, it may result from partial airway obstruction or neuromuscular reflex.
• To detect other breath sounds—such as crackles and rhonchi—or the lack of sound in the lungs, you will need a stethoscope.
• Observe chest movements for depth of respiration. If the patient inhales a small volume of air, record this as shallow; if he inhales a large volume, record this as deep.
• Watch chest movements and listen to breathing *to determine the rhythm and sound of respiration.* (See *Identifying respiratory patterns.*)

Special considerations
Respiratory rates below 8 and above 40 breaths/minute usually are considered abnormal; report the sudden onset of such rates promptly. Observe for signs of dyspnea, such as an anxious facial expression, flaring nostrils, a heaving chest wall, and cyanosis. To detect cyanosis, look for characteristic bluish discoloration in the nail beds or the lips, under the tongue, in the buccal mucosa, or in the conjunctiva.

In assessing the patient's respiratory status, consider his personal and family history. Ask if he smokes and, if so, for how many years and how many packs a day.

A child's respiratory rate may double in response to exercise, illness, or emotion. Normally, the rate for newborns is 30 to 80 breaths/minute; for toddlers, 20 to 40;

Identifying respiratory patterns

TYPE	CHARACTERISTICS	PATTERN	POSSIBLE CAUSES
Apnea	Periodic absence of breathing		• Mechanical airway obstruction • Conditions affecting the brain's respiratory center in the lateral medulla oblongata
Apneustic	Prolonged, gasping inspiration, followed by extremely short, inefficient expiration		• Lesions of the respiratory center
Bradypnea	Slow, regular respirations of equal depth		• Normal pattern during sleep • Conditions affecting the respiratory center: tumors, metabolic disorders, respiratory decompensation; use of opiates and alcohol
Cheyne-Stokes	Fast, deep respirations of 30 to 170 seconds punctuated by periods of apnea lasting 20 to 60 seconds		• Increased intracranial pressure, severe congestive heart failure, renal failure, meningitis, drug overdose, cerebral anoxia
Eupnea	Normal rate and rhythm		• Normal respiration
Kussmaul's	Fast (over 20 breaths/minute), deep (resembling sighs), labored respirations without pause		• Renal failure or metabolic acidosis, particularly diabetic ketoacidosis
Tachypnea	Rapid respirations. Rate rises with body temperature—about four breaths/minute for every degree Fahrenheit above normal		• Pneumonia, compensatory respiratory alkalosis, respiratory insufficiency, lesions of the respiratory center, and salicylate poisoning

and for children of school age and older, 15 to 25. Children usually reach the adult rate (12 to 20) at about age 15.

Documentation
Record the rate, depth, rhythm, and sound of the patient's respirations.

Blood pressure

Defined as the lateral force exerted by blood on the arterial walls, blood pressure depends on the force of ventricular contractions, arterial wall elasticity, peripheral vascular resistance, and blood volume and viscosity. Systolic, or maximum, pressure occurs during left ventricular contraction and reflects the integrity of the heart, arteries, and arterioles. Diastolic, or minimum, pressure occurs during left ventricular relaxation and directly indicates blood vessel resistance.

Pulse pressure, the difference between systolic and diastolic pressures, varies inversely with arterial elasticity. Rigid vessels, incapable of distention and recoil, produce high systolic pressure and low diastolic pressure. Normally, systolic pressure exceeds diastolic pressure by about 40 mm Hg. Narrowed pulse pressure—a difference of less than 30 mm Hg—occurs when systolic pressure falls and diastolic pressure remains constant, when diastolic pressure rises and systolic pressure stays constant, or when systolic pressure falls and diastolic pressure rises. These changes reflect reduced stroke volume, increased peripheral resistance, or both. Widened pulse pressure—a difference of more than 50 mm Hg between systolic and diastolic blood pressures—occurs when systolic pressure rises and diastolic pressure remains constant, when diastolic pressure falls and systolic pressure remains constant, or when systolic pressure rises and diastolic pressure falls. These changes reflect increased stroke volume, decreased peripheral resistance, or both.

Blood pressure is measured in millimeters of mercury with a sphygmomanometer and a stethoscope, usually at the brachial artery (less often at the popliteal or radial artery). Lowest in the neonate, blood pressure rises with age, weight gain, prolonged stress, and anxiety. (See *Effects of age on blood pressure.)*

Frequent blood pressure measurement is critical after serious injury, surgery, or anesthesia and during any illness or condition that threatens cardiovascular stability. (This may be done with an automated vital signs monitor.) Regular measurement is indicated for patients with a history of hypertension or hypotension, and yearly screening is recommended for all adults.

Equipment

Mercury or aneroid sphygmomanometer ▪ stethoscope ▪ alcohol sponge ▪ automated vital signs monitor (if available).

The sphygmomanometer consists of an inflatable compression cuff linked to a manual air pump and a mercury manometer or an aneroid gauge. The mercury sphygmomanometer is more accurate and requires calibration less frequently than the aneroid model but is larger and heavier. To obtain an accurate reading, you must rest its gauge on a level surface and view the meniscus at eye level; you can rest an aneroid gauge in any position but must view it directly from the front. Some mercury manometers have specially designed cases that open to form a level surface; others must be attached to a wall or to a base unit that stands on the floor.

Hook, bandage, snap, or Velcro cuffs come in six standard sizes ranging from newborn to extra-large adult. Disposable cuffs are available.

The automated vital signs monitor is a noninvasive device that measures pulse rate, systolic and diastolic pressures, and mean arterial pressure at preset intervals. (See *Using an electronic vital signs monitor.)*

Preparation of equipment

Carefully choose a cuff of appropriate size for the patient. *An excessively narrow cuff may cause a falsely high pressure reading; an excessively wide one, a falsely low reading.* If you're not using your own stethoscope, disinfect the earpieces with an alcohol sponge before placing them in your ears *to avoid cross-contamination.*

To use an automated vital signs monitor, collect the monitor, dual air hose, and pressure cuff. Then make sure the monitor unit is firmly positioned near the patient's bed.

Implementation

- Tell the patient that you're going to take his blood pressure.
- The patient can lie supine or sit erect during blood pressure measurement. His arm should be extended at

Effects of age on blood pressure

AGE	BLOOD PRESSURE (mm Hg)
Neonate	systolic: 50 to 52 diastolic: 25 to 30 mean: 35 to 40
3 years	systolic: 78 to 114 diastolic: 46 to 78
10 years	systolic: 90 to 132 diastolic: 56 to 86
16 years	systolic: 104 to 108 diastolic: 60 to 92
Adult	systolic: 95 to 140 diastolic: 60 to 90
Older adult	systolic: 140 to 160 diastolic: 70 to 90

Using an electronic vital signs monitor

An electronic vital signs monitor allows you to track a patient's vital signs continually, without having to reapply a blood pressure cuff each time. What's more, the patient won't need an invasive arterial line to gather similar data. The machine shown here is a Dinamap VS Monitor 8100, but these steps can be followed with most other monitors.

Some automated vital signs monitors, such as the Dinamap, are lightweight and battery-operated, and can be attached to an I.V. pole for continual monitoring, even during patient transfers. Make sure you know the capacity of the monitor's battery, and plug the machine in whenever possible to keep it charged.

Before using any monitor, check its accuracy. Determine the patient's pulse rate and blood pressure manually, using the same arm you'll use for the monitor cuff. Compare your results when you get initial readings from the monitor. If the results differ, call your supply department or the manufacturer's representative.

Preparing the device
• Explain the procedure to the patient. Describe the alarm system *so he won't be frightened if it's triggered.*
• Make sure the power switch is off. Then plug the monitor into a properly grounded wall outlet. Next, secure the dual air hose to the front of the monitor.
• Connect the pressure cuff's tubing into the other ends of the dual air hose, and tighten connections *to prevent air leaks.* Keep the air hose away from the patient *to avoid accidental dislodgment.*
• Squeeze all air from the cuff, and wrap it loosely around the patient's arm or leg, allowing 2 fingerbreadths between cuff and arm or leg. Never apply the cuff to a limb that has an I.V. line in place. Position the cuff's "artery" arrow over the palpated brachial artery. Then secure the cuff for a snug fit.

Selecting parameters
• When you turn on the monitor, it will default to a manual mode. (In this mode, you can obtain vital signs yourself before switching to the automatic mode.) Press the "auto/manual" button to select the automatic mode. The monitor will give you baseline data for the pulse rate, systolic and diastolic pressures, and mean arterial pressure.
• Compare your previous manual results with these baseline data. If they match, you're ready to set the

alarm parameters. Press the "select" button to blank all displays except systolic pressure.
• Use the "high" and "low" limit buttons to set the specific parameters for systolic pressure. (These limits range from a high of 240 to a low of 0.) You'll also do this three more times for mean arterial pressure, pulse rate, and diastolic pressure. After you've set the parameters for diastolic pressure, press the "select" button again to display all current data. Even if you forget to do this last step, the monitor will automatically display current data 10 seconds after you set the last parameters.

Collecting data
• You also need to tell the monitor how often to obtain data. Press the "set" button until you reach the desired time interval in minutes. If you've chosen the automatic mode, the monitor will display a default cycle time of 3 minutes. You can override the default cycle time to set the interval you prefer.
• You can obtain a set of vital signs at any time by pressing the "start" button. Also, pressing the "cancel" button will stop the interval and deflate the cuff. You can retrieve stored data by pressing the "prior data" button. The monitor will display the last data obtained along with the time elapsed since then. Scrolling backward, you can retrieve data from the previous 99 minutes.

Positioning the blood pressure cuff

Wrap the cuff snugly around the upper arm above the antecubital area (the inner aspect of the elbow). When measuring an adult, place the lower border of the cuff about 1″ (2.5 cm) above the antecubital space. The center of the bladder should rest directly over the medial aspect of the arm. Most cuffs have an arrow for you to position over the brachial artery. Then, place the bell of the stethoscope on the brachial artery at the point where you hear the strongest beats.

Brachial artery

heart level and be well supported. *If the artery is below heart level, the blood pressure may read falsely high.* Be sure the patient is relaxed and comfortable when you take his blood pressure *so it stays at its normal level.*

• Wrap the deflated cuff snugly around the upper arm. (See *Positioning the blood pressure cuff* for specific instructions.)

• If necessary, connect the appropriate tube to the rubber bulb of the air pump and the other tube to the manometer. Then insert the stethoscope earpieces into your ears.

• Locate the brachial artery by palpation. Center the bell of the stethoscope over the part of the artery where you detect the strongest beats, and hold it in place with one hand. *The bell of the stethoscope transmits low-pitched arterial blood sounds more effectively than the diaphragm.*

• Using the thumb and index finger of your other hand, turn the thumbscrew on the rubber bulb of the air pump clockwise to close the valve.

• Then pump air into the cuff while auscultating the sound over the brachial artery *to compress and, eventually, occlude arterial blood flow.* Pump air until the mercury column or aneroid gauge registers 160 mm Hg or at least 10 mm Hg above the level of the last audible sound.

• Carefully open the valve of the air pump and slowly deflate the cuff—no faster than 5 mm Hg/second. While releasing air, watch the mercury column or aneroid gauge and auscultate the sound over the artery.

• When you hear the first beat or clear tapping sound, note the pressure on the column or gauge. This is the systolic pressure. (The beat or tapping sound is the first of five Korotkoff sounds. The second sound resembles a murmur or swish; the third sound, crisp tapping; the fourth sound, a soft, muffled tone; and the fifth, the last sound heard.)

• Continue to release air gradually while auscultating the sound over the artery.

• Note the diastolic pressure—the fourth Korotkoff sound. If you continue to hear sounds as the column or gauge falls to zero (common in children), record the pressure at the beginning of the fourth sound. This is important *because, in some patients, a distinct fifth sound is absent.*

• Rapidly deflate the cuff. Record the pressure, wait 15 to 30 seconds, then repeat the procedure and record the pressures *to confirm your original findings.* After doing so, remove and fold the cuff, and return it to storage.

Special considerations

If you can't auscultate blood pressure, you may estimate systolic pressure. To do this, first palpate the brachial or radial pulse. Then inflate the cuff until you no longer detect the pulse. Slowly deflate the cuff and, when you detect the pulse again, record the pressure as the palpated systolic pressure. When measuring blood pressure in the popliteal artery, position the patient on his abdomen; wrap a cuff around the middle of the thigh, and proceed with blood pressure measurement.

Palpation of systolic blood pressure also may be important *to avoid underestimating blood pressure in patients with an auscultatory gap.* This gap is a loss of sound between the first and second Korotkoff sounds that may be as great as 40 mm Hg. You may find this in patients with venous congestion or hypotension.

If your patient is crying or anxious, delay blood pressure measurement, if possible, until the patient becomes calm *to avoid falsely elevated readings.*

If your hospital considers the fourth and fifth Korotkoff sounds as the first and second diastolic pressures, record both pressures.

Remember that malfunction in an aneroid sphygmomanometer can be identified only by checking it against a mercury manometer of known accuracy. Be sure to check your aneroid manometer this way periodically. Malfunction in a mercury manometer is evident in abnormal behavior of the mercury column. Don't attempt to repair either type of sphygmomanometer yourself; instead, send

auscultate — listen

Correcting problems of blood pressure measurement

PROBLEM AND POSSIBLE CAUSE	NURSING ACTION
False-high reading	
• Cuff too small	• Make sure the cuff bladder is 20% wider than the circumference of the arm or leg being used for measurement.
• Cuff wrapped too loosely, reducing its effective width	• Tighten the cuff.
• Slow cuff deflation, causing venous congestion in the arm or leg	• Never deflate the cuff more slowly than 2 mm Hg/heartbeat.
• Tilted mercury column	• Read pressures with the mercury column vertical.
• Poorly timed measurement—after patient has eaten, ambulated, appeared anxious, or flexed arm muscles	• Postpone blood pressure measurement or help the patient relax before taking pressures.
False-low reading	
• Incorrect position of arm or leg	• Make sure the arm or leg is level with the patient's heart.
• Mercury column below eye level	• Read the mercury column at eye level.
• Failure to notice auscultatory gap (sound fades out for 10 to 15 mm Hg, then returns)	• Estimate systolic pressure by palpation before actually measuring it. Then check this pressure against the measured pressure.
• Inaudible low-volume sounds	• Before reinflating the cuff, instruct the patient to raise the arm or leg to decrease venous pressure and amplify low-volume sounds. After inflating the cuff, tell the patient to lower the arm or leg. Then deflate the cuff and listen. If you still fail to detect low-volume sounds, chart the palpated systolic pressure.

it to the appropriate service department. (See *Correcting problems of blood pressure measurement.)*

Occasionally, blood pressure must be measured in both arms or with the patient in two different positions (such as lying and standing, or sitting and standing). In such cases, observe and record any significant difference between the two readings and record the blood pressure, the extremity, and the position used.

Complications

Don't take blood pressure in the arm on the affected side of a mastectomy *because it may decrease already compromised lymphatic circulation, worsen edema, and damage the arm.* Likewise, don't take blood pressure on the same

arm of an arteriovenous fistula or hemodialysis shunt *because blood flow through the vascular device may be compromised.*

Documentation

On the patient's chart, record blood pressure as systolic over diastolic pressures, such as 120/78 mm Hg; if necessary, record systolic over the two diastolic pressures, such as 120/78/20 mm Hg. Chart an auscultatory gap if present. If required by your hospital, chart blood pressures on a graph, using dots or checkmarks. Also, document the extremity used and the patient's position.

Types of scales

For ambulatory patients

Standing scale

For acutely ill or debilitated patients

Chair scale

Bed scale

Height and weight

Height and weight are routinely measured for most patients during admission to the hospital. An accurate record of the patient's height and weight is essential for calculating dosages of drugs, anesthetics, and contrast agents; assessing the patient's nutritional status; and determining the height-weight ratio. And because body weight provides the best overall picture of fluid status, monitoring it daily proves important for patients receiving sodium-retaining or diuretic medications. Rapid weight gain may signal fluid retention; rapid weight loss may indicate diuresis.

Weight can be measured with a standing scale, chair scale, or bed scale; height can be measured with the measuring bar on a standing scale or with a tape measure for a supine patient.

Equipment
Scale—standing (with measuring bar), chair, or bed ■ wheelchair (if needed to transport patient) ■ tape measure if needed.

Preparation of equipment
Select the appropriate scale—usually, a standing scale for an ambulatory patient or a chair or bed scale for an acutely ill or debilitated patient. (See *Types of scales.*) Then check scale balance. Standing scales and, to a lesser extent, bed scales may become unbalanced when transported.

Implementation
• Explain the procedure to the patient. Refer to a chart of suggested healthy weight ranges *to determine norms for your patient's height and weight.* (See *Suggested weights for adults.)*

Suggested weights for adults

This chart provides a guideline for determining healthy weights. Higher weights in each category typically apply to men, who average more muscle and bone; lower weights usually apply to women, who have less muscle and bone. Suggested weights for people age 35 and over are higher than those for younger adults because recent research shows that older people can carry somewhat more weight without impairing their health. Height is measured without shoes; weight is measured without clothes.

HEIGHT	WEIGHT (LB)		HEIGHT	WEIGHT (LB)	
	Age 19 to 34	Age 35 and over		Age 19 to 34	Age 35 and over
5'0"	97 to 128	108 to 138	5'10"	132 to 174	146 to 188
5'1"	101 to 132	111 to 143	5'11"	136 to 179	151 to 194
5'2"	104 to 137	115 to 148	6'0"	140 to 184	155 to 199
5'3"	107 to 141	119 to 152	6'1"	144 to 189	159 to 205
5'4"	111 to 146	122 to 157	6'2"	148 to 195	164 to 210
5'5"	114 to 150	126 to 162	6'3"	152 to 200	168 to 216
5'6"	118 to 155	130 to 167	6'4"	156 to 205	173 to 222
5'7"	121 to 160	134 to 172	6'5"	160 to 211	177 to 228
5'8"	125 to 164	138 to 178	6'6"	164 to 216	182 to 234
5'9"	129 to 169	142 to 183			

Source: U.S. Department of Agriculture, U.S. Department of Health and Human Services. *Nutrition and Your Health: Dietary Guidelines for Americans,* 3rd ed. Washington, D.C., 1990.

Using a standing scale
• Place a paper towel on the scale's platform.
• Tell the patient to remove his robe and slippers or shoes *to ensure accurate measurement of height and weight.* If the scale has wheels, lock them before the patient steps on. Assist the patient onto the scale *to prevent falls.* Remain close to the patient *so you can steady him if necessary.*
• If you're using an upright balance (gravity) scale, slide the lower rider to the groove representing the largest increment below the patient's estimated weight. Grooves represent 50, 100, 150, and 200 lb (23, 45, 68, and 91 kg). Then slide the small upper rider until the beam balances. Add the upper and lower rider figures *to de-* termine the weight. (The upper rider is calibrated to eighths of a pound.)
• If you're using a multiple-weight scale, move the appropriate ratio weights onto the weight holder to balance the scale; ratio weights are labeled 50, 100, and 200 lb. Add ratio weights until the next weight causes the main beam to fall. Then adjust the main beam poise until the scale balances. Next, add the sum of the ratio weights to the figure on the main beam *to obtain the patient's weight.*
• Return ratio weights to their rack and the weight holder to its proper place.

• If you use a scale with a digital display, make sure the display reads 0 before use. Read the display with the patient on the scale and standing as still as possible.

• If you're measuring height, tell the patient to stand erect on the platform of the scale. Raise the measuring bar beyond the top of the patient's head, extend the horizontal arm, and lower the bar until it touches the top of the patient's head. Then read the patient's height.

• Help the patient off the scale, and give him his robe and slippers or shoes. Then return the measuring bar to its initial position.

Using a chair scale
• Transport the patient to the weighing area or the scale to the patient's bedside.

• Lock the scale in place *to prevent it from moving accidentally.*

• If you're using a scale with a swing-away chair arm, unlock the arm. When unlocked, the arm swings back 180 degrees to permit easy patient access.

• Position the scale beside the patient's bed or wheelchair with the chair arm open. Transfer the patient onto the scale, swing the chair arm to the front of the scale, and lock it in place.

• Weigh the patient by adding ratio weights and adjusting the main beam poise. Then unlock the swing-away chair arm as before, and transfer the patient back to his bed or wheelchair.

• Lock the main beam *to avoid damaging the scale during transport.* Unlock the wheels and remove the scale from the patient's room.

Using a multiple-weight bed scale
• Provide privacy, and tell the patient that you're going to weigh him on a special bed scale.

• Position the scale next to the patient's bed and lock the scale's wheels. Then turn the patient on his side, facing away from the scale.

• Release the stretcher frame to the horizontal position, and pump the hand lever until the stretcher is positioned over the mattress. Lower the stretcher onto the mattress, and roll the patient onto the stretcher.

• Raise the stretcher 2″ (5 cm) above the mattress. Then add ratio weights, and adjust the main beam poise as for the standing and chair scales.

• After weighing the patient, lower the stretcher onto the mattress, turn the patient on his side, and remove the stretcher. Be sure to leave the patient in a comfortable position.

Using a digital bed scale
• Provide privacy, and tell the patient that you're going to weigh him on a special bed scale. If the patient is being weighed for the first time, demonstrate the scale's operation.

• Release the stretcher to the horizontal position, then lock it in place. Turn the patient on his side, facing away from the scale.

• Roll the base of the scale under the patient's bed. Adjust the lever *to widen the base of the scale, providing stability.* After doing so, lock the scale's wheels.

• Center the stretcher above the bed, lower it onto the mattress, and roll the patient onto the stretcher. Then position the circular weighing arms of the scale over the patient, and attach them securely to the stretcher bars.

• Pump the handle with long, slow strokes *to raise the patient a few inches off the bed.* Ensure that the patient doesn't lean on or touch the headboard, side rails, or other bed equipment *because this will affect weight measurement.*

• Depress the operate button, and read the patient's weight on the digital display panel. Then press in the scale's handle *to lower the patient onto the bed.*

• Detach the circular weighing arms from the stretcher bars, roll the patient off the stretcher and remove it, and position him comfortably in bed.

• Release the wheel lock and withdraw the scale. Return the stretcher to its vertical position for storage.

Special considerations
Reassure and steady patients who are at risk for losing their balance on a scale.

Weigh the patient at the same time each day (usually before breakfast), in similar clothing, and using the same scale. If the patient uses crutches, weigh him with the crutches. Then weigh the crutches and any heavy clothing and subtract their weight from the total to determine the patient's weight. If the patient is markedly obese, check scale capacity. (Although some newer scales can measure up to 600 lb [272 kg], most scales can measure a maximum of 250 lb [113 kg].) You may have to weigh the patient on a large commercial scale (usually located on the loading dock or in the dietary department).

Before using a bed scale, cover its stretcher with a drawsheet *to avoid stains from perspiration, drainage, or excretions.* Balance the scale with the drawsheet in place *to ensure accurate weighing.*

When rolling the patient onto the stretcher, be careful not to dislodge I.V. lines, indwelling catheters, and other supportive equipment.

Documentation
Record the patient's height and weight on the nursing assessment form and other medical records, as required by your hospital.

Assessment techniques

To perform physical assessment, a nurse uses four basic techniques: inspection, palpation, percussion, and auscultation. Performing these techniques correctly helps elicit valuable information about the patient's condition.

Inspection requires the use of vision, hearing, touch, and smell. Special lighting and various equipment — such as an otosocope, a tongue blade, or an ophthalmoscope — may be used to enhance vision or examine an otherwise hidden area. Inspection begins during the first patient contact and continues throughout the assessment.

Palpation usually follows inspection, except when examining the abdomen or assessing infants and children. Palpation involves touching the body to determine the size, shape, and position of structures; to detect and evaluate temperature, pulsations, and other movement; and to elicit tenderness.

The four palpation techniques include light palpation, deep palpation, light ballottement, and deep ballottement. Ballottement is the palpation technique used to evaluate a floating or movable structure; the nurse gently bounces the structure being assessed by applying pressure against it; she then waits to feel it rebound. This technique may be used, for example, to check the position of an organ or a fetus.

Percussion uses quick, sharp tapping of the fingers or hands against body surfaces to produce sounds, detect tenderness, or assess reflexes. Percussing for sound helps locate organ borders, identify organ shape and position, and determine if an organ is solid or filled with fluid or gas.

Organs and tissues produce sounds of varying loudness, pitch, and duration, depending on their density. For example, air-filled cavities, such as the lungs, produce markedly different sounds from those produced by the liver and other dense tissues. Percussion techniques include indirect percussion, direct percussion, and blunt percussion.

Auscultation involves listening to various body sounds — particularly those produced by the heart, lungs, vessels, stomach, and intestines. Most auscultated sounds result from the movement of air or fluid through these structures.

Usually, the nurse auscultates after performing the other assessment techniques. When examining the abdomen, however, auscultation should occur after inspection but before percussion and palpation. This way, bowel sounds can be heard before palpation disrupts them. Auscultation is best performed first on infants and young children, who may start to cry when palpated or per-cussed. Auscultation is most successful when performed in a quiet environment with a properly fitted stethoscope.

Equipment
Flashlight or gooseneck lamp, as appropriate ■ ophthalmoscope ■ otoscope ■ stethoscope.

Implementation
● Explain the procedure to the patient, have him undress, and drape him appropriately.
● Make sure the room is warm and adequately lit *to make the patient comfortable and aid visual inspection.*
● Warm your hands and the stethoscope.

Inspection
● Focus on areas related to the patient's chief complaint. Use your eyes, ears, and sense of smell to observe the patient.
● To inspect a specific body area, first make sure the area is sufficiently exposed and adequately lit. Then survey the entire area, noting key landmarks and checking its overall condition. Next, focus on specifics — color, shape, texture, size, and movement. Note any unusual findings as well as predictable ones.

Palpation
● Explain the procedure to the patient, and tell him what to expect, such as occasional discomfort as pressure is applied. Encourage him to relax *because muscle tension or guarding can interfere with performance and results of palpation.*
● Choose the area of your hands and fingers that will provide the best assessment *because all areas aren't equally sensitive to all sensations.* For example, use the fingertips to assess the texture of a rash, or the back of the hand to assess the temperature of a joint. (See *Using your hands in palpation,* page 24.)
● Provide just enough pressure to assess the tissue beneath one or both hands. Then release pressure and gently move to the next area, systematically covering the entire surface to be assessed.
● To perform light palpation, depress the skin, indenting it ½″ to ¾″ (1 to 2 cm). Use the lightest touch possible *because excessive pressure blunts your sensitivity.*
● If the patient tolerates light palpation and you need to assess deeper structures, increase your fingertip pressure, indenting the skin about 1½″ (4 cm). Place your other hand on top of the palpating hand *to control and guide your movements.*
● To perform light ballottement, apply light, rapid pressure from quadrant to quadrant on the patient's abdomen. Keep your hand on the skin to detect tissue rebound.

Using your hands in palpation

To enhance palpation technique, take advantage of the tactile sensitivity specific to each hand region. You can use your whole hand to test handgrip strength.

The tips and pads of the fingers can best distinguish texture and shape.

A single finger or nail tip can best stroke the skin when attempting to elicit the cremasteric (testicular refraction) or abdominal reflex during the neurologic examination.

The thumb and index finger can best assess hair texture, grasp tissues, and feel for lymph node enlargement.

The flattened fingerpads can best palpate tender tissues, feel for crepitus (crackling) at joints, and lightly probe the abdomen.

The back, or dorsal surface, of the hand can best feel for warmth.

The ulnar surface of the hand (at the base of the fingers on the palmar side) can best feel thrills (fine vibrations over the precordium) and fremitus (tremulous vibrations over the chest wall) as well as vocal vibrations through the chest wall.

• To perform deep ballottement, apply abrupt, deep pressure and then release it. Maintain fingertip contact.

• Use both hands (bimanual palpation) to trap a deep, underlying, hard-to-palpate organ (such as the kidney or spleen) or to fix or stabilize an organ (such as the uterus) with one hand while you palpate it with the other.

Percussion

• First, decide which of the percussion techniques best suits your assessment needs. Indirect percussion helps reveal the size and density of underlying thoracic and abdominal organs and tissues. Direct percussion helps assess an adult's sinuses for tenderness and elicits sounds in a child's thorax. Blunt percussion aims to elicit tenderness over organs such as the kidneys, gallbladder, or liver. When percussing, note the characteristic sounds produced. (See *Identifying percussion sounds.*)

• To perform indirect percussion, place one hand on the patient and tap the middle finger with the middle finger of the other hand. (See *Performing indirect percussion,* page 26.)

• To perform direct percussion, tap your hand or fingertip directly against the body surface.

• To perform blunt percussion, strike the ulnar surface of your fist against the body surface. Or place the palm of one hand against the body, make a fist with the other hand, and strike the back of the first hand.

Auscultation

• First, determine whether to use the bell or diaphragm of your stethoscope. Use the diaphragm to detect high-pitched sounds, such as breath and bowel sounds. Use the bell to detect lower-pitched sounds, such as heart and vascular sounds.

• Place the diaphragm or bell of the stethoscope over the appropriate area of the patient's body. Place the earpieces in your ears, listen intently to individual sounds, and try to identify their characteristics. Determine the intensity, pitch, and duration of each sound, and check the frequency of recurring sounds.

Special considerations

Avoid palpating or percussing an area of the body known to be tender at the start of your examination. Instead, work around the area; then gently palpate or percuss it at the end of the examination. *This progression minimizes your patient's discomfort and apprehension.*

To pinpont an inflamed area deep within the patient's body, perform a variation on deep palpation: Press firmly with one hand over the area you suspect is involved, and then lift your hand away quickly. If the patient reports that pain increases when you release the pressure, then you have identified rebound tenderness. (Suspect peritonitis if you elicit rebound tenderness when examining the abdomen.)

If you cannot palpate because the patient fears pain, try distracting him with conversation. Then perform aus-

Identifying percussion sounds

Percussion produces sounds that vary according to the tissue being percussed. This chart lists important percussion sounds along with their characteristics and typical sources.

SOUND	INTENSITY	PITCH	DURATION	QUALITY	SOURCE
Resonance	Moderate to loud	Low	Long	Hollow	Normal lung
Tympany	Loud	High	Moderate	Drumlike	Gastric air bubble, intestinal air
Dullness	Soft to moderate	High	Moderate	Thudlike	Liver, full bladder, pregnant uterus
Hyperresonance	Very loud	Very low	Long	Booming	Hyperinflated lung (as in emphysema)
Flatness	Soft	High	Short	Flat	Muscle

Performing indirect percussion

To perform indirect percussion, use the middle finger of your nondominant hand as the pleximeter (the mediating device used to receive the taps) and the middle finger of your dominant hand as the plexor (the device used to tap the pleximeter). Place the pleximeter finger firmly against a body surface, such as the upper back. With your wrist flexed loosely, use the tip of your plexor finger to deliver a crisp blow just beneath the distal joint of the pleximeter. Be sure to hold the plexor perpendicular to the pleximeter. Tap lightly and quickly, removing the plexor as soon as you have delivered each blow. Move your nondominant hand to cover the entire area to be percussed.

cultation and gently press your stethoscope into the affected area *to try to elicit tenderness.*

Complications
Palpation may cause an enlarged spleen or infected appendix to rupture.

Documentation
Document your assessment findings and the technique used to elicit those findings—for example, "right lower quadrant tenderness on deep palpation, no rebound tenderness."

Physical assessment

Nurses perform a complete physical assessment when the patient is admitted to the hospital and partial reassessments as the patient's condition warrants. A complete assessment includes a thorough health history and physical examination. The health history includes the chief complaint, a history of the present illness, general medical and surgical histories, a family history, a social history, and a review of systems.

Typically, physical examination follows a methodical, head-to-toe format. Patient preparation includes a clear explanation of the examination, and proper positioning and draping before and during the examination. During this procedure, the nurse must make every effort to recognize and respect the patient's feelings (particularly of embarrassment and anxiety) as well as to provide comfort measures and follow appropriate safety precautions.

Equipment
Although equipment varies with the examination's focus, the following may be included: scale with height measurement bar ▪ urine specimen container and laboratory request form (if ordered) ▪ sphygmomanometer ▪ watch with second hand ▪ stethoscope ▪ thermometer ▪ gown (for patient) ▪ examining table (with stirrups if necessary) ▪ gloves ▪ drapes (sheet, bath blanket, or towel, as needed) ▪ adhesive tape ▪ spotlight or gooseneck lamp ▪ flashlight ▪ laryngeal mirror ▪ tongue blades ▪ percussion (reflex) hammer ▪ otoscope ▪ tuning fork ▪ ear specula ▪ tape measure ▪ visual acuity chart ▪ ophthalmoscope ▪ test tubes of hot and cold water ▪ containers of odorous materials (such as coffee, chocolate) ▪ substances for taste assessment (sugar, salt, vinegar) ▪ coin ▪ pin and cotton ▪ paper clip ▪ fecal occult blood test kit ▪ linen-saver pad ▪ water-soluble lubricant ▪ facial tissues ▪ cotton-tipped applicators ▪ nursing assessment form.

Preparation of equipment
Adjust the temperature in the examining room and close the doors *to prevent drafts.* Cover the examining table with a clean sheet or disposable paper. Then assemble the appropriate equipment for the examination.

Implementation
● Review the patient's health history *to obtain subjective data about the patient and insight into problem areas and subtle physical changes.* Investigate the patient's chief complaint. (See *Exploring a patient's symptoms.)*
● Obtain biographical data, including the patient's name; address; telephone number; contact person; sex; age and

Exploring a patient's symptoms

Essential to a complete physical assessment is a clear understanding of your patient's symptoms. One method for gaining that understanding involves using the mnemonic device PQRST as a guide.

Provocative or palliative
What causes the symptom? What makes it better or worse?
• What were you doing when you first noticed it?
• What seems to trigger it? Stress? Position? Certain activities? An argument? (For a sign, such as an eye discharge: What seems to cause it or make it worse? For a psychological symptom such as depression: Does the depression occur after specific events?)
• What relieves the symptom? Changing diet? Changing position? Taking medication? Being active?
• What makes the symptom worse?

Quality or quantity
How does the symptom feel, look, or sound? How much of it are you experiencing now?
• How would you describe the symptom—how it feels, looks, or sounds?
• How much are you experiencing now? Is it so much that it prevents you from performing any activities? Is it more or less than you experienced at any other time?

Region or radiation
Where is the symptom located? Does it spread?
• Where does the symptom occur?
• In the case of pain, does it travel down your back or arms, up your neck, or down your legs?

Severity
How does the symptom rate on a scale of 1 to 10, with 10 being the most severe?
• How bad is the symptom at its worst? Does it force you to lie down, sit down, or slow down?
• Does the symptom seem to be getting better, getting worse, or staying about the same?

Timing
When did the symptom begin? How often does it occur? Is it sudden or gradual?
• On what date and time did the symptom first occur?
• How did the symptom start? Suddenly? Gradually?
• How often do you experience the symptom? Hourly? Daily? Weekly? Monthly?
• When do you usually experience the symptom? During the day? At night? In the early morning? Does it awaken you? Does it occur before, during, or after meals? Does it occur seasonally?
• How long does an episode of the symptom last?

birth date; birthplace; Social Security number; race, nationality, and cultural background; marital status and names of persons living with the patient; education; religion; and occupation.
• Ask about health and illness patterns, the reason for seeking health care, current and past health status, family health status, and condition of body systems.
• Ask about health promotion and protection patterns, including health beliefs, personal habits, sleep and wake cycles, exercise, recreation, nutrition, stress level and coping skills, socioeconomic status, environmental health conditions, and occupational health hazards.
• Explore the patient's role and relationship patterns, including self-concept, cultural and religious influences, family roles and relationships, sexuality and reproductive patterns, social support systems, and any other psychosocial considerations.
• Explain the physical examination and answer questions.
• Instruct the patient to void if possible. Collect a urine specimen if ordered. *Emptying the bladder increases patient comfort during the examination.*

• Help the patient undress, and provide a gown. Then measure and record height, weight, and vital signs.
• Assist the patient onto the examination table. Requirements for positioning and draping vary with the body system and region being assessed. To examine the head, neck, and anterior and posterior thorax, have the patient sit on the edge of the examination table or the bed. For the abdomen and cardiovascular system, place the patient in a supine position and stand to his right. For a female patient, place a towel over her breasts and upper thorax during abdominal assessment. Pull the sheet down as far as her symphysis pubis, but no farther.
• Perform a physical examination as outlined in *Performing a head-to-toe assessment,* pages 28 to 38.

Documentation
Document significant normal and abnormal findings in an organized manner according to body systems.

(Text continues on page 39.)

Performing a head-to-toe assessment

The chart on the following pages provides guidelines for a systematic head-to-toe assessment. It groups assessment techniques by body region and nurse-patient positioning to make the assessment as efficient as possible and to avoid tiring the patient. The first column describes the assessment technique to use for each body system or region. The second column lists normal findings for adults. The third column reviews special considerations, including the purpose of the technique as well as nursing and developmental considerations.

TECHNIQUE	NORMAL FINDINGS	SPECIAL CONSIDERATIONS
Head and neck		
Inspect the patient's head. Note hair color, texture, and distribution. Palpate from the forehead to the posterior triangle of the neck for the posterior cervical lymph nodes.	Symmetrical, rounded normocephalic head positioned at midline and erect with no lumps or ridges	• This technique can detect asymmetry, size changes, enlarged lymph nodes, and tenderness. • Wear gloves for palpation if the patient has scalp lesions. • Inspect and gently palpate the fontanels and sutures in an infant.
Palpate in front of and behind the ears, under the chin, and in the anterior triangle for the anterior cervical lymph nodes.	Nonpalpable lymph nodes or small, round, soft, mobile, nontender lymph nodes	• This technique can detect enlarged lymph nodes. • Palpable lymph nodes may be normal in a patient under age 12.
Palpate the left and then the right carotid artery.	Bilateral equality in pulse amplitude and rhythm	• This technique evaluates circulation through the carotid pulse.
Auscultate the carotid arteries.	No bruit on auscultation	• Auscultation in this area can detect a bruit, a sign of turbulent blood flow.
Palpate the trachea.	Straight, midline trachea	• This technique evaluates trachea position.
Palpate the suprasternal notch.	Palpable pulsations with an even rhythm	• Palpation in this area allows evaluation of aortic arch pulsations.
Palpate the supraclavicular area.	Nonpalpable lymph nodes	• This technique can detect enlarged lymph nodes.
Palpate the thyroid gland and auscultate for bruits.	Thin, mobile thyroid isthmus; nonpalpable thyroid lobes	• Palpation detects thyroid enlargement, tenderness, or nodules.
Have the patient touch his chin to his chest and to each shoulder, each ear to the corresponding shoulder, then tip his head back as far as possible.	Symmetrical strength and movement of neck muscles	• These maneuvers evaluate range of motion (ROM) in the neck.

Performing a head-to-toe assessment *(continued)*

TECHNIQUE	NORMAL FINDINGS	SPECIAL CONSIDERATIONS
Head and neck *(continued)*		
Place your hands on the patient's shoulders while the patient shrugs them against resistance. Then place your hand on the patient's left cheek, then the right, and have the patient push against it.	Symmetrical strength and movement of neck muscles	• This procedure checks cranial nerve XI (accessory nerve) functioning and trapezius and sternocleidomastoid muscle strength.
Have the patient smile, frown, wrinkle the forehead, and puff out the cheeks.	Symmetrical smile, frown, and forehead wrinkles; equal puffing out of the cheeks	• This maneuver evaluates the motor portion of cranial nerve VII (facial nerve).
Occlude one nostril externally with your finger while the patient breathes through the other. Repeat on the other nostril.	Patent nostrils	• This technique checks the patency of the nasal passages.
Inspect the internal nostrils using a nasal speculum or an ophthalmoscope handle with a nasal attachment.	Moist, pink to red nasal mucosa without deviated septum, lesions, or polyps	• This technique can detect edema, inflammation, and excessive drainage. • Use only a flashlight to inspect an infant's or toddler's nostrils; a nasal speculum is too sharp.
Palpate the nose.	No bumps, lesions, edema, or tenderness	• This technique assesses for structural abnormalities in the nose. • An infant's nose usually is slightly flattened.
Palpate and percuss the frontal and maxillary sinuses. If palpation and percussion elicit tenderness, assess further by transilluminating the sinuses.	No tenderness on palpation or percussion	• These techniques are used to elicit tenderness, which may indicate sinus congestion or infection. • In a child under age 8, frontal sinuses commonly are too small to assess.
Palpate the temporomandibular joints as the patient opens and closes the jaws.	Smooth joint movement without pain; correct approximation	• This action assesses the temporomandibular joints and the motor portion of cranial nerve V (trigeminal nerve).
Inspect the oral mucosa, gingivae, teeth, and salivary gland openings, using a tongue blade and a penlight.	Pink, moist, smooth oral mucosa without lesions or inflammation; pink, moist slightly irregular gingivae without sponginess or edema; 32 teeth with correct occlusion	• This technique evaluates the condition of several oral structures. • A child may have up to 20 temporary (baby) teeth. • Slight gingival swelling may be normal during pregnancy.

(continued)

Performing a head-to-toe assessment *(continued)*

TECHNIQUE	NORMAL FINDINGS	SPECIAL CONSIDERATIONS
Head and neck *(continued)*		
Observe the tongue and the hard and soft palates.	Pink, slightly rough tongue with a midline depression; pink to light red palates with symmetrical lines	• Observation provides information about the patient's hydration status and the condition of these oral structures.
Ask the patient to stick out his tongue.	Midline tongue without tremors	• This procedure tests cranial nerve XII (hypoglossal nerve).
Ask the patient to say "Ahh" while sticking out his tongue. Inspect the visible oral structures.	Symmetrical rise in soft palate and uvula during phonation; pink, midline, cone-shaped uvula; +1 tonsils (both tonsils behind the pillars)	• Phonation ("Ahh") checks portions of cranial nerves IX and X (glossopharyngeal and vagus nerves). Lowering the tongue aids viewing.
Test the gag reflex using a tongue blade.	Gagging	• Gagging during this procedure indicates that cranial nerves IX and X are intact.
Place the tongue blade at the side of the tongue while the patient pushes it to the left and right with the tongue.	Symmetrical ability to push tongue blade to left and right	• This action tests cranial nerve XII.
Test the sense of smell using a test tube of coffee, chocolate, or another familiar substance.	Correct identification of smells in both nostrils	• This action tests cranial nerve I (olfactory nerve). • Make sure the patient keeps both eyes closed during the test.
Eyes and ears		
Perform a visual acuity test using the standard Snellen eye chart or another visual acuity chart, with the patient wearing corrective lenses if needed.	20/20 vision	• This test assesses the patient's distance vision (central vision) and evaluates cranial nerve II (optic nerve).
Ask the patient to identify the pattern in a specially prepared page of color dots or plates.	Correct identification of pattern	• This test assesses the patient's color perception.
Test the six cardinal positions of gaze.	Bilaterally equal eye movement without nystagmus	• This test evaluates the function of each of the six extraocular muscles and tests cranial nerves III, IV, and VI (oculomotor, trochlear, and abducens nerves).
Inspect the external structures of the eyeball (eyelids, eyelashes, and lacrimal apparatus).	Bright, clear, symmetrical eyes free of nystagmus; eyelids close completely; no lesions, scaling, or inflammation	• This inspection allows detection of such problems as ptosis, ectropion (outward-turning eyelids), entropion (inward-turning eyelids), and styes.

Performing a head-to-toe assessment *(continued)*

TECHNIQUE	NORMAL FINDINGS	SPECIAL CONSIDERATIONS
Eyes and ears *(continued)*		
Inspect the conjunctiva and sclera.	Pink palpebral conjunctiva and clear bulbar conjunctiva without swelling, drainage, or hyperemic blood vessels; white, clear sclera	• Inspection detects conjunctivitis and the scleral color changes that may occur with systemic disorders.
Inspect the cornea, iris, and anterior chamber by shining a penlight tangentially across the eye.	Clear, transparent cornea and anterior chamber; illumination of total iris	• This technique assesses anterior chamber depth and the condition of the cornea and iris. • An elderly patient may exhibit a thin, grayish ring in the cornea (called arcus senilis).
Examine the pupils for equality of size, shape, reaction to light, and accommodation.	Pupils equal, round, reactive to light and accommodation (PERRLA), directly and consensually	• Testing the pupillary response to light and accommodation assesses cranial nerves III, IV, and VI.
Observe the red reflex using an ophthalmoscope.	Sharp, distinct orange-red glow	• Presence of the red reflex indicates that the cornea, anterior chamber, and lens are free from opacity and clouding.
Inspect the ear. Perform an otoscopic examination if indicated.	Nearly vertically positioned ears that line up with the eye, match the facial color, are similarly shaped, and are in proportion to the face; no drainage, nodules, or lesions	• A dark-skinned patient may have darker orange or brown cerumen (earwax); a fair-skinned patient typically will have yellow cerumen.
Palpate the ear and mastoid process.	No pain, swelling, nodules, or lesions	• This assessment technique can detect inflammation or infection. It may also uncover other abnormalities, such as nodules or lesions.
Perform the whispered voice test or the watch-tick test on one ear at a time.	Whispered voice heard at a distance of 1′ to 2′ (30 to 61 cm); watch-tick heard at a distance of 5″ (13 cm)	• This test grossly assesses cranial nerve VIII (acoustic nerve).
Perform Weber's test using a 512 or 1024 Hertz (Hz) tuning fork.	Tuning fork vibrations heard equally in both ears or in the middle of the head	• This test differentiates conductive from sensorineural hearing loss. • The sound is heard best in the ear with a conductive loss.
Perform the Rinne test using a 512 or 1024 Hz tuning fork.	Tuning fork vibrations heard in front of the ear for as long as they are heard on the mastoid process	• This test helps differentiate conductive from sensorineural hearing loss.

(continued)

Performing a head-to-toe assessment *(continued)*

TECHNIQUE	NORMAL FINDINGS	SPECIAL CONSIDERATIONS
Posterior thorax		
Observe the skin, bones, and muscles of the spine, shoulder blades, and back as well as symmetry of expansion and accessory muscle use.	Even skin tone; symmetrical placement of all structures; bilaterally equal shoulder height; symmetrical expansion with inhalation; no accessory muscle use	• Observation provides information about lung expansion and accessory muscle use during respiration. It may also detect a deformity that can alter ventilation, such as scoliosis.
Assess the anteroposterior and lateral diameters of the thorax.	Lateral diameter up to twice the anteroposterior diameter (2:1)	• This assessment may detect abnormalities, such as an increased anteroposterior diameter (barrel chest may be as low as 1:1). • Normal anteroposterior diameters vary with age. • Measure an infant's chest circumference at the nipple line.
Palpate down the spine.	Properly aligned spinous processes without lesions or tenderness; firm, symmetrical, evenly spaced muscles	• This technique detects pain in the spine and paraspinous muscles. It also evaluates the muscles' consistency.
Palpate over the posterior thorax.	Smooth surface; no lesions, lumps, or pain	• This technique helps detect musculoskeletal inflammation.
Assess respiratory excursion.	Symmetrical expansion and contraction of the thorax	• This technique checks for equal expansion of the lungs.
Palpate for tactile fremitus as the patient repeats the word "ninety-nine."	Equally intense vibrations of both sides of the chest	• Palpation provides information about the content of the lungs; vibrations increase over consolidated or fluid-filled areas and decrease over gas-filled areas.
Percuss over the posterior and lateral lung fields.	Resonant percussion note over the lungs that changes to a dull note at the diaphragm	• This technique helps identify the density and location of the lungs, diaphragm, and other anatomic structures. • Percussion may produce hyperresonant sounds in a patient with chronic obstructive pulmonary disease or an elderly patient because of hyperinflation of lung tissue.
Percuss for diaphragmatic excursion on each side of the posterior thorax.	Excursion from 1¼″ to 2¼″ (3 to 6 cm)	• This technique evaluates diaphragm movement during respiration.

Performing a head-to-toe assessment *(continued)*

TECHNIQUE	NORMAL FINDINGS	SPECIAL CONSIDERATIONS
Posterior thorax *(continued)*		
Auscultate the lungs through the posterior thorax as the patient breathes slowly and deeply through the mouth. Also auscultate lateral areas.	Bronchovesicular sounds (soft, breezy sounds) between the scapulae; vesicular sounds (soft, swishy sounds about two notes lower than bronchovesicular sounds) in the lung periphery	• Lung auscultation helps detect abnormal fluid or mucus accumulation as well as obstructed passages. • Auscultate a child's lungs before performing other assessment techniques that may cause crying, which increases the respiratory rate and interferes with clear auscultation. • A child's breath sounds are normally harsher or more bronchial than an adult's.
Anterior thorax		
Observe the skin, bones, and muscles of the anterior thoracic structures as well as symmetry of expansion and accessory muscle use during respiration.	Even skin tone; symmetrical placement of all structures; symmetrical costal angle of less than 90 degrees; symmetrical expansion with inhalation; no accessory muscle use	• Observation provides information about lung expansion and accessory muscle use. It may also detect a deformity that can prevent full lung expansion, such as pigeon chest.
Inspect the anterior thorax for lifts, heaves, or thrusts. Also check for the apical impulse.	No lifts, heaves, or thrusts; apical impulse not usually visible	• Apical impulse may be visible in a thin or young patient.
Palpate over the anterior thorax.	Smooth surface; no lesions, lumps, or pain	• This technique helps detect musculoskeletal inflammation.
Assess respiratory excursion.	Symmetrical expansion and contraction of the thorax	• This technique checks for equal expansion of the lungs.
Palpate for tactile fremitus as the patient repeats the word "ninety-nine."	Equally intense vibrations of both sides of the chest, with more vibrations in the upper chest than in the lower chest	• Palpation provides information about the content of the lungs.
Percuss over the anterior thorax.	Resonant percussion note over lung fields that changes to a dull note over ribs and other bones	• This technique helps identify the density and location of the lungs, diaphragm, and other anatomic structures. • Percussion is unreliable in an infant because of the infant's small chest size. • Percussion may produce hyperresonant sounds in an elderly patient because of hyperinflation of lung tissue.

(continued)

Performing a head-to-toe assessment *(continued)*

TECHNIQUE	NORMAL FINDINGS	SPECIAL CONSIDERATIONS
Anterior thorax *(continued)*		
Auscultate the lungs through the posterior thorax as the patient breathes slowly and deeply through the mouth. Also auscultate lateral areas.	Bronchovesicular sounds (soft, breezy sounds) between the scapulae; vesicular sounds (soft, swishy sounds about two notes lower than bronchovesicular sounds) in the lung periphery	• Lung auscultation helps detect abnormal fluid or mucus accumulation. • Auscultate a child's lungs before performing other assessment techniques that may cause crying. • Breath sounds are normally harsher or more bronchial in a child.
Inspect the breasts and axillae with the patient's hands resting at the sides of the body, placed on the hips, and raised above the head.	Symmetrical, convex, similar-looking breasts with soft, smooth skin and bilaterally similar venous patterns; symmetrical axillae with varying amounts of hair, but no lesions; nipples at same level on chest and of same color	• This technique evaluates the general condition of the breasts and axillae and detects such abnormalities as retraction, dimpling, and flattening. • Expect to see enlarged breasts with darkened nipples and areolae and purplish linear streaks if the patient is pregnant.
Palpate the axillae with the patient's arms resting against the side of the body.	Nonpalpable nodes	• This technique detects nodular enlargements and other abnormalities.
Palpate the breasts and nipples with patient lying supine.	Smooth, relatively elastic tissue without masses, cracks, fissures, areas of induration (hardness), or discharge	• This technique evaluates the consistency and elasticity of the breasts and nipples and may detect nipple discharge. • The premenstrual patient may exhibit breast tenderness, nodularity, and fullness. • A pregnant patient may discharge colostrum from the nipple and may exhibit nodular breasts with prominent venous patterns.
Inspect the neck for jugular vein distention with patient lying supine at a 45-degree angle.	No visible pulsations	• This technique assesses right-sided heart pressure.
Palpate the precordium for the apical impulse.	Apical impulse present in the apical area (fifth intercostal space at the midclavicular line)	• This action evaluates the size and location of the left ventricle.

Performing a head-to-toe assessment *(continued)*

TECHNIQUE	NORMAL FINDINGS	SPECIAL CONSIDERATIONS
Anterior thorax *(continued)*		
Auscultate the aortic, pulmonic, tricuspid, and mitral areas for heart sounds.	S_1 and S_2 heart sounds with a regular rhythm and an age-appropriate rate	• Auscultation over the precordium evaluates the heart rate and rhythm and can detect extra sounds, murmurs, and other abnormal heart sounds. • A child may have functional (innocent) heart murmurs.
Abdomen		
Observe the abdominal contour.	Symmetrical flat or rounded contour	• This technique determines whether the abdomen is distended or scaphoid. • An infant or a toddler will have a rounded abdomen.
Inspect the abdomen for skin characteristics, symmetry, contour, peristalsis, and pulsations.	Symmetrical contour with no lesions, striae, rash, or visible peristaltic waves	• Inspection can detect an incisional or umbilical hernia, or an abnormality caused by bowel obstruction.
Auscultate all four quadrants of the abdomen.	Normal bowel sounds in all four quadrants; no bruits	• Abdominal auscultation can detect abnormal bowel sounds.
Percuss from below the right breast to the inguinal area down the right midclavicular line.	Dull percussion note over the liver; tympanic note over the rest of the abdomen	• Percussion in this area helps evaluate the size of the liver.
Percuss from below the left breast to the inguinal area down the left midclavicular line.	Tympanic percussion note	• Percussion in this area that elicits a dull note can detect an enlarged spleen.
Palpate all four abdominal quadrants.	Nontender organs without masses	• Palpation provides information about the location, size, and condition of the underlying structures.
Palpate for the kidneys on each side of the abdomen.	Nonpalpable kidneys or solid, firm, smooth kidneys (if palpable)	• This technique evaluates the general condition of the kidneys.
Palpate the liver at the right costal border.	Nonpalpable liver or smooth, firm, nontender liver with a rounded, regular edge (if palpable)	• This technique evaluates the general condition of the liver.
Palpate for the spleen at the left costal border.	Nonpalpable spleen	• This procedure detects any splenomegaly (spleen enlargement).
Palpate the femoral pulses in the groin.	Strong, regular pulse	• Palpation assesses vascular patency.

(continued)

Performing a head-to-toe assessment *(continued)*

TECHNIQUE	NORMAL FINDINGS	SPECIAL CONSIDERATIONS
Upper extremities		
Observe the skin and muscle mass of the arms and hands.	Uniform color and texture with no lesions; elastic turgor; bilaterally equal muscle mass	• The skin provides information about hydration and circulation. Muscle mass provides information about injuries and neuromuscular disease.
Ask the patient to extend the arms forward and then rapidly turn the palms up and down.	Steady hands with no tremor or pronator drift	• This maneuver tests proprioception and cerebellar function.
Place your hands on the patient's upturned forearms while the patient pushes up against resistance. Then place your hands under the forearms while the patient pushes down.	Symmetrical strength and ability to push up and down against resistance	• This procedure checks the muscle strength of the arms.
Inspect and palpate the fingers, wrists, and elbow joints.	Smooth, freely movable joints with no swelling	• An elderly patient may exhibit osteoarthritic changes.
Palpate the patient's hands to assess skin temperature.	Warm, moist skin with bilaterally even temperature	• Skin temperature assessment provides data about circulation to the area.
Palpate the radial and brachial pulses.	Bilaterally equal rate and rhythm	• Palpation of pulses helps evaluate peripheral vascular status.
Inspect the color, shape, and condition of the patient's fingernails, and test for capillary refill.	Pink nail beds with smooth, rounded nails; brisk capillary refill; no clubbing	• Nail assessment provides data about the integumentary, cardiovascular, and respiratory systems.
Place two fingers in each of the patient's palms while the patient squeezes your fingers.	Bilaterally equal hand strength	• This maneuver tests muscle strength in the hands.
Lower extremities		
Inspect the legs and feet for color, lesions, varicosities, hair growth, nail growth, edema, and muscle mass.	Even skin color; symmetrical hair and nail growth; no lesions, varicosities, or edema; bilaterally equal muscle mass	• Inspection assesses adequate circulatory function.
Test for pitting edema in the pretibial area.	No pitting edema	• This test assesses for excess interstitial fluid.
Palpate for pulses and skin temperature in the posterior tibial, dorsalis pedis, and popliteal areas.	Bilaterally even pulse rate, rhythm, and skin temperature	• Palpation of pulses and temperature in these areas evaluates the patient's peripheral vascular status.

Performing a head-to-toe assessment *(continued)*

TECHNIQUE	NORMAL FINDINGS	SPECIAL CONSIDERATIONS
Lower extremities *(continued)*		
Perform the straight leg test on one leg at a time.	Painless leg lifting	• This test checks for vertebral disk problems.
Palpate for crepitus as the patient abducts and adducts the hip. Repeat on the opposite leg.	No crepitus; full ROM without pain	• Perform Ortolani's maneuver on an infant to assess hip abduction and adduction.
Ask the patient to raise his thigh against the resistance of your hands. Repeat this procedure on the opposite thigh.	Each thigh lifts easily against resistance	• This maneuver tests the motor strength of the upper legs.
Ask the patient to push outward against the resistance of your hands.	Each leg pushes easily against resistance	• This maneuver tests the motor strength of the lower legs.
Ask the patient to pull backward against the resistance of your hands.	Each leg pulls easily against resistance	• This maneuver tests the motor strength of the lower legs.
Nervous system		
Lightly touch the ophthalmic, maxillary, and mandibular areas on each side of the patient's face with a cotton-tipped applicator and a pin.	Correct identification of sensation and location	• This test evaluates the function of cranial nerve V (trigeminal nerve).
Touch the dorsal and palmar surfaces of the arms, hands, and fingers with a cotton-tipped applicator and pin.	Correct identification of sensation and location	• This test evaluates the function of the ulnar, radial, and medial nerves.
Touch several nerve distribution areas on the legs, feet, and toes with a cotton-tipped applicator and pin.	Correct identification of sensation and location	• This test evaluates the function of the dermatome areas randomly.
Place your fingers above the patient's wrist and tap them with a reflex hammer. Repeat on the other arm.	Normal reflex reaction	• This procedure elicits the brachioradialis deep tendon reflex (DTR).
Place your fingers over the antecubital fossa and tap them with a reflex hammer. Repeat on the other arm.	Normal reflex reaction	• This procedure elicits the biceps DTR.
Place your fingers over the triceps tendon area and tap them with a reflex hammer. Repeat on the other arm.	Normal reflex reaction	• This procedure elicits the triceps DTR.

(continued)

Performing a head-to-toe assessment *(continued)*

TECHNIQUE	NORMAL FINDINGS	SPECIAL CONSIDERATIONS
Nervous system *(continued)*		
Tap just below the patella with a reflex hammer. Repeat this procedure on the opposite patella.	Normal reflex reaction	• This procedure elicits the patellar DTR.
Tap over the Achilles tendon area with a reflex hammer. Repeat this procedure on the opposite ankle.	Normal reflex reaction	• This procedure elicits the Achilles DTR.
Stroke the sole of the patient's foot with the end of the reflex hammer handle.	Plantar reflex	• This procedure elicits plantar flexion of all toes. • Expect Babinski's sign in children age 2 and under.
Ask the patient to demonstrate dorsi-flexion by bending both feet upward against resistance.	Both feet lift easily against resistance	• This procedure tests foot strength and ROM.
Ask the patient to demonstrate plantar flexion by bending both feet downward against resistance.	Both feet push down easily against resistance	• This procedure tests foot strength and ROM.
Inspect the feet and toes for lesions and lumps.	No lesions or lumps	• Condition of the feet and toes helps evaluate peripheral vascular status.
Using your finger, trace a one-digit number in the palm of the patient's hand.	Correct identification of number	• This procedure evaluates the patient's tactile discrimination through graphes-thesia.
Place a familiar object, such as a key or a coin, in the patient's hand.	Correct identification of object	• This procedure evaluates the patient's tactile discrimination.
Observe the patient while he walks with a regular gait, on the toes, on the heels, and heel-to-toe.	Steady gait, good balance, and no signs of muscle weakness or pain in any style of walking	• This technique evaluates the cerebellum and motor system and checks for verte-bral disk problems.
Inspect the scapulae, spine, back, and hips as the patient bends forward, backward, and from side to side.	Full ROM, easy flexibility, and no signs of scoliosis or varicosities	• Inspection evaluates the patient's ROM and detects musculoskeletal abnormali-ties, such as scoliosis.
Perform the Romberg test. Ask the pa-tient to stand straight with both eyes closed and both arms extended, with hands palms up.	Steady stance with minimal weaving	• This test checks cerebellar functioning and evaluates balance and coordination.

Preparation of a nursing care plan

A care plan directs the patient's nursing care from admission to discharge. This written action plan is based on nursing diagnoses that have been formulated after reviewing assessment findings. (See *Elements of a nursing diagnosis.*) The care plan consists of three parts: *goals* or *expected outcomes*, which describe behaviors or results to be achieved within a specified time; appropriate *nursing actions* or *interventions* needed to achieve these goals; and *evaluations* of the established goals.

A nursing care plan should be written for each patient, preferably within 24 hours of admission. It's usually begun by the patient's primary nurse or the nurse who admits the patient. If the care plan contains more than one nursing diagnosis, the nurse must assign priorities to each one and implement those with the highest priority first. Nurses update and revise the plan throughout the patient's stay, and the document becomes part of the permanent patient record.

Some health care facilities use standardized care plans that can be modified to serve many patients. Others use computer programs to facilitate nursing care plan development. Most have preprinted care plan forms, often on the nursing Kardex, that can be filled in as needed.

Besides guiding patient care, a nursing care plan serves as a database when planning assignments, giving change-of-shift reports, conferring with the doctor or other members of the health care team, planning patient discharge, and documenting patient care. In addition, the care plan can be used as a management tool to determine staffing needs and assignments.

Equipment

Preprinted nursing care plan form ■ computer program for nursing care plan development if appropriate ■ patient record, including nursing assessment.

Implementation

● Review the patient record, especially the nursing assessment completed on admission. Obtain from the patient any additional subjective or objective information needed to complete your assessment. Review diagnostic test results, the medical plan, and other information that may affect patient care. If the patient has just been admitted, complete a nursing history and physical assessment and add it to the patient's record.
● Based on an analysis of the data, determine which nursing diagnoses will guide your patient care. Be sure to address all of the patient's significant needs when determining nursing diagnoses.

Elements of a nursing diagnosis

The following summary presents the key elements of a nursing diagnosis.

Human response or problem
After analyzing the patient's condition, choose a diagnostic label from a hospital-sanctioned list or create a label specific to the patient. For consistency, most hospitals use NANDA's list of nursing diagnoses. An example of a diagnostic label is *Fluid volume excess.*

Related factors
The second part of the nursing diagnosis lists factors that seem to influence the patient in a way that pertains to the diagnostic label. Connect these factors to the diagnostic label with the phrase *related to* or the abbreviation *R/T.* The previous example could read, *Fluid volume excess R/T increased sodium intake.*

Signs and symptoms
To complete the nursing diagnosis, list signs and symptoms uncovered during assessment that help define the diagnostic label. You may list them beneath the diagnosis and related factors. Or you may add them to the diagnostic statement and connect them with the phrase *as evidenced by* or the abbreviation *AEB.* The example could read, *Fluid volume excess R/T increased sodium intake AEB edema, weight gain, shortness of breath, and S_3 heart sounds.*

● Work with the patient to identify individualized short-term and long-term goals (expected outcomes) for each nursing diagnosis. Short-term goals include those of immediate concern that can be achieved quickly. Long-term goals take more time to achieve and usually involve prevention, patient teaching, and rehabilitation.

A correctly written goal expresses the desired patient behavior, criteria for measurement, appropriate time, and conditions under which the behavior will occur. For example, a goal containing all these elements might read: "Using crutches, Mary Ballin will walk to the end of the hall and back by Monday." *Goals (or expected outcomes) serve as the basis for evaluating the effectiveness of your nursing interventions.*
● Select interventions that will help the patient achieve the stated goals for each nursing diagnosis. Include spe-

Tips for writing an effective patient care plan

How do you write a care plan that's realistic, accurate, and helpful? Here are some guidelines.

Be systematic
Avoid setting an initial goal that's impossible to achieve. For example, suppose the goal for a newly admitted patient with a cerebrovascular accident was "Patient will ambulate without assistance." Although this goal is certainly appropriate in the long term, several short-term goals, such as "Patient maintains joint range-of-motion," need to be achieved first.

Be realistic
The nursing intervention should match staff resources and capabilities. For example, "Passive range-of-motion exercises to all extremities every 2 hours" may not be reasonable given the unit's staffing pattern and care requirements. The goals you set to correct a patient's problem should reflect what's reasonably possible in your setting—for example, "Passive range-of-motion exercises with a.m. care, p.m. care, and once at night."

Be clear
Remember, you'll use goals to evaluate the effectiveness of the care plan, so it's important to express them clearly.

Be specific
"Give plenty of fluids" doesn't indicate much; the directive is nonspecific. In contrast, an intervention that says "Force fluids—1,000 ml/day shift, 1,000 ml/evening shift, 500 ml/night shift" allows another nurse to carry out the intervention with some assurance of having done what you ordered.

Be brief
An intervention that says "Follow turning schedule posted at bedside" is more readable and useful than having the entire schedule written on the nursing care plan.

---

cific information, such as the frequency or particular intervention technique. *Goals specify what you and your patient would like to have happen and establish criteria against which you'll judge further nursing actions.* (See *Tips for writing an effective patient care plan.*)

Special considerations
Always fill out the nursing care plan in ink *because the document is part of the permanent medical record.* If you must revise your plan as the patient's condition changes, fill out a new care plan and add it to the medical record.

Sign and date the care plan whenever you make new entries *to keep the plan current and to maintain accountability for planning the patient's care.*

Be aware that using a standardized care plan risks "standardizing" your patient's care, too. Customize the standardized plan as needed *to address your patient's individual concerns.*

Because long-term goals may not be met during hospitalization, your planning should address postdischarge and home care needs as well. Interventions may include coordinating home care services.

Documentation
Documentation of the patient's progress (or lack of it) is required by the Joint Commission on Accreditation of Health Care Organizations and other regulatory agencies that monitor health care quality. Document all pertinent nursing diagnoses, expected outcomes, nursing interventions, and evaluations of expected outcomes. Write the care plan clearly and concisely, so other members of the health care team can understand it.

SAFETY AND MOBILITY
Restraints

Various soft restraints limit movement to prevent the confused, disoriented, or combative patient from injuring himself or others. Vest and belt restraints, used to prevent falls from a bed or a chair, permit full movement of arms and legs. Limb restraints, used to prevent removal of supportive equipment—such as I.V. lines, indwelling catheters, and nasogastric tubes—allow only slight limb motion. Like limb restraints, mitts prevent removal of supportive equipment, keep the patient from scratching rashes or sores, and prevent the combative patient from injuring himself or others. Body restraints, used to control the combative or hysterical patient, immobilize all or most of the body.

When soft restraints aren't sufficient and sedation is dangerous or ineffective, leather restraints can be used. Depending on the patient's behavior, leather restraints may be applied to all limbs (four-point restraints) or to one arm and one leg (two-point restraints). The duration of such restraint is governed by state law and by hospital policy.

Because a patient rarely submits readily to leather restraints, safe and speedy application requires team-work by several staff members, the availability of all equipment, proper patient positioning, and a brief, clear explanation of the procedure to the patient.

Restraints must be used cautiously in seizure-prone patients because they increase the risk of fracture and trauma. And because restraints can cause skin irritation and restrict blood flow, they shouldn't be applied directly over wounds or I.V. catheters. Vest restraints should be used with caution in patients who have congestive heart failure or respiratory disorders. Such restraints can tighten with movement, further limiting circulation and respiratory function.

Equipment
For soft restraints: restraint (vest, limb, mitt, belt, or body, as needed) ∎ gauze pads if needed.

For leather restraints: two wrist and two ankle leather restraints ∎ four straps ∎ key ∎ large gauze pads to cushion each extremity.

Preparation of equipment
Before entering the patient's room, make sure the restraints are the correct size, using the patient's build and weight as a guide. (For children, who typically are too small for standard restraints, see *Types of child restraints,* page 42.) If the restraints are too loose and you can't obtain smaller ones, build them up with gauze pads or washcloths and tape them down securely. If you use leather restraints, be sure the straps are unlocked and the key fits the locks.

Implementation
• Obtain a doctor's order for the restraint if required. However, never leave a confused or combative patient unattended or unrestrained while attempting to secure the order.
• If necessary, obtain adequate assistance to restrain the patient before entering his room. Enlist the aid of several co-workers and organize their effort, giving each person a specific task; for example, one person explains the procedure to the patient and applies the restraints while the others immobilize the patient's arms and legs.

• Tell the patient what you're about to do and describe the restraints to him. Assure him that they are being used to protect him from injury rather than to punish him.

Applying a vest restraint
• Assist the patient to a sitting position if his condition permits. Then slip the vest over his gown. Crisscross the cloth flaps at the front, placing the V-shaped opening at the patient's throat. Never crisscross the flaps in the back *because this may cause the patient to choke if he tries to squirm out of the vest.*
• Pass the tab on one flap through the slot on the opposite flap. Then adjust the vest for the patient's comfort. You should be able to slip your fist between the vest and the patient. Avoid wrapping the vest too tightly *because it may restrict respiration.*
• Tie all restraints securely to the frame of the bed, chair, or wheelchair and out of the patient's reach. Use a bow or a knot that can be released quickly and easily in an emergency. (See *Knots for securing soft restraints,* page 43.) Never tie a regular knot to secure the straps. Leave 1″ to 2″ (2.5 to 5 cm) of slack in the straps *to allow room for movement.*
• After applying the vest, check the patient's respiratory rate and breath sounds regularly. Be alert for signs of respiratory distress. Also, make sure the vest hasn't tightened with the patient's movement. Loosen the vest frequently, if possible, *so the patient can stretch, turn, and breathe deeply.*

Applying a limb restraint
• Wrap the patient's wrist or ankle with gauze pads *to reduce friction between the patient's skin and the restraint, helping to prevent irritation and skin breakdown.* Then wrap the restraint around the gauze pads.
• Pass the strap on the narrow end of the restraint through the slot in the broad end, and adjust for a snug fit. Or fasten the buckle or Velcro cuffs to fit the restraint. You should be able to slip one or two fingers between the restraint and the patient's skin. Avoid applying the restraint too tightly *because it may impair circulation distal to the restraint.*
• Tie the restraint as above.
• After applying limb restraints, be alert for signs of impaired circulation in the extremity distal to the restraint. If the skin appears blue or feels cold, or if the patient complains of a tingling sensation or numbness, loosen the restraint. Perform range-of-motion (ROM) exercises regularly *to stimulate circulation and prevent contractures and resultant loss of mobility.*

Types of child restraints

You may need to restrain an infant or a child to prevent injury or to facilitate examination, diagnostic tests, or treatment. If so, follow these steps:
• Provide a simple explanation, reassurance, and constant observation to minimize the child's fear.
• Explain the restraint to the parents and enlist their help. Reassure them that it will not hurt the child.
• Make sure restraint ties or safety pins are secured outside the child's reach to prevent injury.
• When using a mummy restraint, secure the infant's arms in proper alignment with the body to avoid dislocation and other injuries.

Vest

Elbow

Mummy

Belt

Limb

Crib with net

Mitt

Restraining board

Applying a mitt restraint
- Wash and dry the patient's hands.
- Roll up a washcloth or gauze pad, and place it in the patient's palm. Have him form a loose fist, if possible, then pull the mitt over it and secure the closure.
- *To restrict the patient's arm movement,* attach the strap to the mitt and tie it securely, using a bow or a knot that can be released quickly and easily in an emergency.
- When using mitts made of transparent mesh, check hand movement and skin color frequently *to assess circulation.* Remove the mitts regularly *to stimulate circulation,* and perform passive ROM exercises *to prevent contractures.*

Applying a belt restraint
- Center the flannel pad of the belt on the bed. Then wrap the short strap of the belt around the bed frame and fasten it under the bed.
- Position the patient on the pad. Then have him roll slightly to one side while you guide the long strap around his waist and through the slot in the pad.
- Wrap the long strap around the bed frame and fasten it under the bed.
- After applying the belt, slip your hand between the patient and the belt *to ensure a secure but comfortable fit. A loose belt can be raised to chest level; a tight one can cause abdominal discomfort.*

Applying a body (Posey net) restraint
- Place the restraint flat on the bed, with arm and wrist cuffs facing down and the V at the head of the bed.
- Place the patient in the prone position on top of the restraint.
- Lift the V over the patient's head. Thread the chest belt through one of the loops in the V *to ensure a snug fit.*
- Secure the straps around the patient's chest, thighs, and legs. Then turn the patient on his back.
- Secure the straps to the bed frame *to anchor the restraint.* Then secure the straps around the patient's arms and wrists.

Applying leather restraints
- Position the patient supine on the bed, with each arm and leg securely held down *to minimize combative behavior and to prevent injury to the patient and others.* Immobilize the patient's arms and legs at the joints—knee, ankle, shoulder, and wrist—*to minimize his movement without exerting excessive force.*
- Apply pads to the patient's wrists and ankles *to reduce friction between his skin and the leather, preventing skin irritation and breakdown.*
- Wrap the restraint around the gauze pads. Then insert the metal loop through the hole that gives the best fit.

Knots for securing soft restraints

When securing soft restraints, use knots that can be released quickly and easily, like those shown below. Remember, never secure restraints to the bed's side rails.

Magnus hitch

Clove hitch

Loop

Reverse clove hitch

Apply the restraints securely but not too tightly. You should be able to slip one or two fingers between the restraint and the patient's skin. *A tight restraint can compromise circulation; a loose one can slip off or move up the patient's arm or leg, causing skin irritation and breakdown.*
- Thread the strap through the metal loop on the restraint, close the metal loop, and secure the strap to the bed frame, out of the patient's reach.
- Lock the restraint by pushing in the button on the side of the metal loop, and tug it gently to be sure it's secure. Once the restraint is secure, a co-worker can release the arm or leg. Flex the patient's arm or leg slightly before locking the strap *to allow room for movement and to prevent frozen joints and dislocations.*
- Place the key in an accessible location at the nurse's station.
- After applying leather restraints, observe the patient regularly *to give emotional support and to reassess the need*

for continued use of the restraint. Check his pulse rate and vital signs at least every 2 hours. Remove or loosen the restraints one at a time, every 2 hours, and perform passive ROM exercises if possible. Watch for signs of impaired peripheral circulation, such as cool, cyanotic skin. To unlock the restraint, insert the key into the metal loop, opposite the locking button. This releases the lock, and the metal loop can be opened.

Special considerations

Because the authority to use restraints varies among hospitals, you should know your hospital's policy. You may be able to apply restraints without a doctor's order in an emergency. Also, be sure to know your state's regulations governing such restraints. For example, some states prohibit the use of four-point restraints.

When the patient is at high risk for aspiration, restrain him on his side. Never secure all four restraints to one side of the bed *because the patient may fall out of bed.*

When loosening restraints, have a co-worker on hand to assist in restraining the patient if necessary.

After assessing the patient's behavior and condition, you may decide to use a two-point restraint, which should restrain one arm and the opposite leg—for example, the right arm and the left leg. Never restrain the arm and leg on the same side *because the patient may fall out of bed.*

Don't apply a limb restraint above an I.V. site *because the constriction may occlude the infusion or cause infiltration into surrounding tissue.*

Never secure restraints to the side rails *because someone might inadvertently lower the rail before noticing the attached restraint. This may jerk the patient's limb or body, causing him discomfort and trauma.*

Don't restrain a patient in the prone position. *This position limits his field of vision, intensifies feelings of helplessness and vulnerability, and impairs respiration, especially if the patient has been sedated.*

Because the restrained patient has limited mobility, his nutrition, elimination, and positioning become your responsibility. *To prevent pressure ulcers,* reposition the patient regularly, and massage and pad bony prominences and other vulnerable areas.

When using washable restraints, place them in the laundry as your hospital directs. Many hospitals separate restraints from other linens to avoid losing them.

Complications

Excessively tight limb restraints can reduce peripheral circulation; tight vest restraints can impair respiration. Apply restraints carefully and check them regularly.

Skin breakdown can also occur under limb restraints. To prevent this, pad the patient's wrists and ankles, loosen or remove the restraints frequently, and provide regular skin care.

Long periods of immobility can predispose the patient to pneumonia, urine retention, constipation, and sensory deprivation. Reposition the patient and attend to his elimination requirements as needed.

Some patients resist restraints by biting, kicking, scratching, or head butting, possibly injuring themselves or others.

Documentation

Record the behavior that necessitated restraints, when the restraints were applied and removed, and the type of restraints used. If you expect a continued need for restraints, document their use in the Kardex.

Record vital signs, skin condition, respiratory status, peripheral circulation, and mental status.

Devices to maintain alignment and reduce pressure

Various assistive devices can be used to maintain correct body positioning and to help prevent complications that commonly arise when a patient must be on prolonged bed rest. These devices include cradle boots to protect the heels and help prevent skin breakdown, footdrop, and external hip rotation; abduction pillows to help prevent internal hip rotation after femoral fracture, hip fracture, or surgery; trochanter rolls to help prevent external hip rotation; and hand rolls to help prevent hand contractures.

Several of these devices—cradle boots, trochanter rolls, and hand rolls—are especially useful when caring for patients who have a loss of sensation, mobility, or consciousness.

Equipment

Cradle boots or substitute ■ abduction pillow ■ trochanter rolls ■ hand rolls. (See *Common preventive devices.*)

Cradle boots are made of sponge rubber and have space cut out to enclose the ankle and foot. Other commercial boots are available, but not all help to prevent external hip rotation. Footboards with antirotation blocks help prevent footdrop and external hip rotation but don't prevent heel pressure. High-topped sneakers may be used to help prevent footdrop, but they don't prevent external hip rotation or heel pressure.

The abduction pillow is a wedge-shaped piece of sponge rubber with lateral indentations for the patient's thighs.

Common preventive devices

Hand roll: prevents hand contractures

Cradle boot: prevents footdrop, skin breakdown, and external hip rotation

Abduction pillow: prevents internal hip rotation

Trochanter roll: prevents external hip rotation

Its straps wrap around the thighs to maintain correct positioning. Although a properly shaped bed pillow may temporarily substitute for the commercial abduction pillow, it's difficult to apply and fails to maintain the correct lateral alignment.

The commercial trochanter roll is made of sponge rubber but can also be improvised from a rolled blanket or towel. The hand roll, available in hard and soft materials, is held in place by fixed or adjustable straps. It can be improvised from a rolled washcloth secured with roller gauze and adhesive tape.

Preparation of equipment
If you're using a device that's available in different sizes, select the appropriate size for the patient.

Implementation
• Explain the purpose and steps of the procedure to the patient.

Applying cradle boots
• Open the slit on the superior surface of the boot. Then place the patient's heel in the circular cutout area. If the patient is positioned laterally, you may apply the boot only to the bottom foot and support the flexed top foot with a pillow.
• If appropriate, insert the other heel in the second boot.
• Position the patient's legs properly *to prevent strain on hip ligaments and pressure on bony prominences.*

Applying an abduction pillow

• Place the pillow between the supine patient's legs. Slide it toward the groin so that it touches the legs all along its length.
• Place the upper part of both legs in the pillow's lateral indentations, and secure the straps *to prevent the pillow from slipping.*

Applying trochanter rolls

• Position one roll along the outside of the thigh, from the iliac crest to midthigh. Then place another roll along the other thigh. Make sure neither roll extends as far as the knee *to avoid peroneal nerve compression and palsy, which can lead to footdrop.*
• If you've fashioned trochanter rolls from a towel, leave several inches unrolled and tuck this under the patient's thigh *to hold the device in place and maintain the patient's position.*

Applying hand rolls

• Place one roll in the patient's hand to maintain the neutral position. Then secure the strap, if present, or apply roller gauze and secure with nonallergenic or adhesive tape.
• Place another roll in the other hand.

Special considerations

Remember that the use of assistive devices doesn't preclude regularly scheduled patient positioning, range-of-motion exercises, and skin care.

Home care

Explain the use of appropriate devices to the patient and caregiver. Demonstrate how to use each device, emphasizing proper alignment of extremities, and have the patient or caregiver give a return demonstration so you can check for proper technique. Emphasize measures needed to prevent pressure ulcers.

Complications

Contractures and pressure ulcers may occur with use of a hand roll and possibly with other assistive devices. To avoid these problems, remove a soft hand roll every 4 hours (every 2 hours if the patient has hand spasticity); remove a hard hand roll every 2 hours.

Documentation

Record the use of these devices in the patient's chart and the nursing care plan, and indicate assessment for complications. Reevaluate your patient care goals as needed.

 # Passive range-of-motion exercises

Used to move the patient's joints through as full a range of motion as possible, passive range-of-motion (ROM) exercises improve or maintain joint mobility and help prevent contractures. Performed by a nurse, a physical therapist, or a caregiver of the patient's choosing, these exercises are indicated for the patient with temporary or permanent loss of mobility, sensation, or consciousness. Performed properly, passive ROM exercises require recognition of the patient's limits of motion and support of all joints during movement.

Passive ROM exercises are contraindicated in patients with septic joints, acute thrombophlebitis, severe arthritic joint inflammation, or recent trauma with possible hidden fractures or internal injuries.

Implementation

• Determine the joints that need ROM exercises, and consult the doctor or physical therapist about limitations or precautions for specific exercises. The exercises below treat all joints, but they don't have to be performed in the order given or all at once. You can schedule them over the course of a day, whenever the patient is in the most convenient position. Remember to perform all exercises slowly, gently, and to the end of the normal range of motion or to the point of pain, but no further. (See *Glossary of joint movements* to review ROM terminology.)
• Before you begin, raise the bed to a comfortable working height.

Exercising the neck

• Support the patient's head with your hands and extend the neck, flex the chin to the chest, and tilt the head laterally toward each shoulder.
• Rotate the head from right to left.

Exercising the shoulders

• Support the patient's arm in an extended, neutral position, then extend the forearm and flex it back. Abduct the arm outward from the side of the body, and adduct it back to the side.
• Rotate the shoulder so that the arm crosses the midline, and bend the elbow so that the hand touches the opposite shoulder, then touches the mattress of the bed for complete internal rotation.
• Return the shoulder to a neutral position and, with elbow bent, push the arm backward so that the back of the hand touches the mattress for complete external rotation.

Glossary of joint movements

Abduction

Adduction

Dorsiflexion

Plantar flexion

Extension

Flexion

External rotation

Internal rotation

Eversion

Inversion

Supination

Pronation

Exercising the elbow
- Place the patient's arm at his side with his palm facing up.
- Flex and extend the arm at the elbow.

Exercising the forearm
- Stabilize the patient's elbow, and then twist the hand to bring the palm up (supination).
- Twist it back again to bring the palm down (pronation).

Exercising the wrist
- Stabilize the forearm and flex and extend the wrist.
- Then rock the hand sideways for lateral flexion and rotate the hand in a circular motion.

Exercising the fingers and thumb
- Extend the patient's fingers, and then flex the hand into a fist; repeat extension and flexion of each joint of each finger and thumb separately.
- Spread two adjoining fingers apart (abduction) and then bring them together (adduction).
- Oppose each fingertip to the thumb, and rotate the thumb and each finger in a circle.

Exercising the hip and knee
- Fully extend the patient's leg, and then bend the hip and knee toward the chest, allowing full joint flexion.
- Next, move the straight leg sideways, out and away from the other leg (abduction), and then back, over, and across it (adduction).
- Rotate the straight leg internally toward the midline, and then externally away from the midline.

Exercising the ankle
- Bend the patient's foot so that the toes push upward (dorsiflexion), and then bend the foot so that the toes push downward (plantar flexion).
- Rotate the ankle in a circular motion.
- Invert the ankle so that the sole of the foot faces the midline, and evert the ankle so that the sole faces away from the midline.

Exercising the toes
- Flex the patient's toes toward the sole of the foot, and then extend them back toward the top of the foot.
- Spread two adjoining toes apart (abduction) and bring them together (adduction).

Special considerations
Because joints begin to stiffen within 24 hours of disuse, start passive ROM exercises as soon as possible, and perform them at least once a shift, particularly while bathing or turning the patient. Use proper body mechanics, and repeat each exercise at least three times.

Patients who experience prolonged bed rest or limited activity without profound weakness can also be taught to perform ROM exercises on their own (called active ROM) or may benefit from isometric exercises. (See *Learning about isometric exercises.*)

If the disabled patient requires long-term rehabilitation after discharge, consult with a physical therapist and teach a family member or caregiver to perform passive ROM exercises.

Documentation
Record the joints exercised, the presence of edema or pressure areas, any pain resulting from the exercises, any limitation of ROM, and the patient's tolerance of the exercises.

Progressive ambulation

After surgery or a period of bed rest, patients must begin the gradual return to full ambulation. When begun promptly and properly, this process — called progressive ambulation — thwarts many of the complications of prolonged inactivity.

Complications prevented by early progressive ambulation include respiratory stasis and hypostatic pneumonia; circulatory stasis, thrombophlebitis, and emboli; urine retention, urinary tract infection, and urinary stasis and calculus formation; abdominal distention, constipation, and decreased appetite; and sensory deprivation. Progressive ambulation also helps restore the patient's sense of equilibrium and enhances his self-confidence and self-image.

Progressive ambulation begins with dangling the patient's feet over the edge of the bed and progresses to seating him in an armchair or wheelchair, walking around the room with him, and then walking with him in the halls until he can walk by himself. The patient's progress depends on his physical condition and his tolerance. Successful return to full ambulation requires correct body mechanics, careful patient observation, and open communication between patient, doctor, and nurse.

Equipment
Robe ▪ chair or wheelchair ▪ slippers for sitting, hard-soled shoes for walking ▪ assistive device (cane, crutches, walker) if necessary ▪ optional: walking belt.

Learning about isometric exercises

Patients can strengthen and increase muscle tone by contracting muscles against resistance (from other muscles or from a stationary object, such as a bed or a wall) without joint movement. These exercises require only a comfortable position—standing, sitting, or lying down—and proper body alignment. For each exercise, instruct the patient to hold each contraction for 2 to 5 seconds and to repeat it three to four times daily, below peak contraction level for the first week and at peak level thereafter.

Neck rotators
The patient places the heel of his hand above one ear. Then he pushes his head toward the hand as forcefully as possible, without moving the head, neck, or arm. He repeats the exercise on the other side.

Neck flexors
The patient places both palms on his forehead. Without moving his neck, he pushes the head forward while resisting with the palms.

Neck extensors
The patient clasps his fingers behind his head, then pushes the head against the clasped hands without moving his neck.

Shoulder elevators
Holding the right arm straight down at the side, the patient grasps his right wrist with his left hand. He then tries to shrug his right shoulder, but prevents it from moving by holding his arm in place. He repeats this exercise, alternating arms.

Shoulder, chest, and scapular musculature
The patient places his right fist in his left palm and raises both arms to shoulder height. He pushes the fist into the palm as forcefully as possible without moving either arm. Then, with his arms in the same position, he clasps the fingers and tries to pull the hands apart. He repeats the pattern, beginning with the left fist in the right palm.

Elbow flexors and extensors
With his right elbow bent 90 degrees and his right palm facing upward, the patient places his left fist against his right palm. He tries to bend the right elbow further while resisting with the left fist. He repeats the pattern, bending the left elbow.

Abdomen
The patient assumes a sitting position and bends slightly forward, with his hands in front of the middle of his thighs. He tries to bend forward further, resisting by pressing the palms against the thighs.

Alternatively, in the supine position, he clasps his hands behind his head. Then he raises his shoulders about 1″ (2.5 cm), holding this position for a few seconds.

Back extensors
In a sitting position, the patient bends forward and places his hands under his buttocks. He tries to stand up, resisting with both hands.

Hip abductors
While standing, the patient squeezes his inner thighs together as tightly as possible. Placing a pillow between the knees supplies resistance and increases the effectiveness of this exercise.

Hip extensors
The patient squeezes his buttocks together as tightly as possible.

Knee extensors
The patient straightens his knee fully. Then he vigorously tightens the muscle above the knee so that it moves the kneecap upward. He repeats this exercise, alternating legs.

Ankle flexors and extensors
The patient pulls his toes upward, holding briefly. Then he pushes them down as far as possible, again holding briefly.

Preparation of equipment
If the patient requires an assistive device, the physical therapist usually selects the appropriate one and teaches its use.

Implementation
• Check the patient's history, diagnosis, and therapeutic regimen. Ask him if he feels pain or weakness; if necessary, give medication for pain and wait 30 to 60 minutes for it to take effect before attempting ambulation. Re-

Helping the patient regain mobility

Dangling legs
To help the patient support himself in a dangling position, move an overbed table in front of him and place a pillow on it.

Sitting
Seat the patient in a chair with armrests and a straight back, with his lower back against the rear of the chair, feet flat on the floor, hips and knees at right angles, and upper body straight. Rest his forearms on the armrests.

Walking
Provide a path unimpeded by equipment and other objects, and avoid overexertion. If necessary, hold the patient so you can control his upper and lower body and any lateral movements.

member that the medicated patient may overestimate his capabilities or develop hypotension, dizziness, or drowsiness.

• Explain the immediate goal of ambulation and the way you'll help him achieve it. (See *Helping the patient regain mobility.*) Provide encouragement *because he may be hesitant or fearful;* reassure him that he need not attempt more than he can reasonably do. If he fears pain in an incision, show him how to support it by placing a hand alongside or gently over the dressing site, or splint the incision for him.

• Remove equipment or other objects *to provide a clear path and prevent falls.*

Dangle the patient's legs
• Position the bed horizontally and the patient laterally, facing you. Move his legs over the side of the bed and grasp his shoulders, standing with your feet apart so you have a wide base of support. Ask the patient to help by pushing up from the bed with his arms. Then shift your weight from the foot closest to the patient's head to the other foot as you steadily and deliberately raise the patient to the sitting position. Pull with your whole body, not just your arms, *to avoid straining your back and jostling the patient.*

Alternatively, you can raise the head of the bed to a 45-degree angle *to allow easier elevation of the patient.* Don't use this method if the patient has trouble balancing

himself while sitting *because he could fall.* Ask a co-worker for assistance whenever necessary.
• While the patient adjusts to an upright position, continue to stand facing him *to keep him from falling,* and observe him closely. Be alert for signs and symptoms of orthostatic hypotension, such as fainting, dizziness, and complaints of blurred vision. If desired, check the patient's pulse rate and blood pressure. If the pulse rate increases more than 20 beats/minute, allow the patient to rest before progressing slowly.

Assist the patient to stand
• After the patient can dangle his legs successfully and can support his weight on them, attempt the standing position.
• Help the patient put on a robe and slippers or shoes. If you plan to use a walking belt, apply it now. Do not allow a robe, a urinary catheter's drainage tube, or anything else to dangle around the patient's feet.
• If the patient is alert and has fair to good strength, place his feet flat on the floor and allow him to stand by himself. As he stands, place one hand under his axilla and the other hand around his waist *to prevent falls.* Help him stand fully erect *to promote good balance and correct breathing.* Encourage him to look forward and not at the floor *to help maintain his balance.*
• If the patient needs help standing up, position your knees at either side of his. Bend your knees, put your arms around his waist, and instruct him to push up from the bed with his arms. Then straighten your knees and pull the patient with you while rising to an erect position. *This technique helps you avoid back muscle strain.*

Help the patient sit or walk
• Once the patient stands, you can pivot and lower him into an armchair or wheelchair, or you can begin to walk with him.
• If you've decided to seat him, make sure the chair is secure and won't slip as you lower the patient into it. Place his lower back against the rear of the chair and his feet flat on the floor. Position his hips and knees at right angles, and keep his upper body straight. Then flex his elbows and place his forearms on the arms of the chair.
• If the patient can walk safely only with your assistance, stand behind him, placing one hand under his axilla and the other hand around his waist. *This allows you to control the upper and lower body as well as lateral deviation.*
• If you can't support the patient, ask a co-worker to help you. Stand to one side of the patient and place your hand under his arm or on his elbow, or grasp the walking belt. Standing on the other side of the patient, the assisting co-worker should support the patient in the same way.

• Give the patient verbal and tactile cues *to encourage him during walking.* Stay close to a railed wall or another supportive structure and, if necessary, allow the patient to rest in a chair before attempting to walk back to his room. If he can't walk back, tell him to remain seated while you summon assistance or obtain a wheelchair. Don't leave the patient unattended if you have any reason to think he may fall. If you can't find a chair nearby, have the patient lean against the wall and call for assistance as you help support him. If necessary, steady him as he slides down the wall to sit on the floor.

Special considerations
If early ambulation is impossible, encourage bed exercises. Don't let the use of catheters and infusion bottles discourage ambulation; secure these devices so they are easily portable, and check dressings and tubes carefully afterward for proper position and changes in drainage. If appropriate, measure pulse, respiratory rate, and blood pressure. When leaving the patient sitting up in a chair, make certain he has a call button or signal device. Restrain the confused patient to prevent falls.
   If the patient begins to fall, don't try to catch him. Instead, do your best to break his fall by easing him to the bed, chair, or floor, making sure he doesn't strike his head. Then summon help. Don't leave the patient alone—he needs your comfort and reassurance.
   If the patient experiences dyspnea, diaphoresis, or orthostatic hypotension, stabilize his position and take vital signs. Place him in semi-Fowler's position to facilitate breathing. If his condition doesn't improve rapidly, notify the doctor.

Documentation
Record the type of transfer and assistance required; the duration of sitting, standing, or walking; the distance walked, if appropriate; the patient's response to ambulation; and any significant changes in blood pressure, pulse, and respiration.

 ## Tilt table

The tilt table, a padded table or bed-length board that can be raised gradually from a horizontal to a vertical position, can help prevent the complications of prolonged bed rest. Used for the patient with a spinal cord injury, brain damage, orthostatic hypotension, or any other condition that prevents free standing, the tilt table increases tolerance of the upright position, conditions the cardiovascular system, stretches muscles, and helps prevent contractures, bone demineralization, and urinary calculus formation.

Equipment
Tilt table with footboard and restraining straps ■ sphygmomanometer ■ stethoscope ■ antiembolism stockings or elastic bandages ■ optional: abdominal binder.

Preparation of equipment
Common types of tilt tables include the electric table, which moves at a slow, steady rate; the manual table, which is raised by a handle; and the spring-assisted table, which is raised by a pedal. Familiarize yourself with operating instructions for the model you'll be using.

Implementation
• Explain the use and benefits of the tilt table to the patient.
• Apply antiembolism stockings *to restrict vessel walls and help prevent blood pooling and edema.* If necessary, apply an abdominal binder *to avoid pooling of blood in the splanchnic region, which contributes to insufficient cerebral circulation and orthostatic hypotension.*
• Make sure the tilt table is locked in the horizontal position. Then summon assistance and transfer the patient to the table, placing him in the supine position with feet flat against the footboard.
• If the patient can't bear weight on one leg, place a wooden block between the footboard and the weight-bearing foot, permitting the non-weight-bearing leg to dangle freely.
• Fasten the safety straps, then take the patient's blood pressure and pulse rate.
• Tilt the table slowly in 15- to 30-degree increments, evaluating the patient constantly. Take his blood pressure every 3 to 5 minutes *because movement from the supine to the upright position decreases systolic pressure.* Be alert for signs and symptoms of insufficient cerebral circulation: dizziness, nausea, pallor, diaphoresis, tachycardia, or a change in mental status. If the patient experiences any of these signs or symptoms, or hypotension or seizures, return the table immediately to the horizontal position.
• If the patient tolerates the position shift, continue to tilt the table until reaching the desired angle, usually between 45 degrees and 80 degrees. A 60-degree tilt gives the patient the physiologic effects and sensations of standing upright.
• Gradually return the patient to the horizontal position, and check his vital signs. Then obtain assistance and transfer the patient onto the stretcher for transport back to his room.

Special considerations
Let the patient's response determine the angle of tilt and duration of elevation, but avoid prolonged upright positioning *because it may lead to venous stasis.*
◆ *Nursing alert.* Never leave the patient unattended on the tilt table *because marked physiologic changes, such as hypotension or severe headache, can occur suddenly.* ◆

Complications
Use of a tilt table can lead to sudden hypotension, severe headache, and other dramatic physiologic changes.

Documentation
Record the angle and duration of elevation; changes in the patient's pulse rate, blood pressure, and physical and mental status; and his response to treatment.

Canes

Indicated for the patient with one-sided weakness or injury, occasional loss of balance, or increased joint pressure, a cane provides balance and support for walking and reduces fatigue and strain on weight-bearing joints. Available in various sizes, the cane should extend from the greater trochanter to the floor and have a rubber tip to prevent slipping. Canes are contraindicated for the patient with bilateral weakness; such a patient should use crutches or a walker.

Equipment
Rubber-tipped cane ■ optional: walking belt.
　　Although wooden canes are available, three types of aluminum canes are used most frequently. The standard aluminum cane—used by the patient who needs only slight assistance to walk—provides the least support; its half-circle handle allows it to be hooked over chairs. The T-handle cane—used by the patient with hand weakness—has a straight, shaped handle with grips and a bent shaft. It provides greater stability than the standard cane. The quad (broad-based) cane is used by the patient with poor balance or one-sided weakness and an inability to hold onto a walker with both hands stemming from a cerebrovascular accident. The base of this type of cane splits into four short, splayed legs in a rectangular array. The quad cane provides greater stability than a standard cane but considerably less than a walker.

Preparation of equipment
Ask the patient to hold the cane on the uninvolved side 4″ to 6″ (10 to 15 cm) from the base of the little toe. If

the cane is made of aluminum, adjust its height by pushing in the metal button on the shaft and raising or lowering the shaft; it it's wood, the rubber tip can be removed and excess length sawed off. At the correct height, the handle of the cane is level with the greater trochanter and allows approximately 15-degree flexion at the elbow. If the cane is too short, the patient will have to drop his shoulder to lean on it; if it's too long, he'll have to raise his shoulder and will have difficulty supporting his weight.

Implementation

• Explain the mechanics of cane walking to the patient. Demonstrate the technique, then have the patient return the demonstration. Coordinate practice sessions in the physical therapy department if necessary.
• Tell the patient to hold the cane on the uninvolved side *to promote a reciprocal gait pattern and to distribute weight away from the involved side.*
• Instruct the patient to hold the cane close to his body *to prevent leaning,* and to move the cane and the involved leg simultaneously, followed by the uninvolved leg.
• Encourage the patient to keep the stride length of each leg and the timing of each step (cadence) equal.

Negotiating stairs

• Instruct the patient to always use a railing, if present, when going up or down stairs. Tell him to hold the cane with the other hand or to keep it in the hand grasping the railing. To ascend stairs, the patient should lead with the uninvolved leg and follow with the involved leg; to descend, he should lead with the involved leg and follow with the uninvolved one. Help the patient remember by telling him to use this mnemonic device: "The good goes up, and the bad goes down."
• To negotiate stairs without a railing, the patient should use the walking technique to ascend and descend the stairs but should move the cane just before the involved leg. Thus, to ascend stairs, the patient should hold the cane on the uninvolved side, step with the uninvolved leg, advance the cane, then move the involved leg. To descend, he should hold the cane on the uninvolved side, lead with the cane, then advance the involved leg and, finally, the uninvolved leg.

Using a chair

• To teach the patient to sit down, stand by his affected side and tell him to place the backs of his legs against the edge of the chair seat. Then tell him to move the cane out from his side and to reach back with both hands to grasp the chair's armrests. Supporting his weight on the armrests, he can then lower himself onto the seat. While he's seated, he should keep the cane hooked on the armrest or the chair back.

• To teach the patient to get up, stand by his affected side and tell him to unhook the cane from the chair and hold it in his stronger hand as he grasps the armrests. Then tell him to move his uninvolved foot slightly forward, to lean slightly forward, and to push against the armrests to raise himself upright.
• Warn the patient not to lean on the cane when sitting or rising from the chair *to prevent falls.*
• Supervise your patient each time he gets in or out of a chair until you're both certain he can do it alone.

Special considerations

To prevent falls during the learning period, guard the patient carefully by standing behind him slightly to his stronger side and putting one foot between his feet and your other foot to the outside of the uninvolved leg. If necessary, use a walking belt.

Complications

A poorly fitted cane can cause the patient to lose his balance and fall.

Documentation

Record the type of cane used, the amount of guarding required, the distance walked, and the patient's understanding and tolerance of cane walking.

Crutches

Crutches remove weight from one or both legs, enabling the patient to support himself with his hands and arms. Typically prescribed for the patient with lower-extremity injury or weakness, crutches require balance, stamina, and upper-body strength for successful use. Crutch selection and walking gait depend on the patient's condition. The patient who can't use crutches may be able to use a walker.

Equipment

Crutches with axillary pads, handgrips, and rubber suction tips ■ optional: walking belt.

Three types of crutches are commonly used. Standard aluminum or wooden crutches are used by the patient with a sprain, strain, or cast. They require stamina and upper-body strength. Aluminum forearm crutches are used by the paraplegic or other patient using the swing-through gait. They have a collar that fits around the forearm and a horizontal handgrip that provides support. Platform crutches are used by the arthritic patient who has an upper-extremity deficit that prevents weight bear-

Fitting a patient for a crutch

Position the crutch so that it extends from a point 4″ to 6″ (10 to 15 cm) to the side and 4″ to 6″ in front of the patient's feet to 1½″ to 2″ (4 to 5 cm) below the axillae (about the width of two fingers). Then adjust the handgrips so that the patient's elbows are flexed at a 15-degree angle when he's standing with the crutches in the resting position.

ing through the wrist. They provide padded surfaces for the upper extremities.

Preparation of equipment

After choosing the appropriate crutches, adjust their height with the patient standing or, if necessary, recumbent. (See *Fitting a patient for a crutch* for specific instructions.)

Implementation

• Consult with the patient's doctor and physical therapist *to coordinate rehabilitation orders and teaching.*
• Describe the gait you will teach and the reason for your choice. Then demonstrate the gait, as necessary. Have the patient give a return demonstration.
• Place a walking belt around the patient's waist, if necessary, *to help prevent falls.* Tell the patient to position the crutches and to shift his weight from side to side. Then place the patient in front of a full-length mirror *to facilitate learning and coordination.*
• Teach the four-point gait to the patient who can bear weight on both legs. Although this is the safest gait, *because three points are always in contact with the floor,* it requires greater coordination than others *because of its constant shifting of weight.* Use this sequence: right crutch, left foot, left crutch, right foot. Suggest counting *to help develop rhythm,* and make sure each short step is of equal length. If the patient gains proficiency at this gait, teach the faster two-point gait.
• Teach the two-point gait to the patient with weak legs but good coordination and arm strength. This is the most natural crutch-walking gait *because it mimics walking, with alternating swings of the arms and legs.* Instruct the patient to advance the right crutch and left foot simultaneously, followed by the left crutch and right foot.
• Teach the three-point gait to the patient who can bear only partial or no weight on one leg. Instruct him to advance both crutches 6″ to 8″ (15 to 20 cm) along with the involved leg. Then tell him to bring the uninvolved leg forward and to bear the bulk of his weight on the crutches but some of it on the involved leg, if possible. Stress the importance of taking steps of equal length and duration with no pauses.
• Teach the swing-to or swing-through gaits—the fastest ones—to the patient with complete paralysis of the hips and legs. Instruct the patient to advance both crutches simultaneously and to swing the legs parallel to (swing-to) or beyond the crutches (swing-through).
• To teach the patient who uses crutches to get up from a chair, tell him to hold both crutches in one hand, with the tips resting firmly on the floor. Then instruct him to push up from the chair with his free hand, supporting himself with the crutches.
• To sit down, the patient reverses the process: Tell him to support himself with the crutches in one hand and to lower himself with the other.
• To teach the patient to ascend stairs using the three-point gait, tell him to lead with the uninvolved leg and to follow with both the crutches and the involved leg. To descend stairs, he should lead with the crutches and the involved leg and follow with the good leg. He may find

it helpful to remember "The good goes up, the bad goes down."

Special considerations

Encourage arm- and shoulder-strengthening exercises to prepare the patient for crutch walking. If possible, teach two techniques—one fast and one slow—*so the patient can alternate between them to prevent excessive muscle fatigue and can adjust more easily to various walking conditions.*

Complications

When used with chronic conditions, the swing-to and swing-through gaits can lead to atrophy of the hips and legs if appropriate therapeutic exercises are not performed routinely. Warn the patient against habitually leaning on his crutches *because prolonged pressure on the axillae can damage the brachial nerves, causing brachial nerve palsy.*

Documentation

Record the type of gait the patient used, the amount of assistance required, the distance walked, and the patient's tolerance of the crutches and gait.

Walkers

A walker consists of a metal frame with handgrips and four legs that buttresses the patient on three sides. One side remains open. Because this device provides greater stability and security than other ambulatory aids, it's recommended for the patient with insufficient strength and balance to use crutches or a cane, or with weakness requiring frequent rest periods. Attachments for standard walkers and modified walkers help meet special needs.

Equipment

Walker ■ platform or wheel attachments, as necessary.

Various types of walkers are available. The standard walker is used by the patient with unilateral or bilateral weakness or an inability to bear weight on one leg. It requires arm strength and balance. Platform attachments may be added to this walker for the patient with arthritic arms or a casted arm, who can't bear weight directly on his hand, wrist, or forearm. With the doctor's approval, wheels may be placed on the front legs of the standard walker to allow the extremely weak or poorly coordinated patient to roll the device forward, instead of lifting it. However, wheels are applied infrequently *because they may be a safety hazard.*

The stair walker—used by the patient who must negotiate stairs without bilateral handrails—requires good arm strength and balance. Its extra set of handles extends toward the patient on the open side. The rolling walker—used by the patient with very weak legs—has four wheels and a seat. The reciprocal walker—used by the patient with very weak arms—allows one side to be advanced ahead of the other.

Preparation of equipment

Obtain the appropriate walker with the advice of a physical therapist, and adjust it to the patient's height: His elbows should be flexed at a 15-degree angle when standing comfortably within the walker with his hands on the grips. To adjust the walker, turn it upside down, and change the leg length by pushing in the button on each shaft and releasing it when the leg is in the correct position. Make sure the walker is level before the patient attempts to use it.

Implementation

• Help the patient stand within the walker, and instruct him to hold the handgrips firmly and equally. Stand behind him, closer to the involved leg.
• If the patient has one-sided leg weakness, tell him to advance the walker 6″ to 8″ (15 to 20 cm) and to step forward with the involved leg and follow with the uninvolved leg, supporting himself on his arms. Encourage him to take equal strides. If he has equal strength in both legs, instruct him to advance the walker 6″ to 8″ and to step forward with either leg. If he can't use one leg, tell him to advance the walker 6″ to 8″ and to swing onto it, supporting his weight on his arms.
• If the patient is using a reciprocal walker, teach him the two-point or four-point gait (see "Crutches" in this chapter). If the patient is using a wheeled or stair walker, reinforce the physical therapist's instructions. Stress the need for caution when using a stair walker.
• Teach the patient how to use a chair safely. (See *Teaching safe use of a walker,* page 56.)

Special considerations

If the patient starts to fall, support his hips and shoulders *to help maintain an upright position if possible.*

Documentation

Record the type of walker and attachments used, the degree of guarding required, the distance walked, and the patient's tolerance of ambulation.

Teaching safe use of a walker

Sitting down

• First, tell the patient to stand with the back of his stronger leg against the front of the chair, his weaker leg slightly off the floor, and the walker directly in front.

• Tell him to grasp the armrests on the chair one arm at a time while supporting most of his weight on the stronger leg. (In the illustrations below, the patient has left leg weakness.)

• Tell the patient to lower himself into the chair and slide backward. After he is seated, he should place the walker beside the chair.

Getting up

• After bringing the walker back to the front of his chair, tell the patient to slide forward in the chair. Placing the back of his stronger leg against the seat, he should then advance the weaker leg.

• Next, with both hands on the armrests, the patient can push himself to a standing position. Supporting himself with the stronger leg and the opposite hand, the patient should grasp the walker's handgrip with his free hand.

• Then have the patient grasp the free handgrip with his other hand.

Supplemental bed equipment

Certain equipment can promote the bedridden patient's comfort and help prevent pressure ulcers and other complications of immobility. A wood or hard plastic footboard prevents footdrop by maintaining proper alignment. It also raises bed linens off of the patient's feet. The foot cradle — a horizontal or arched bar over the end of the bed — keeps bed linens off of the patient's feet, preventing skin irritation and breakdown, especially in patients with peripheral vascular disease or neuropathy. The bed board, made of wood or wood covered with canvas, firms the mattress and is especially useful for the patient with spinal injuries. The metal basic frame and the metal trapeze (a triangular piece attached to this frame) allow the patient with arm mobility and strength to lift himself off the bed, facilitating bed making and bedpan positioning. The metal overbed cradle, a cagelike frame positioned on top of the mattress, keeps bed linens off of the patient with burns, open wounds, or a wet cast.

The vinyl water mattress and the foam mattress, used to prevent or treat pressure ulcers, exert less pressure on the skin than the standard hospital mattress. Although the alternating pressure pad (a vinyl pad divided into chambers filled with air or water and attached to an electric pump) serves the same purpose, it also stimulates circulation by alternately inflating and deflating its chambers.

All supplemental bed equipment is optional, depending on the patient's needs. Reusable and disposable water mattresses are available. The reusable water mattress replaces the standard hospital mattress and rests on a sheet of heavy cardboard placed over the bedsprings; the smaller, less bulky disposable mattress rests on top of the standard hospital mattress. (See *Types of supplemental bed equipment*, page 58.)

Equipment
Footboard and cover ■ drawsheet ■ bath blanket ■ foot cradle ■ bed board ■ basic frame with trapeze ■ overbed cradle ■ roller gauze ■ water mattress ■ stretcher ■ alternating pressure pad ■ pump and tubing ■ footstool ■ linen-saver pad ■ foam mattress (such as a convoluted foam mattress) ■ safety pins ■ plastic protective sleeve for foam mattress (partial or full length).

Preparation of equipment
If you're preparing a footboard for use, place a cover over it to provide padding. Or pad it with a folded drawsheet or bath blanket: Bring the top and side edges of the sheet or blanket to the back of the footboard, miter the corners, and secure them at the center with safety pins. *Padding cushions the patient's feet against pressure from the hard footboard, helping to prevent skin irritation and breakdown.* Avoid wrinkles *to prevent skin irritation.*

Implementation
● Tell the patient what you're going to do and describe the equipment.
● Wash your hands.

Using a footboard
● Move the patient up in bed *to allow room for the footboard.* Loosen the top linens at the foot of the bed, and then fold them back over the patient *to expose his feet.*
● Lift the mattress at the foot of the bed, and place the lip of the footboard between the mattress and the bedsprings. Or secure the footboard under both sides of the mattress.

● Adjust the footboard so that the patient's feet rest comfortably against it. If the footboard isn't adjustable, tuck a folded bath blanket between the board and the patient's feet.
● Unless the footboard has side supports, place a sandbag, a folded bath blanket, or a pillow alongside each foot *to maintain 90-degree foot alignment.*
● Fold the top linens over the footboard, tuck them under the mattress, and miter the corners.

Using a foot cradle
● Loosen the top linens at the foot of the bed, and fold them over the patient or to one side.
● When using a one-piece cradle, place one side arm under the mattress, carefully extend the arch over the bed, and place the other side arm under the mattress on the opposite side. Then adjust the tension rods *so that they rest securely over the edge of the mattress.*
● When using a sectional cradle with two side arms, first place the side arms under the mattress. Secure the tension rods over the edge of the mattress. Then carefully place the arch over the bed and connect it to the side arms.

When using a sectional cradle with one side arm, connect the side arm and horizontal cradle bar before placement. Then place the side arm under the mattress on one side of the bed.
● Cover the cradle with the top linens, tuck them under the mattress at the foot of the bed, and miter the corners.

Using a bed board
● Transfer the patient from his bed to a stretcher or a chair. Obtain assistance if necessary.
● Strip the linens from the bed. If you plan to reuse them, fold each piece neatly and hang it over the back of a chair. Otherwise, place soiled linens in a laundry bag.
● If the bed board consists of wooden slats encased in canvas, lift the mattress at the head of the bed and center the board over the bedsprings *to prevent it from jutting out and causing accidental injury.* Unroll the slats to cover the bedsprings at the head of the bed. Then lift the mattress at the foot of the bed and unroll the remaining slats.

If the bed board consists of one solid or two hinged pieces of wood, lift the mattress on one side of the bed and center the board over the bedsprings.
● After positioning the bed board, replace the linens. Then return the patient to bed.

Using a basic frame with trapeze
● If an orthopedic technician isn't available to secure the frame and trapeze to the patient's bed, get assistance to

Types of supplemental bed equipment

Sectional cradle with two side arms

One-piece cradle

L-shaped footboard

Adjustable footboard

Sectional cradle with one side arm

Overbed cradle

Convoluted foam mattress

Trapeze and basic frame

Alternating pressure pad

attach these devices to the bed, as necessary. Be sure to hang the trapeze within the patient's easy reach so he won't need to strain to reach it.

Using an overbed cradle
• Loosen and remove the top linens.
• Carefully lower the cradle onto the patient's bed and secure it in place. Wrap roller gauze around both sides

of the cradle. Then pull the gauze taut and attach it to the bedsprings.
• Cover the cradle with the top linens, tuck them under the mattress at the foot of the bed, and miter the corners.

Using a portable water mattress
• This mattress is heavy and bulky, so you'll need several co-workers *to help you transfer it from the stretcher to the patient's bed.* Check with the maintenance department before transferring the mattress *because its weight may rule out use on some electric beds.* Also, ensure that the patient isn't prone to motion sickness *because the movement of the water in the mattress may cause nausea.*
• Position the mattress on the bed, and place the protective cover over it. Then place a bottom sheet over the cover and tuck it in loosely.
• Place a sheepskin, linen-saver pad, or drawsheet over the bottom sheet, as needed. Adding these items doesn't decrease the effectiveness of this mattress.
• Position the patient comfortably on the mattress. Then cover him with the top linens, and tuck them in loosely.
• Check the water mattress daily *to ensure adequate flotation.* To do so, place your hand under the patient's thighs. If you can feel the bottom of the mattress, arrange to have water added.

Using an alternating pressure pad
• If possible, transfer the patient from his bed to a chair or stretcher. Get help if necessary.
• Strip the linens from the bed. Then inspect the plug and electrical cord of the alternating pressure pad for defects. Don't use the unit if it appears damaged.
• Unfold the pad on top of the mattress with the appropriate side facing up.
• Place the motor on a linen-saver pad on the floor or on a footstool near the mattress outlets. Connect the tubing securely to the motor and to the mattress outlets, and plug the cord into an electrical outlet. Turn the motor on.
• After several minutes, observe the emptying and filling of the pad's chambers, and check the tubing for kinks *because they could interfere with the pad's function.*
• Place a bottom sheet over the pad, and tuck it in loosely. *To avoid tube constriction,* don't miter the corner where the tubing is attached.
• Position the patient comfortably on the pad, cover him with the top linens, and tuck them in loosely.
• If the pad becomes soiled, clean it with a damp cloth and mild soap, then dry it well. *To avoid damaging the pad's surface,* don't use alcohol.
• When the patient no longer needs the pad or is discharged, turn the motor off, disconnect the tubing, and unplug the cord from the wall outlet. Remove the pad

from the patient's bed, and fold and discard it. Or, if applicable, give the pad to the patient to take home. Inform him that the motor needed to power the pad can usually be rented from a surgical supply store. Explain to the patient or a caregiver how to operate the pad at home.
• Coil the tubing and electrical cord, and then strap them to the motor. Return the motor unit to the central supply department.

Using a convoluted foam mattress
• If possible, transfer the patient from his bed to a chair or stretcher. Get help if necessary.
• Strip the linens from the bed. Then place the foam mattress on top of the standard mattress, wavy side up.
• Slip the protective sleeve over the foam mattress at the patient's buttock level *to prevent leakage of excretions into the mattress.* If necessary, use a full-length sleeve.
• Place a bottom sheet over the foam mattress, and tuck it in loosely. *Tucking it too tightly can decrease the cushioning effect.*
• Position the patient comfortably on the mattress. Then cover him with the top linens and tuck them in loosely.
• When the patient no longer needs the mattress or is discharged, discard the mattress or let him take it home. (See *Helping patients improvise assistive devices at home,* page 60.)

Special considerations
Place the patient in bed before positioning and securing an overbed or foot cradle *to ensure its proper placement and to prevent patient injury.* Similarly, remove the cradle before the patient gets out of bed. When turning or positioning the patient on his side, be sure the foot cradle's tension rod doesn't rest against his skin *because this may cause pressure and predispose him to skin breakdown.*

Exercise caution when turning the obese patient on a water mattress *because turning displaces a large volume of water.* Be sure to keep the side rails raised during turning *to prevent falls.*

Avoid placing excessive layers of drawsheets or linen-saver pads between the alternating pressure pad and the patient, *because these decrease the pad's effectiveness.* Avoid using pins or sharp instruments near an alternating pressure pad or water mattress *to prevent accidental puncture.*

Use up to three foam mattresses on the bed, as the patient's condition requires. Place one mattress on the bed to prevent pressure ulcers, two or three mattresses to treat them. You can decrease the pressure exerted on the bony prominences by increasing the number of mattresses.

◆ *Nursing alert.* Because a plastic-covered mattress slides off a bed board easily, be sure a co-worker is standing

Helping patients improvise assistive devices at home

Assistive devices can increase patient comfort and improve care given in the home. This equipment need not be expensive. If the patient's illness is brief or financial constraints exist, teach patients and caregivers to improvise assistive devices with common household items. For example:

• Side rails can be made by placing kitchen chairs along the sides of a bed and securing their legs to the bed frame.

• Linen-saver pads can be fashioned from shower curtains, plastic tablecloths, a plastic raincoat, or trash bags.

• Absorbent pads can be made by placing sheets of newspaper and a bottom layer of plastic inside a pillowcase. When damp, discard the newspaper and wash the pillowcase.

• An ironing board, a wooden crate with two sides removed, a child's table, or a sturdy cardboard box can serve as an over-the-bed table or a bed cradle.

• Backrests can be fashioned from a large item such as a cutting board padded on top and supported underneath by pillows.

• A pull rope to assist the patient in turning or sitting up can be made by braiding nylon stockings together and fastening the rope to the side or end of the bed.

on the opposite side of the bed when you're transferring the patient from stretcher to bed.◆

If the bottom sheet isn't wide enough to cover both the standard and foam mattresses, use two bottom sheets. Cover the standard mattress with one sheet, then cover the foam mattress with a second sheet and tuck it between the standard and foam mattresses. Two top sheets may be needed to cover the patient when using a footboard, foot cradle, or bed cradle.

Because a foam mattress is tightly rolled for storage, it may need to be unrolled on a clean empty bed and allowed to recover its original springiness before use.

Don't use a foam mattress to lift the patient *because the mattress may tear, causing the patient to fall.*

Documentation

In your notes and care plan, record the type of supplemental bed equipment used, the time and date of use, and the patient's response to treatment.

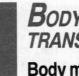

BODY MECHANICS AND TRANSFER TECHNIQUES

Body mechanics

Many patient care activities require the nurse to push, pull, lift, and carry. By using proper body mechanics, the nurse can avoid musculoskeletal injury and fatigue, and reduce the risk of injuring patients. Correct body mechanics can be summed up in three principles, as presented below.

Keep a low center of gravity by flexing the hips and knees instead of bending at the waist. This position distributes weight evenly between the upper and lower body and helps maintain balance.

Create a wide base of support by spreading the feet apart. This tactic provides lateral stability and lowers the body's center of gravity.

Maintain proper body alignment and keep the body's center of gravity directly over the base of support by moving the feet rather than twisting and bending at the waist.

Implementation

Follow the directions below to push, pull, stoop, lift, and carry correctly.

Pushing and pulling correctly

• Stand close to the object and place one foot slightly ahead of the other, as in a walking position. Tighten the leg muscles and set the pelvis by simultaneously contracting the abdominal and gluteal muscles.

• To push, place your hands on the object and flex your elbows. Lean into the object by shifting weight from the back leg to the front leg, and apply smooth, continuous pressure.

• To pull, grasp the object and flex your elbows. Lean away from the object by shifting weight from the front leg to the back leg. Pull smoothly, avoiding sudden, jerky movements.

• After you've started to move the object, keep it in motion; *stopping and starting uses more energy.*

Stooping correctly

• Stand with your feet 10″ to 12″ (25 to 30 cm) apart and one foot slightly ahead of the other *to widen the base of support.*

• Lower yourself by flexing your knees, and place more weight on the front foot than on the back foot. Keep the upper body straight by not bending at the waist.

• To stand up again, straighten the knees and keep the back straight.

Lifting and carrying correctly
• Assume the stooping position directly in front of the object *to minimize back flexion and avoid spinal rotation when lifting.*
• Grasp the object, and tighten your abdominal muscles.
• Stand up by straightening the knees, using the leg and hip muscles. Always keep your back straight *to maintain a fixed center of gravity.*
• Carry the object close to your body at waist height — near the body's center of gravity — *to avoid straining the back muscles.*

Special considerations
Wear shoes with low heels, flexible nonslip soles, and closed backs *to promote correct body alignment, facilitate proper body mechanics, and prevent accidents.* When possible, pull rather than push an object *because the elbow flexors are stronger than the extensors.* When doing heavy lifting or moving, remember to use assistive or mechanical devices, if available, or obtain assistance from co-workers; know your limitations and use sound judgment.

 # Patient transfer from bed to stretcher

Transfer from bed to stretcher, one of the most common transfers, can require the help of one or more co-workers, depending on the patient's size and condition and the primary nurse's physical abilities. Techniques for achieving this transfer include the straight lift, carry lift, lift sheet, and roller board.

In the straight (or patient-assisted) lift — used to move the pediatric or very light patient, or the patient who can assist transfer — the members of the transfer team place their hands and arms beneath the patient's buttocks and, if necessary, his shoulders. Other patients may require a four-person straight lift, detailed below. In the carry lift, team members roll the patient onto their upper arms and hold him against their chests. In the lift sheet transfer, they place a sheet under the patient and lift or slide him onto the stretcher. In the roller board transfer, two team members slide the patient onto the stretcher.

Equipment
Stretcher ■ roller board or lift sheet if necessary.

Preparation of equipment
Adjust the bed to the same height as the stretcher.

Implementation
• Tell the patient that you're going to move him from the bed to the stretcher and place him in the supine position.
• Ask team members to remove their rings and watches *to avoid scratching the patient during transfer.*

Four-person straight lift
• Place the stretcher parallel to the bed, and lock the wheels of both *to ensure the patient's safety.*
• Stand at the center of the stretcher, and have another team member stand at the patient's head. The two other team members should stand next to the bed, on the other side — one at the center and the other at the patient's feet.
• Slide your arms, palms up, beneath the patient, while the other team members do the same. In this position, you and the team member directly opposite support the patient's buttocks and hips; the team member at the head of the bed supports the patient's head and shoulders; the one at the foot supports the patient's legs and feet.
• On a count of three, the team members lift the patient several inches, move him onto the stretcher, and slide their arms out from under him. Keep movements smooth *to minimize patient discomfort and avoid muscle strain by team members.*

Four-person carry lift
• Place the stretcher perpendicular to the bed, with the head of the stretcher at the foot of the bed. Lock the bed and stretcher wheels *to ensure the patient's safety.*
• Raise the bed to a comfortable working height.
• Line up all four team members on the same side of the bed as the stretcher, with the tallest member at the patient's head and the shortest at his feet. The member at the patient's head is the leader of the team and gives the lift signals.
• Tell the team members to flex their knees and slide their hands, palms up, under the patient until he rests securely on their upper arms. Make sure the patient is adequately supported at the head and shoulders, buttocks and hips, and legs and feet.
• On a count of three, the team members straighten their knees and roll the patient onto his side, against their chests. *This reduces strain on the lifters* and allows them to hold the patient for several minutes if necessary.
• Together, the team members step back, with the member supporting the feet moving the farthest. The team members move forward to the stretcher's edge and, on a count of three, lower the patient onto the stretcher by bending

at the knees and sliding their arms out from under the patient.

Four-person lift sheet transfer

• Position the bed, stretcher, and team members for the straight lift. Then instruct the team to hold the edges of the sheet under the patient, grasping them close to the patient *to obtain a firm grip, provide stability, and spare the patient undue feelings of instability.*
• On a count of three, the team members lift or slide the patient onto the stretcher in a smooth, continuous motion *to avoid muscle strain and minimize patient discomfort.*

Roller board transfer

• Place the stretcher parallel to the bed, and lock the wheels of both *to ensure the patient's safety.*
• Stand next to the bed, and instruct a co-worker to stand next to the stretcher.
• Reach over the patient and pull the far side of the bedsheet toward you to turn the patient slightly on his side. Your co-worker then places the roller board beneath the patient, making sure the board bridges the gap between stretcher and bed.
• Ease the patient onto the roller board and release the sheet. Your co-worker then grasps the near side of the sheet at the patient's hips and shoulders and pulls him onto the stretcher in a smooth, continuous motion. She then reaches over the patient, grasps the far side of the sheet, and logrolls him toward her.
• Remove the roller board as your co-worker returns the patient to the supine position.

After all transfers

• Position the patient comfortably on the stretcher, apply safety straps, and raise and secure the side rails.

Special considerations

When transferring a helpless or markedly obese patient from bed to stretcher, first lift and move the patient, in increments, to the edge of the bed. Then rest for a few seconds, repositioning the patient if necessary, and lift him onto the stretcher. If the patient can bear weight on his arms or legs, two or three co-workers can perform this transfer: One co-worker can support the buttocks and guide the patient, another can stabilize the stretcher by leaning over it and guiding the patient into position, and a third can transfer any attached equipment. If a team member isn't available to guide equipment, move I.V. lines and other tubing first *to make sure they're out of the way and not in danger of pulling loose,* or disconnect tubes if possible. If the patient is light, three co-workers can perform the carry lift; however, no matter how many team members are present, one must stabilize the head

if the patient can't support it himself, has cervical instability or injury, or has undergone surgery.

Depending on the patient's size and condition, lift sheet transfer can require two to seven co-workers.

Documentation

Record the time and, if necessary, the type of transfer in your notes. Complete other required forms, as necessary.

Patient transfer from bed to wheelchair

For the patient with diminished or absent lower-body sensation or one-sided weakness, immobility, or injury, transfer from bed to wheelchair may require partial support to full assistance—initially by at least two persons. Subsequent transfer of the patient with generalized weakness may be performed by one nurse. After transfer, proper positioning helps prevent excessive pressure on bony prominences, which predisposes the patient to skin breakdown.

Equipment

Wheelchair with locks (or sturdy chair) ■ pajama bottoms (or robe) ■ shoes or slippers with nonslip soles ■ optional: transfer board if appropriate. (See *Teaching the patient to use a transfer board.)*

Implementation

• Explain the procedure to the patient and demonstrate his role.
• Place the wheelchair parallel to the bed, facing the foot of the bed, and lock its wheels. Make sure the bed wheels are also locked. Raise the footrests *to avoid interfering with the transfer.*
• Check pulse rate and blood pressure with the patient supine *to obtain a baseline.* Then help him put on the pajama bottoms and slippers or shoes with nonslip soles *to prevent falls.*
• Raise the head of the bed and allow the patient to rest briefly *to adjust to posture changes.* Then, bring him to the dangling position (see "Progressive ambulation" in this chapter). Recheck pulse rate and blood pressure if you suspect cardiovascular instability. Don't proceed until the patient's pulse rate and blood pressure are stabilized *to prevent falls.*
• Tell the patient to move toward the edge of the bed and, if possible, to place his feet flat on the floor. Stand

Teaching the patient to use a transfer board

For the patient who can't stand, a transfer board allows safe transfer from bed to wheelchair. To perform this transfer, take the following steps.

• First explain and demonstrate the procedure. Eventually, the patient may become proficient enough to transfer himself independently or with some supervision.

• Help the patient put on pajama bottoms or a robe, and shoes or slippers.

• Place the wheelchair parallel to and facing the foot of the bed. Lock the wheels, and remove the armrest closest to the patient. Make sure the bed is flat, and adjust its height so that it's level with the wheelchair seat.

• Assist the patient to a sitting position on the edge of the bed, with his feet resting on the floor. Make sure the front edge of the wheelchair seat is aligned with the back of the patient's knees as shown in the illustration below. *Although it's important that the patient have an even surface on which to transfer, he may find it easier to transfer to a slightly lower surface.*

• Ask the patient to lean away from the wheelchair while you slide one end of the transfer board under him.

• Now place the other end of the transfer board on the wheelchair seat, and help the patient return to the upright position.

• Stand in front of the patient *to prevent him from sliding forward.* Tell him to push down with both arms, lifting the buttocks up and onto the transfer board. The patient then repeats this maneuver, edging along the board, until he's seated in the wheelchair. If the patient can't use his arms to assist with the transfer, stand in front of him, put your arms around him, and—if he's able—have him put his arms around you. Gradually slide him across the board until he's safely in the chair as shown below.

• Once the patient is in the chair, fasten a seat belt, if necessary, *to prevent falls.*

• Then remove the transfer board, replace the wheelchair armrest, and reposition the patient in the chair.

in front of the patient, blocking his toes with your feet and his knees with yours *to prevent his knees from buckling.*

• Flex your knees slightly, place your arms around the patient's waist, and tell him to place his hands on the edge of the bed. Avoid bending at your waist *to prevent back strain.*

• Ask the patient to push himself off the bed and to support as much of his own weight as possible. At the same time, straighten your knees and hips, raising the patient as you straighten your body.

• Supporting the patient as needed, pivot toward the wheelchair, keeping your knees next to his. Tell the patient to grasp the farthest armrest of the wheelchair with his closest hand.

• Help the patient lower himself into the wheelchair by flexing your hips and knees, but not your back. Instruct him to reach back and grasp the other wheelchair armrest as he sits *to avoid abrupt contact with the seat.* Fasten the seat belt *to prevent falls* and, if necessary, check pulse rate and blood pressure *to assess cardiovascular stability.* If the pulse rate is 20 beats or more above baseline, stay with the patient and monitor him closely until it returns to normal *because he is experiencing orthostatic hypotension.*

• If the patient can't position himself correctly, help him move his buttocks against the back of the chair *so the ischial tuberosities, not the sacrum, provide the base of support.*

• Place the patient's feet flat on the footrests, pointed straight ahead. Then position the knees and hips with the correct amount of flexion and in appropriate alignment. If appropriate, use elevating leg rests to flex the patient's hips at more than 90 degrees; *this position relieves pressure on the popliteal space and places more weight on the ischial tuberosities.*

• Position the patient's arms on the wheelchair's armrests with shoulders abducted, elbows slightly flexed, forearms pronated, and wrists and hands in the neutral position. If necessary, support or elevate the patient's hands and forearms with a pillow *to prevent dependent edema.*

Special considerations

If the patient starts to fall during transfer, ease him to the closest surface — bed, floor, or chair. Never stretch to finish the transfer. Doing so can cause loss of balance, falls, muscle strain, and other injuries — to you and the patient.

If the patient has one-sided weakness, follow the preceding steps, but place the wheelchair on the patient's unaffected side. Instruct the patient to pivot and bear as much weight as possible on the unaffected side. Support the affected side *because the patient will tend to lean*

to this side. Use pillows to support the hemiplegic patient's affected side *to prevent slumping in the wheelchair.*

Documentation

If necessary, record the time of transfer and the extent of assistance in your notes, and note how the patient tolerated the activity.

Patient transfer with a hydraulic lift

Using a hydraulic lift to raise the immobile patient from the supine to the sitting position allows safe, comfortable transfer between bed and chair. It's indicated for the obese or immobile patient for whom manual transfer poses the potential for nurse or patient injury. Although most hydraulic lift models can be operated by one person, it's better to have two staff members present during transfer to stabilize and support the patient.

Equipment

Hydraulic lift, with sling, chains or straps, and hooks ▪ chair or wheelchair.

Preparation of equipment

Because hydraulic lift models may vary in weight capacity, check the manufacturer's specifications before attempting patient transfer. Make sure the bed and wheelchair wheels are locked before beginning the transfer.

Implementation

• Explain the procedure to the patient, and reassure him that the hydraulic lift can safely support his weight and won't tip over.

• Make sure the side rail opposite you is raised and secure. Then roll the patient toward you, onto his side, and raise the side rail. Walk to the opposite side of the bed and lower the side rail.

• Place the sling under the patient's buttocks with its lower edge below the greater trochanter. Then fanfold the far side of the sling against the back and buttocks.

• Roll the patient toward you onto the sling, and raise the side rail. Then lower the opposite side rail.

• Slide your hands under the patient and pull the sling from beneath him, smoothing out all wrinkles. Then roll the patient onto his back and center him on the sling.

• Place the appropriate chair next to the head of the bed, facing the foot.

• Lower the side rail next to the chair, and raise the bed only until the base of the lift can extend under the bed.

Using a hydraulic lift

After placing the patient supine in the center of the sling, position the hydraulic lift above him, as shown here. Then attach the chains to the hooks on the sling.

Turn the lift handle clockwise to raise the patient to the sitting position. If he's positioned properly, continue to raise him until he's suspended just above the bed.

After positioning the patient above the wheelchair, turn the lift handle counterclockwise to lower him onto the seat. When the chains become slack, stop turning and unhook the sling from the lift.

To avoid alarming and endangering the patient, don't raise the bed completely.
• Set the lift's adjustable base to its widest position *to ensure the highest level of stability.* Then move the lift so that its arm lies perpendicular to the bed, directly over the patient.
• Connect one end of the chains (or straps) to the side arms on the lift; connect the other, hooked end to the sling. Face the hooks away from the patient *to prevent them from slipping and to avoid the risk of their pointed edges injuring the patient.* The patient may place his arms inside or outside the chains (or straps) or he may grasp them once the slack is gone (to avoid injury). (See *Using a hydraulic lift.*)
• Tighten the turnscrew on the lift. Then, depending on the type of lift you're using, pump the handle or turn it clockwise until the patient has assumed a sitting position and his buttocks clear the bed surface by 1″ or 2″ (2.5 or 5 cm). Momentarily suspend the patient above the bed *until he feels secure in the lift and sees that it can bear his weight.*
• Steady the patient as you move the lift or, preferably, have another co-worker guide the patient's body while you move the lift. Depending on the type of lift you're using, the arm should now rest in front or to one side of the chair.

• Release the turnscrew. Then depress the handle or turn it counterclockwise *to lower the patient into the chair.* While lowering the patient, push gently on his knees *to maintain the correct sitting posture.* After lowering the patient into the chair, fasten the seat belt *to ensure his safety.*
• Remove the hooks or straps from the sling, but leave the sling in place under the patient so you'll be able to transfer him back to the bed from the chair. Then move the lift away from the patient.
• To return the patient to bed, reverse the procedure.

Special considerations
If the patient has an altered center of gravity (caused by a halo vest or a lower-extremity cast, for example), obtain help from a co-worker before transferring him with a hydraulic lift.

If the patient will require use of a hydraulic lift for transfers after discharge, teach his family how to use this device correctly and allow them to practice with supervision.

Documentation
If necessary, record the time of transfer in your notes.

Operating a Stryker wedge frame

First, obtain the help of a co-worker. Then remove the armboards from the frame. Arrange the anterior frame over the patient and lock it at the head end. Replace the anterior half of the ring, if removed, and close it over the patient until it locks automatically.

Then place the patient's arms around the anterior frame if he is able to grasp it. Otherwise, use safety straps to keep his arms in place. Pull out the locking pin, release the lock and, with a co-worker's help, turn the patient. Always turn the patient in the direction of the narrow wedge to minimize his risk of falling.

SPECIAL BEDS
Turning frames

When a patient must remain immobile, such as after spinal injury or surgery, use of a turning frame allows repeated changes between the supine and prone positions without disturbing spinal alignment. The turning frame includes an anterior section and a posterior section, with the patient secured between them. The anterior and posterior sections pivot as one unit; the patient lies on the anterior frame in the prone position and on the posterior frame in the supine position.

One type of turning frame, the Stryker frame, accommodates cervical traction. (See *Operating a Stryker wedge frame.*) Another type, made by the Orthopedic Equipment Company, accommodates cervical and pelvic traction.

Operating either frame requires training and experience for at least one member of the turning team. Use of these frames may be contraindicated in obese patients.

Equipment
Turning frames with safety straps ▪ armboards ▪ special sheets (with ties) for each frame ▪ fresh linens ▪ pillow or sheepskin ▪ hand rolls or cradle boots ▪ footboard.

Preparation of equipment
Place sheets on the anterior and posterior frames. Tie the sheet corners to the frame, and secure the remainder of each sheet to the nearest fastener. Make sure the posterior frame's perineal opening is in the correct position. Secure the posterior frame to the bed and lock it in place. Then, turn the bed *to check that it's working properly.* Next, lock its wheels.

Implementation
• Obtain assistance from several co-workers for the initial transfer of the patient to the frame.
• Explain the use of the turning frame to the patient. Tell him that he may feel confined when the frames are in place, and that he may experience a floating sensation during turning. Reassure him that the frames will hold him securely and that the top frame will be removed after he is turned.
• Check to see that the posterior frame is locked into position.
• Transfer the patient in the supine position to the posterior frame, taking care to maintain spinal alignment. Attach and adjust the armboards *for comfort and support.* Make sure the patient's hands are in a functional position *to prevent deformity.*

Using the CircOlectric bed

This type of bed allows you to rotate the patient 180 degrees to a prone or supine position. It is fitted with safety stops that prevent it from being rotated more than 210 degrees. During operation, one nurse reassures the patient and ensures his safety while the other turns the bed.

an elevator or the patient's room. To do so, simply remove the connecting bolts; after the bed is in the patient's room, reassemble the frame.

Place a specially fitted sheet over the turning frame and the bottom mattress *to ensure the patient's comfort and help prevent pressure ulcers.* If necessary, secure a bedpan below the perineal opening of the bottom mattress.

Before placing the patient in the bed, examine its electrical cord and plug for defects, and place the cord where it won't be caught or severed during turning. Then plug the cord into an electrical outlet and check the bed's mechanical function. Lock the bed's wheels before transferring the patient.

Implementation

• *Because the size and appearance of the CircOlectric bed may initially alarm the patient,* describe the bed's advantages and the turning procedure to the patient beforehand. Reassure him that the bed will hold him securely.
• After obtaining assistance from co-workers, transfer the patient to the bed, taking care to position him correctly over the perineal opening.
• Position the bed's footboard against his feet *to help prevent footdrop and promote body alignment.* To secure the footboard, press the buttons and slide the unit toward his feet until it reaches the desired position. When turning the frame, press the buttons and slide the footboard toward the end of the bed.
• Place sheepskin under the patient's heels *to help prevent pressure ulcers.* If necessary, place supports under the patient's lower legs *to raise his heels off the bed.*
• Install the canvas-covered side rails *to ensure the patient's safety and promote a sense of security.* Loosen the stabilizing bolts in the square holders on either side of the bed. Then select the correct counterpiece on the side rail: The straight counterpiece keeps the side rail upright for protection at night and during supine positioning, while the 90-degree angle counterpiece keeps it level for prone positioning and for use as an armrest. After each side rail is in position, tighten its stabilizing bolt.

Turning to the prone position

• Before turning the patient, straighten the bed and its wheels as needed *to prevent unwanted movement.* Then release the footboard and move it away from the patient's feet. Leave enough room for placement of a footboard on the turning frame.
• If the patient is in traction, secure the traction guide equipment to the mobile portion of the frame. Because the weights will hang freely on the side of the circular frame, they won't be affected by turning.
• With the assistance of a co-worker, lift the turning frame over the patient. Remove the nuts on the bolts at both ends of the mattress. Slip the holes in the turning frame over the bolts and replace the nuts, turning them as tightly as possible. If you can't secure the nuts tightly by hand, place a turning key in the small holes of the nuts and then tighten them.
• Pad and position the footboard on the turning frame. Depress the buttons to adjust it properly. Be sure the footboard rests securely against the patient's feet *because it will bear his weight when he's upright.*
• Apply the head restraint *to support and immobilize the head during the turning and prone positioning.* Make sure the restraint is sufficiently padded *to help prevent facial pressure ulcers. Check for pressure areas to determine the best position for the head support because some beds have*

slings instead of metal bars. Secure the headrest by adjusting the clamps.

• Tuck in the sheets at the head of the mattress *so they don't rub against the patient's neck, causing ulcerations or occluding a tracheostomy.* Tell the patient to cross his hands over his chest or to grasp the sides of the turning frame *to protect his hands.* If the patient is paralyzed, place his arms at the sides and fasten the safety straps around the turning and posterior frames. *This promotes the patient's safety and keeps his arms at his sides and between the frames during turning.*

• Remove the bedpan if it's in place. Free I.V. lines, traction weights, any indwelling catheter drainage bag, or other attachments, and reposition them *to prevent dislodgement, entanglement, or complications during turning.*

• Unclamp the control switch from the bed frame. Hold it so you can operate the switch with your thumb. While a co-worker watches and reassures the patient, turn the bed using steady, continuous pressure on the control switch *to minimize the patient's nausea and vertigo.* Safety latches prevent the bed from turning too far in either direction.

• After the patient is positioned correctly, release the nut from the front of the main mattress. Free the mattress frame from the bolt and replace the nut. Pull forward on the release bar at the top of the frame. A series of springs raises the mattress up and off the patient's back, and a catch in the frame locks the mattress in the raised position. While the patient is prone, provide back care and change the sheets on the main mattress. If the patient's feet are lower than his head, check his feet and ankles for dependent edema.

Returning to the supine position

• Release the catch by pulling the release bar forward. Pull the mattress into place and bolt it.

• Remove the armrests and bedpan. Correctly position I.V. lines, traction weights, any indwelling catheter drainage bag, and other tubing or attachments before turning. Hold the control switch in the reverse position until the bed is level.

• When the bed is in position, release the nuts, remove the turning frame, and replace the nuts. Position the patient comfortably and adjust the footboard appropriately.

• If the patient is at a stage of rehabilitation requiring periodic standing, flip the safety latch forward *to stop the bed in the upright position.* Be sure to release the latch before returning the patient to horizontal.

• If the patient needs to sit up periodically, push forward on the lever at the side of the mattress. Apply safety belts, if necessary. To return the patient to the supine position, pull back on the lever.

Special considerations

Provide extra skin care and padding for the feet, occiput, chin, and forehead *because these areas endure added pressure.* If the patient has a tracheostomy and is connected to a mechanical ventilator, use a hand-held resuscitation bag, such as an Ambu bag, during turning. If the patient is receiving oxygen, temporarily disconnect it during turning.

The patient may experience nausea, vertigo, fear of falling, or spatial disorientation during turning. *To minimize nausea and vertigo,* be sure to complete the turn slowly and without interruption. *To minimize spatial disorientation,* place an overbed table within the patient's field of vision.

Watch carefully for signs of cardiac arrest, particularly during the patient's first few turnings. If the patient has neurologic damage, a doctor should be present the first few times.

After turning and positioning are completed, provide prism glasses or attach a mirror to the upper part of the bed *to increase the patient's field of vision.*

If the electricity fails, you can turn the bed with the hand crank stored in the tray at the head of the bed. Keep the end stud nuts on the appropriate frame bar when not in use *to avoid misplacing them.*

Complications

Pressure ulcers may form on the feet, occiput, chin, and forehead after a prolonged period, and on the heels of a patient with diminished sensation in his legs.

Documentation

Record the date and time the patient was transferred to the bed, the frequency of turning, and the patient's response to the maneuver.

Rotation beds

Because of their constant motion, rotation beds—such as the Roto Rest—promote postural drainage and peristalsis and help prevent the complications of immobility, including pressure ulcers, deep vein thrombi, orthostatic hypotension, bone demineralization, and formation of renal calculi. The bed rotates from side to side in a cradlelike motion, achieving a maximum elevation of 62 degrees and full side-to-side turning approximately every 4½ minutes.

Because the bed holds the patient motionless, it's especially helpful for patients with spinal cord injury, multiple trauma, cerebrovascular accident, multiple scle-

Understanding the Roto Rest bed

Driven by a silent motor, this bed turns the immobilized patient slowly and continuously, more than 300 times daily. The motion provides constant passive exercise and peristaltic stimulation without depriving the patient of sleep or risking further injury. The bed is radiolucent, permitting X-rays to be taken through it without moving the patient. It also has a built-in cooling fan, and allows access for surgery on multiple-trauma patients without disrupting spinal alignment or traction.

The bed's hatches give access to various parts of the patient's body. Arm hatches permit full range of motion and have holes for chest tubes. Leg hatches allow full hip extension. The perineal hatch provides access for bowel and bladder care, the thoracic hatch for chest auscultation and lumbar puncture, and the cervical hatch for wound care, bathing, and shampooing.

Top view

Arm hatch

Leg hatch

Back view

Perineal hatch — Cervical hatch

Thoracic hatch

---

rosis, coma, severe burns, hypostatic pneumonia, atelectasis, or other unilateral lung involvement causing poor ventilation and perfusion.

Rotation beds can accommodate cervical traction devices and tongs. One type of Roto Rest bed has an access hatch underneath for the perineal area; another type has access hatches for the perineal, cervical, and thoracic areas. Both have arm and leg hatches that fold down to allow range-of-motion exercises. Other features include variable angles of rotation, a fan, access for X-rays, and supports and clips for chest tubes, catheters, and drains. Racks beneath the bed hold X-ray plates in place for chest and spinal films. (See *Understanding the Roto Rest bed.*)

Rotation beds are contraindicated for the patient who has severe claustrophobia or who has an unstable cervical fracture without neurologic deficit and the complications of immobility. Patient transfer and positioning on the bed should be performed by at least two persons to ensure his safety.

The instructions given below apply to the Roto Rest bed.

Equipment
Rotation bed with appropriate accessories ■ pillowcases or linen-saver pads ■ flat sheet or padding.

Preparation of equipment
When using the Roto Rest bed, carefully inspect the bed and run it through a complete cycle in both automatic and manual modes *to ensure that it's working properly.* If you're using the Mark I model, check the tightness of the set screws at the head of the bed.

To prepare the bed for the patient, remove the counterbalance weights from the keel and place them in the base frame's storage area. Release the connecting arm by pulling down on the cam handle and depressing the lower side of the footboard. Next, lock the table in the horizontal position, and place all side supports in the extreme lateral position by loosening the cam handles on the underside of the table. Slide the supports off the bed. Note that all supports and packs are labeled *right* or *left* on the bottom *to facilitate reassembly.*

Remove the knee packs by depressing the snap button and rotating and pulling the packs from the tube. Then remove the abductor packs (the Mark III model has only one) by depressing and sliding them toward the head of the bed. Next, loosen the foot and knee assemblies by lifting the cam handle at its base, and slide them to the foot of the bed. Finally, loosen the shoulder clamp assembly and knobs, swing the shoulder clamps to the vertical position, and retighten them.

If you're using the Mark I model, remove the cervical, thoracic, and perineal packs. Cover them with pillowcases or linen-saver pads, smooth all wrinkles, and replace the packs. If you're using the Mark III model, remove the perineal pack, cover, and replace. Cover the upper half of the bed, which is a solid unit, with padding or a sheet. Install new disposable foam cushions for the patient's head, shoulders, and feet.

Implementation

- If possible, show the patient the bed before use. Explain and demonstrate its operation and reassure the patient that the bed will hold him securely.
- Before positioning the patient on the bed, make sure it's turned off. Then, place and lock the bed in horizontal position, out of gear. Latch all hatches and lock the wheels.
- Obtain assistance and transfer the patient. Move him gently to the center of the bed *to prevent contact with the pillar posts and to ensure proper balance during bed operation.* Smooth the pillowcase or linen-saver pad beneath his hips. Then, place any tubes through the appropriate notches in the hatches and ensure that any traction weights hang freely.
- Insert the thoracic side supports in their posts. Adjust the patient's longitudinal position to allow a 1" (2.5 cm) space between the axillae and the supports, *thereby avoiding pressure on the axillary blood vessels and the brachial plexus.* Push the supports against his chest and lock the cam arms securely *to provide support and ensure patient safety.*
- Place the disposable supports under his legs *to remove pressure from his heels and prevent pressure ulcers.*
- Install and adjust the foot supports so his feet lie in the normal anatomic position, *thereby helping to prevent footdrop.* The foot supports should be in position for only 2 hours of every shift *to prevent excessive pressure on the soles and toes.*
- Place the abductor packs in the appropriate supports, allowing a 6" (15 cm) space between the packs and the patient's groin. Tighten the knobs on the bed's underside at the base of the support tubes.
- Install the leg side supports snugly against the patient's hips, and tighten the cam arms. Position the knee assemblies slightly above his knees and tighten the cam arms. Then place your hand on the patient's knee and move the knee pack until it rests lightly on the top of your hand. Repeat for the other knee.
- Loosen the retaining rings on the crossbar, and slide the head and shoulder assembly laterally. *The retaining rings maintain correct lateral position of the shoulder clamp assembly and head support pack.*
- Carefully lower the head and shoulder assembly into place and slide it to touch the patient's head.
- Place your hand on the patient's shoulder, and move the shoulder pack until it touches your hand. Tighten it in place. Repeat for the other shoulder. *The 1" clearance between the shoulders and the packs prevents excess pressure, which can lead to pressure ulcers.*
- Place the head pack close to, but not touching, the patient's ears (or tongs).
- Tighten the head and shoulder assembly securely *so it won't lift off the bed.* Position the restraining rings next to the shoulder assembly bracket and tighten them.
- Place the patient's arms on the disposable supports. Install the side arm supports and secure the safety straps, placing one across the shoulder assembly and the other over the thoracic supports. If necessary, cover the patient with a flat sheet.

Balancing the bed

- Place one hand on the footboard *to prevent the bed from turning rapidly if it's unbalanced.* Then remove the locking pin. If the bed rotates to one side, reposition the patient in its center; if it tilts to the right, gently turn it slightly to the left and slide the packs on the right side toward the patient; if it tilts to the left, reverse the process. If a large imbalance exists, you may have to adjust the packs on both sides.
- After the patient is centered, gently turn the bed to the 62-degree position.
- Measure the space between the patient's chest, hip, and thighs and the inside of the packs. If this space exceeds ½" (1.3 cm) for the Mark III model or 1" for the Mark I, return the bed to horizontal position, lock it in place, and slide the packs inward on both sides. If the space appears too tight, proceed as above but slide both packs outward. *Excessively loose packs cause the patient to slide from side to side during turning, possibly resulting in unnecessary movement at fracture sites, skin irritation from shearing force, and bed imbalance. Overly tight packs can place pressure on the patient during turning.*

• After adjusting the packs, check the bed; balance it and make any necessary adjustments.

• If you're using the Mark III model bed and the patient weighs more than 160 lb (72 kg), the bed may become top-heavy. To correct this, place counterbalance weights in the appropriate slots in the keel of the bed. Add one weight for every 20 lb (9 kg) over 160, but remember that placement of weights doesn't replace correct patient positioning.

• If you're using the Mark I model, it may be necessary to add weights for the patient weighing less than 160 lb. Place one weight for each 20 lb less than 160 in the proper bracket at the foot of the bed.

Initiating automatic bed rotation

• Ensure that all packs are securely in place. Then hold the footboard firmly and remove the locking pin *to start the bed's motor.* The bed will continue to rotate until the pin is reinserted.

• Raise the connecting arm cam handle until the connecting assembly snaps into place, locking the bed into automatic rotation.

• Remain with the patient for at least three complete turns from side to side *to evaluate his comfort and safety.* Observe his response and offer him emotional support.

Special considerations

If the patient develops cardiac arrest while on the bed, perform cardiopulmonary resuscitation after taking the bed out of gear, locking it in horizontal position, removing the side arm support and the thoracic pack, lifting the shoulder assembly, and dropping the arm pack. Doing all these steps takes only 5 to 10 seconds. *You won't need a cardiac board because of the bed's firm surface.*

If the electricity fails, lock the bed in horizontal or lateral position and rotate it manually every 30 minutes *to prevent pressure ulcers.* If cervical traction causes the patient to slide upward, place the bed in reverse Trendelenburg's position; if extremity traction causes the patient to migrate toward the foot of the bed, use Trendelenburg's position.

Lock the bed in the extreme lateral position for access to the back of the head, thorax, and buttocks through the appropriate hatches. Clean the mattress and nondisposable packs during patient care, and rinse them thoroughly *to remove all soap residue.* When replacing the packs and hatches, take care not to pinch the patient's skin between the packs. *This can cause pain and tissue necrosis.*

Expect increased drainage from any pressure ulcers for the first few days the patient is on the bed *because the motion helps debride necrotic tissue and improves local circulation.*

Perform or schedule daily range-of-motion exercises, as ordered, *because the bed allows full access to all extremities without disturbing spinal alignment.* Drop the arm hatch for shoulder rotation, remove the thoracic packs for shoulder abduction, and drop the leg hatch and remove leg and knee packs for hip rotation and full leg motion.

For female patients, tape an indwelling urinary catheter to the thigh before bringing it through the perineal hatch. For the male patient with spinal cord lesions, tape the catheter to the abdomen and then to the thigh *to facilitate gravity drainage.* Hang the drainage bag on the clips provided, and make sure it doesn't become caught between the bed frames during rotation.

If the patient has a tracheal or endotracheal tube and is on mechanical ventilation, attach the tube support bracket between the cervical pack and the arm packs. Tape the connecting T tubing to the support and run it beside the patient's head and off the center of the table *to help prevent reflux of condensation.* For a patient with pulmonary congestion or pneumonia, suction secretions more often during the first 12 to 24 hours on the bed *because the motion will increase drainage.* A vibrator is available for use under the thoracic hatch of the Mark I to help mobilize pulmonary secretions more quickly.

Documentation

Record changes in the patient's condition and his response to therapy in your progress notes. Note turning times and ongoing care on the flowchart.

 Clinitron therapy bed

Originally called the air-fluidized bed and designed for managing burns, the Clinitron therapy bed is now used for patients with various debilities. The bed is actually a large tub that supports the patient on a thick layer of silicone-coated microspheres of lime glass. A monofilament polyester filter sheet covers the microsphere-filled tub. Warmed air, propelled by a blower beneath the bed, passes through it. The resulting fluidlike surface reduces pressure on the skin sufficiently to avoid obstructing capillary blood flow, thereby helping to prevent pressure ulcers and to promote wound healing. The bed's air temperature can be adjusted to help control hypothermia and hyperthermia. (See *A look at the Clinitron therapy bed.*)

Small amounts of wound drainage can flow into the microspheres, eliminating the need for most dressings. In addition, use of this therapy permits harmless contact between the bed's surface and grafted sites, promoting comfort and healing. In addition, when the air pressure

A look at the Clinitron therapy bed

The Clinitron therapy bed is a large tub filled with microspheres that are suspended by air pressure and give the patient fluidlike support. The bed provides the advantages of flotation without the disadvantages of instability, patient positioning difficulties, and immobility.

Diffuser board
Temperature probe
Removable sieve
Polyester filter sheet

Control panel

Microsphere-filled tank

---

is turned off, the bed forms a firm surface that molds to the shape of the patient's body, allowing the nurse to move the patient or change his position.

The Clinitron therapy bed may be contraindicated for the patient unable to mobilize and expel pulmonary secretions because the lack of back support impairs productive coughing. Patients who have skin problems may benefit from an air therapy bed instead of a Clinitron bed. (See *Air therapy beds,* page 74.) Because operation of the Clinitron therapy bed is complex, it requires special training.

Equipment
Clinitron therapy bed with microspheres (about 1,650 lb [750 kg]) ■ filter sheet ■ six aluminum rails (for restraining and sealing filter sheet) ■ flat sheet ■ elastic cord.

Preparation of equipment
Normally, a manufacturer's representative or a trained hospital staff member prepares the bed for use. If you must help with the preparation, be sure the microspheres reach to within ½″ (1.3 cm) of the top of the tank. Then position the filter sheet on the bed with its printed side facing up. Match the holes in the sheet to the holes in the edge of the bed's frame. Place the aluminum rails on

the frame, with the studs in the proper holes. Depress the rails firmly, and secure them by tightening the knurled knobs to seal the filter sheet. Place a flat hospital sheet over the filter sheet, and secure it with the elastic cord *to prevent billowing.* Turn on the air current *to activate the microspheres.* Then turn it off *to ensure that the bed's working properly.*

Implementation
● Explain and, if possible, demonstrate the operation of the Clinitron therapy bed for the patient. Tell him the reason for its use and that he'll feel as though he's floating on air. Then turn off the air pressure.
● With the help of three or more co-workers, transfer the patient to the bed using a lift sheet.
● Turn on the air pressure to activate the bed, and remove the lift sheet.
● Adjust the air temperature as necessary. Because the bed usually operates within 10° to 12° F (5.5° to 6.7° C) of ambient air temperature, set the room temperature to 75° F (24° C). If microsphere temperature reaches 105° F (41° C), the bed automatically shuts off. It restarts automatically after 30 minutes.

Air therapy beds

Patients who have or risk skin breakdown may benefit from an alternative to the Clinitron therapy bed: an air therapy bed without the microspheres. This type of bed has air-filled compartments that can be inflated to varying degrees, thus providing different levels of support to different body parts.

Optional in some air therapy beds is a pulsating or rotating motion that stimulates capillary blood flow, prevents venous stasis, increases peristalsis, and improves pulmonary hygiene. Because ordinary linen-saver pads block air flow, you'll need to use air-permeable pads that are available from the manufacturer.

Special considerations

Monitor the patient's fluid and electrolyte status *because the warm, dry air circulated by the Clinitron therapy bed increases evaporative water loss, possibly requiring modifications in oral or I.V. fluid intake.* Because of this drying effect, always cover a mesh graft for the first 2 to 8 days, as ordered. If the patient experiences excessive dryness of the upper respiratory tract, use a humidifier and mask, as ordered. Encourage coughing and deep breathing *to help prevent pulmonary complications.* After prolonged use of a Clinitron therapy bed, watch for hypocalcemia and hypophosphoremia.

Any copiously draining wound should be covered with a porous dressing *to absorb some of the drainage.* Cover petroleum-jelly or silver-based topical applications with an impervious dressing *to minimize or prevent their ab-*sorption by the microspheres. Avoid using wet dressings or soaks *because the excess fluid causes the microspheres to clump, impairing the fluid support effect.* The bed restarts automatically if shut off for 30 minutes, so unplug it to perform longer procedures.

To position a bedpan, roll the patient away from you, place the bedpan on the flat sheet, and push it into the microspheres. Then reposition the patient. To remove the bedpan, hold it steady and roll the patient away from you. Turn off the air pressure and remove the bedpan. Then turn the air on and reposition the patient.

Don't wear a watch when handling the microspheres *because they are small enough to penetrate the watch and damage the mechanism.* Don't secure the filter sheet with pins or clamps, *which may puncture the sheet and release microspheres.* Take care to avoid puncturing the bed when giving injections. Repair any holes or tears with iron-on patching tape. Sieve the microspheres monthly or between patients *to remove any clumped microspheres.* Handle them carefully to avoid spills, because they will make floors slippery and may cause falls. Treat a soiled filter sheet and clumped microspheres as contaminated items and handle according to hospital policy. Change the filter sheet and operate the unit unoccupied for 24 hours between patients.

Documentation

Record the duration of therapy and the patient's response to it. Document the condition of the patient's skin, pressure ulcers, and any other wounds.

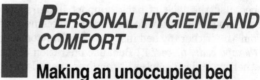

PERSONAL HYGIENE AND COMFORT

Making an unoccupied bed

Although considered routine, daily changing and periodic straightening of bed linens promotes patient comfort and prevents skin breakdown. When preceded by thorough hand washing, performed using clean technique, and followed by proper handling and disposal of soiled linens, this procedure helps control nosocomial infections. In *open-bed technique,* performed during the ambulatory patient's hospitalization, bedmaking entails folding top linens to the foot of the bed to permit easy patient access. In *closed-bed technique,* performed after the patient's discharge, bedmaking entails keeping top linens unfolded and even with the top of the mattress until the next patient's admission.

Equipment

Two sheets (one fitted, if available) ■ pillowcase ■ bedspread ■ gloves, if the patient has open lesions or has been incontinent ■ optional: bath blanket, laundry bag, linen-saver pads, drawsheet.

Preparation of equipment

Obtain clean linen, which should be folded in half lengthwise and then folded again, creating a center crease that makes it easier to position the sheet on the bed. If the linen is folded incorrectly, refold it before attempting to make the bed. The bottom sheet should be folded so the rough side of the hem is facedown when placed on the bed; *this helps prevent skin irritation caused by the rough hem edge rubbing against the patient's heels.* The top sheet should be folded similarly, so the smooth side of the hem is faceup when folded over the spread, *giving the bed a finished appearance.*

Implementation

• Wash your hands thoroughly, don gloves if the patient has lesions or has been incontinent, and bring clean linen to the patient's bedside. If the patient is present, tell him that you're going to change his bed. Help him to a chair if necessary.
• Move any furniture away from the bed *to provide ample working space.*
• Lower the head of the bed *to make the mattress level and ensure tight-fitting, wrinkle-free linens.* Then, raise the bed to a comfortable working height *to prevent back strain.*
• When stripping the bed, watch for the patient's eyeglasses, dentures, or other belongings that may have fallen among the linens.
• Remove the pillowcase and place it in the laundry bag, or use the pillowcase, hooked over the back of a chair, as a laundry bag. Set the pillow aside.
• Lift the mattress edge slightly and work around the bed, untucking the linens. If you plan to reuse the top linens, fold the top hem of the spread down to the bottom hem. Then pick up the hemmed corners, fold the spread into quarters, and hang it over the back of the chair. Do the same for the top sheet. Otherwise, carefully remove and place the top linens in the laundry bag or pillowcase. *To avoid spreading microorganisms,* don't fan the linen, hold it against your clothing, or place it on the floor.
• Remove the soiled bottom linens, and place them in the laundry bag.
• If the mattress has slid downward, push it to the head of the bed; *adjusting it after bedmaking loosens the linens.*
• Place the bottom sheet with its center fold in the middle of the mattress. For a fitted sheet, secure the top and bottom corners over the mattress corners on the side of the bed nearest you. For a flat sheet, align the end of the sheet with the foot of the mattress, and miter the top corner *to keep the sheet firmly tucked under the mattress.* To miter the corner, first tuck the top end of the sheet evenly under the mattress at the head of the bed. Then lift the side edge of the sheet about 12″ (30 cm) from the mattress corner and hold it at a right angle to the mattress. Tuck in the bottom edge of the sheet hanging below the mattress. Finally, drop the top edge and tuck it under the mattress.
• After tucking under one side of the bottom sheet, place the drawsheet (if needed) about 15″ (38 cm) from the top of the bed, with its center fold in the middle of the bed. Then tuck in the entire edge of the drawsheet on the side of the bed nearest you.
• Place the top sheet with its center fold in the middle of the bed and its wide hem even with the top of the bed. Position the rough side of the hem faceup, *so the smooth side shows after folding.* Allow enough sheet at the top of the bed to form a cuff over the spread.
• Place the spread over the top sheet, with its center fold in the middle of the bed. (If the patient will be returning from surgery, follow an alternate technique as described in *Making a surgical bed,* page 76.)
• Make a 3″ (7.6 cm) toe pleat, or vertical tuck, in the top linens *to allow room for the patient's feet and to prevent pressure that can cause discomfort, skin breakdown, and footdrop.*
• Tuck the top sheet and spread under the foot of the mattress. Then, miter the bottom corners.
• Move to the opposite side of the bed and repeat the procedure.
• After fitting all corners of the bottom sheet or tucking them under the mattress, pull the sheet at an angle from the head toward the foot of the bed. *This tightens the linens, making the bottom sheet taut and wrinkle-free and promoting patient comfort.*
• Fold the top sheet over the spread at the head of the bed *to form a cuff and to give the bed a finished appearance.* When making an open bed, fanfold the top linens to the foot of the bed *to allow easy patient access.* If a linen-saver pad is needed, place it on top of the bottom sheets.
• Slip the pillow into a clean case, tucking its corners well into the case *to ensure a smooth fit.* Then place the pillow with its seam toward the top of the bed *to prevent it from rubbing against the patient's neck, causing irritation,* and its open edge facing away from the door *to give the bed a finished appearance.*
• Lower the bed and lock its wheels *to ensure patient safety.*
• Return furniture to its proper place, and place the call button within the patient's easy reach. Carry soiled linens from the room in outstretched arms *to avoid contaminating your uniform.*

Making a surgical bed

Preparation of a surgical bed permits easy patient transfer from surgery and promotes cleanliness and comfort. To make such a bed, take the following steps:

• Assemble linens as you would for making an unoccupied bed, including two clean sheets (one fitted, if available), a drawsheet, a bath blanket, a spread or sheet, a pillowcase, facial tissues, a trash bag, and linen-saver pads. Raise the bed to a comfortable working height *to prevent back strain.*

• Slip the pillow into a clean pillowcase and place it on a nearby table or chair.

• Make the foundation of the bed using the bottom sheet and drawsheet.

• Place an open bath blanket about 15″ (38 cm) from the head of the bed with its center fold positioned in the middle of the bed. *The blanket warms the patient and counteracts the decreased body temperature caused by anesthesia.*

• Place a top sheet or spread on the bath blanket, and position it as you did the blanket. Then fold the blanket and sheet back from the top, so that the blanket shows over the sheet. Similarly, fold the sheet and blanket up from the bottom, as shown below.

• On the side of the bed where you'll receive the patient (usually nearest the door), fold up the two outer corners of the sheet and blanket so they meet in the middle of the bed, as shown at the top of the next column.

• Pick up the point hanging over this side of the bed, and fanfold the linens back to the opposite side of the bed *so the linens won't interfere with patient transfer from the stretcher to the bed.*

• Raise the bed to the high position if you haven't already. Then lock the wheels and lower the side rails. Be sure the side rails work properly. Move the bedside stand and other objects out of the stretcher's path *to facilitate easy transfer when the patient arrives.*

• After the patient is transferred to the bed, position the pillow for his comfort and safety. Cover him by pulling the top point of the sheet and blanket over him and opening the folds. After covering the patient, tuck in the linens at the foot of the bed and miter the corners.

• After disposing of the linens, remove gloves if used and wash your hands thoroughly *to prevent the spread of microorganisms.*

Special considerations

Because a hospital mattress is usually covered with plastic to protect it and to facilitate cleaning between patients, a flat bottom sheet tends to loosen and become untucked. Use a fitted sheet, if available, to prevent this.

If a fitted sheet is not available, the top corners of a flat sheet may be tied together under the top of the mattress to prevent the sheet from becoming dislodged. A bath blanket placed on top of the mattress, under the bottom sheet, helps to absorb moisture and prevent dislodgement of the bottom sheet.

Documentation
Although linen changes aren't usually documented, record their dates and times in your notes for patients with incontinence, excessive wound drainage, or diaphoresis.

Making an occupied bed

For the bedridden patient, daily linen changes promote comfort and help prevent skin breakdown and nosocomial infection. Such changes necessitate the use of side rails to prevent the patient from rolling out of bed and, depending on his condition, the use of a turning sheet to move him from side to side.

Making an occupied bed may require more than one person. It also entails loosening the bottom sheet on one side and fanfolding it to the center of the mattress instead of loosening the bottom sheet on both sides and removing it, as in an unoccupied bed. Also, the foundation of the bed must be made before applying the top sheet instead of making both the foundation and top on one side before completing them on the other side. (See *Making a traction bed,* page 78, for a specialized technique.)

Equipment
Two sheets (one fitted, if available) ▪ pillowcase ▪ one or two drawsheets ▪ spread ▪ one or two bath blankets ▪ gloves, if the patient has open lesions or has been incontinent ▪ sheepskin or other comfort-enhancing device, as needed ▪ optional: laundry bag, linen-saver pad.

Preparation of equipment
Obtain clean linen and be sure it's folded properly, as for an unoccupied bed.

Implementation
• Wash your hands, don gloves if necessary, and bring clean linen to the patient's room.
• Identify the patient and tell him you will be changing his bed linens. Explain how he can help if he is able, adjusting the plan according to his abilities and needs. Provide privacy.
• Move any furniture away from the bed *to ensure ample working space.*
• Raise the side rail on the far side of the bed *to prevent falls.* Adjust the bed to a comfortable working height *to prevent back strain.*

• If the patient's condition permits, lower the head of the bed *to ensure tight-fitting, wrinkle-free linens.*
• When stripping the bed, watch for the patient's eyeglasses, dentures, and other belongings that may have fallen among the linens.
• Cover the patient with a bath blanket *to avoid exposure and provide warmth and privacy.* Then fanfold the top sheet and spread from beneath the bath blanket, and bring them back over the blanket. Loosen the top linens at the foot of the bed and remove them separately. If you plan to reuse the top linens, fold each piece neatly and hang it over the back of the chair. Otherwise, place it in the laundry bag. *To avoid dispersing microorganisms,* don't fan the linens, hold them against your clothing, or place them on the floor.
• If the mattress slides down when the head of the bed is raised, pull it up toward the head of the bed. *Adjusting the mattress after the bed is made loosens the linens.* If the patient is able, ask him to grasp the head of the bed and pull with you; otherwise, ask a co-worker to help you.
• Roll the patient to the far side of the bed, and position the pillow lengthwise under his head *to support his neck.* Ask the patient to help (if he's able) by grasping the far side rail as he turns *so that he's positioned at the far side of the bed.*
• Loosen the soiled bottom linens on the side of the bed nearest you. Then roll the linens toward the patient's back in the middle of the bed.
• Place a clean bottom sheet on the bed, with its center fold in the middle of the mattress. If you're using a fitted sheet, secure the top and bottom corners over the side of the mattress nearest you. If you're using a flat sheet, place its end even with the foot of the mattress. Miter the top corner as you would for an unoccupied bed *to keep linens firmly tucked under the mattress, preventing wrinkling.*
• Fanfold the remaining clean bottom sheet toward the patient, and place the drawsheet, if needed, about 15" (38 cm) from the top of the bed, with its center fold in the middle of the mattress. Tuck in the entire edge of the drawsheet on the side nearest you. Fanfold the remaining drawsheet toward the patient.
• If necessary, position a linen-saver pad on the drawsheet *to absorb excretions or surgical drainage,* and fanfold it toward the patient.
• Raise the other side rail, and roll the patient over the soiled and fanfolded linen to the clean side of the bed. Ask the patient to help (if he's able) by grasping the rail.
• Move to the unfinished side of the bed and lower the side rail nearest you. Then loosen and remove the soiled bottom linens separately and place them in the laundry bag.

Making a traction bed

For a patient in traction, obtain help from a co-worker to make the bed. Work from head to toe *to minimize the risk of traction misalignment.*

Preparation
• Wash your hands. Put on gloves if the patient has open lesions or has been incontinent. Bring clean linen to the patient's room, and arrange the linen in the order of use on the bedside stand or a chair.
• Explain the procedure to the patient, provide privacy, and remove unnecessary furniture and equipment from around the bed.

Change the linens
• Lower the side rails on both sides of the bed. Stand near the headboard on one side, and have a co-worker stand near the headboard on the opposite side, facing you.
• Gently pull the mattress to the head of the bed. Avoid sudden movements *because they can misalign traction and cause patient discomfort.*
• Remove the pillow from the bed. Loosen the bottom linens, and roll them from the headboard toward the patient's head. Then, remove the soiled pillowcase and replace it with a clean one.
• Fold a clean bottom sheet crosswise with the rough side of the hem facedown. Then place the sheet across the head of the bed. Tell the patient to raise her head and upper shoulders by grasping the trapeze above the bed. With your co-worker, quickly fanfold the bottom

sheet from the head of the bed under the patient's shoulders, so that it meets the soiled linen. Tuck at least 12″ (30 cm) of the bottom sheet tightly under the head of the mattress. Miter the corners and tuck in the sides as far down as possible.
• Tell the patient to raise her buttocks by grasping the trapeze. As a team, move toward the foot of the bed and, in one movement, quickly and carefully roll soiled linens and clean linens under the patient's buttocks, as shown in the illustration.
• Instruct the patient to release the trapeze and to rest. Place a pillow under her head for comfort.
• If allowed, remove any pillows from under the patient's extremity. If pillow removal is contraindicated, continue to move linens toward the foot of the bed and under the patient's legs and traction while your co-worker lifts the pillows and supports the patient's extremity.
• Put soiled linens in a laundry bag or pillowcase.
• Tuck the remaining loose linens securely under the mattress. To ensure a tight-fitting bottom sheet, have the patient raise her weight off the bed by simultaneously grasping the trapeze and raising her buttocks while you pull the sheet tight. As needed, place a drawsheet, linen-saver pad, or sheepskin under the patient's buttocks. After the foundation is made, you can complete the bedmaking alone.
• If the bottom sheet doesn't cover the foot of the mattress, use a drawsheet to cover it. Miter its corners and tuck in the sides.
• Replace the pillows under the patient's extremity, then cover her with a clean top sheet. Fold over the top hem of the sheet approximately 8″ (20 cm). If one or both legs are in traction, fit the lower end of the sheet loosely over the traction apparatus; avoid applying unnecessary pressure to the traction ropes. To secure the sheet, tuck in the corner opposite the traction under the foot of the bed and miter the corner. Neatly tuck in the lower corner of the sheet on the traction side *to expose the leg and foot.*
• If the traction equipment exposes the patient's sides, place a drawsheet across the bed. Avoid using a full sheet or spread *because either one will be too cumbersome.*
• Lower the bed but don't allow the traction weights to touch the floor. Raise the side rails *to prevent falls.* If allowed, leave one side rail down so the patient can reach the bedside stand.

• Pull the clean bottom sheet taut. Secure a fitted sheet over the mattress corners or place the end of a flat sheet even with the foot of the bed, and miter the top corner. Pull the drawsheet taut and tuck it tightly under the mattress. Unfold and smooth the linen-saver pad, if used.

• Assist the patient to the supine position if his condition permits.

• Remove the soiled pillowcase, and place it in the laundry bag. Then slip the pillow into a clean pillowcase, tucking its corners well into the case *to ensure a smooth fit.* Place the pillow beneath the patient's head, with its seam toward the top of the bed *to prevent it from rubbing against the patient's neck, causing irritation.* Place the pillow's open edge away from the door *to give the bed a finished appearance.*

• Unfold the clean top sheet over the patient with the rough side of the hem facing away from the bed *to avoid irritating the patient's skin.* Allow enough sheet at the top of the bed to form a cuff over the spread.

• Remove the bath blanket from beneath the sheet, and center the spread over the top sheet.

• Make a 3″ (7.6 cm) toe pleat, or vertical tuck, in the top linens *to allow room for the patient's feet and prevent pressure that can cause discomfort, skin breakdown, and footdrop.*

• Tuck the top sheet and spread under the foot of the bed, and miter the bottom corners. Fold the top sheet over the spread *to give the bed a finished appearance.*

• Raise the head of the bed to a comfortable position for the patient, make sure both side rails are raised, and then lower the bed and lock its wheels *to ensure the patient's safety.* Assess the patient's body alignment and his mental and emotional status.

• Return furniture to its proper place, and place the call button within the patient's easy reach. Remove the laundry bag from the room.

• Remove and discard gloves, if used, and wash your hands thoroughly *to prevent the spread of nosocomial infections.*

Special considerations
Use a fitted bottom sheet, when available, because a flat sheet slips out from under the mattress easily, especially if the mattress is plastic-coated.

Prevent the patient from sliding down in bed by tucking a tightly rolled pillow under the top linens at the foot of the bed. Provide additional comfort for the diaphoretic or bedridden patient by folding a bath blanket in half lengthwise and placing it between the bottom sheet and the plastic mattress cover; the blanket acts as a cushion and helps absorb moisture. *To help prevent sheet burns on the heels, elbows, and bony prominences,* center a bath

blanket or sheepskin over the bottom sheet, and tuck the blanket securely under the mattress.

If the patient can't help you to move or turn him, devise a turning sheet *to facilitate bedmaking and repositioning.* To do this, first fold a drawsheet or bath blanket and place it under the patient's buttocks. Make sure the sheet extends from shoulders to knees *so that it supports most of the patient's weight.* Roll the sides of the sheet to form handles. Next, ask a co-worker to help you lift and move the patient. With one person holding each side of the sheet, you can move the patient without wrinkling the bottom linens. If you can't get help and must turn the patient yourself, stand at the side of the bed. Turn the patient toward the rail and, if he's able, ask him to grasp the rail to assist in turning. Then reach over the patient and firmly grasp the opposite rolled edge of the turning sheet. Pull the rolled edge carefully toward you and turn the patient.

Documentation
Although linen changes aren't usually documented, record their dates and times in your notes for patients with incontinence, excessive wound drainage, pressure ulcers, or diaphoresis.

 Bed bath

A complete bed bath cleans the skin, stimulates circulation, provides mild exercise, and promotes comfort. Bathing also allows assessment of skin condition, joint mobility, and muscle strength. Depending on the patient's overall condition and duration of hospitalization, he may have a complete or partial bath daily. A partial bath — including hands, face, axillae, back, genitalia, and anal region — can replace the complete bath for the patient with dry, fragile skin or extreme weakness, and can supplement the complete bath for the diaphoretic or incontinent patient.

Equipment
Bath basin ■ bath blanket ■ soap ■ towel ■ washcloth ■ skin lotion ■ orangewood stick ■ gloves, if the patient has open lesions or has been incontinent ■ deodorant ■ optional: bath oil, perineal pad, ABD pad, linen-saver pad.

Preparation of equipment
Adjust the temperature of the patient's room, and close any doors or windows to prevent drafts. Determine the patient's preference for soap or other hygiene aids *because*

some patients are allergic to soap or prefer bath oil or lotions. Assemble the equipment on an overbed table or bedside stand.

Implementation

• Tell the patient you'll be giving him a bath, and provide privacy. If the patient's condition permits, encourage him to assist with bathing *to provide exercise and promote independence.*

• Raise the patient's bed to a comfortable working height *to avoid back strain.* Offer him a bedpan or urinal.

• Fill the bath basin two-thirds full of warm water (about 115° F [46° C]) and bring it to the patient's bedside. If a bath thermometer isn't available, test the water temperature carefully with your elbow *to avoid scalding or chilling the patient;* the water should feel comfortably warm.

• If the bed will be changed after the bath, remove the top linen. If not, fanfold it to the foot of the bed.

• Don gloves if necessary. Position the patient supine, if possible.

• Remove the patient's gown and other articles, such as elastic stockings, elastic bandages, and restraints (as ordered). Cover him with a bath blanket *to provide warmth and privacy.*

• Place a towel under the patient's chin. To wash his face, begin with the eyes, working from the inner to the outer canthus without soap. Use a separate section of the washcloth for each eye *to avoid spreading ocular infection.*

• If the patient tolerates soap, apply it to the cloth, and wash the rest of his face, ears, and neck, using firm, gentle strokes. Rinse thoroughly *because residual soap can cause itching and dryness.* Then dry the area thoroughly. Observe the skin for irritation, scaling, or other abnormalities.

• Turn down the bath blanket, and drape the patient's chest with a bath towel. While washing, rinsing, and drying the chest and axillae, observe the patient's respirations. Use firm strokes *to avoid tickling the patient.* If the patient tolerates deodorant, apply it.

• Place a bath towel beneath the patient's arm farthest from you. Then bathe his arm, using long, smooth strokes and moving from wrist to shoulder, *to stimulate venous circulation.* If possible, soak the patient's hand in the basin *to remove dirt and soften nails.* Clean the patient's fingernails with the orangewood stick, if necessary. Observe the color of his hand and nail beds to *assess peripheral circulation.* Follow the same procedure for the other arm and hand.

• Turn down the bath blanket to expose the patient's abdomen and groin, keeping a bath towel across his chest *to prevent chills.* Bathe, rinse, and dry the abdomen and groin while checking for abdominal distention or tenderness. Then turn back the bath blanket to cover the patient's chest and abdomen.

• Uncover the leg farthest from you, and place a bath towel under it. Flex this leg and bathe it, moving from ankle to hip *to stimulate venous circulation.* Do not massage the leg, however, *to avoid dislodging any existing thrombus, possibly causing a pulmonary embolus.* Rinse and dry the leg.

• If possible, place a basin on the patient's bed, flex the leg at the knee, and place the foot in the basin. Soak the foot, and then wash and rinse it thoroughly. Remove the foot from the basin, dry it, and clean the toenails. Observe skin condition and color during cleaning *to assess peripheral circulation.* Repeat the procedure for the other leg and foot.

• Cover the patient with the bath blanket *to prevent chilling.* Then lower the bed and raise the side rails *to ensure patient safety* while you change the bath water.

• When you return, roll the patient on his side or stomach, place a towel beneath him, and cover him *to prevent chilling.* Bathe, rinse, and dry his back and buttocks.

• Massage the patient's back with lotion, giving attention to bony prominences. Check for redness, abrasions, and pressure ulcers.

• Bathe the anal area from front to back *to avoid contaminating the perineum.* Rinse and dry the area well.

• After lowering the bed and raising the side rails *to ensure the patient's safety,* change the bath water again. Then turn the patient on his back and bathe the genital area thoroughly but gently, using a different section of the washcloth for each downward stroke. Bathe from front to back, avoiding the anal area. Rinse thoroughly and pat dry.

• If applicable, perform indwelling catheter care. Apply perineal pads or scrotal supports, as needed.

• Dress the patient in a clean gown, and reapply any elastic bandages, elastic stockings, or restraints removed before the bath.

• Remake the bed or change the linens, and remove the bath blanket.

• Place a bath towel beneath the patient's head *to catch loose hair,* and then brush and comb his hair.

• Return the bed to its original position and make the patient comfortable.

• Carry soiled linens to the hamper with outstretched arms. *To avoid spreading microorganisms,* don't let soiled linens touch your clothing. Remove gloves, if applicable.

Special considerations

Fold the washcloth around your hand to form a mitt while bathing the patient. *This keeps the cloth warm longer and avoids dribbling water on the patient from the cloth's loose ends.* Change the water as often as necessary to keep it warm and clean.

Carefully dry creased skin-fold areas—for example, under breasts, in the groin area, and between fingers, toes, and buttocks. Dust these areas lightly with powder after drying *to reduce friction.* Use powder sparingly *to avoid caking and irritation, and to avoid provoking coughing in patients with respiratory disorders.*

If the patient has very dry skin, use bath oil instead of soap. No rinsing is necessary. Warm the lotion before using it for back massage *because cold lotion can startle the patient and induce muscle tension and vasoconstriction.* (See "Back care" in this chapter.) *To improve circulation, maintain joint mobility, and preserve muscle tone,* move the body joints through their full range of motion during the bath.

If the patient is incontinent, loosely tuck an ABD pad between his buttocks and place a linen-saver pad under him *to absorb fecal drainage.* Together these pads will help prevent skin irritation and reduce the number of linen changes.

Documentation
Record the date and time of the bed bath on the flowchart. Note the patient's tolerance for the bath, his range of motion, and his self-care abilities, and report any unusual findings.

Tub baths and showers

Tub baths and showers provide personal hygiene, stimulate circulation, and reduce tension for the patient. They also allow you to observe skin conditions and assess joint mobility and muscle strength. If not precluded by the patient's condition or safety considerations, privacy during bathing promotes the patient's sense of well-being by allowing him to assume responsibility for his own care.

Patients who are recovering from recent surgery, who are emotionally unstable, or who have casted extremities or dressings in place usually require the doctor's permission for a tub bath or shower. (For an alternate bathing method, see *Using the hydraulic bath lift.)*

Equipment
One or two washcloths ▪ bath towel ▪ bath blanket ▪ soap (or nonallergenic equivalent) ▪ nonskid bath mat, if tub lacks nonskid strips ▪ towel mat ▪ bath thermometer ▪ clean clothing or hospital gown ▪ optional: chair, shower cap, bath oil, shampoo, or mild castile soap.

Using the hydraulic bath lift

For the debilitated patient who is unable to ambulate to the shower or tub, a hydraulic bath lift can facilitate transfer and eliminate strain on the nurse's back. The bath lift typically is used in a rehabilitation or geriatric setting.

To accomplish patient transfer, lower the lift (a chair or stretcher) to the patient's bed level. Suspend the patient, position him above a height-adjustable tub set to your most comfortable working height, and then lower him into the tub. Because the patient remains on the lift throughout his bath, simply reverse the procedure when taking the patient out of the tub.

When using a hydraulic lift for the first time, most patients feel somewhat insecure and fearful. With experience, however, most find the bathing system comfortable and relaxing.

Preparation of equipment
Prepare the bathing area before the patient arrives. Close any doors or windows and adjust the room temperature *to avoid chilling the patient.* Check that the bathtub or shower is clean. Then assemble bathing articles and observe appropriate safety measures.

For a bath: Position a chair next to the tub *to help the patient get in and out and to provide a seat if he becomes weak.* Place a bath blanket over the chair *to cover the patient if he becomes chilled.* Fill the tub halfway with water, and test the temperature with a bath thermometer. The temperature should range from 100° to 110° F (38° to 43° C). If you don't have a bath thermometer, test the temperature by immersing your elbow in the water; it should feel comfortable to the touch. Besides the obvious risk of scalding the patient, excessively hot water can cause cutaneous vasodilation, *which alters blood flow to the brain and may lead to dizziness or fainting.*

For a shower: Place a nonskid chair in the shower *to provide support.* The chair also allows the patient to sit down while washing his legs and feet, *reducing the risk of falling.*

Cover the floor of the shower with a nonskid mat unless it already has nonskid strips. Next, place a towel mat next to the bathing area. Remove electrical appliances, such as hair driers and heaters, from the patient's reach *to prevent electrical accidents.* Adjust water flow and temperature just before the patient gets into the shower.

Implementation
• Escort the patient to the bathing area, explain the procedure, and help him undress as necessary. Offer him a shower cap if he wants to keep his hair dry. Otherwise, provide shampoo or mild castile soap.
• Help the patient into the tub or shower. Provide washcloths and soap. If he has dry skin, add bath oil to the water. Wait until after he gets into the tub before adding bath oil *because oil makes the tub slick and increases the risk of falling.*
• Taking care to respect his privacy, help the patient bathe, as needed; he may appreciate help washing his back. If you can safely leave the patient alone, place the call button within easy reach and show him how to use it.
• Tell the patient to leave the door unlocked for his own safety, but assure him that you'll post an OCCUPIED sign on the door. Stay nearby in case of emergency, and check on the patient every 5 to 10 minutes.
• When the patient finishes bathing, drain the tub or turn off the shower.
• Assist the patient onto the bath mat *to prevent him from falling.* Then help him to dry off and don a clean gown or other clothing, as appropriate.
• Escort the patient to his room or to his bed.
• Dry the floor of the bathing area well *to prevent slipping.* Ensure that the tub or shower is cleaned and disinfected.
• Dispose of soiled towels and return the patient's personal belongings to his bedside.

Special considerations
If you're giving a tub bath to a patient with a cast or dressing on an arm or leg, wrap the extremity in a clear plastic bag. Secure the bag with tape, being careful not to constrict circulation. Instruct the patient to dangle the arm or leg over the edge of the tub, and keep it out of the water.

Encourage the patient to use safety devices, bars, and rails when bathing. *Because bathing in warm water causes vasodilation,* the patient may feel faint. If so, open the drain or turn off the shower. Cover the patient's shoulders and back with a bath towel, and instruct him to lean forward in the tub and to lower his head. Alternatively, assist him out of the shower onto a chair, lower his head, and summon help. If you have an ampule of aromatic spirits of ammonia readily available, break it open and wave it under the patient's nostrils. Never leave the patient unattended to obtain an ampule. When the patient recovers, escort him to bed and monitor vital signs.

Documentation
Describe the patient's skin condition and record any discoloration or redness in your notes.

Hair care

Hair care includes combing, brushing, and shampooing. Combing and brushing stimulates scalp circulation, removes dead cells and debris, and distributes hair oils to produce a healthy sheen. Shampooing removes dirt and old oils and helps prevent skin irritation.

Frequency of hair care depends on the length and texture of the patient's hair, the duration of hospitalization, and the patient's condition. Usually, hair should be combed and brushed daily, and shampooed according to the patient's normal routine. Typically, no more than 1 week, or perhaps 2, should elapse between washings. Shampooing is contraindicated in patients with recent craniotomy, depressed skull fracture, conditions necessitating intracranial pressure monitoring, or other cranial involvement.

Equipment
Comb and brush ■ hand towel ■ liquid shampoo (or mild soap, such as castile) ■ shampoo tray with tubing ■ washcloth ■ three bath towels ■ two bath blankets ■ cotton ■ pail or plastic wastebasket ■ two large pitchers or other large containers ■ one small pitcher or beaker ■ basin ■ linen-saver pads ■ gloves, if the patient has open scalp lesions ■ optional: hair conditioner or rinse, alcohol, oil, hair ties, footstool, drawsheet.

Preparation of equipment
The comb and brush should be clean. If necessary, wash them in hot, soapy water. The comb should have dull, even teeth *to prevent scratching the scalp.* The brush should have stiff bristles *to enhance vigorous brushing and stimulation of circulation.*

Before shampooing the patient's hair, adjust room temperature and eliminate drafts *to prevent chilling the patient.* Next, obtain a shampoo tray or devise a trough, if necessary. (For instructions, see *How to make a shampoo trough.*)

Implementation
• Assemble the equipment on the patient's bedside stand.

Combing and brushing
• Tell the patient you're going to comb and brush his hair. If possible, encourage him to do this himself, assisting him as necessary.
• Adjust the bed to a comfortable working height *to prevent back strain.* If the patient's condition allows, help him to a sitting position by raising the head of the bed.

• Support the patient's feet in the correct position with a footboard *to prevent footdrop.*
• Make sure all tubes are positioned properly *to maintain their function.*
• Retain the help of one or more co-workers before you turn the patient.
• To turn the patient from supine to prone, remove the top sheet, if present. Then, place a pillow or sheepskin lengthwise over the patient's legs, chest, or other areas *to promote comfort and act as a pad during turning.*
• Detach the armboards and store them on the shelf under the bed.
• Carefully remove the nuts at both ends of the posterior frame, and position the anterior frame so its face support fits over the patient's face and its upper portion extends from the shoulders to the symphysis pubis, with the 4″ (10 cm) opening over the perineum. Make sure the lower portion of the frame extends to the ankles, allowing the feet to extend over the end of the frame in the prone position. Check that the patient is in proper alignment.
• After adjusting the anterior frame, securely lock it in place at both ends.
• Place the patient's arms at his sides or, if possible, have him put them around and grasp the anterior frame *for a sense of security during turning.*
• Place two or three safety straps around the turning frames *to promote the patient's safety and prevent his arms and legs from slipping during turning.* If necessary, reposition the I.V., indwelling urinary catheter, or chest tubing appropriately *to prevent dislodgement or entanglement during turning.*
• In wedge-shaped frames, always turn the patient in the direction of the narrow wedge *to minimize the risk of falling.* Tell the patient which direction he'll be turning.
• With one co-worker positioned at each end of the bed, simultaneously remove the locking pins and release the bed turning locks. Then, on the count of three, turn the patient quickly and smoothly, maintaining cervical traction. If extra co-workers are present, ask them to stand beside the frame during the turn *to reassure the patient, who may be anxious and afraid of falling.*
• Close both locks and replace the pins before releasing your grip on the frame. Then remove the safety straps and the posterior frame.
• Position the patient properly. Make sure all tubing and equipment are properly positioned and adjusted.
• Replace and adjust the armboards and change the linens if necessary.
• Assess the patient's level of consciousness, mobility, and sensation. Assess the skin for redness or pressure areas, and provide skin care or other prescribed treatments.

• Evaluate the patient's tolerance for the prone and supine positions.
• Follow the same procedure to return the patient to the supine position.

Special considerations

Turn the patient at least every 2 hours. Between turnings, perform appropriate range-of-motion exercises, as ordered. If the patient finds the prone position uncomfortable, administer prescribed pain medication before turning. If he has skull tongs in place, turn him cautiously *to avoid dislodging them.* If he's connected to a mechanical ventilator, disconnect the device immediately before turning and reconnect it immediately afterward. Hand rolls and cradle boots can be used during turning *to help keep the patient's hands and feet comfortable.*

Remove the perineal section of the frame for bedpan use, but always replace it immediately afterward *to prevent spinal misalignment from inadequate support of the patient's buttocks in the supine position.* Provide appropriate diversion and encourage the patient's family and friends to do so *to counteract boredom.* Adjust the reading board for meals and reading, and provide adequate light *to prevent eyestrain.*

Documentation

Record the time of turning, the patient's reaction during turning, any treatments administered, and your observations concerning the patient's skin condition and overall status.

CircOlectric bed

This bed permits frequent turning of the severely injured or immobilized patient with minimal trauma or extraneous movement. Its multiple intermediate positions help prevent and treat pressure ulcers and respiratory and circulatory complications. The bed's narrow mattress permits close proximity between patient and nurse, allowing better body mechanics and preventing back strain. Because this bed is portable, it eliminates potentially traumatic patient transfer. Safe operation requires at least two persons. (See *Using the CircOlectric bed,* page 68.)

Equipment

CircOlectric bed ▪ fitted sheets ▪ sheepskin ▪ bedpan.

Preparation of equipment

In some hospitals with low doorways, you may need to remove the upper half of the frame to get the bed into

• Provide privacy, and drape a bath towel over the patient's pillow and shoulders *to catch loose hair and dirt.* Don gloves if the patient has open scalp lesions.

• For short hair, comb and brush one side at a time. For long or curly hair, turn the patient's head away from you, and then part his hair down the middle from front to back. If the hair is tangled, rub alcohol or oil on the hair strands to loosen them. Comb and vigorously brush the hair on the side facing you. Then turn the patient's head and comb and brush the opposite side. Part hair into small sections for easier handling. Comb one section at a time, working from the ends toward the scalp to remove tangles. Anchor each section of hair above the area being combed *to avoid hurting the patient.* After combing, brush vigorously.

• Style the hair as the patient prefers. Braiding long or curly hair helps prevent snarling. To braid, part hair down the middle of the scalp and begin braiding near the face. Don't braid too tightly *to avoid patient discomfort.* Fasten the ends of the braids with hair ties. Pin the braids across the top of the patient's head or let them hang, as the patient desires, *so the finished braids don't press against the patient's scalp.*

• After styling the hair, carefully remove the towel by folding it inward. *This prevents loose hairs and debris from falling onto the pillow or into the patient's bed.*

Shampooing a bedridden patient's hair

• Cover the patient with a bath blanket. Then fanfold the linens to the foot of the bed, or remove them if they're scheduled to be changed.

• Place a wastebasket on a linen-saver pad on the floor or on a footstool near the head of the bed. The pail or container catches wastewater from the shampoo tray.

• Fill large pitchers or containers with comfortably warm water and place them on the overbed table.

• Lower the head of the bed until it's horizontal, and remove the patient's pillow, if allowed.

• Fold the second bath blanket and tuck it under the patient's shoulders *to improve water drainage.*

• Cover the bath blanket and the head of the bed with a linen-saver pad *to protect them from moisture.*

• Place a bath towel and linen-saver pad together, and position them around the patient's neck and over his shoulders. *This protects the patient from moisture and pads his neck against the pressure of the shampoo tray.*

• Place the shampoo tray under the patient's head with his neck in the U-shaped opening. Arrange the bath blanket and towel so the patient is comfortable.

• Adjust the shampoo tray to carry wastewater away from the patient's head, and place the drainage tubing in the pail. Tuck a folded towel or drawsheet under the opposite

side of the shampoo tray *to promote drainage, if necessary.* Don gloves if the patient has open scalp lesions.

• When shampooing, place cotton in the patient's ears *to prevent moisture from collecting in the ear canals.*

• Fill the small pitcher or beaker by dipping it into the large pitcher. Carefully pour water over the patient's hair. *To avoid spills,* don't overfill the shampoo tray.

• Then, with your fingertips, rub shampoo into the patient's hair. Massage his scalp well *to emulsify hair oils. Vigorous rubbing stimulates the scalp and also helps the patient relax.*

• Using the small pitcher or beaker, pour water over the patient's hair until it's free of shampoo. Then reapply shampoo and rinse again. Apply conditioner or a rinse, if desired.

• Remove the shampoo tray, and wrap the patient's hair in a towel. Remove the linen-saver pad from the bed, and return the bed to its original position.

• Dry the patient's hair by gently rubbing it with a towel. Then comb, brush, and style it.

• Remake the bed or change the linens, if needed, and remove the bath blanket.

• Reposition the patient comfortably.

• Remove and empty the pail. Clean the shampoo tray, and return it to storage. Remove pitchers from the bedside, and return the shampoo to the bedside stand.

Special considerations

When giving hair care, check the patient's scalp carefully for signs of scalp disorders or skin breakdown, particularly if the patient is bedridden. Make sure each patient has his own comb and brush *to avoid cross-contamination.*

If you don't have a shampoo tray and can't devise a trough, place pillows under the patient's shoulders to elevate his head, and use a basin. Because a standard basin doesn't have a drainage spout, empty it frequently *to prevent overflow.*

Documentation

Record the date, time, and patient's response to the shampoo on the flowchart. Describe any scalp abnormalities in your notes.

Shaving

Performed with a straight, safety, or electric razor, shaving is part of the male patient's usual daily care. Besides reducing bacterial growth on the face, shaving promotes patient comfort by removing whiskers that can itch and irritate the skin and produce an unkempt appearance. Because nicks and cuts occur most frequently with a straight or a safety razor, shaving with an electric razor is indicated for the patient with a clotting disorder or the patient undergoing anticoagulant therapy. Shaving may be contraindicated in the patient with a facial skin disorder or wound.

Equipment

For a straight or a safety razor: Shaving kit containing a straight razor and soap container, or a safety razor ■ gloves ■ soap or shaving cream ■ towel ■ washcloth ■ basin ■ optional: after-shave lotion, talcum powder.

For an electric razor: Bath towel ■ optional: pre-shave and after-shave lotions, mirror, grounded three-pronged plug.

Preparation of equipment

With a straight or a safety razor, make sure the blade is sharp, clean, even, and rust-free. If necessary, insert a new blade securely into the razor. A razor may be used more than once, but only by the same patient. If the patient is bedridden, assemble the equipment on the bedside stand or overbed table; if he's ambulatory, assemble it at the sink. When the patient is ready to shave, fill the basin or sink with warm water.

If you're using an electric razor, check its cord for fraying or other damage that could create an electrical hazard. If the razor isn't double-insulated or battery-operated, use a grounded three-pronged plug. Examine the razor head for sharp edges and dirt. Read the manufacturer's instructions, if available, and assemble the equipment at the bedside.

Implementation

● Tell the patient that you're going to shave him, and provide privacy. Ask him to assist you as much as possible *to promote his independence.*

● Unless contraindicated, place the conscious patient in the high Fowler's or semi-Fowler's position. If the patient is unconscious, elevate his head *to prevent soap and water from running behind it.*

● Direct bright light onto the patient's face, but not into his eyes.

Using a straight or a safety razor

● Drape a bath towel around the patient's shoulders, and tuck it under his chin *to protect the bed from moisture and to catch falling whiskers.*

● Put on gloves, and fill the basin with warm water. Using the washcloth, wet the patient's entire beard with warm water. Let the warm cloth soak the beard for at least 1 minute *to soften whiskers.*

● Apply shaving cream to the beard. Or, if you're using soap, rub to form a lather.

● Gently stretch the patient's skin taut with one hand and shave with the other, holding the razor firmly. Ask the patient to puff his cheeks or turn his head, as necessary, to shave hard-to-reach areas.

● Begin at the sideburns and work toward the chin using short, firm, downward strokes in the direction of hair growth. *This reduces skin irritation and helps prevent nicks and cuts.*

● Rinse the razor often *to remove whiskers.* Apply more warm water or shaving cream to the face, as needed, *to maintain adequate lather.*

● Shave across the chin and up the neck and throat. Use short, gentle strokes for the neck and the area around the nose and mouth *to avoid skin irritation.*

● Change the water, and rinse any remaining lather and whiskers from the patient's face. Then dry his face with a bath towel and, if the patient desires, apply after-shave lotion or talcum powder.

● Rinse the razor and basin, and then return the razor to its storage area.

Using an electric razor

● Plug in the razor, and apply pre-shave lotion, if available, *to remove skin oils.* If the razor head is adjustable, select the appropriate setting.

• Using a circular motion and pressing the razor firmly against the skin, shave each area of the patient's face until smooth.

• If the patient desires, apply talcum powder or after-shave lotion.

• Clean the razor head, and return the razor to its storage area.

Special considerations

If the patient is conscious, find out his usual shaving routine. Although shaving in the direction of hair growth is most common, the patient may prefer the opposite direction.

Don't interchange patients' shaving equipment *to prevent cross-contamination.*

Complications

Cuts and abrasions are the most common complications of shaving and can require application of antiseptic lotion.

Documentation

If applicable, record nicks or cuts resulting from shaving.

Eye care

When paralysis or coma impairs or eliminates the corneal reflex, frequent eye care aims to keep the exposed cornea moist, preventing ulceration and inflammation. Application of saline-saturated gauze pads over the eyelids moistens the eyes. Commercially available eye ointments and artificial tears also lubricate the corneas, but a doctor's order is required for their use.

Although eye care isn't a sterile procedure, asepsis should be maintained as much as possible.

Equipment

Sterile basin ■ gloves ■ sterile towel ■ sterile normal saline solution ■ sterile cotton balls ■ mineral oil ■ artificial tears or eye ointment (if ordered) ■ gauze or eyepads ■ nonallergenic tape.

Preparation of equipment

Assemble the equipment at the patient's bedside. Pour a small amount of saline solution into the basin.

Implementation

• Wash your hands thoroughly, put on gloves, and tell the patient what you're about to do, even if he is comatose or appears unresponsive.

• To remove secretions or crusts adhering to the eyelids and eyelashes, first soak a cotton ball in sterile normal saline solution. Then gently wipe the patient's eye with the moistened cotton ball, working from the inner canthus to the outer canthus *to prevent debris and fluid from entering the nasolacrimal duct.*

• *To prevent cross-contamination,* use a fresh cotton ball for each wipe until the eye is clean. *To prevent irritation,* avoid using soap for cleaning the eyes. Repeat the procedure for the other eye.

• After cleaning the eyes, instill artificial tears or apply eye ointment, as ordered, *to keep them moist.*

• Close the patient's eyelids. Dab a small amount of mineral oil on each lid *to lubricate and protect fragile skin.*

• Soak gauze or eyepads in sterile normal saline solution, place them over the eyelids, and secure with nonallergenic tape. Change gauze pads, as necessary, *to keep them well saturated.*

• After giving eye care, cover the basin with a sterile towel and dispose of gloves. Change the eye care setup (basin, towel, and normal saline solution) at least daily.

Documentation

Record the time and type of eye care in your notes. If applicable, chart administration of eyedrops or ointment in the patient's medication record. Document unusual crusting or excessive or colored drainage.

Contact lens care

Illness or emergency treatment may require that you insert or remove and store a patient's contact lenses. Proper handling and lens care techniques help prevent eye injury and infection as well as lens loss or damage. Appropriate lens-handling techniques depend in large part on what type of lenses the patient wears.

All contact lenses float on the corneal tear layer. Rigid lenses typically have a smaller diameter than the cornea; soft lens diameter typically exceeds that of the cornea. Because they're larger and more pliable, soft lenses tend to mold themselves more closely to the eye for a more stable fit than rigid lenses.

Modes of lens wear vary widely. Although most patients remove and clean their lenses daily, some wear lenses overnight or for several days (sometimes up to a month) without removing them for cleaning. Still other patients wear disposable lenses, which means that they replace old lenses with new ones at regular intervals (a few days to a few months), possibly without removing them for cleaning between replacements.

Keep in mind that lenses handled improperly can provide a direct source of contamination to the eye.

Equipment

Lens storage case or two small medicine cups and adhesive tape ■ gloves ■ patient's equipment for contact lens care, if available ■ sterile normal saline solution or soaking solution ■ flashlight, if needed ■ optional: suction cup.

Preparation of equipment

If a commercial lens storage case isn't available, place enough sterile normal saline solution into two small medicine cups to submerge a lens in each one. To avoid confusing the left and right lenses, which may have different prescriptions, mark one cup "L" and the other cup "R" and place the corresponding lens in each cup.

Implementation

• Tell the patient what you're about to do, wash your hands, and put on gloves *to help prevent ocular infection.*

Inserting rigid lenses

• Wet one lens with solution, and gently rub it between your thumb and index finger, or place it on your palm and rub it with your opposite index finger. Rinse well with the solution, leaving a small amount in the lens.
• Place the lens, convex side down, on the tip of the index finger of your dominant hand.
• Instruct the patient to gaze upward slightly. Separate the eyelids with your other thumb and index finger, and place the lens directly and gently on the cornea. You need not press it to the eye; the tear film will attract it naturally at the first touch. Using the same procedure, insert the opposite lens.

Inserting soft lenses

• To see if the lens is inside out, bend it between your thumb and index finger or fill it with saline or soaking solution. If the lens tends to roll inward or the edge points slightly inward, it's oriented correctly. If the edge points outward or the lens tends to collapse over your fingertip, it's probably inside out and should be reversed.
• Wet the lens with fresh normal saline solution, and rub it gently between your thumb and index finger, or place it on your palm and rub it with your opposite index finger. Rinse well.
• Place the lens, convex side down, on the tip of the index finger of your dominant hand.
• Instruct the patient to gaze upward slightly. Separate the eyelids with your other thumb and index finger, and place the lens on the sclera, just below the cornea. Then, slide the lens gently upward with your finger until it centers on the cornea. Using the same procedure, insert the opposite lens.

Removing rigid lenses

• Before removing a lens, position the patient supine *to prevent the lens from popping out onto the floor, risking loss or damage.*
• Place one thumb against the patient's upper eyelid and the other thumb against the lower eyelid. Move the lids toward each other while gently pressing inward against the eye *to trap the lens edge and break the suction.* Extract the lens from the patient's eyelashes. (See *Removing a patient's contact lenses.*)
• Depending on the lens type and thickness, it may pop out when the suction breaks. You may want to try to break the suction with one hand while cupping the other hand below the patient's eye *to catch the lens as it falls.*
• Sometimes the lens will pop out on its own if you ask the patient to blink after stretching the corner of the eyelids toward the temporal bone, thus tightening the lid edges against the globe of the eye.
• After removal, place the lens in the proper well of the storage case (L or R) with enough of the appropriate storage solution to cover it. Alternatively, place the lens in a labeled medicine cup with solution, and secure adhesive tape over the top of the cup *to prevent loss of the lens.*
• Remove and care for the opposite lens using the same technique.

Removing soft lenses

• Position the patient supine. Using your nondominant hand, raise the patient's upper eyelid and hold it against the orbital rim.
• Lightly place the forefinger of your other hand on the lens and move it down onto the sclera below the cornea. Then pinch the lens between your forefinger and thumb; it should pop off.
• Place the lens in the proper well of the storage case with enough of the appropriate storage solution to cover it. Alternatively, place the lens in a labeled medicine cup with solution, and secure adhesive tape over the top of the cup *to prevent loss of the lens.*
• Remove and care for the other lens using the same technique.

Cleaning lenses

• Because lens-cleaning steps vary with lens type and with each manufacturer's and doctor's instructions, ask the patient to guide you step-by-step through his normal cleaning routine.

Removing a patient's contact lenses

Contact lens removal techniques depend largely on the type of lenses the patient wears and how readily they come off the eye. For successful removal of soft and rigid lenses, follow the steps outlined below. If you have trouble removing lenses manually, try using a specially-made suction cup.

Soft lenses
With the patient looking up and her upper lid raised, use your dominant index finger to slide the lens onto the lower cornea. Pinch the lens between your index finger and thumb to remove it.

Rigid lenses
Place one thumb on each eyelid and move the lids toward each other, pressing gently against the eyeball. When the lids meet the lens edges, the suction breaks and the lens is released, as shown at the top of the next column. Catch the lens in your lower hand or remove it from the patient's lashes.

Using a suction cup
Separate the lids with your nondominant hand. Squeeze the suction cup with your dominant hand, and place it gently against the lens. Open your fingers slightly to create suction between the lens and the cup. Rock the lens gently to remove it.

• If the patient is unable to tell you how to clean his lenses properly, remember that all lens types require two steps: cleaning and disinfection.

• Cleaning involves rubbing the lens with a surfactant solution designed to remove most surface deposits. For most patients, especially those who wear soft lenses, the cleaning step also may include use of an enzyme agent to remove protein deposits against which surfactant cleaners typically are ineffective. Enzyme cleaning involves soaking the lenses overnight in a solution in which you've dissolved special enzyme tablets.

• Disinfection, which doesn't require rubbing, may be accomplished through chemical means or by heat. This step aims to rid the lens of infectious organisms.

• If you must clean a patient's lenses, use only his own solutions. *This minimizes the risk of allergic reactions to substances included in other solution brands.* Never touch the nozzle opening of a solution bottle to the lens, your fingers, or anything else *to avoid contaminating solution remaining in the bottle.*

Special considerations
If the patient's eyes appear dry or you have trouble moving the lens on the eye, instill several drops of sterile normal saline solution, and wait a few minutes before trying again to remove the lens *to prevent corneal damage.* If you still can't remove the lens easily, notify the doctor. Avoid instillation of eye medication while the patient is

wearing lenses. The lenses can trap the medication, possibly causing eye irritation or lens damage.

Don't allow soft lenses, which are 40% to 60% water, to dry out. If they do, soak them in sterile normal saline solution and they may return to their natural shape.

If an unconscious patient is admitted to the emergency department, check for contact lenses by opening each eyelid and searching with a small flashlight. If you detect lenses, remove them immediately *because tears cannot circulate freely beneath the lenses with eyelids closed, possibly leading to corneal oxygen depletion or infection.*

Advise contact lens wearers to carry appropriate identification to speed lens removal and ensure proper care in an emergency.

If a patient cannot provide adequate care for his lenses during hospitalization, encourage him to send them home with a family member. If you aren't sure how to care for the lenses in the interim, store them in sterile normal saline solution until the family member can take them home.

Documentation
Record eye condition before and after removal of lenses; the time of lens insertion, removal, and cleaning; the location of stored lenses; and, if applicable, the removal of lenses from the hospital by a family member.

 Mouth care

Given in the morning, at bedtime, or after meals, mouth care entails brushing and flossing the teeth and inspecting the mouth. It removes soft plaque deposits and calculus from the teeth, cleans and massages the gums, reduces mouth odor, and helps prevent infection. By freshening the patient's mouth, mouth care also enhances appreciation of food, thereby aiding appetite and nutrition.

Although the ambulatory patient can usually perform mouth care alone, the bedridden patient may require partial or full assistance. The comatose patient requires use of suction equipment to prevent aspiration during oral care.

Equipment
Towel or facial tissues ■ emesis basin ■ trash bag ■ mouthwash ■ toothbrush and toothpaste ■ pitcher and glass ■ drinking straw ■ dental floss ■ gloves ■ dental floss holder, if available ■ small mirror, if necessary ■ optional: oral irrigating device.

For the comatose or debilitated patient, as needed: Linen-saver pad ■ bite-block ■ petroleum jelly ■ hydrogen peroxide ■ mineral oil ■ cotton-tipped mouth swab ■ oral suction equipment or gauze pads ■ optional: lemon-glycerin swabs or mouth-care kit, tongue blade, 4" × 4" gauze pads, adhesive tape.

Preparation of equipment
Fill a pitcher with water and bring it and other equipment to the patient's bedside. If you'll be using oral suction equipment, connect the tubing to the suction bottle and suction catheter, insert the plug into an outlet, and check for correct operation. If necessary, devise a bite-block to protect yourself from being bitten during the procedure. Wrap a gauze pad over the end of a tongue blade, fold the edge in, and secure it with adhesive tape.

Implementation
● Wash your hands thoroughly, put on gloves, explain the procedure to the patient, and provide privacy.

Supervising mouth care
● For the bedridden patient capable of self-care, encourage him to perform his own mouth care.
● If allowed, place the patient in Fowler's position. Place the overbed table in front of the patient, and arrange the equipment on it. Open the table and set up the built-in mirror, if available, or position a small mirror on the table.
● Drape a towel over the patient's chest to protect his gown. Instruct him to floss his teeth while looking into the mirror.
● Observe the patient *to be sure he's flossing correctly,* and correct him if necessary. Tell him to wrap the floss around the second or third fingers of both hands. Starting with his back teeth and without injuring the gums, he should insert the floss as far as possible into the space between each pair of teeth. Then he should clean the surfaces of adjacent teeth by pulling the floss up and down against the side of each tooth. After the patient flosses a pair of teeth, remind him to use a clean 1" (2.5-cm) section of floss for the next pair.
● After the patient flosses, mix mouthwash and water in a glass, place a straw in the glass, and position the emesis basin nearby. Then instruct the patient to brush his teeth and gums while looking into the mirror. Encourage him to rinse frequently during brushing, and provide facial tissues for him to wipe his mouth.

Performing mouth care
● For the comatose patient or the conscious patient incapable of self-care, you'll perform mouth care. If the patient wears dentures, clean them thoroughly. (See

Dealing with dentures

Prostheses made of plastic or vulcanite, dentures replace some or all of the patient's natural teeth. Dentures require proper care to remove soft plaque deposits and calculus and to reduce mouth odor. Such care involves removing and rinsing dentures after meals, daily brushing and removal of tenacious deposits, and soaking in a commercial denture cleaner. Dentures must be removed from the comatose or presurgical patient to prevent possible airway obstruction.

Preparation
Start by assembling the following equipment at the patient's bedside: emesis basin ■ labeled denture cup ■ toothbrush or denture brush ■ gloves ■ toothpaste ■ commercial denture cleaner ■ paper towel ■ cotton-tipped mouth swab ■ mouthwash ■ gauze ■ optional: adhesive denture liner.
   Wash your hands and put on gloves.

Removing dentures
• To remove a full upper denture, grasp the front and palatal surfaces of the denture with your thumb and forefinger. Position the index finger of your opposite hand over the upper border of the denture, and press *to break the seal between denture and palate.* Grasp the denture with gauze *because saliva can make it slippery.*
• To remove a full lower denture, grasp the front and lingual surfaces of the denture with your thumb and index finger, and gently lift up.
• To remove partial dentures, exert equal pressure on the border of each side of the denture. Avoid lifting the clasps, *which easily bend or break.*

Oral and denture care
• After removing dentures, place them in a properly labeled denture cup. Add warm water and a commercial denture cleaner *to remove stains and hardened deposits.* Follow package directions. Avoid soaking dentures overnight if they have metal parts *because corrosion may result.* Also, avoid soaking dentures in mouthwash *because it may pit the denture material.*
• Instruct the patient to rinse with mouthwash *to remove food particles and reduce mouth odor.* Then stroke the palate, buccal surfaces, gums, and tongue with a soft toothbrush or cotton-tipped mouth swab *to clean the mucosa and stimulate circulation.* Inspect for irritated areas or sores *because they may indicate a poorly fitting denture.*
• Carry the denture cup, emesis basin, toothbrush, and toothpaste to the sink. After lining the basin with a paper towel, fill it with water *to cushion the dentures in case you drop them.* Hold the dentures over the basin, wet them with warm water, and apply toothpaste to a denture brush or long-bristled toothbrush. Clean the dentures using only moderate pressure *to prevent scratches* and warm water *to prevent distortion.*
• Clean the denture cup, and place the dentures in it. Rinse the brush, and clean and dry the emesis basin. Return all equipment to the patient's bedside stand.

Inserting dentures
• If the patient desires, apply adhesive liner to the dentures. Moisten them with water, if necessary, *to reduce friction and ease insertion.*
• Encourage the patient to wear his dentures *to enhance his appearance, facilitate eating and speaking, and prevent changes in the gum line that may affect denture fit.*

Dealing with dentures.) Some patients may benefit from using an oral irrigating device, such as a Water Pik. (See *Using an oral irrigating device,* page 90.)
• Raise the bed to a comfortable working height *to prevent back strain.* Then lower the head of the bed, and position the patient on his side, with his face extended over the edge of the pillow *to facilitate drainage and prevent fluid aspiration.*
• Arrange the equipment on the overbed table or bedside stand, including the oral suction equipment, if necessary. Turn on the machine. If a suction machine isn't available, wipe the inside of the patient's mouth frequently with a gauze pad.

• Place a linen-saver pad under the patient's chin and an emesis basin near his cheek *to absorb or catch drainage.*
• Lubricate the patient's lips with petroleum jelly *to prevent dryness and cracking.* Reapply lubricant, as needed, during oral care.
• If necessary, insert the bite-block *to hold the patient's mouth open during oral care.*
• Using a dental floss holder, hold the floss against each tooth and direct it as close to the gum as possible without injuring the sensitive tissues around the tooth.
• After flossing the patient's teeth, mix mouthwash and water in a glass and place the straw in it.

Using an oral irrigating device

An oral irrigating device, such as the Water Pik, directs a pulsating jet of water around the teeth to massage gums and remove debris and food particles. It's especially useful for cleaning areas missed by brushing, such as around bridgework, crowns, and dental wires. Because this device enhances oral hygiene, it benefits patients undergoing head and neck irradiation, which can damage teeth and cause severe caries. The device also maintains oral hygiene in a patient with a fractured jaw or with mouth injuries that limit standard mouth care.

Equipment

To use the device, first assemble the following equipment: oral irrigating device ■ towel ■ emesis basin ■ pharyngeal suction apparatus ■ salt solution or mouthwash, if ordered ■ soap.

Implementation

• Turn the patient to his side *to prevent aspiration of water.* Then, place a towel under his chin and an emesis basin next to his cheek *to absorb or catch drainage.*
• Insert the oral irrigating device's plug into a nearby electrical outlet. Remove the device's cover, turn it upside down, and fill it with lukewarm water or with a mouthwash or salt solution, as ordered. When using a salt solution, dissolve the salt beforehand in a separate container. Then pour the solution into the cover.
• Secure the cover to the base of the device. Remove the water hose handle from the base, and snap the jet tip into place. If necessary, wet the grooved end of the tip *to ease insertion.* Adjust the pressure dial to the setting most comfortable for the patient. If his gums are tender and prone to bleed, choose a low setting.
• Adjust the knurled knob on the handle *to direct the water jet,* place the jet tip in the patient's mouth, and turn on the device. Instruct the alert patient to keep his lips partially closed *to avoid spraying water.*
• Direct the water at a right angle to the gum line of each tooth and between teeth. Avoid directing water under the patient's tongue *because this may injure sensitive tissue.*

After irrigating each tooth, pause briefly and instruct the patient to expectorate the water or solution into the emesis basin. If he's unable to do so, suction it from the sides of the mouth with the pharyngeal suction apparatus. After irrigating all teeth, turn off the device, and remove the jet tip from the patient's mouth.
• Empty the remaining water or solution from the cover, remove the jet tip from the handle, and return the handle to the base. Clean the jet tip with soap and water, rinse the cover, and dry them both and return them to storage.

• Wet the toothbrush with water. If necessary, use hot water *to soften the bristles.* Apply toothpaste.
• Brush the patient's lower teeth from the gum line up; the upper teeth, from the gum line down. Place the brush at a 45-degree angle to the gum line, and press the bristles gently into the gingival sulcus. Using short, gentle strokes *to prevent gum damage,* brush the facial surfaces (toward the cheek) and the lingual surfaces (toward the tongue) of the bottom teeth. Use just the tip of the brush for the lingual surfaces of the front teeth. Then, using the same technique, brush the facial and lingual surfaces of the top teeth. Next, brush the biting surfaces of the bottom and top teeth, using a back and forth motion. If possible, ask the patient to rinse frequently during brushing by taking the mouthwash solution through the straw. Hold the emesis basin steady under the patient's cheek, and wipe his mouth and cheeks with facial tissues, as needed.
• After brushing the patient's teeth, dip a cotton-tipped mouth swab into the mouthwash solution. Press the swab against the side of the glass to remove excess moisture. Gently stroke the gums, buccal surfaces, palate, and

tongue *to clean the mucosa and stimulate circulation.* Replace the swab as necessary for thorough cleaning. Avoid inserting the swab too deeply *to prevent gagging and vomiting.*

After mouth care

• Assess the patient's mouth for cleanliness and tooth and tissue condition. Then remove your gloves, rinse the toothbrush, and clean the emesis basin and glass. Empty and clean the suction bottle, if used, and place a clean suction catheter on the tubing. Return reusable equipment to the appropriate storage location and properly discard disposable equipment in the trash bag.

Special considerations

Use cotton-tipped mouth swabs to clean the teeth of a patient with sensitive gums. *These swabs produce less friction than a toothbrush but don't clean as well.*

Clean the mouth of a toothless comatose patient by wrapping a gauze pad around your index finger, moistening it with mouthwash, and gently swabbing the oral tissues. If necessary, moisten gauze pads in an equal mixture of hydrogen peroxide and water *to remove tenacious mucus.*

Remember that mucous membranes dry quickly in the patient breathing through his mouth or receiving oxygen therapy. Moisten his mouth and lips regularly with mineral oil, lemon-glycerin swabs, or water. If you use water as the lubricant, place a short straw in a glass of water and stop the open end with your finger. Remove the straw from the water and, with your finger in place, position it in the patient's mouth. Release your finger slightly to let the water flow out gradually. If the patient is comatose, suction excess water *to prevent aspiration.*

Documentation

Record the date and time of mouth care in your notes. Also document any unusual conditions, such as bleeding, edema, mouth odor, excessive secretions, or plaque on the tongue.

Back care

Regular bathing and massage of the neck, back, buttocks, and upper arms promotes patient relaxation and allows assessment of skin condition. Particularly important for the bedridden patient, massage causes cutaneous vasodilation, helping to prevent pressure ulcers caused by prolonged pressure on bony prominences or by perspiration. Gentle back massage can be performed after myo-cardial infarction but may be contraindicated in patients with rib fractures, surgical incisions, or other recent traumatic injury to the back.

Equipment

Basin ■ soap ■ bath blanket ■ bath towel ■ washcloth ■ back lotion with lanolin base ■ gloves, if the patient has open lesions or has been incontinent ■ optional: talcum powder.

Preparation of equipment

Fill the basin two-thirds full with warm water. Place the lotion bottle in the basin to warm it. *Application of warmed lotion prevents chilling or startling the patient, thereby reducing muscle tension and vasoconstriction.*

Implementation

• Assemble the equipment at the patient's bedside.
• Explain the procedure to the patient, and provide privacy. Ask him to tell you if you're applying too much or too little pressure.
• Adjust the bed to a comfortable working height and lower the head of the bed, if allowed. Wash your hands and put on gloves, if applicable.
• Place the patient in the prone position, if possible, or on his side. Position him along the edge of the bed nearest you *to prevent back strain.*
• Untie the patient's gown, and expose his back, shoulders, and buttocks. Then drape the patient with a bath blanket *to prevent chills and minimize exposure.* Place a bath towel next to or under the patient's side *to protect bed linens from moisture.*
• Fold the washcloth around your hand to form a mitt. *This prevents the loose ends of the cloth from dripping water onto the patient, and also keeps the cloth warm longer.* Then, work up a lather with soap.
• Using long, firm strokes, bathe the patient's back, beginning at the neck and shoulders and moving downward to the buttocks. Rinse and dry well *because moisture trapped between the buttocks can cause chafing and predispose the patient to formation of pressure ulcers.* While giving back care, closely examine the patient's skin, especially the bony prominences of the shoulders, the scapulae, and the coccyx, for redness or abrasions.
• Remove the warmed lotion bottle from the basin, and pour a small amount of lotion into your palm. Rub your hands together *to distribute the lotion.* Then, apply the lotion to the patient's back, using long, firm strokes. *The lotion reduces friction, making back massage easier.*
• Massage the patient's back, beginning at the base of the spine and moving upward to the shoulders. For a relaxing effect, massage slowly; for a stimulating effect, massage quickly. Alternate the three basic strokes: ef-

How to give a back massage

Three strokes used commonly when giving a back massage are effleurage, friction, and petrissage. Start with effleurage and go on to friction and then to petrissage. Perform each stroke at least six times before moving on to the next, and then repeat the whole series if desired. When performing effleurage and friction, keep your hands parallel to the vertebrae to avoid tickling the patient. For all three strokes, maintain a regular rhythm and steady contact with the patient's back to help him relax.

Effleurage
Using your palm, stroke from the buttocks up to the shoulders, over the upper arms, and back to the buttocks. Use slightly less pressure on the downward strokes.

Friction
Use circular thumb strokes to move from buttocks to shoulders; then, using a smooth stroke, return to the buttocks, as shown at the top of the next column.

Petrissage
Using your thumb to oppose your fingers, knead and stroke half the back and upper arms, starting at the buttocks and moving toward the shoulder. Then knead and stroke the other half of the back, rhythmically alternating your hands.

fleurage, friction, and petrissage, as shown in *How to give a back massage*. Add lotion, as needed, keeping one hand on the patient's back *to avoid interrupting the massage.*
• Compress, squeeze, and lift the trapezius muscle *to help relax the patient.*
• Finish the massage by using long, firm strokes, and blot any excess lotion from the patient's back with a towel. Then, retie the patient's gown and straighten or change the bed linens, as necessary.

• Return the bed to its original position, and make the patient comfortable. Empty and clean the basin. Dispose of gloves, if used, and return equipment to the appropriate storage area.

Special considerations
Before giving back care, assess the patient's body structure and skin condition, and tailor the duration and intensity of the massage accordingly. If you're giving back

care at bedtime, have the patient ready for bed beforehand, so the massage can help him fall asleep.

Use separate lotion for each patient *to prevent cross-contamination.* If the patient has oily skin, substitute a talcum powder or lotion of the patient's choice. However, don't use powder if the patient has an endotracheal or tracheal tube in place *to avoid aspiration.* Also, avoid using powder and lotion together *because this may lead to skin maceration.*

When massaging the patient's back, stand with one foot slightly forward and your knees slightly bent *to allow effective use of your arm and shoulder muscles.* Give special attention to bony prominences *because these areas are disposed to formation of pressure ulcers.* Don't massage the patient's legs unless ordered *because reddened legs can signal clot formation, and massage can dislodge the clot, causing an embolus.* Develop a turning schedule and give back care at each position change.

Documentation
Chart back care on the flowchart. Record redness, abrasion, or change in skin condition in your notes.

Foot care

Daily bathing of feet and regular trimming of toenails promotes cleanliness, prevents infection, stimulates peripheral circulation, and controls odor by removing debris from between toes and under toenails. It's particularly important for bedridden patients and those especially susceptible to foot infection. Increased susceptibility may be caused by peripheral vascular disease, diabetes mellitus, poor nutritional status, arthritis, or any condition that impairs peripheral circulation. In such patients, proper foot care should include meticulous cleanliness and regular observation for signs of skin breakdown. (See *Foot care for diabetic patients* for additional instructions.)

Toenail trimming is contraindicated in patients with toe infections, diabetes mellitus, neurologic disorders, renal failure, or peripheral vascular disease, unless performed by a doctor or podiatrist.

Equipment
Bath blanket ■ large basin ■ soap ■ towel ■ linen-saver pad ■ pillow ■ washcloth ■ toenail clippers ■ orangewood stick ■ emery board ■ cotton-tipped applicator ■ cotton ■ lotion ■ water-absorbent powder ■ bath thermometer ■ gloves, if the patient has open lesions.

Foot care for diabetic patients

Because diabetes mellitus can reduce blood supply to the feet, normally minor foot injuries can lead to dangerous infection. When caring for a diabetic patient, keep these foot care guidelines in mind:
• Exercising the feet daily can help improve circulation. While the patient is sitting on the edge of the bed, ask him to point his toes upward, then downward, 10 times. Then have him make a circle with each foot 10 times.
• A diabetic's shoes must fit properly. Instruct the patient to break in new shoes gradually by increasing wearing time by 30 minutes each day. Also tell him to check his old shoes frequently in case they develop rough spots in the lining.
• Tell the patient to wear clean socks daily and to avoid socks with holes, darned spots, or rough, irritating seams.
• Advise the patient to see a doctor if he has corns or calluses.
• Tell the patient to wear warm socks or slippers and use extra blankets to avoid cold feet. He should not use heating pads and hot water bottles because these may cause burns.
• Teach the patient to regularly inspect the skin on his feet for cuts, cracks, blisters, or red, swollen areas. Even slight cuts on the feet should receive a doctor's attention. As a first-aid measure, tell him to wash the cut thoroughly and apply a mild antiseptic. Urge him to avoid harsh antiseptics, such as iodine, because they can damage tissue.
• Advise the diabetic patient to avoid tight-fitting garments or activities that can decrease circulation. The patient should especially avoid wearing elastic garters, sitting with knees crossed, picking at sores or rough spots on the feet, walking barefoot, or applying adhesive tape to the skin on his feet.

Preparation of equipment
Fill the basin halfway with warm water. Test water temperature with a bath thermometer *because patients with diminished peripheral sensation could burn their feet in excessively hot water (over 105° F [40.6° C]) without feeling any warning pain.* If a bath thermometer is unavailable, test the water by inserting your elbow. The water temperature should feel comfortably warm.

Implementation

• Assemble equipment at the patient's bedside. Wash your hands and put on gloves, if necessary.
• Tell the patient that you'll wash his feet and provide foot and toenail care.
• Cover the patient with a bath blanket. Fanfold the top linen to the foot of the bed.
• Place a linen-saver pad and a towel under the patient's feet *to keep the bottom linen dry.* Then position the basin on the pad.
• Insert a pillow beneath the patient's knee *to provide support,* and cushion the rim of the basin with the edge of the towel *to prevent pressure.*
• Immerse one foot in the basin. Wash it with soap, then allow it to soak for about 10 minutes. *Soaking softens the skin and toenails, loosens debris under toenails, and comforts and refreshes the patient.*
• After soaking the foot, rinse it with a washcloth, remove it from the basin, and place it on the towel.
• Dry the foot thoroughly, especially between the toes, *to avoid skin breakdown.* Blot gently to dry *because harsh rubbing may damage the skin.*
• Empty the basin, refill it with warm water, and clean and soak the other foot.
• While the second foot is soaking, give the first one a pedicure. Using the cotton-tipped applicator, carefully clean the toenails. Using an orangewood stick, gently remove any dirt beneath the toenails; avoid injuring subungual skin.
• Trim nails with toenail clippers, if needed, by cutting straight across *to prevent ingrown toenails.* Clip small sections of the nail at a time, starting at one edge and working across. File trimmed toenails with an emery board to smooth rough edges. *Keeping toenails trimmed and filed prevents scratching and injury to the skin on the opposite leg.*
• Rinse the foot that has been soaking, dry it thoroughly, and give it a pedicure.
• Apply lotion *to moisten dry skin,* or lightly dust water-absorbent powder between the toes *to absorb moisture.*
• Remove and clean all equipment and dispose of gloves.

Special considerations

While providing foot care, observe the color, shape, and texture of the toenails. If you see redness, drying, cracking, blisters, discoloration, or other signs of traumatic injury, especially in patients with impaired peripheral circulation, notify the doctor. *Because such patients are vulnerable to infection and gangrene,* they need prompt treatment.

If a patient's toenail grows inward at the corners, tuck a wisp of cotton under it *to relieve pressure on the toe.*

When giving the bedridden patient foot care, unless contraindicated, perform range-of-motion exercises *to stimulate circulation and prevent foot contractures or muscle atrophy.* Tuck folded 2″ × 2″ gauze pads between overlapping toes *to protect the skin from the toenails.* Apply heel protectors *to prevent skin breakdown.*

Documentation

Record the date and time of bathing and toenail trimming in your notes. Record and report any abnormal findings and any nursing actions you take.

Perineal care

Perineal care, including the external genitalia and the anal area, should be performed during the daily bath and, if necessary, at bedtime and after urination and bowel movements. The procedure promotes cleanliness and prevents infection. It also removes irritating and odorous secretions, such as smegma, a cheeselike substance that collects under the foreskin of the penis and on the inner surface of the labia. For the patient with perineal skin breakdown, frequent bathing followed by application of an ointment or cream aids healing.

Universal precautions must be followed when providing perineal care, with due consideration given to the patient's privacy.

Equipment

Gloves ▪ washcloths ▪ clean basin ▪ mild soap ▪ bath towel ▪ bath blanket ▪ toilet tissue ▪ linen-saver pad ▪ trash bag ▪ optional: bedpan, peri bottle, antiseptic soap, petroleum jelly, zinc oxide cream, vitamin A and D ointment, and an ABD pad.

Following genital or rectal surgery, you may need to use sterile supplies, including sterile gloves, gauze, and cotton balls.

Preparation of equipment

Obtain ointment or cream, as needed. Fill the basin two-thirds full with warm water. Also, fill the peri bottle with warm water, if needed.

Implementation

• Assemble equipment at the patient's bedside. Provide privacy.
• Wash your hands thoroughly, put on gloves, and tell the patient what you're about to do.
• Adjust the bed to a comfortable working height *to prevent back strain,* and lower the head of the bed, if allowed.

• Provide privacy and help the patient to a supine position. Place a linen-saver pad under the patient's buttocks *to protect the bed from stains and moisture.*

Perineal care for the female patient
• To minimize the patient's exposure and embarrassment, place the bath blanket over her with corners head to foot and side to side. Wrap each leg with a side corner, tucking it under the hip. Then fold back the corner between the legs to expose the perineum.
• Ask the patient to bend her knees slightly and to spread her legs. Separate her labia with one hand and wash with the other, using gentle downward strokes from the front to the back of the perineum *to prevent intestinal organisms from contaminating the urethra or vagina.* Avoid the area around the anus, and use a clean section of washcloth for each stroke by folding each used section inward. *This prevents the spread of contaminated secretions or discharge.*
• Using a clean washcloth, rinse thoroughly from front to back *because soap residue can cause skin irritation.* Pat the area dry with a bath towel *because moisture can also cause skin irritation and discomfort.*
• Apply ordered ointments or creams.
• Turn the patient on her side to Sims' position, if possible, *to expose the anal area.*
• Clean, rinse, and dry the anal area, starting at the posterior vaginal opening and wiping from front to back.

Perineal care for the male patient
• Drape the patient's legs *to minimize exposure and embarrassment* and expose the genital area.
• Hold the shaft of the penis with one hand and wash with the other, beginning at the tip and working in a circular motion from the center to the periphery *to avoid introducing microorganisms into the urethra.* Use a clean section of washcloth for each stroke *to prevent the spread of contaminated secretions or discharge.*
• Rinse thoroughly, using the same circular motion.
• For the uncircumcised patient, gently retract the foreskin and clean beneath it. Rinse well but don't dry *because moisture provides lubrication and prevents friction when replacing the foreskin.* Replace the foreskin *to avoid constriction of the penis, which causes edema and tissue damage.*
• Wash the rest of the penis, using downward strokes toward the scrotum. Rinse well and pat dry with a bath towel.
• Clean the top and sides of the scrotum; rinse thoroughly and pat dry. Handle the scrotum gently *to avoid causing discomfort.*
• Turn the patient on his side. Clean the bottom of the scrotum and the anal area. Rinse well and pat dry.

After providing perineal care
• Reposition the patient and make him comfortable. Remove the bath blanket and linen-saver pad, and then replace the bed linens.
• Clean and return the basin and dispose of soiled articles including gloves.

Special considerations
Give perineal care to a patient of the opposite sex in a matter-of-fact way *to minimize embarrassment.*

If the patient is incontinent, first remove excess feces with toilet tissue. Then position him on a bedpan, and add a small amount of antiseptic soap to a peri bottle *to eliminate odor.* Irrigate the perineal area *to remove any remaining fecal matter.*

After cleaning the perineum, apply ointment or cream (petroleum jelly, zinc oxide cream, or vitamin A and D ointment) *to prevent skin breakdown by providing a barrier between the skin and excretions.*

To reduce the number of linen changes, tuck an ABD pad between the patient's buttocks *to absorb oozing feces.*

Documentation
Record perineal care and any special treatment in your notes. Document the need for continued treatment, if necessary, in your care plan. Describe perineal skin condition and any odor or discharge.

 Hour of sleep care

Hour of sleep (h.s.) care meets the patient's physical and psychological needs in preparation for sleep. It includes providing for the patient's hygiene, making the bed clean and comfortable, and ensuring safety. For example, raising the bed's side rails can prevent the drowsy or sedated patient from falling out. Bedtime care also provides an opportunity to answer the patient's questions about the next day's tests and procedures and to discuss his worries and concerns.

Effective h.s. care prepares the patient for a good night's sleep. Ineffective care may contribute to sleeplessness, which can intensify patient anxiety and interfere with treatment and recuperation.

Equipment
Bedpan, urinal, or commode ■ basin ■ soap ■ towel ■ washcloth ■ toothbrush and toothpaste ■ denture cup and commercial denture cleaner, if necessary ■ lotion ■ clean linens, if necessary ■ blankets ■ facial tissues ■ soft restraints, if necessary.

Recording fluid intake and output

Accurate intake and output records help evaluate a patient's fluid and electrolyte balance, suggest various diagnoses, and influence the choice of fluid therapy. These records are mandatory for patients with burns, renal failure, electrolyte imbalance, recent surgical procedures, congestive heart failure, or severe vomiting and diarrhea, and for those patients receiving diuretics or corticosteroids. Intake and output records are also significant in monitoring patients with nasogastric tubes, drainage collection devices, or those receiving I.V. therapy.

Fluid intake comprises all fluid entering the patient's body, including beverages, fluids contained in solid foods taken by mouth, and foods that are liquid at room temperature, such as flavored gelatin, custard, ice cream, and some beverages. Additional intake includes G.I. instillations, bladder irrigations, and I.V. fluids.

Fluid output includes all fluid that leaves the patient's body, including urine, loose stools, vomitus, aspirated fluid loss, and drainage from surgical drains, nasogastric tubes, and chest tubes.

When recording fluid intake and output, enlist the patient's help if possible. Record amounts in cubic centimeters (cc) or milliliters (ml). Measure, don't estimate. For a small child, weigh diapers if appropriate. Monitor intake and output during each shift, and notify the doctor if amounts differ significantly over a 24-hour period. Document your findings in the appropriate location; describe any fluid restrictions and the patient's compliance.

Preparation of equipment
Assemble the equipment at the patient's bedside. For the ambulatory patient who is capable of self-care, assemble soap, a washcloth, a towel, and oral hygiene items at the sink.

Implementation
• Tell the patient you will help him prepare for sleep, and provide privacy.
• Offer the patient on bed rest a bedpan, urinal, or commode. Otherwise, assist the ambulatory patient to the bathroom.
• Fill the basin with warm water and bring it to the patient's bedside. Immerse the lotion in the basin *to warm it for back massage.* Then wash the patient's face and hands and dry them well. Encourage the patient to do this himself, if possible, *to promote independence.*
• Provide toothpaste or a properly labeled denture cup and commercial denture cleaner. Assist the patient with oral hygiene, as necessary. (See "Mouth care" in this chapter.) If the patient prefers to wear dentures until bedtime, leave denture-care items within easy reach.
• After providing mouth care, turn the patient on his side or stomach. Wash, rinse, and dry the patient's back and buttocks. Massage well with lotion *to help relax the patient.* (See "Back care" in this chapter for complete information on massage.) While providing back care, observe the skin for redness, cracking, or other signs of breakdown. If the patient's gown is soiled or damp, provide a clean one and help him put it on, if necessary.
• Check dressings, binders, antiembolism stockings, or other aids, changing or readjusting them as needed.
• Refill the water container, and place it and a box of facial tissues within the patient's easy reach *to prevent falls if patient needs to reach for these items.*
• Straighten or change bed linens, as necessary, and fluff the patient's pillow. Cover him with a blanket or place one within his easy reach *to prevent chills during the night.* Then position him comfortably. If he appears distressed, restless, or in pain, give ordered drugs, as needed.
• After making the patient comfortable, evaluate his mental and physical condition. Then, if ordered and in accord with hospital policy, apply soft restraints *to prevent falls.* Place the bed in a low position and raise the side rails. Place the call button within the patient's easy reach, and instruct him to call you whenever necessary. Next, tidy the patient's environment: Move all breakables from the overbed table out of his reach, and remove any equipment and supplies that could cause falls should the patient get up during the night. Finally, turn off the overhead light and put on the night-light.

Special considerations
Ask the patient about his sleep routine at home and, whenever possible, let him follow it. Also try to observe certain rituals, such as a bedtime snack, *which can aid sleep.* A back massage, a tub bath, or a shower also help relax the patient and promote a restful night. If the patient normally bathes or showers before bedtime, let him do so in the hospital if his condition and doctor's orders permit it.

Documentation
Record the time and type of h.s. care in your notes. Include application of soft restraints or any other special procedures.

NUTRITION AND ELIMINATION
Feeding

Confusion, arm or hand immobility, injury, weakness, or restrictions on activities or positions may prevent a patient from feeding himself. Feeding the patient then becomes a key nursing responsibility. Injured or debilitated patients may experience depression and subsequent anorexia. Meeting such patients' nutritional needs requires determining food preferences, conducting the feeding in a friendly, unhurried manner, encouraging self-feeding to promote independence and dignity, and documenting intake and output. (See *Recording fluid intake and output.*)

Equipment
Meal tray ■ overbed table ■ linen-saver pad or towels ■ clean linens ■ flexible straws ■ basin of water ■ feeding syringe ■ assistive feeding devices, if necessary.

Implementation
• *Because many adults consider being fed demeaning,* be sure to allow the patient some control over mealtime. For example, let the patient set the pace of the meal or determine the order in which he eats the various foods.
• Raise the head of the bed if allowed. *Fowler's or semi-Fowler's position makes swallowing easier and reduces the risk of aspiration and choking.*
• Before the meal tray arrives, give the patient soap, a basin of water or a wet washcloth, and a hand towel *to clean his hands.* If necessary, you may wash his hands for him.
• Wipe the overbed table with soap and water or alcohol, especially if a urinal or bedpan had been placed on it.
• When the meal tray arrives, compare the name on the tray with the name on the patient's wristband. Check the tray to be sure it contains foods appropriate for the patient's condition.
• Encourage the patient to feed himself if he's able. If the patient is restricted to the prone or the supine position but can use his arms and hands, encourage him to try foods he can pick up, such as sandwiches. If he can assume the Fowler's or semi-Fowler's position but has limited use of his arms or hands, instruct him in the use of assistive feeding devices. (See *Using assistive feeding devices,* page 98.)
• If necessary, tuck a napkin or towel under his chin *to protect his gown from spills.* Use a linen-saver pad or towel *to protect bed linens.*
• Position a chair next to the patient's bed *so you can sit comfortably if you need to feed him yourself.*

Arranging food for the visually impaired patient

To help the blind or visually impaired patient feed himself, tell him that placement of various foods on his plate corresponds to the hours on a clock face. Maintain consistent placement for subsequent meals. The illustration shows meat at 12 o'clock, a vegetable at 6 o'clock, and rice at 9 o'clock.

• Set up the patient's tray, remove the plate from the tray warmer, and discard all plastic wrappings. Then cut the food into bite-sized pieces and prepare it, as necessary. Arrange food on the plate, if necessary. (See *Arranging food for the visually impaired patient.*)
• Ask the patient which food he prefers to eat first *to promote his sense of control over the meal.* Some patients prefer to eat one food at a time, while others prefer to alternate foods.
• If the patient has difficulty swallowing, offer liquids carefully with a spoon or feeding syringe *to help prevent aspiration.* Pureed or soft foods, such as custard or flavored gelatin, may be easier to swallow than liquids. If the patient doesn't have difficulty swallowing, use a flexible straw *to reduce the risk of spills.*
• Ask the patient to indicate when he's ready for another mouthful. Pause between courses and whenever the patient wants to rest. During the meal, wipe the patient's mouth and chin, as necessary.
• When the patient finishes eating, remove the tray. If necessary, clean up spills and change the bed linens. Provide mouth care.

Using assistive feeding devices

Various feeding devices can help the patient who has limited arm mobility, grasp, range of motion, or coordination. Before introducing your patient to an assistive feeding device, assess his ability to master it. Don't introduce a device he can't manage. If his condition is progressively disabling, encourage him to use the device only until his mastery of it falters.

Introduce the assistive device before mealtime, with the patient seated in a natural position. Explain its purpose, show the patient how to use it, and encourage him to practice. After meals, wash the device thoroughly and store it in the patient's bedside stand. Document the patient's progress and share it with staff and family members to help reinforce the patient's independence. Specific devices include the following:

Plate guard

This device blocks food from spilling off the plate. Attach the guard to the side of the plate opposite the hand the patient uses to feed himself. Guiding the patient's hand, show him how to push food against the guard to secure it on the utensil. Then have him try again with food of a different consistency. When the patient tires, feed him the rest of the meal. At subsequent meals, encourage the patient to feed himself for progressively longer periods until he can feed himself an entire meal.

Swivel spoon

This utensil helps the patient with limited range of motion in his forearm and will fit in universal cuffs.

Universal cuffs

These flexible bands help the patient with flail hands or diminished grasp. Each cuff contains a slot that holds a fork or spoon. Attach the cuff to the hand the patient uses to feed himself. Then place the fork or spoon in the cuff slot. Bend the utensil to facilitate feeding.

Long-handled utensils

These utensils have jointed stems to help the patient with limited range of motion in his elbow and shoulder.

Utensils with built-up handles

These utensils can help the patient with diminished grasp. They can be purchased or can be improvised by wrapping tape around the handles.

Special considerations

Don't feed the patient too quickly *because this can upset him and impair digestion.*

If the patient is restricted to the prone position, give foods that he can chew easily. If he's restricted to the supine position, feed him liquids carefully and only after he has swallowed any food in his mouth *to reduce the risk of aspiration.*

If the patient's food intake is inadequate because of chronic poor eating habits or anorexia, offer small, frequent meals *to provide a well-balanced diet.* If the patient won't eat, try to find out why. For example, confirm his food preferences. Also, make sure the patient isn't in pain at mealtimes or that he hasn't received any treatments immediately before a meal that could upset or nauseate him. Find out if any of his medications cause anorexia, nausea, or sedation. Of course, clear the bedside of emesis basins, urinals, bedpans, and similar distractions at mealtimes.

Establish a pattern for feeding the patient, and share this information with the rest of the nursing staff *so the patient doesn't need to repeatedly instruct staff members about the best way to feed him.*

If the patient and his family are willing, suggest that family members assist with feeding. This will make the patient feel more comfortable at mealtimes and may facilitate discharge planning.

Complications

Choking and aspiration of food can occur if the patient is fed too quickly or is given excessively large mouthfuls.

Documentation

Describe the feeding technique used in the nursing care plan to ensure continuity of care. In your notes, record the amount of food and fluid consumed; also note the fluids consumed on the intake and output record, if required. Note which foods the patient consistently fails to eat, then try to find the reason. Record the patient's level of independence. For the blind patient, record the pattern of feeding on the nursing care plan.

Bedpan and urinal

These devices permit elimination by the bedridden patient and accurate observation and measurement of urine and stool by the nurse. A bedpan is used by the female patient for defecation and urination and by the male patient for defecation; a urinal is used by the male patient for urination. Either device should be offered fre-

quently — before meals, visiting hours, morning and evening care, and before any treatments or procedures. Whenever possible, allow the patient to use a bedpan or urinal in privacy.

Equipment

Bedpan or urinal with cover ∎ toilet tissue ∎ two washcloths ∎ soap ∎ gloves ∎ towel ∎ linen-saver pad ∎ bath blanket ∎ pillow ∎ optional: air freshener, talcum powder.

Available in adult and pediatric sizes, the bedpan may be disposable or reusable (the latter can be sterilized). The fracture pan, a type of bedpan, is used when spinal injuries, body or leg casts, or other conditions prohibit or restrict turning the patient. Like the bedpan, the urinal may be disposable or reusable.

Preparation of equipment

Obtain the appropriate bedpan or urinal. If you're using a metal bedpan, warm it under running water *to avoid startling the patient and stimulating muscle contraction, which hinders elimination.* Dry the bedpan thoroughly and test its temperature *because metal retains heat.* If necessary, lightly sprinkle talcum powder on the edge of the bedpan *to reduce friction during placement and removal.* For a thin patient, place a linen-saver pad at the edge of the bedpan *to minimize pressure on the coccyx.*

Implementation

• If the patient's condition permits, provide privacy. Put on gloves *to prevent contact with body fluids and comply with universal precautions.*

To place a bedpan

• If allowed, elevate the head of the bed slightly *to prevent hyperextension of the spine when the patient raises the buttocks.*

• Rest the bedpan on the edge of the bed. Then, turn down the corner of the top linens and draw up the patient's gown. Ask him to raise the buttocks by flexing his knees and pushing down on his heels. While supporting the patient's lower back with one hand, center the curved, smooth edge of the bedpan beneath the buttocks.

• If the patient cannot raise his buttocks, lower the head of the bed to horizontal and help the patient roll onto one side, with buttocks toward you. Position the bedpan properly against the buttocks, and then help the patient roll back onto the bedpan. Once the patient is positioned comfortably, raise the head of the bed as indicated.

• After positioning the bedpan, elevate the head of the bed further, if allowed, until the patient is sitting erect. *Because this position resembles the normal elimination posture, it aids in defecation and urination.* (See *Using a com-*

Using a commode

An alternative to a bedpan, a commode is a portable chair made of wood, plastic, or metal, with a large opening in the center of the seat. It may have a bedpan or bucket that slides underneath the opening, or it may slide directly over the toilet, adding height to the standard toilet seat. Unlike a bedpan, a commode allows the patient to assume his normal elimination posture, which aids in defecation.

Before the patient uses it, inspect the commode's condition and make sure it is clean. Roll or carry the commode to the patient's room. Place it parallel and as close as possible to the patient's bed, and secure its brakes or wheel locks. If necessary, block its wheels with sandbags. Assist the patient onto the commode, provide toilet tissue, and place the call button within his reach. Instruct the patient to push the call button when he has finished.

If necessary, assist the patient with cleaning. Help him into bed and make him comfortable. Offer the patient soap, water, and a towel to wash his hands. Then close the lid of the commode or cover the bucket. Roll the commode or carry the bucket to the bathroom or hopper room. If ordered, observe and measure the contents before disposal. Rinse and clean the bucket, and then spray or wipe the bucket and commode seat with disinfectant. Use an air freshener if appropriate.

mode for another implement that permits normal elimination posture.)

• If elevation of the head of the bed is contraindicated, tuck a small pillow or folded bath blanket under the patient's back *to cushion the sacrum against the edge of the bedpan and support the lumbar region.*

• If the patient can be left alone, place the bed in a low position and raise the side rails *to ensure his safety.* Place toilet tissue and the call button within the patient's reach, and instruct him to push the button after elimination. If the patient is weak or disoriented, remain with him.

• Before removing the bedpan, lower the head of the bed slightly. Then ask the patient to raise his buttocks off the bed. Support the lower back with one hand, and gently remove the bedpan with the other *to avoid skin injury caused by friction.* If the patient cannot raise his buttocks, ask him to roll off the pan while you assist with one

hand. Hold the pan firmly with the other hand to avoid spills. Cover the bedpan and place it on the chair.

• Assist with cleaning the anal and perineal area, as necessary, *to prevent irritation and infection.* Turn the patient on his side, wipe carefully with toilet tissue, clean the area with a damp washcloth and soap, and dry well with a towel. For the female patient, clean from front to back *to avoid introducing rectal contaminants into the vaginal or urethral openings.*

To place a urinal

• Lift the corner of the top linens, hand the urinal to the patient, and allow him to position it.

• If the patient can't position the urinal himself, spread his legs slightly and hold the urinal in place *to prevent spills.*

• After the patient voids, carefully withdraw the urinal.

After use of a bedpan or urinal

• Give the patient a clean, damp, warm washcloth for his hands. Check the bed linens for wetness or soiling, and straighten or change them, if needed. Make the patient comfortable. Place the bed in the low position and raise the side rails.

• Take the bedpan or urinal to the bathroom or hopper room. Observe the color, odor, amount, and consistency of its contents. If ordered, measure urine output or liquid stool, or obtain a specimen for laboratory analysis.

• Empty the bedpan or urinal into the toilet or hopper. Rinse with cold water and clean it thoroughly, using a disinfectant solution. Dry and return it to the patient's bedside stand.

• Use an air freshener, if necessary, *to eliminate offensive odors and reduce the patient's embarrassment.*

• Remove gloves and wash your hands.

Special considerations

Explain to the patient that drug treatment and changes in his environment, diet, and activities may disrupt his usual elimination schedule. Try to anticipate elimination needs, and offer the bedpan or urinal frequently *to help reduce embarrassment and minimize the risk of incontinence.* Avoid placing a bedpan or urinal on top of the bedside stand or overbed table *to avoid contamination of clean equipment and food trays.* Similarly, avoid placing it on the floor *to prevent the spread of microorganisms from the floor to the patient's bed linens when the device is used.*

If the patient feels pain during turning or feels uncomfortable on a standard bedpan, use a fracture pan. Unlike the standard bedpan, the fracture pan is slipped under the buttocks from the front rather than the side. Because it's shallower than the standard bedpan, you need only lift the patient slightly to position it. If the patient is obese or otherwise difficult to lift, ask a co-worker to help you.

If the patient has an indwelling urinary catheter in place, carefully position and remove the bedpan *to avoid tension on the catheter, which could dislodge it or irritate the urethra.* After the patient defecates, wipe, clean, and dry the anal region, taking care to avoid catheter contamination. If necessary, clean the urinary meatus with povidone-iodine solution.

Documentation

Record the time, date, and type of elimination on the flowchart and the amount of urine output or liquid stool on the intake and output record, as needed. In your notes, document the presence of blood, pus, or other abnormal characteristics in urine or stool.

Male incontinence device

Many patients don't require an indwelling urinary catheter to manage their incontinence. For male patients, a male incontinence device reduces the risk of urinary tract infection from catheterization, promotes bladder retraining when possible, helps prevent skin breakdown, and improves the patient's self-image. The device consists of a condom catheter secured to the shaft of the penis and connected to a leg bag or drainage bag. It has no contraindications, but can cause skin irritation and edema.

Equipment

Condom catheter ▪ drainage bag ▪ extension tubing ▪ nonallergenic tape or incontinence sheath holder ▪ commercial adhesive strip or skin-bond cement ▪ elastic adhesive or Velcro, if needed ▪ gloves ▪ razor, if needed ▪ basin ▪ soap ▪ washcloth ▪ towel.

Preparation of equipment

Fill the basin with lukewarm water. Then, bring the basin and the remaining equipment to the patient's bedside.

Implementation

• Explain the procedure to the patient, wash your hands thoroughly, put on gloves, and provide privacy.

Applying the device

• If the patient is circumcised, wash the penis with soap and water, rinse well, and pat dry with a towel. If the patient is uncircumcised, gently retract the foreskin and clean beneath it. Rinse well but don't dry *because moisture provides lubrication and prevents friction during foreskin*

replacement. Replace the foreskin *to avoid penile constriction.* Then, if necessary, shave the base and shaft of the penis *to prevent the adhesive strip or skin-bond cement from pulling pubic hair.*

• If you're using a precut commercial adhesive strip, insert the glans penis through its opening, and position the strip 1″ (2.5 cm) from the scrotal area. If you're using uncut adhesive, cut a strip to fit around the shaft of the penis. Remove the protective covering from one side of the adhesive strip and press this side firmly to the penis *to enhance adhesion.* Then remove the covering from the other side of the strip. If a commercial adhesive strip isn't available, apply skin-bond cement and let it dry for a few minutes.

• Position the rolled condom catheter at the tip of the penis, with its drainage opening at the urinary meatus.

• Unroll the catheter upward, past the adhesive strip on the shaft of the penis. Then gently press the sheath against the strip until it adheres. (See *How to apply a condom catheter,* page 102.)

• After the condom catheter is in place, secure it with hypoallergenic tape or an incontinence sheath holder.

• Using extension tubing, connect the condom catheter to the leg bag or drainage bag. Remove and discard your gloves.

Removing the device

• Don gloves and simultaneously roll the condom catheter and adhesive strip off the penis and discard them. If you've used skin-bond cement rather than an adhesive strip, remove it with solvent. Also remove and discard the nonallergenic tape or incontinence sheath holder.

• Clean the penis with lukewarm water, rinse thoroughly, and dry. Check for swelling or signs of skin breakdown.

• Remove the leg bag by closing the drain clamp, unlatching the leg straps, and disconnecting the extension tubing at the top of the bag. Discard your gloves.

Special considerations

If nonallergenic tape or an incontinence sheath holder isn't available, secure the condom with a strip of elastic adhesive or Velcro. Apply the strip snugly — but not too tightly — *to prevent circulatory constriction.*

Inspect the condom catheter for twists and the extension tubing for kinks *to prevent obstruction of urine flow, which could cause the condom to balloon, eventually dislodging it.*

Documentation

Record the date and time of application and removal of the incontinence device. Also note skin condition and the patient's response to the device, including voiding pattern, to assist with bladder retraining.

How to apply a condom catheter

Apply an adhesive strip to the shaft of the penis about 1″ (2.5 cm) from the scrotal area.

Then roll the condom catheter onto the penis past the adhesive strip, leaving about ½″ (1.3 cm) of clearance at the end. Press the sheath gently against the strip until it adheres.

Credé's maneuver

When lower motor neuron damage impairs the voiding reflex, the urinary bladder may become flaccid or areflexic. Because the bladder fails to contract properly, urine collects inside it, causing distention. Credé's maneuver—application of manual pressure over the lower abdomen—promotes complete emptying of the bladder. After appropriate instruction, the patient can perform this maneuver himself, unless he cannot reach his lower abdomen or lacks sufficient strength and dexterity. Even when performed properly, however, Credé's maneuver isn't always successful and doesn't always eliminate the need for catheterization.

Credé's maneuver cannot be used after abdominal surgery if the incision is not completely healed. When using Credé's maneuver, close monitoring of urine output is necessary to help detect possible infection from accumulation of residual urine.

Equipment
Bedpan, urinal, or bedside commode.

Implementation
• Explain the procedure to the patient and wash your hands.
• If allowed, place the patient in Fowler's position and position the bedpan or urinal. Alternatively, if the patient's condition permits, assist him onto the bedside commode.
• Place your hands flat on the patient's abdomen just below the umbilicus. Ask the female patient to bend forward from the hips. Then, firmly stroke downward toward the bladder about six times *to stimulate the voiding reflex.*
• Place one hand on top of the other above the pubic arch. Press firmly inward and downward *to compress the bladder and expel residual urine.*

Special considerations
After the patient has learned the procedure and can use Credé's maneuver successfully, measuring the expelled urine may not be necessary. The patient may then use the maneuver to void directly into the toilet.

Documentation
Record the date and time of the procedure and the amount of urine expelled.

Digital removal of fecal impaction

Fecal impaction—a large, hard, dry mass of stool in the folds of the rectum and, at times, in the sigmoid colon—results from prolonged retention and accumulation of stool. Common causes include poor bowel habits, inactivity, dehydration, improper diet (especially inadequate fluid intake), constipation-inducing drugs, and incomplete bowel cleaning after a barium enema or barium swallow. Digital removal of fecal impaction, which is used when oil retention and cleansing enemas, suppositories, and laxatives fail to clear the impaction, may require a doctor's order.

This procedure is contraindicated during pregnancy; after rectal, genitourinary, abdominal, perineal, or gynecologic reconstructive surgery; in patients with myocardial infarction, coronary insufficiency, pulmonary embolus, congestive heart failure, heart block, and Stokes-Adams syndrome (without pacemaker treatment); and in patients with GI or vaginal bleeding, hemorrhoids, rectal polyps, or blood dyscrasias.

Equipment
Gloves (2 pairs) ■ linen-saver pad ■ bedpan ■ plastic disposal bag ■ soap ■ water-filled basin ■ towel ■ water-soluble lubricant ■ washcloth.

Implementation
• Explain the procedure to the patient and provide privacy.
• Position the patient on his left side and flex his knees *to allow easier access to the sigmoid colon and rectum.* Drape the patient, and place a linen-saver pad beneath the buttocks *to prevent soiling the bed linens.*
• Put on gloves, and moisten an index finger with water-soluble lubricant *to reduce friction during insertion, thereby avoiding injury to sensitive tissue.*
• Instruct the patient to breathe deeply *to promote relaxation.* Then gently insert the lubricated index finger beyond the anal sphincter until you touch the impaction. Rotate the finger gently around the stool *to dislodge and break it into small fragments.* Then work the fragments downward to the end of the rectum, and remove each one separately.
• Before removing the finger, gently stimulate the anal sphincter with a circular motion two or three times *to increase peristalsis and encourage evacuation.*
• Remove the finger and change your gloves. Then clean the anal area with soap and a basin of water and lightly pat dry with a towel.
• Offer the patient the bedpan or commode *because digital manipulation stimulates the urge to defecate.*
• Place disposable items in the plastic bag and discard properly. If necessary, clean the bedpan and return it to the bedside stand.
• Wash your hands.

Special considerations
If the patient experiences pain, nausea, rectal bleeding, changes in pulse rate or skin color, diaphoresis, or syncope, stop immediately and notify the doctor.

Complications
Digital removal of fecal impaction can stimulate the vagus nerve and may decrease heart rate and cause syncope.

Documentation
Record the time and date of the procedure, the patient's response, and stool color, consistency, and odor.

CARE OF THE SURGICAL PATIENT
Preoperative care

Preoperative care begins when the patient's surgery is planned and ends with the administration of anesthesia. This phase of care includes a preoperative interview and assessment to collect baseline subjective and objective data from the patient and his family; diagnostic tests such as urinalysis, electrocardiogram, and chest radiography; preoperative teaching; securing informed consent from the patient; and physical preparation.

Equipment
Gloves ■ thermometer ■ sphygmomanometer ■ stethoscope ■ watch with second hand ■ weight scale ■ tape measure.

Preparation of equipment
Assemble all equipment needed at the patient's bedside or in the admission area.

Implementation
• Obtain a health history and assess the patient's knowledge, perceptions, and expectations about his surgery. Ask about previous medical and surgical interventions. Also determine the patient's psychosocial needs; ask about occupational well-being, financial matters, support systems, mental status, and cultural beliefs. Use your institution's preoperative surgical assessment data base, if available, to gather this information. Obtain a drug history. Ask about current prescription and over-the-counter medications, and about known allergies to foods and drugs.
• Measure the patient's height, weight, and vital signs.
• Identify risk factors that may interfere with a positive expected outcome. Be sure to consider age, general health, medications, mobility, nutritional status, fluid and electrolyte disturbances, and life-style. Also consider the

Obtaining informed consent

Informed consent means that the patient is entitled to a full explanation of the procedure, its risks and complications, and the risk if the procedure isn't performed at this time. Although obtaining informed consent is the doctor's responsibility, the nurse is responsible for verifying that this step has been taken.

You may be asked to witness the patient's signature. However, if you didn't hear the doctor's explanation to the patient, you must sign that you are witnessing the patient's signature only.

Consent forms must be signed before the patient receives his preoperative medication because forms signed after sedatives are given are legally invalid. Adults and emancipated minors can sign their own consent forms. Children's consent forms, or those of adults with impaired mental status, must be signed by a parent or guardian.

primary disorder's duration, location, and nature, and the extent of the surgical procedure.
• Explain preoperative procedures to the patient. Include typical events that the patient can expect. Discuss equipment that may be used postoperatively, such as nasogastric tubes and I.V. equipment. Explain the typical incision, dressings, and staples or sutures that will be used. *Preoperative teaching can help reduce postoperative anxiety and pain, increase patient compliance, hasten recovery, and decrease length of hospital stay.*
• Talk the patient through the sequence of events from operating room to recovery room (postanesthesia care unit or PACU) back to patient's room. Some patients may be transferred from the PACU to an intensive care unit or surgical care unit. Your patient may also benefit from a tour of the areas he will see during the perioperative events.
• Tell the patient about exercises that he may be expected to perform after surgery, such as deep breathing, coughing (while splinting the incision if necessary), extremity exercises, and movement and ambulation *to minimize respiratory and circulatory complications.* If the patient will undergo ophthalmic or neurologic surgery, he won't be asked to cough *because coughing increases intracranial pressure.*
• If the patient is to receive patient-controlled anesthesia (PCA) postoperatively, teach him about the technique. Urge him to push the medication button on the unit only when he feels pain — not when he is tired, sleepy, or is pain-free. (See "Use of I.V. controllers and pumps," Chapter 6, for more information on PCA.)
• On the day of surgery, important interventions include giving morning care, verifying that the patient has signed an informed consent form (see *Obtaining informed consent*), administering ordered preoperative medications, completing the preoperative checklist and chart, and providing support to the patient and his family.
• Other immediate preoperative interventions may include preparing the GI tract (restricting food and fluids for about 8 hours before surgery) *to reduce vomiting and the risk of aspiration,* cleaning the lower GI tract of fecal material by enemas before abdominal or GI surgery, and giving antibiotics for 2 or 3 days preoperatively *to prevent contamination of the peritoneal cavity by GI bacteria.*
• Just before the patient is moved to the surgical area, make sure he's wearing a hospital gown, has his identification band in place, and has his vital signs recorded. Check to see that hairpins, nail polish, and jewelry have been removed. Note whether dentures, contact lenses, or prosthetic devices have been removed or left in place.

Special considerations

Preoperative medications must be given on time *to enhance the effect of ordered anesthesia.* The patient should take nothing by mouth preoperatively. Do not give oral medications unless ordered. Be sure to raise the bed's side rails immediately after giving preoperative medications.

If family or others are present, direct them to the appropriate waiting area and offer support as needed.

Documentation

Complete the preoperative checklist used by your hospital. Record all nursing care measures and preoperative medications, results of diagnostic tests, and the time the patient is transferred to the surgical area. The chart and the surgical checklist must accompany the patient to surgery.

Skin preparation

Proper preparation of the patient's skin for surgery renders it as free as possible from microorganisms, thereby reducing the risk of infection at the incision site. It does not duplicate or replace the full sterile preparation that immediately precedes surgery. Rather, it may involve a bath, shower, or local scrub with an antiseptic detergent solution, and hair removal. (See *Where to remove hair for surgery,* pages 106 and 107.)

The Association of Operating Room Nurses (AORN) recommends that hair not be removed from the area surrounding the operative site unless it's thick enough to interfere with surgery because hair removal may increase the risk of infection. Each hospital has a hair removal policy.

The area of preparation always exceeds that of the expected incision to minimize the number of microorganisms in the areas adjacent to the proposed incision and to allow surgical draping of the patient without contamination.

Equipment
Antiseptic soap solution ■ tap water ■ bath blanket ■ two clean basins ■ linen-saver pad ■ adjustable light ■ sterile razor with sharp new blade, if needed ■ scissors ■ optional: 4" × 4" gauze pads, cotton-tipped applicators, acetone or nail polish remover, orangewood stick, trash bag, towel, gloves.

Preparation of equipment
Use warm tap water *because heat reduces the skin's surface tension and facilitates removal of soil and hair.* Dilute the antiseptic detergent solution with warm tap water in one basin *for washing,* and pour plain warm water into the second basin *for rinsing.*

Implementation
● Check the doctor's order and explain the procedure to the patient, including the reason for the extensive preparations *to avoid causing undue anxiety.* Provide privacy, wash your hands thoroughly, and don gloves.
● Place the patient in a comfortable position, drape him with the bath blanket, and expose the preparation area. For most surgeries, this area extends 12" (30 cm) in each direction from the expected incision site. However, *to ensure privacy and avoid chilling the patient,* expose only one small area at a time while performing skin preparation.
● Position a linen-saver pad beneath the patient *to catch spills and avoid linen changes.* Adjust the light to illuminate the preparation area.
● Assess skin condition in the preparation area and report any rash, abrasion, or laceration to the doctor before beginning the procedure. *Any break in the skin increases the risk of infection and could cause cancellation of planned surgery.*
● Have the patient remove all jewelry in or near the operative site.
● As ordered, don gloves and begin removing hair from the preparation area by clipping any long hairs with scissors. If ordered, shave all remaining hair within the area *to remove microorganisms.* Perform the procedure as

near to the time of surgery as possible *so that microorganisms will have minimal time to proliferate.* Use only a sterilized or sterile disposable razor with a sharp new blade *to avoid the risk of infection from a contaminated razor.*
● Use a gauze pad to spread liquid soap over the shave site, or use the pad provided in the disposable kit.
● Pull the skin taut in the direction opposite the direction of hair growth *because this makes the hair rise and facilitates shaving.*
● Holding the razor at a 45-degree angle, shave with short strokes in the direction of hair growth *to avoid skin irritation and achieve a smooth clean shave.*
● If possible, avoid lifting the razor from the skin and placing it down again *to minimize the risk of lacerations.* Also avoid applying pressure *because this can cause abrasions, particularly over bony prominences.*
● Rinse the razor frequently and reapply liquid soap to the skin as needed *to keep the area moist.*
● Change the rinse water if necessary. Then rinse the soap solution and loose hair from the preparation area, and inspect the skin. Immediately notify the doctor of any new nicks, lacerations, or abrasions, and file a report if your institution requires it.
● Proceed with a 10-minute scrub *to ensure a clean preparation area.* Wash the area with a gauze pad dipped in the antiseptic soap solution. Using a circular motion, start at the expected incision site and work outward toward the periphery of the area *to avoid recontaminating the clean area.* Apply light friction while washing *to improve the antiseptic effect of the solution.* Replace the gauze pad as necessary.
● Carefully clean skin folds and crevices *because they harbor greater numbers of microorganisms.* Scrub the perineal area last, if it's part of the preparation area, for the same reason. Pull loose skin taut. If necessary, use cotton-tipped applicators to clean the umbilicus and an orangewood stick to clean under nails. Be sure to remove any nail polish *because the anesthetist uses nail bed color to determine adequate oxygenation and may place a probe on the nail to measure oxygen saturation.*
● Dry the area with a clean towel and remove the linen-saver pad.
● Give the patient any special instructions for care of the prepared area, and remind him to keep the area clean for surgery. Make sure the patient is comfortable.
● Properly dispose of solutions and trash bag, and clean or dispose of soiled equipment and supplies according to hospital policy.

Special considerations
Avoid shaving facial or neck hair on women and children unless ordered. Never shave eyebrows *because this dis-*

(Text continues on page 108.)

Where to remove hair for surgery

Shoulder and upper arm
On operative side, from fingertips to hairline and center chest to center spine, extending to iliac crest and including the axilla.

Forearm, elbow, and hand
On operative side, from fingertips to shoulder. Include the axilla unless surgery is for hand. Trim and clean fingernails.

Thigh
On operative side, from toes to 3″ (7.6 cm) above umbilicus and from midline front to midline back, including pubis. Clean and trim toenails.

Chest
From chin to iliac crests and nipple on unaffected side to midline of back on operative side (2″ [5 cm] beyond midline of back for thoracotomy). Include axilla and entire arm to elbow on operative side.

Abdomen
From 3″ above the nipples to upper thighs, including the pubis.

Lower abdomen
From 2″ above umbilicus to midthigh, including pubic area. For femoral ligation, to midline of thigh in back. For herniaplasty and embolectomy, to costal margin and down to knee.

Where to remove hair for surgery *(continued)*

Hip
On operative side, from toes to nipples and at least 3″ (7.6 cm) beyond midline back and front, including the pubis. Clean and trim toenails.

Knee and lower leg
On operative side, remove hair from toes to groin. Clean and trim toenails.

Ankle and foot
On operative side, remove hair from toes to 3″ above the knee. Clean and trim toenails.

Flank
On operative side, remove hair from nipples to pubis, 3″ beyond midline in back, 2″ past abdominal midline. Include pubic area and, on affected side, upper thigh and axilla.

Perineum
From pubis, perineum, and perianal area, and from the waist to at least 3″ below the groin in front and at least 3″ below the buttocks in back.

Spine
Remove hair from entire back, including shoulders and neck to hairline, and down to both knees. Include axillae.

rupts *normal hair growth and the new growth may prove unsightly.* Scalp shaving is usually performed in the operating room, but if you're required to prepare the patient's scalp, put all hair in a plastic or paper bag and store with the patient's possessions.

If the patient won't hold still for shaving, remove hair with a depilatory cream. Although this method produces clean, intact skin without risking lacerations or abrasions, it can cause skin irritation or rash, especially in the groin area. If possible, cut long hairs with scissors before applying the cream *because removal of remaining hair then requires less cream.* Then use a glove to apply the cream in a layer ½″ (1.3 cm) thick. After about 10 minutes, remove the cream with moist gauze pads. Next, wash the area with antiseptic soap solution, rinse, and pat dry.

Complications
Rashes, nicks, lacerations, and abrasions are the most common complications of skin preparation. They also increase the risk of postoperative infection.

Documentation
Record the date, time, and area of preparation; skin condition before and after preparation; any complications; and the patient's tolerance. If your hospital requires it, complete an incident report if the patient suffers nicks, lacerations, or abrasions during skin preparation.

Postoperative care

This phase of care begins when the patient arrives in the post-anesthesia care unit (PACU) and continues as he moves on to the short procedure unit, medical-surgical unit, or critical care area. Postoperative care aims to minimize postoperative complications by early detection and prompt treatment. The patient recovering from anesthesia may be experiencing pain, inadequate oxygenation, or adverse physiologic effects of sudden movement.

Recovery from general anesthesia takes longer than induction because the anesthetic is retained in fat and muscle. Fat has a meager blood supply; thus, it releases the anesthetic slowly, providing enough anesthesia to maintain adequate blood and brain levels during surgery. The patient's recovery time varies with his amount of body fat, his overall condition, his premedication regimen, and the type, dosage, and duration of anesthesia.

Equipment
Thermometer ■ watch with second hand ■ stethoscope ■ sphygmomanometer ■ postoperative flowchart or other documentation tool.

Preparation of equipment
Assemble equipment at the patient's bedside.

Implementation
● Obtain the patient's record from the PACU nurse. This should include a summary of operative procedures and pertinent findings; type of anesthesia; vital signs (preoperative, intraoperative and postoperative); medical history; medication history, including preoperative, intraoperative, and postoperative medications; fluid therapy, including estimated blood loss, type and number of drains, catheters, and characteristics of drainage; and notes on the condition of the surgical wound. *If the patient had vascular surgery, for example , knowing the location and duration of blood vessel clamping is important for preventing postoperative complications.*

● Transfer the patient from the PACU stretcher to the bed and position him properly. Get a co-worker to help, if necessary. When moving the patient, keep transfer movements smooth *to minimize pain and postoperative complications and avoid back strain by team members.*

● If the patient has had orthopedic surgery, always get a co-worker to help transfer him. Ask the co-worker to move only the affected extremity.

● If the patient is in skeletal traction, you may have to follow special orders for moving him. If you must move him, have a co-worker move the weights as you and another co-worker move the patient.

● Make the patient comfortable and raise the bed's side rails *to ensure the patient's safety.*

● Assess the patient's level of consciousness, skin color, and mucous membranes.

● Monitor the patient's respiratory status by assessing his airway. Note breathing rate and depth, and auscultate breath sounds. Administer oxygen and initiate oximetry *to monitor oxygen saturation* if ordered.

● Monitor the patient's pulse rate. It should be strong and easily palpable. The postoperative heart rate should be within 20% of the preoperative heart rate.

● Compare postoperative blood pressure to preoperative blood pressure. It should be within 20% of the preoperative level unless the patient suffered a hypotensive episode during surgery.

● Assess the patient's temperature *because anesthesia lowers body temperature.* Body temperature should be at least 95° F (35° C). If it's lower, apply blankets *to warm the patient.*

• Assess the patient's infusion sites for redness, pain, swelling, or drainage.

• Assess surgical wound dressings. Dressings should be clean and dry. If they're soiled, assess the characteristics of the drainage and outline the soiled area. Note the date and time of assessment on the dressing. Assess the soiled area frequently; if it enlarges, reinforce the dressing and alert the doctor.

• Note the presence and condition of any drains and tubes. Note the color, type, odor, and amount of drainage. Make sure all drains are properly connected and free of kinks and obstructions.

• If the patient has had vascular or orthopedic surgery, assess the appropriate extremity — or all extremities, depending on the surgical procedure. Assess color, temperature, sensation, movement, and presence and quality of pulses, and notify the doctor of any abnormalities.

• As the patient recovers from anesthesia, monitor his respiratory and cardiovascular status closely. Be alert for signs of airway obstruction and hypoventilation caused by laryngospasm, or for sedation, which can lead to hypoxemia. Cardiovascular complications — such as arrhythmias and hypotension — may result from the anesthetic agent or the operative procedure.

• Encourage coughing and deep-breathing exercises. Don't encourage them if the patient has just had nasal, ophthalmic, or neurologic surgery *to avoid increasing intracranial pressure.*

• Administer postoperative medications, such as antibiotics, analgesics, antiemetics, or reversal agents, as ordered and appropriate.

• Remove all fluids from the patient's bedside until he is alert enough to eat and drink. Before giving him liquids, assess his gag reflex *to prevent aspiration.* To do this, lightly touch the back of the patient's throat with a cotton swab — the patient will gag if the reflex has returned. Do this test quickly *to prevent a vagal reaction.*

Special considerations

Fear, pain, anxiety, hypothermia, confusion, and immobility can upset the patient and jeopardize his safety and postoperative status. Offer emotional support to the patient and his family. Keep in mind that the patient who has lost a body part or who has been diagnosed with an incurable disease will need ongoing emotional support. Refer him and his family to appropriate clerical or psychological counseling.

As the patient recovers from general anesthesia, reflexes appear in reverse order to that in which they disappeared. Hearing recovers first, so avoid holding inappropriate conversations near the patient.

The patient under general anesthesia can't protect his own airway because of muscle relaxation. As he recovers, his cough and gag reflexes reappear. If he can lift his head without assistance, he's usually able to breathe on his own and protect his airway.

If the patient received spinal anesthesia, he will need to remain supine with the bed adjusted to between 0 degrees and 20 degrees for at least 6 hours *to reduce the risk of spinal headache from leakage of cerebrospinal fluid.* The patient will also be unable to move his legs so be sure to explain this to him, and reassure him that sensation and mobility will return.

If patient has had epidural anesthesia for postoperative pain control, monitor his respiratory status closely. *Respiratory arrest may result from paralysis of the diaphragm by the anesthetic.* The patient may also experience nausea, vomiting, or itching.

If the patient will be using a patient-controlled anesthesia (PCA) unit, make sure he understands how to use it. Caution him to activate it only when he has pain, not when he feels sleepy or is pain-free. Review your hospital criteria for PCA.

Complications

Postoperative complications may include arrhythmias, hypotension, hypovolemia, septicemia, septic shock, atelectasis, pneumonia, thrombophlebitis, pulmonary embolism, urine retention, wound infection, wound dehiscence, evisceration, abdominal distention, paralytic ileus, constipation, altered body image, and postoperative psychosis.

Documentation

Document vital signs on the appropriate flowchart. Record the condition of dressings, and drains, and characteristics of drainage. Document all interventions taken to alleviate pain and anxiety and the patient's responses to them. Document any complications that may have occurred and interventions taken.

SPIRITUAL AND TERMINAL CARE

Spiritual care

Religious beliefs can profoundly influence a patient's recovery rate, attitude toward treatment, and overall response to hospitalization. In certain religious groups, beliefs can preclude diagnostic tests and therapeutic treatments, demand dietary restrictions, and prohibit organ donation and artificial prolongation of life. (See *Beliefs and practices of selected religions,* pages 110 to 112.)

Beliefs and practices of selected religions

A patient's religious beliefs can affect his attitudes toward illness and traditional medicine. By trying to accommodate the patient's religious beliefs and practices in your care plan, you can increase his willingness to learn and comply with treatment regimens. Because religious beliefs may vary within particular sects, individual practices may differ from those described here.

RELIGION	BIRTH AND DEATH RITUALS	DIETARY RESTRICTIONS	PRACTICES IN HEALTH CRISIS
Adventist	None (baptism of adults only)	Alcohol, coffee, tea, narcotics, stimulants; in many groups, meat prohibited also	Communion and baptism performed. Some members believe in divine healing, anointing with oil, and prayer. Some regard Saturday as the Sabbath.
Baptist	At birth, none (baptism of believers only); before death, counseling by clergy member and prayer	Alcohol; in some groups, coffee and tea prohibited also	Some believe in healing by laying on of hands. Resistance to medical therapy occasionally approved.
Christian Scientist	At birth, none; before death, counseling by a Christian Science practitioner	Alcohol, coffee, and tobacco prohibited	Many members refuse all treatment, including drugs, biopsies, physical examination, and blood transfusions and permit vaccination only when required by law. Alteration of thoughts is believed to cure illness. Hypnotism and psychotherapy are prohibited. (Christian Science nurses and nursing homes honor these beliefs.)
Church of Christ	None (baptism at age 8 or older)	Alcohol discouraged	Communion, anointing with oil, laying on of hands, and counseling by a minister.
Eastern Orthodox	At birth, baptism and confirmation; before death, last rites. For members of the Russian Orthodox Church, arms are crossed after death, fingers set in cross, and unembalmed body clothed in natural fiber.	For members of the Russian Orthodox Church and usually the Greek Orthodox Church, no meat or dairy products on Wednesday, Friday, and during Lent	Anointing of the sick. For members of the Russian Orthodox Church, cross necklace is replaced immediately after surgery and shaving of male patients is not allowed except in preparation for surgery. For members of the Greek Orthodox Church, communion and Sacrament of Holy Unction.
Episcopalian	At birth, baptism; before death, occasional last rites	For some members, abstention from meat on Friday, fasting before communion (which may be daily)	Communion, prayer, and counseling by a minister.

Beliefs and practices of selected religions *(continued)*

RELIGION	BIRTH AND DEATH RITUALS	DIETARY RESTRICTIONS	PRACTICES IN HEALTH CRISIS
Jehovah's Witnesses	None	Abstention from foods to which blood has been added	Typically, no blood transfusions are permitted; may require a court order for emergency transfusion.
Judaism	Ritual circumcision on eighth day after birth; burial of dead fetus; ritual washing of dead; burial (including organs and other body tissues) occurs as soon as possible; no autopsy or embalming	For Orthodox and Conservative Jews, kosher dietary laws (for example, pork and shellfish prohibited); for Reform Jews, usually no restrictions	Donation or transplantation of organs requires rabbinical consultation. For Orthodox and Conservative Jews, medical procedures may be prohibited on Sabbath—from sundown Friday to sundown Saturday—and special holidays.
Lutheran	Baptism usually performed 6 to 8 weeks after birth	None	Communion, prayer, and counseling by a minister.
Mormon	At birth, none (baptism at age 8 or older); before death, baptism and gospel preaching	Alcohol, tobacco, tea, and coffee prohibited; meat intake limited	Divine healing through the laying on of hands; communion on Sunday; some members may refuse medical treatment. Many wear a special undergarment.
Moslem	If abortion occurs before 130 days, fetus treated as discarded tissue; after 130 days, as a human being. Before death, confession of sins with family present; after death, only relatives or friends may touch the body.	Pork prohibited; daylight fasting during ninth month of Muhammadan calendar	Faith healing for the patient's morale only; conservative members reject medical therapy.
Orthodox Presbyterian	Infant baptism; scripture reading and prayer before death	None	Communion, prayer, and counseling by a minister.
Pentecostal Assembly of God, Foursquare Church	None (baptism only after age of accountability)	Abstention from alcohol, tobacco, meat slaughtered by strangling, any food to which blood has been added, and sometimes pork	Divine healing through prayer, anointing with oil, and laying on of hands.

(continued)

Beliefs and practices of selected religions *(continued)*

RELIGION	BIRTH AND DEATH RITUALS	DIETARY RESTRICTIONS	PRACTICES IN HEALTH CRISIS
Roman Catholic	Infant baptism, including baptism of aborted fetus without sign of clinical death (tissue necrosis); before death, anointing of the sick	Fasting or abstention from meat on Ash Wednesday and on Fridays during Lent; this practice usually waived for the hospitalized	Burial of major amputated limb (sometimes) in consecrated ground; donation or transplantation of organs allowed if the benefit to recipient outweighs the donor's potential harm.
United Methodist	None (baptism of children and adults only)	None	Communion before surgery or similar crisis; donation of body parts encouraged.

Consequently, effective patient care requires recognition and respect for the patient's religious beliefs. Recognizing his beliefs and need for spiritual care may require close attention to the patient's nonverbal cues or seemingly casual remarks that express his spiritual concerns. Respecting his beliefs may require setting aside one's own to help the patient follow his. Providing spiritual care may require contacting an appropriate member of the clergy in the hospital or community; assisting him in performing rites and administering sacraments by gathering the necessary equipment; and preparing the patient for the pastoral visit.

Equipment
Clean towels (one or two) ■ teaspoon, or 1-oz (30 ml) medicine cup (for baptism) ■ container of water (for emergency baptism).

Some hospitals, particularly those with a religious affiliation, provide baptismal trays. The clergy member may bring holy water, holy oil, or other religious articles to minister to the patient.

Preparation of equipment
For baptism, cover a small table with a clean towel. Fold a second towel and place it on the table, along with the teaspoon or medicine cup. For communion and anointing, cover the bedside stand with a clean towel. For religious circumcision, sterilize the ceremonial instruments, if requested to do so by the participating clergy member. (In Jewish practice, a *mohel* is a specialist certified by rabbinical authorities to perform circumcision.)

Implementation
● Check the patient's admission record *to determine religious affiliation.* Remember that the patient may claim no religious beliefs. If a patient states that he is agnostic, this may not rule out his desire for spiritual or pastoral care. Such patients may also wish to speak with a clergy member, so watch and listen carefully for subtle expressions of this desire.
● Evaluate the patient's behavior for signs of loneliness, anxiety, or fear—*emotions that may signal his need for spiritual counsel.* Also consider whether the patient is facing a health crisis, which may occur before childbirth, surgery, chronic illness, or impending death. Remember that a patient may feel acutely distressed because of his inability to participate in religious observances. Help such a patient verbalize his beliefs *to relieve stress.* Listen to the patient and let him express his concerns, but carefully refrain from imposing your beliefs on him *to avoid conflict and further stress.* If the patient requests, arrange a visit by an appropriate member of the clergy. Consult this clergy member if you need more information about the patient's beliefs.
● If your patient faces the possibility of abortion, amputation, transfusion, or other medical procedures with important religious significance or implications, try to discover his or her spiritual attitude. Also, try to determine your patient's attitude toward the importance of laying on of hands, confession, communion, observance of holy days (such as the Sabbath), and restrictions in diet or physical appearance. Helping the patient continue his normal religious practices during hospitalization *can help reduce stress.*

• If the patient is pregnant, find out her beliefs concerning infant baptism and circumcision, and comply with them after delivery.

• If a neonate is in critical condition, call an appropriate clergy member immediately. To administer emergency baptism, the official pours a small amount of holy water into a teaspoon or a medicine cup and sprinkles a few drops of water over the infant's head while saying, "(Name of child), I baptize you in the name of the Father, the Son, and the Holy Spirit. Amen." In an extreme emergency, you can perform a Roman Catholic baptism, using a container of any available water. If you do so, be sure to notify the priest *because this sacrament must be administered only once.*

• If a Jewish woman delivers a male infant prematurely or by cesarean birth, ask her if she plans to observe the rite of circumcision or *bris,* a significant ceremony performed on the eighth day after birth. (Because a patient who delivers a healthy, full-term baby vaginally is usually discharged quickly, this ceremony is normally performed outside the hospital.) For a *bris,* ensure privacy and, if requested, sterilize the instruments.

• If the patient requests communion, prepare him for it before the clergy member arrives. First, place him in Fowler's or semi-Fowler's position, if his condition permits. Otherwise, allow him to remain supine. Tuck a clean towel under his chin and straighten the bed linens.

• If a terminally ill patient requests the Sacrament of the Sick (Last Rites) or special treatment of his body after death, call an appropriate clergy member. For the Roman Catholic patient, call a Roman Catholic priest to administer the sacrament, even if the patient is unresponsive or comatose. To prepare the patient for this sacrament, uncover the arms and fold back the top linens to expose the feet. After the clergy member anoints the patient's forehead, eyes, nose, mouth, hands, and feet, straighten and retuck the bed linens.

Special considerations

Handle the patient's religious articles carefully to avoid damage or loss. Become familiar with religious resources in your hospital. Some hospitals employ one or more clergy members who counsel patients and staff and link patients to other pastoral resources.

If the patient tries to convert you to his personal beliefs, tell him that you respect his beliefs but are content with your own. Likewise, avoid attempts to convert the patient to your personal beliefs.

Documentation

Complete a baptismal form and attach it to the patient's record; send a copy of the form to the appropriate clergy member. Record the rites of circumcision and Last Rites

in your notes. Also, record Last Rites in red on the Kardex so it won't be repeated unnecessarily.

 ## Care of the dying patient

A patient needs intensive physical support and emotional comfort as he approaches death. Signs and symptoms of impending death include reduced respiratory rate and depth, decreased or absent blood pressure, weak or erratic pulse rate, lowered skin temperature, decreased level of consciousness (LOC), diminished sensorium and neuromuscular control, diaphoresis, pallor, cyanosis, and mottling.

Emotional support for the dying patient and his family most often means simple reassurance and the nurse's physical presence to help ease fear and loneliness. More intense emotional support is important at much earlier stages, especially for patients with long-term progressive illnesses, who can work through the stages of dying. (See *Five stages of dying,* page 114.)

Emotional care also requires respect for the patient's wishes about extraordinary means of supporting life. The patient may have signed a living will. This document, legally binding in most states, declares the patient's desire for a natural death unimpeded by the artificial support of defibrillators, respirators, auxiliary hearts, life-sustaining drugs, and so on. If the patient has signed such a document, the nurse must respect his wishes and communicate the doctor's "no code" order to all staff members.

Equipment

Clean bed linens ▪ clean gowns ▪ gloves ▪ water-filled basin ▪ soap ▪ washcloth ▪ towels ▪ lotion ▪ linen-saver pads ▪ petroleum jelly ▪ lemon-glycerin swabs ▪ suction and resuscitation equipment, as necessary ▪ optional: indwelling urinary catheter.

Implementation

• Assemble equipment at the patient's bedside, as needed.

Meeting physical needs

• Take vital signs often, and observe for pallor, diaphoresis, and decreased LOC.

• Reposition the patient in bed at least every 2 hours, *because sensation, reflexes, and mobility diminish first in the legs and gradually in the arms.* Make sure the bed sheets cover him loosely *to reduce discomfort caused by pressure on arms and legs.*

Five stages of dying

According to Elisabeth Kübler-Ross, author of *On Death and Dying,* the dying patient may progress through five psychological stages in preparation for death. Although each patient experiences these stages differently, and not necessarily in this order, understanding them will help you meet your patient's needs.

Denial
When the patient first learns of his terminal illness, he'll refuse to accept the diagnosis. He may experience physical symptoms similar to a stress reaction—shock, fainting, pallor, sweating, tachycardia, nausea, and GI disorders. During this stage, be honest with the patient but not blunt or callous. Maintain communication with him so he can discuss his feelings when he accepts the reality of death. Don't force the patient to confront this reality.

Anger
Once the patient stops denying his death, he may show deep resentment toward those who will live on after he dies—to you, to the hospital staff, and to his own family. Although you may instinctively draw back from the patient or even resent him for his behavior, remember that he is dying and has a right to be angry. After you accept his anger, you can help him find different ways to express it and can help his family to understand it.

Bargaining
Although the patient accepts impending death, he attempts to bargain for more time with God or fate. He will probably strike this bargain secretly. If he does confide in you, don't urge him to keep his promises.

Depression
First, the patient may experience regrets about his past; then he grieves about his current condition. He may withdraw from his friends, family, doctor, and from you. He may suffer from anorexia, increased fatigue, self-neglect. You may find him sitting alone, in tears. Accept the patient's sorrow, and if he talks to you, listen. Provide comfort by touch, as appropriate. Resist the temptation to make optimistic remarks or cheerful small talk.

Acceptance
In this last stage, the patient accepts the inevitability and imminence of his death—without emotion. He may simply desire the quiet company of a family member or friend. If, for some reason, a family member or friend can't be present, stay with the patient to satisfy his final need. Remember that many patients die before reaching this stage.

• When the patient's vision and hearing start to fail, turn his head toward the light and speak to him from near the head of the bed. *Because hearing may be acute despite loss of consciousness,* avoid whispering or speaking inappropriately about the patient in his presence.

• Change the bed linens and the patient's gown as needed. Provide skin care during gown changes, and adjust the room temperature for patient comfort, if necessary.

• Observe for incontinence or anuria, *the result of diminished neuromuscular control or decreased renal function.* If necessary, obtain an order to catheterize the patient, or place linen-saver pads beneath the patient's buttocks. Don gloves and provide perineal care with soap, a washcloth and towels *to prevent irritation and discomfort.*

• With suction equipment, suction the patient's mouth and upper airway *to remove secretions.* Elevate the head of the bed *to decrease respiratory resistance.* As the patient's condition deteriorates, he may breathe mostly through his mouth.

• Offer fluids frequently, and lubricate the patient's lips and mouth with petroleum jelly or lemon-glycerin swabs *to counteract dryness.*

• If the comatose patient's eyes are open, provide appropriate eye care *to prevent corneal ulceration.* Such ulceration can cause blindness and prevent the use of these tissues for transplantation should the patient die. (See *Understanding organ and tissue donation.*)

• Provide ordered pain medication as needed. Keep in mind that, as circulation diminishes, medications given intramuscularly will be poorly absorbed. Medications should be given intravenously, if possible, *for optimum results.*

Meeting emotional needs
• Fully explain all care and treatments to the patient even if he's unconscious *because he may still be able to hear.* Answer the conscious patient's questions as candidly as possible, without sounding calloused or blunt.

slightly *to prevent discoloration from blood settling in the face.*

• If the patient wore dentures and hospital policy permits, gently insert them; then close the mouth. Close the eyes by gently pressing on the lids with your fingertips. If they don't stay closed, place moist cotton balls on the eyelids for a few minutes, and then try again to close them. Place a folded towel under the chin *to keep the jaw closed.*

• Remove all indwelling catheters, tubes, and tape, and apply adhesive bandages to puncture sites. Replace soiled dressings.

• Collect all the patient's valuables *to prevent loss.* If you're unable to remove a ring, cover it with gauze, tape it in place, and tie the gauze to the wrist *to prevent slippage and subsequent loss.*

• Clean the body thoroughly, using soap, a basin and washcloths. Place one or more ABD pads between the buttocks *to absorb rectal discharge or drainage.*

• Cover the body up to the chin with a clean sheet.

• Offer comfort and emotional support to the family and intimate friends. Ask if they wish to see the body. If they do, allow them to do so in privacy. Ask if they would prefer to leave the patient's jewelry on the body.

• After the family leaves, remove the towel from under the chin of the deceased patient. Pad the chin, and wrap chin straps under the chin and tie them loosely on top of the head. Then, pad the wrists and ankles *to prevent bruises,* and tie them together with gauze or soft string ties.

• Fill out the three identification tags. Each tag should include the deceased patient's name, room and bed numbers, date and time of death, and doctor's name. Tie one tag to the deceased patient's hand or foot, but don't remove his hospital identification bracelet *to ensure correct identification.*

• Place the shroud or body wrap on the morgue stretcher and, after obtaining assistance, transfer the body to the stretcher. Wrap the body, and tie the shroud or wrap with the string provided. Then, attach another identification tag, and cover the shroud or wrap with a clean sheet. If a shroud or wrap isn't available, dress the deceased patient in a clean gown and cover the body with a sheet.

• Place the deceased patient's personal belongings, including valuables, in a bag and attach the third identification tag to it.

• If the patient died of an infectious disease, label the body according to your hospital's policy.

• Close the doors of adjoining rooms, if possible. Then take the body to the morgue. Use corridors that aren't crowded and, if possible, use a service elevator.

Special considerations

Give the deceased patient's personal belongings to his family or bring them to the morgue. If you give the family jewelry or money, make sure a co-worker is present as a witness. Obtain the signature of an adult family member *to verify receipt of valuables or to state their preference that jewelry remain on the patient.*

Offer emotional support to the deceased patient's family and friends, and to the patient's hospital roommate, if appropriate.

Documentation

Although the extent of documentation varies among hospitals, always record the disposition of the patient's possessions, especially jewelry and money. Also note the date and time the deceased patient was transported to the morgue.

Selected references

Association of Operating Room Nurses. *AORN Standards and Recommended Practices for Preoperative Nursing.* Denver: Association of Operating Room Nurses, Inc., 1989.

Barnum, B. *Nursing Theory: Analysis, Application, Evaluation.* Glenview, Ill.: Scott, Foresman & Co., 1990.

Barris, R., et al. *Occupational Therapy in Psychosocial Practice.* Thorofare, N.J.: Charles B. Slack, Inc., 1988.

Basmajian, J. *Therapeutic Exercise,* 5th ed. Baltimore: Williams & Wilkins Co., 1989.

Baum, C., et al. *Human Performance Deficits: Occupational Therapy Assessment and Intervention.* Thorofare, N.J.: Charles B. Slack, Inc., 1989.

Bomar, P. *Nurses and Family Health Promotions: Concepts, Assessment, and Interventions.* Baltimore: Williams & Wilkins Co., 1989.

Carpenito, L.J. *Nursing Diagnosis: Application to Clinical Practice,* 2nd ed. Philadelphia: J.B. Lippincott Co., 1988.

Doenges, M., et al. *Nursing Care Plans: Guidelines for Planning Patient Care,* 2nd ed. Philadelphia: F.A. Davis Co., 1989.

Doughty, D., et al. "Your Patient: Which Therapy?" *Journal of Enterostomal Therapy* 17(4):154-59, July-August 1990.

Fraulini, K. *After Anesthesia: A Guide for PACU, ICU and Medical-Surgical Nurses.* Norwalk, Conn.: Appleton & Lange, 1987.

Guzzetta, C. *Assessment Tools for Clinical Practice.* St. Louis: C.V. Mosby Co., March 1989.

Henderson, V. "Nursing Process—A Critique," *Holistic Nursing Practice* 1(3):7-18, 1987.

Illustrated Manual of Nursing Practice. Springhouse, Pa.: Springhouse Corp., 1991.

Kemp, B., et al. *Fundamentals of Nursing: A Framework for Practice,* 2nd ed. Glenview, Ill.: Scott, Foresman & Co., 1989.

Kneedler, J., and Dodge, G. *Perioperative Patient Care: The Nursing Perspective,* 2nd ed. St. Louis: C.V. Mosby Co., 1987.

Kozier, B., and Erb, G. *Techniques in Clinical Nursing,* 3rd ed. Reading, Mass.: Addison-Wesley Publishing Co., 1989.

Leuner, J., et al. *Mastering the Nursing Process: A Case Method Approach.* Philadelphia: F.A. Davis Co., 1989.

Lovell, H., and Anderson, C. "Put Your Patient on the Right Bed," *RN* 53(5):66-72, May 1990.

Morton, P. *Health Assessment in Nursing.* Springhouse, Pa.: Springhouse Corp., 1989.

Norton, D. "Helping Patients Give the Gift of Life," *RN* 53(12):30-34, December 1990.

Nurse's Handbook of Law and Ethics. Springhouse, Pa.: Springhouse Corp., 1992.

Pender, N. *Health Promotion in Nursing Practice,* 2nd ed. East Norwalk, Conn.: Appleton & Lange, 1987.

Potter, P., and Perry, A. *Fundamentals of Nursing: Concepts, Process and Practice,* 2nd ed. St. Louis: Mosby-Year Book, Inc., 1989.

Sparks, S., and Taylor, C. *Nursing Diagnosis Reference Manual.* Springhouse, Pa.: Springhouse Corp., 1991.

Stevens, S., and Becker, K. "A Simple, Step-by-Step Approach to Neurological Assessment," Part 1. *Nursing88* 18(9):53-61, September 1988.

Sutton, S. *Home Health Nursing: Clinical Procedures.* Baltimore: Williams & Wilkins Co., 1988.

Taylor, M., et al. *Fundamentals of Nursing: The Art and Science of Nursing Care.* Philadelphia: J.B. Lippincott Co., 1989.

Yura, H., and Walsh, M. *The Nursing Process: Assessing, Planning, Implementing, Evaluating,* 5th ed. Norwalk, Conn.: Appleton & Lange, 1987.

CHAPTER 2

INFECTION CONTROL

KAREN M.J. McCLEAVE, RN, MS, CFNP, CIC

Introduction

The mysteries of infection have been unfolding since Koch, Pasteur, and other microbiologists uncovered the link between bacteria and infection in the late 19th century. But despite our increased understanding of infectious diseases and the advent of programs to survey, prevent, identify, and control them, nosocomial infections occur more than 2 million times each year. They raise health care costs by about $2 billion, lengthen hospital stays, and lead directly or indirectly to about 25,000 patient deaths annually.

Not all nosocomial infections can be prevented. Immunodeficient patients, for example, or those receiving immunosuppressive therapy may succumb to nosocomial infection despite all precautions. However, studies have shown that about 400,000 infections could be prevented every year by faithful adherence to infection-control principles. This chapter contains detailed instructions for using these principles effectively.

Causes and incidence

Nosocomial infections result from aerobic and anaerobic bacteria, viruses, parasites, and fungi. The most common nosocomial infections involve the urinary tract, surgical wounds, the lower respiratory tract, and blood.

Urinary tract infections commonly result from catheter insertion or urogenital surgery. Surgical wound infections result from contamination during surgery, skin damage from preoperative hair removal, impaired blood supply, or coexisting medical problems. Lower respiratory tract infections can result from aspiration of oropharyngeal secretions, contaminated ventilation equipment (such as nebulizers), lung seeding by blood-borne pathogens, or airborne spread of pathogens from other patients. Bacteremia may arise as a complication of other nosocomial infections, such as pneumonia and surgical wound infections.

Nosocomial infections are three times more common among surgical patients than nonsurgical patients. The risk of such infections rises with the patient's age and duration of preoperative and total hospitalization.

Infection-control programs

According to recommendations issued in 1958 by the Joint Commission on Accreditation of Hospitals (now the Joint Commission on Accreditation of Healthcare Organizations) and the American Hospital Association, every accredited hospital must have an infection-control committee and a surveillance system as part of a formal infection-control program. Such a program aims to reduce the infection rate by emphasizing to the hospital staff the risk of contagion and by encouraging them to assume responsibility for preventing it. An effective infection-control program can reduce the incidence of nosocomial infections by about 20%.

To guide hospitals in their infection-control efforts, the Centers for Disease Control (CDC) in 1970 published a manual that detailed seven categories of isolation techniques. The recommendations were revised in 1983 to reduce unnecessary procedures and to adapt to the increased use of intensive care units, invasive procedures, and immunosuppressive treatments, and to counter the spread of drug-resistant pathogens. In 1984, a new approach to infection control, known as body substance isolation, called for health care workers to don gloves before contacting mucous membranes and broken skin, and before anticipated contact with any moist body substances. In 1988, the CDC refined this concept in its *universal precautions*, which recommend that health care workers wear gloves and other personal protective equipment (such as a mask, goggles, and a gown) to reduce exposure to blood and body fluids implicated in the transmission of blood-borne infections. Universal precautions may be implemented to replace diagnosis- and disease-specific isolation categories. Alternatively, these latter isolation categories may be used to supplement universal precautions.

In most hospitals, infection-control practitioners—usually registered nurses—assume daily responsibility for surveillance and other aspects of infection control. Although specific responsibilities may vary among hospitals, typical activities include:
• teaching the hospital staff the importance of correct hand washing between patient contacts (the most effective way to reduce infection risk)
• assessing patients for infection and taking proper precautions against contamination and contagion
• showing the staff how to collect and handle laboratory specimens
• developing infection-control guidelines, instructing the staff, and monitoring isolation procedures.

Isolation as prevention

Most isolation procedures aim to prevent transmission of disease from infected patients to other patients, hospital staff, and visitors. In contrast, isolation may also aim to protect immunocompromised patients from exogenous pathogens. Many mysteries must be solved before these and other procedures can reduce the incidence

Proper hand-washing technique

To minimize the spread of infection, follow these basic hand-washing instructions. With your hands angled downward under the faucet, adjust the water temperature until it's comfortably warm.

Work up a generous lather by scrubbing vigorously for 10 seconds. Be sure to clean beneath fingernails, around knuckles, and along the sides of fingers and hands.

Rinse your hands completely to wash away suds and microorganisms. Pat dry with a paper towel. To prevent recontaminating your hands on the faucet handles, cover each one with a dry paper towel when turning off the water.

of nosocomial infections. But for now, strict adherence to your hospital's infection-control policies and the procedures outlined in this chapter can go far toward keeping infection at bay.

GENERAL PRINCIPLES
Hand washing

The hands serve as the conduit for almost every transfer of potential pathogens from one patient to another, from a contaminated object to the patient, or from hospital staff to the patient. Thus, hand washing is the single most important procedure in preventing contagion. To protect patients from nosocomial infections, hand washing must be performed routinely and thoroughly. In effect, clean and healthy hands with smooth skin, short fingernails, and no rings or false fingernails minimize the risk of contamination. Microorganisms are more difficult to remove from rough or chapped hands.

Equipment
Soap or detergent ■ warm running water ■ paper towels ■ optional: antiseptic cleaning agent, fingernail brush, plastic sponge brush or plastic cuticle stick.

Implementation
• Remove rings or false fingernails as your hospital's policy dictates *because they harbor dirt and skin microorganisms.* Remove your watch or wear it well above the wrist.
• Wet your hands and wrists with warm water and apply soap from a dispenser. Don't use bar soap *because it allows cross-contamination.* Hold your hands below elbow level *to prevent water from running up your arms and back down, thus contaminating clean areas.* (See *Proper hand-washing technique.*)
• Work up a generous lather by rubbing your hands together vigorously for about 10 seconds. *Soap and warm water reduce surface tension and this, aided by friction, loosens surface microorganisms, which wash away in the lather.* The more vigorously you rub your hands when washing, the more microorganisms you remove.
• Pay special attention to the area under fingernails and around cuticles, and to the thumbs, knuckles, and sides of the fingers and hands *because microorganisms thrive in these protected or overlooked areas.* If you don't remove your wedding band, move it up and down your finger to clean beneath it.

• Avoid splashing water on yourself or the floor *because microorganisms spread more easily on wet surfaces and because slippery floors are dangerous.* Avoid touching the sink or faucets *because they're considered contaminated.*

• Rinse hands and wrists well *because running water flushes suds, soil, and microorganisms away.*

• Pat hands and wrists dry with a paper towel. Avoid rubbing, *which can cause abrasion and chapping.*

• If the sink is not equipped with knee or foot controls, turn off the faucets by gripping them with a dry paper towel *to avoid recontaminating your hands.*

Special considerations
Before participating in any sterile procedure or whenever your hands are grossly contaminated, wash your forearms also, and clean under the fingernails and in and around the cuticles with a fingernail brush, disposable sponge brush, or plastic cuticle stick. Use these softer implements *because brushes, metal files, or other hard objects may injure your skin and, if reused, may be a source of contamination.*

Follow your hospital's policy concerning when to wash with soap and when to use an antiseptic cleaning agent. Typically, you'll wash with *soap* before coming on duty; before and after direct or indirect patient contact; before and after performing any bodily functions, such as blowing your nose or using the bathroom; before preparing or serving food; before preparing or administering medications; after direct or indirect contact with a patient's excretions, secretions, or blood; and after completing your shift.

Use an *antiseptic* cleaning agent when *you must reliably eliminate microorganisms from your hands,* such as before and after handling invasive devices, performing wound care and dressing changes, and after your hands have been contaminated with virulent pathogens. Antiseptics are also recommended for hand washing in isolation rooms, newborn nurseries, and before caring for any highly susceptible patient. Even if you're putting on clean or sterile gloves, wash before and after with an antiseptic *so microorganisms will not grow under the gloves or in case the gloves are torn or punctured.*

Home care
If you're providing care in the patient's home, bring your own supply of soap and disposable paper towels. If there's no running water, disinfect your hands with alcohol sponges.

Complications
Because it strips natural skin oils, frequent hand washing may result in dryness, cracking, and irritation. These effects are probably more common after repeated use of antiseptic cleaning agents, especially in persons with sensitive skin. Be sure to remove antiseptic residues carefully to help minimize irritation.

If your hands are dry or cracked, or if you develop dermatitis, apply an emollient hand cream after each washing or switch to a different cleaning agent. Don't allow irritated skin to reduce your attention to hand washing; if that happens, your hands could become a conduit of infection.

Isolation equipment use

Isolation procedures may be implemented to prevent the spread of infection from patient to patient, from the patient to health care workers, or from health care workers to the patient. Isolation procedures may also lessen the risk of infection in immunocompromised patients. Central to the success of these procedures are the selection of proper equipment and adequate training of those who use it.

Equipment
Materials required for isolation typically include barrier clothing, an isolation cart or anteroom for storing equipment, and a door card notifying all who enter the room that isolation precautions are in effect.

Barrier clothing includes the following: gowns ■ gloves ■ caps ■ goggles ■ masks. Each staff member must be trained in the proper use of barrier clothing.

Isolation supplies may include the following: labels ■ tape ■ specially marked laundry bags (and water-soluble laundry bags, if used) ■ plastic trash bags.

An isolation cart may be used when the patient's room has no anteroom. The cart can be a covered, wheeled utility table, or it can be specially designed for use during isolation precautions. It should include a work area (such as a pull-out shelf), drawers or a cabinet area for holding isolation supplies and, possibly, a pole on which to hang coats or jackets.

Supplies for the cart or anteroom should be stocked according to the isolation category being used and the patient's individual needs.

Preparation of equipment
Remove the cover from the isolation cart, if necessary, and set up the work area. Check the cart or anteroom *to ensure that correct and sufficient supplies are in place for the designated isolation category.*

Donning a face mask

To avoid spreading airborne particles, wear a face mask—sterile or nonsterile, as indicated. Position the mask to cover your nose and mouth, and secure it high enough to ensure stability. Tie the bottom string first, then pull the mask up over your face and tie the top string.

Adjust the metal nose strip if the mask has one.

Implementation

• Remove your watch or push it well up your arm. Remove your rings according to hospital policy. *These actions help to prevent the spread of microorganisms hidden under your watch or rings.*
• Wash your hands with an antiseptic cleaning agent *to prevent growth of microorganisms under gloves.*

Putting on isolation garb

• Put the gown on and wrap it around the back of your uniform. Tie the strings or fasten the snaps or pressure-sensitive tabs at the neck. Make sure your uniform is completely covered, and secure the gown at the waist.
• Put on a cap and make sure it covers all your hair.
• Place the mask snugly over your nose and mouth. Secure ear loops around your ears or tie the strings behind your head high enough so the mask won't slip off. If the mask has a metal strip, squeeze it to fit your nose firmly but comfortably. (See *Donning a face mask.*) If you wear eyeglasses, tuck the mask under their lower edge.
• Put on the gloves. Cover the edges of the gown's sleeves by pulling the gloves over the cuffs.

Removing isolation garb

• Remember that the outside surfaces of your barrier clothes are contaminated.
• With the gloves on, untie the gown's waist strings, *which are considered contaminated.*
• With your gloved left hand, remove the right glove by pulling on the cuff, turning the glove inside out as you pull. Don't touch any skin with the outside of either glove. (See *Removing contaminated gloves.*) Then, remove the left glove by wedging one or two fingers of your right hand inside the glove and pulling it off, turning it inside out as you remove it. Discard the gloves in the trash container.
• Untie your mask, holding it only by the strings. Discard the mask and cap in the trash container. If the patient has a disease that is spread by airborne pathogens, you may prefer to remove the mask and cap last.
• Untie the neck straps of your gown. Grasp the outside of the gown at the back of the shoulders and pull the gown down over your arms, turning it inside out as you remove it *to ensure containment of the pathogens.*
• Holding the gown well away from your uniform, fold it inside out. Discard it in the laundry or trash container, depending on whether the gown is cloth or paper.
• If the sink is inside the patient's room, wash your hands and forearms with soap or antiseptic before leaving the room. Turn off the faucet using a paper towel and discard the towel in the room. Grasp the door handle with a clean paper towel to open it, and discard the towel in a trash container inside the room. Close the door from the outside with your bare hand.
• If the sink is in an anteroom, wash your hands and forearms with soap or antiseptic after leaving the room.

Special considerations

Use gowns, gloves, caps, goggles and masks only once, and discard them in the appropriate container before leaving a contaminated area. Isolation garb loses its ef-

• Allow the patient to express his feelings, which may range from anger to loneliness. Take time to talk with the patient. When you do, sit near the head of the bed. Avoid looking rushed or unconcerned.

• Notify family members, if they're not present, when the patient wishes to see them. Let the patient and his family discuss death at their own pace. Give them opportunities to express their feelings, but avoid encouraging them if they seem unwilling.

• Offer to contact a member of the clergy or social services department, or other persons as the patient requests, if appropriate.

Special considerations

If the patient has signed a living will, the doctor will write a "no code" order on his progress notes and order sheets. Know your state's policy regarding the living will. If it's legal, transfer the "no code" order to the patient's chart or Kardex and, at the end of your shift, inform the incoming staff of this order.

If family members remain with the patient, show them the location of bathrooms, lounges, and cafeterias. Explain the patient's needs, treatments, and care plan to them. If appropriate, offer to teach them specific skills so they can take part in nursing care. Emphasize that their efforts are important and effective. As the patient's death approaches, give them emotional support.

At an appropriate time, ask the patient's family if they have considered organ and tissue donation. Check the patient's records *to determine if he completed an organ donor card.*

Documentation

Record changes in the patient's vital signs, intake and output, and LOC. Note the times of cardiac arrest and the end of respiration, and notify the doctor when these occur.

Postmortem care

After the patient dies, care includes preparing him for family viewing, arranging transportation to the morgue or funeral home, and determining the disposition of the patient's belongings. In addition, postmortem care entails comforting and supporting the patient's family and friends and providing for their privacy.

Postmortem care usually begins after a doctor certifies the patient's death. If the patient died violently or under suspicious circumstances, postmortem care may

Understanding organ and tissue donation

The federal Required Request Law, enacted in 1986, states that all acute care facilities that receive Medicare funds must ask about organ donation from every eligible donor. According to the American Medical Association, about 25 kinds of organs and tissues are being transplanted. Although donor organ requirements vary, the typical donor must be between ages 6 months and 50 years and free from transmissible disease, cancer, septicemia, diabetes, and hypertension.

Tissue donation requirements are less restrictive. Virtually any patient who dies free from contagious disease or systemic infection can donate tissue, such as skin, corneas, bone, and heart valves. Cancer patients are the exception, to avoid the risk of spreading metastatic cells.

Collection of most organs, such as the heart, liver, kidney, or pancreas, requires that the patient be pronounced brain dead and kept physically alive until the organs are harvested. Tissue such as eyes, skin, bone, and heart valves may be taken after death. Contact your regional organ procurement organization for specific organ donation criteria or to identify a potential donor. If you don't know the regional organ procurement organization in your area, call the United Network for Organ Sharing at (804) 330-8500.

be postponed until the medical examiner completes an autopsy.

Equipment

Gauze or soft string ties ▪ gloves ▪ chin straps ▪ ABD pads ▪ cotton balls ▪ plastic shroud or body wrap ▪ three identification tags ▪ adhesive bandages to cover wounds or punctures ▪ plastic bag for patient's belongings ▪ water-filled basin ▪ soap ▪ towels ▪ washcloths ▪ stretcher.

A commercial morgue pack usually contains gauze or string ties, chin straps, a shroud, and identification tags.

Implementation

• Document any auxiliary equipment, such as a mechanical ventilator, still present. Put on gloves.

• Place the body in the supine position, arms at the sides and head on a pillow. Then elevate the head of the bed

Removing contaminated gloves

Proper removal techniques are essential for preventing the spread of pathogens from gloves to your skin surface. Follow these steps carefully.

1. Using your left hand, pinch the right glove near the top. Avoid allowing the glove's outer surface to buckle inward against your wrist.

2. Pull downward, allowing the glove to turn inside out as it comes off. Keep the right glove in your left hand after removing it.

3. Now insert the first two fingers of your ungloved right hand under the edge of the left glove. Avoid touching the glove's outer surface or folding it against your left wrist.

4. Pull downward, so the glove turns inside out as it comes off. Continue pulling until the left glove completely encloses the right and has its uncontaminated inner surface facing out.

Defining infection-control terms

Although often used interchangeably, three terms have distinctive meanings of great importance in infection control.

Cleaning physically removes dirt and debris from a surface, usually with water and with or without detergents. Microorganisms removed by cleaning are not killed. Equipment must be cleaned before disinfection or sterilization.

Disinfecting serves as an intermediate state between clean and sterile because it kills certain kinds of microorganisms but not spores. Equipment can be disinfected by pasteurization, by exposure to ultraviolet rays, or by soaking in a disinfectant solution. Before disinfection, equipment must be clean of organic debris because disinfectants can't penetrate pus, blood, or other organic substances and may even be neutralized by them.

Sterilizing destroys all microorganisms — bacteria, viruses, fungi, parasites, and their spores — through the use of pressurized steam, gas (ethylene oxide), liquid (actuated glutaraldehyde), or dry heat. Because boiling water doesn't kill spores, it can't be used for sterilization.

fectiveness when wet *because moisture permits organisms to seep through the material.* Change masks and gowns as soon as moisture is noticeable or according to manufacturer's recommendations or hospital policy.

At the end of your shift, restock used items *to ensure an adequate supply for the next person.* When the patient is transferred to another unit or is discharged, return the isolation cart to the appropriate area for cleaning and restocking of supplies. An isolation room or other room prepared for isolation purposes must be thoroughly cleaned and disinfected before use by another patient. (See *Defining infection-control terms.*)

 Reportable diseases

Certain contagious diseases must be reported to local and state public health officials and, ultimately, to the Centers for Disease Control (CDC). Typically, these diseases fit one of two categories: those reported individually on definitive or suspected diagnosis, and those reported by the number of cases per week. The most

commonly reported diseases include hepatitis, measles, viral meningitis, salmonellosis, shigellosis, syphilis, and gonorrhea. (See *Checklist of reportable diseases* for an extensive listing.)

In most states, the patient's doctor must report communicable diseases to health officials. In hospitals, the infection-control practitioner or epidemiologist reports them. However, you should know the reporting requirements and procedure. Fast, accurate reporting helps identify and control infection sources, prevent epidemics, and guide public health planning and policy.

Equipment
Nursing procedure or infection-control manual ■ disease-reporting form, if available.

Implementation
• Make sure reportable diseases are listed and that the list is available to all shifts.
• Know your hospital's protocol for reporting diseases. Typically, you'll contact the infection-control practitioner or epidemiologist. If this person isn't available, contact your supervisor or the infectious-disease doctor on call.

Documentation
Document any disease reported to the infection-control practitioner, the practitioner's name, and the date and time of the report.

 *G*UIDELINES

Universal precautions

Universal precautions were developed by the Centers for Disease Control (CDC) in response to the increasing incidence of human immunodeficiency virus (HIV), hepatitis B virus (HBV), and other blood-borne diseases. CDC officials recommend that caregivers handle all blood and potentially bloody body substances and tissues as if they're infectious, regardless of the patient's diagnosis.

Universal precautions encompass most of the individual blood and body fluid isolation precautions previously recommended by the CDC for patients with known or suspected blood-borne pathogens. Universal precautions are meant to be combined with other category- or disease-specific isolation precautions, such as disease-specific isolation for highly contagious and resistant organisms (methicillin-resistant *Staphylococcus aureus,* for example).

Checklist of reportable diseases

Because disease reporting laws vary from state to state, this list isn't conclusive, and may be changed periodically. Local agencies report certain diseases to their state health departments, which in turn determine which diseases are reported to the CDC.

- ☐ Acquired immunodeficiency syndrome (AIDS)
- ☐ Amebiasis
- ☐ Animal bites
- ☐ Anthrax (cutaneous or pulmonary)
- ☐ Aseptic meningitis
- ☐ Botulism (food-borne, infant)
- ☐ Brucellosis
- ☐ Cholera
- ☐ Diphtheria (cutaneous or pharyngeal)
- ☐ Encephalitis (postinfectious or primary)
- ☐ Gastroenteritis (institutional outbreaks)
- ☐ Gonorrhea
- ☐ Group A beta-hemolytic streptococcal infections (including scarlet fever)
- ☐ Guillain-Barré syndrome
- ☐ Hepatitis A (include suspected source)
- ☐ Hepatitis B (include suspected source)
- ☐ Hepatitis C, also called non-A, non-B (include suspected source)
- ☐ Hepatitis, unspecified (include suspected source)
- ☐ Influenza
- ☐ Legionellosis (Legionnaires' disease)
- ☐ Leprosy
- ☐ Leptospirosis
- ☐ Malaria
- ☐ Measles (rubeola)
- ☐ Meningitis (specify etiology)

- ☐ Meningococcal disease
- ☐ Mumps
- ☐ Pertussis
- ☐ Plague (bubonic or pneumonic)
- ☐ Poliomyelitis (spinal paralytic)
- ☐ Psittacosis
- ☐ Rabies
- ☐ Reye's syndrome
- ☐ Rheumatic fever
- ☐ Rocky Mountain spotted fever
- ☐ Rubella (congenital syndrome)
- ☐ Rubella (German measles)
- ☐ Salmonellosis (excluding typhoid fever)
- ☐ Shigellosis
- ☐ Smallpox
- ☐ Staphylococcal infections (neonatal)
- ☐ Syphilis (congenital < 1 year)
- ☐ Syphilis (primary or secondary)
- ☐ Tetanus
- ☐ Toxic shock syndrome
- ☐ Trichinosis
- ☐ Tuberculosis
- ☐ Tularemia
- ☐ Typhoid fever
- ☐ Typhus (flea- and tick-borne)
- ☐ Varicella (chicken pox)
- ☐ Yellow fever

The specific body fluids covered by universal precautions include blood; semen; vaginal secretions; cerebrospinal, synovial, pleural, peritoneal, pericardial, and amniotic fluid; bloody saliva; breast milk; and any other body fluid that contains visible blood. Universal precautions don't apply to contact with feces, saliva, nasal secretions, sputum, sweat, tears, vomitus, or urine unless traces of blood are present.

To reduce the risk of spreading nosocomial infections through substances not included in universal precautions, many institutions have adopted an infection-control regimen that combines universal precautions with body substance isolation, a system developed before universal precautions to prevent the spread of nosocomial infections by cross-contamination. Universal precautions recom-mend donning gloves before any exposure to blood and body fluids; body substance isolation recommends donning gloves before contact with blood, all body secretions or excretions, mucous membranes and broken skin, and indwelling device insertion sites. With body substance isolation, respiratory and strict isolation procedures must still be used if an airborne disease is present. Each institution must establish an infection-control policy that lists specific barrier precautions. (See *Guidelines for minimizing infection*, pages 126 to 129, for an example.)

Equipment

Gloves ▪ masks ▪ goggles, glasses, or face shields ▪ gowns or aprons ▪ resuscitation masks ▪ bags for specimens ▪ 1:10 dilution of bleach to water (mixed daily) or hospital-

Guidelines for minimizing infection

The table below lists the minimum requirements for using gloves, gowns, masks, and eye protection to avoid contacting and spreading pathogens. It assumes that thorough hand washing is performed in all cases. Refer to your hospital's guidelines and use your own judgment when assessing the need for barrier protection in specific situations.

PROCEDURE	GLOVES	GOWN	MASK	EYE WEAR
Bathing, for patient with open lesions	✔	–	–	–
Bedding, changing visibly soiled	✔	If soiling likely	–	–
Bleeding or pressure application to control it	✔	If soiling likely	If splattering likely	If splattering likely
Blood glucose (capillary) testing	✔	–	–	–
Breathing treatment, routine	If soiling likely	–	–	–
Cardiopulmonary resuscitation	✔	–	–	–
Central venous line insertion and venesection	✔	–	–	–
Central venous pressure measurement	✔	–	–	–
Cervical cauterization	✔	–	–	–
Chest drainage system change	✔	If splattering likely	–	–
Chest tube insertion	✔	If soiling likely	If splattering likely	If splattering likely
Chest tube removal	✔	If soiling likely	If splattering likely	If splattering likely
Cleaning, anal	✔	–	–	–
Cleaning (feces, spilled blood or body substances, or surfaces contaminated by blood or body fluids)	✔	If soiling likely	–	–
Cleaning, urine	✔	–	–	–
Colonoscopy, flexible sigmoidoscope	✔	✔	–	–
Coughing, frequent and forceful by patient; direct contact with secretions	–	–	✔	✔

Note: ✔ indicates that barrier is necessary; – indicates that barrier typically is not necessary.

Guidelines for minimizing infection *(continued)*

PROCEDURE	GLOVES	GOWN	MASK	EYE WEAR
Dialysis, peritoneal				
Initiation of acute treatment	✔	✔	If splattering likely	If splattering likely
Performing an exchange	✔	✔	If splattering likely	If splattering likely
Termination of acute treatment	✔	✔	If splattering likely	If splattering likely
Dismantling tubing from cycler	✔	✔	If splattering likely	If splattering likely
Discarding peritoneal drainage	✔	✔	If splattering likely	If splattering likely
Irrigating peritoneal catheter	✔	✔	If splattering likely	If splattering likely
Specimen collection	✔	–	–	–
Tubing change	✔	✔	If splattering likely	If splattering likely
Skin care (catheter site)	✔	✔	✔	✔
Assisting with insertion of acute peritoneal catheter (outside sterile field)	✔	✔	If splattering likely	If splattering likely
Dressing change for burns	✔	✔	–	–
Dressing removal or change for wounds with little or no drainage	✔	–	–	–
Dressing removal or change for wounds with large amount of drainage	✔	If soiling likely	–	–
Emptying drainage receptacles, including suction containers, urine receptacles, bedpans, emesis basins	✔	If soiling likely	If splattering likely	If splattering likely
Emptying wastebaskets	✔	–	–	–
Enema	✔	If soiling likely	–	–
Fecal impaction, removal of	✔	–	–	–
Fecal incontinence, placement of indwelling urinary catheter for, and emptying bag	✔	If splattering likely	–	–
Gastric lavage	✔	If soiling likely	–	–
Incision and drainage of abscess	✔	If splattering likely	–	–
Intravenous or intra-arterial line				
Insertion	✔	–	–	–
Removal	✔	–	–	–
Tubing change at catheter hub	✔	–	–	–
Intubation or extubation	✔	If splattering likely	If splattering likely	If splattering likely

(continued)

Guidelines for minimizing infection *(continued)*

PROCEDURE	GLOVES	GOWN	MASK	EYE WEAR
Invasive procedures (lumbar puncture, bone marrow aspiration, paracentesis, liver biopsy) outside sterile field	✔	–	–	–
Irrigation				
Indwelling urinary catheter	✔	–	–	–
Vaginal	✔	If soiling likely	–	–
Wound	✔	If soiling likely	If splattering likely	If splattering likely
Joint or nerve injection	✔	–	–	–
Lesion biopsy or removal	✔	–	–	–
Medication administration				
Eye, ear, and nose drops	✔	–	–	–
I.M. or S.C.	✔	–	–	–
I.V. (direct or into hub of catheter or heparin lock)	✔	–	–	–
Oral	✔	–	–	–
Rectal or vaginal suppository	✔	–	–	–
Topical medication for lesion	✔	–	–	–
Nasogastric tube, insertion or irrigation	✔	If soiling likely	If splattering likely	If splattering likely
Oral and nasal care	✔	–	–	–
Ostomy care, irrigation, and teaching	✔	If soiling likely	–	–
Oxygen tubing, drainage of condensate	✔	–	–	–
Pelvic exam and Pap test	✔	–	–	–
Perineal cleaning	✔	–	–	–
Postmortem care	✔	If soiling likely	–	–
Pressure ulcer care	✔	–	–	–
Shaving	✔	–	–	–
Specimen collection (blood, stool, urine, sputum, wound)	✔	–	–	–

Note: ✔ indicates that barrier is necessary; – indicates that barrier typically is not necessary.

Guidelines for minimizing infection *(continued)*

PROCEDURE	GLOVES	GOWN	MASK	EYE WEAR
Suctioning				
Nasotracheal or endotracheal	✔	If soiling likely	If splattering likely	If splattering likely
Oral or nasal	✔	–	–	–
Temperature, rectal	✔	–	–	–
Tracheostomy suctioning and cannula cleaning	✔	If soiling likely	If splattering likely	If splattering likely
Tracheostomy tube change	✔	–	If splattering likely	If splattering likely
Urine and stool testing	✔	–	–	–
Wound packing	✔	If soiling likely	–	–

Adapted from Pugliese, G., ed. *Universal Precautions: Policies, Procedures, and Resources.* Chicago: American Hospital Publishing, Inc., 1991.

strength disinfectant certified effective against HBV and HIV.

Implementation

• Wash your hands immediately if they become contaminated with blood or body fluids; also wash your hands before and after patient care and after removing gloves. *Hand washing retards the growth of microorganisms on your skin.*

• Wear gloves if you will or could come in contact with blood, specimens, tissue, body fluids or excretions, or contaminated surfaces or objects.

• Change your gloves between patient contacts *to avoid cross-contamination.*

• Wear a gown, face shield, goggles, and a mask during procedures likely to generate droplets of blood or body fluids, such as surgery, endoscopic procedures, or dialysis.

• Handle used needles or other sharp implements carefully. Do not bend, break, reinsert them into their original sheaths, or unnecessarily handle them. Discard them intact immediately after use into an impervious disposal box. *These measures reduce the risk of accidental injury or infection.*

• Immediately notify your employee health provider of all needle-stick accidents, mucosal splashes, or contamination of open wounds with blood or body fluids *to allow investigation of the incident and appropriate care and documentation.*

• Properly label all specimens collected from patients and place them in plastic bags at the collection site.

• Promptly clean all blood and body fluid spills with a 1:10 dilution of bleach to water (mixed daily) or with an approved hospital-strength disinfectant effective against HBV and HIV.

• Disposable food trays and dishes aren't necessary.

• If you have an exudative lesion, avoid all direct patient contact until the condition has resolved and you've been cleared by the employee health provider.

Special considerations

Universal precautions are intended to supplement rather than replace recommendations for routine infection control, such as hand washing and use of gloves.

Keep mouthpieces, resuscitation bags, and other ventilation devices nearby *to minimize the need for emergency mouth-to-mouth resuscitation, thus reducing the risk of exposure to body fluids.*

◆ *Nursing alert.* Because precautions can't be specified for every clinical situation, you must use your judgment in individual cases. What's more, if your work requires you to be exposed to blood, you should receive an HBV vaccine. ◆

Complications

Failure to follow universal precautions may lead to exposure to blood-borne diseases and all the complications they may incur.

Documentation

Record any special needs for universal precautions on the nursing care plan.

Respiratory isolation

This procedure prevents the spread of infectious diseases transmitted by airborne pathogens that are breathed, sneezed, or coughed into the environment. (See *Diseases requiring respiratory precautions.*) This isolation category includes the former categories of acid-fast bacillus (AFB) isolation and strict isolation.

Effective respiratory isolation requires a private room with the door kept closed, the use of masks by anyone entering the room, use of gloves, thorough hand-washing technique, and proper handling and disposal of articles contaminated by respiratory tract secretions. Patients with active tuberculosis or measles must be placed in a room with positive air pressure that is vented directly to the outside of the building.

When handling infants who require respiratory isolation, proper technique requires the use of masks, gloves, and gowns. These barriers prevent contamination of clothing by respiratory tract secretions.

Equipment

Masks ■ gowns, if necessary ■ gloves ■ plastic bags ■ isolation door card ■ isolation tape or labels.

Gather any additional supplies, such as a thermometer, stethoscope, and blood pressure cuff *so that you don't have to leave the isolation room unnecessarily.*

Preparation of equipment

Keep all respiratory isolation supplies outside the patient's room in a cart or anteroom.

Implementation

• Locate the patient in a private room with private toilet facilities and an anteroom, if possible. If necessary, two patients with the same infection may share a room. Explain isolation procedures to the patient *to ease his anxiety and promote cooperation.*

• Keep the patient's door closed at all times *to isolate the patient's airborne secretions.* Put a respiratory isolation card on the door *to notify anyone entering the room.*

• Wash your hands before entering and after leaving the room and during patient care if you handled respiratory tract secretions.

• Pick up your mask by the top strings, adjust it around your nose and mouth, and tie the strings for a comfortable

fit. If the mask has a flexible metal nose strip, adjust it to fit firmly but comfortably. Avoid touching the front of the mask during use *because its surface will have become contaminated.*

• Instruct the patient to cover his mouth with a facial tissue while coughing or sneezing *to control the spread of airborne droplets.*

• Tape an impervious bag to the patient's bedside *so he can dispose of facial tissues correctly.*

• Place all sputum specimens from respiratory isolation patients in impervious, labeled containers and send them to the laboratory.

• Ensure that all visitors wear masks and, if necessary, gowns.

• Place all items that have come in direct contact with the patient—such as linens, trash, and nondisposable utensils or instruments—in a single impervious bag before removal from the room *to prevent contagion.* Place this bag inside a second bag if there is visible outside contamination or if the bag may be punctured.

Special considerations

Before removing your mask, remove your gloves and wash your hands. Untie the strings and dispose of the mask, handling it by the strings only.

If the patient has a highly contagious respiratory disease, you may discard the mask and gloves in a lined, covered receptacle outside the patient's room. Thus, you'll be outside the room (with the door shut behind you) before removing your protective garb.

Remember to discard the mask and gloves right at the door. *Carrying them away from the patient's immediate area promotes contamination.*

Documentation

Record the need for respiratory isolation on the nursing care plan. Document initiation and maintenance of the procedure, the patient's tolerance of the procedure, and any patient teaching. Also document the date isolation was discontinued.

Neutropenic isolation

Unlike other isolation procedures, neutropenic isolation (also known as protective or reverse isolation) guards the patient who is at increased risk of infection against contact with potential pathogens. This procedure is used primarily for patients with extensive noninfected burns and for those who have leukopenia, a depressed immune system, or who are receiving immunosuppressive treat-

Diseases requiring respiratory precautions

DISEASE	PRECAUTIONARY PERIOD
Chicken pox (varicella)	Until lesions become crusted
Diphtheria (pharyngeal)	When nose and throat cultures taken 24 hours after ending treatment are negative for causative organism
Epiglottitis, meningitis, and pneumonia caused by *Haemophilus influenzae*	4 hours after start of effective therapy
Erythema infectiosum	7 days after onset
Hemorrhagic fevers (such as Lassa fever, Marburg virus disease)	Duration of illness
Herpes zoster (shingles)	Duration of illness
Measles (rubeola)	4 days after start of rash (for duration of illness in immunocompromised patients)
Meningitis (*H. influenzae* or *Neisseria meningitidis* known or suspected)	4 hours after start of effective therapy
Meningococcemia	24 hours after start of effective therapy
Mumps	9 days after onset of swelling
Pertussis (whooping cough)	7 days after start of effective therapy or 3 weeks after onset of paroxysms, if untreated
Plague (pneumonic)	3 days after start of effective therapy
Pneumonia (*H. influenzae, N. meningitidis*)	4 hours after start of effective therapy
Rabies	Duration of illness
Rubella (congenital syndrome)	For first year after birth unless nasopharyngeal cultures are negative for causative organism after age 3 months
Rubella (German measles)	7 days after onset of rash
Smallpox (variola)	Duration of illness
Tuberculosis (pulmonary, confirmed or suspected)	Depends on clinical response; usually 10 to 21 days after start of effective therapy

Adapted from Pugliese, G., ed. *Universal Precautions: Policies, Procedures, and Resources*. Chicago: American Hospital Publishing, Inc., 1991.

ments. (See *Conditions or treatments requiring neutropenic isolation* for more information.)

Neutropenic isolation requires a private room equipped with positive air pressure, if possible, to force suspended particles down and out of the room. It also requires use of gowns, gloves, and masks by hospital staff and visitors, and thorough hand-washing technique using an antiseptic cleaning agent.

To care for patients who have temporarily increased susceptibility, such as those who have undergone bone marrow transplantation, neutropenic isolation may also require a patient-isolator unit and the use of sterile linens, gowns, gloves, and head and shoe coverings. In such cases, all other items taken into the room should be sterilized.

Equipment

Gowns ▪ gloves ▪ masks ▪ shoe covers, if required ▪ plastic bags ▪ neutropenic isolation door cards.

Gather any additional supplies, such as a thermometer, stethoscope, and blood pressure cuff *so you don't have to leave the isolation room unnecessarily.*

Preparation of equipment

Keep supplies in a clean enclosed cart or in an anteroom outside the room.

Implementation

• After placing the patient in a private room, explain isolation procedures to him *to ease his anxiety and promote cooperation.*
• Place neutropenic isolation cards on the door *to caution those entering the room.*
• Wash your hands with an antiseptic agent before putting on gloves *to prevent bacterial growth on gloved skin.* Wash your hands again after leaving the room.
• Put on a clean mask each time you enter the patient's room. Use gowns and gloves according to universal precaution recommendations.
• Don't allow visits by anyone known to be infected or ill. Show all visitors how to put on masks before entering the patient's room, and tell them to remove them only after leaving the room.

Special considerations

Don't perform invasive procedures, such as urethral catheterization, unless absolutely necessary *because these procedures risk serious infection in the patient with impaired resistance.* Avoid transporting the patient out of the room; if he must be moved, gown and mask him first.

Instruct the housekeeping staff to put on gowns, gloves, and masks before entering the patient's room; no ill or infected person should enter. The room should be

Conditions or treatments requiring neutropenic isolation

CONDITION OR TREATMENT	PERIOD OF ISOLATION
Acquired immunodeficiency syndrome	Until white blood cell count reaches 1000/mm³ or less, or according to hospital guidelines
Agranulocytosis	Until remission
Burns Noninfected, extensive	Until skin surface heals substantially

Dermatitis
  Noninfected vesicular, bullous, or eczematous disease
  (when severe and extensive)
	Until skin surface heals substantially

Immunosuppressive therapy	Until patient's immunity is adequate
Lymphomas and leukemia Especially in late stages of Hodgkin's disease or acute leukemia	Until clinical improvement is substantial

cleaned with new or scrupulously clean equipment. Because the patient does not have a contagious disease, materials leaving the room need no special precautions, and the room requires no special cleaning after the patient has been discharged.

Documentation

Record the need for neutropenic isolation on the nursing care plan.

Selected references

Centers for Disease Control. "Recommendations for Prevention of HIV Transmission in Health-Care Settings," in *Morbidity and Mortality Weekly Report* 36(Supp. 2S):3S-18S, August 21, 1987.

Centers for Disease Control. "Summary of Notifiable Diseases: United States," in *Morbidity and Mortality Weekly Report* 38(54):3, 10, October 5, 1990.

Centers for Disease Control. "Update: Universal Precautions for Prevention of Transmission of Human Immunodeficiency Virus, Hepatitis B Virus and Other Bloodborne Pathogens in Health-Care Settings," in *Morbidity and Mortality Weekly Report* 37(24):377-88, June 24, 1988.

Department of Labor, Occupational Safety and Health Administration. "Occupational Exposure to Hepatitis B Virus and Human Immunodeficiency Virus, Advance Notice of Proposed Rulemaking" *Federal Register* 52(228):45438-41, November 27, 1987.

Illustrated Manual of Nursing Practice. Springhouse, Pa.: Springhouse Corp., 1991.

Jackson, M.M., et al. "Why Not Treat All Body Substances as Infectious?" *AJN* 87(9):1137-39, September 1987.

Kozier, B., and Erb, G. *Techniques in Clinical Nursing*, 3rd ed. New York: Addison-Wesley Publishing Co., 1989.

Pugliese, Gina, ed. *Universal Precautions: Policies, Procedures, and Resources*. Chicago: American Hospital Publishing, 1991.

Wyngarden, J.B., and Smith, L.B. *Cecil Textbook of Medicine*, 18th ed. Philadelphia: W.B. Saunders Co., 1988.

CHAPTER 3

SPECIMEN COLLECTION AND TESTING

SHERRY BUFFINGTON, RN, CCRN, CLA (ASCP)

Introduction

Collecting specimens promptly and correctly can directly affect a patient's diagnosis, treatment, and recovery. In many cases, the nurse holds sole responsibility for collecting appropriate specimens.

However, even for tests that aren't the nurse's hands-on responsibility, you may be responsible for scheduling them, preparing the patient beforehand, assisting the doctor or other caregiver in performing the test, and caring for the patient afterward. For some tests, you'll teach the patient how to perform the procedure at home — for example, blood glucose tests or fecal occult blood tests. In every case, your nursing responsibilities depend on the clinical setting and your hospital's policies as well as the guidelines provided in your state's or province's nurse practice act.

No matter what part you play in a patient's diagnostic workup, your role always is pivotal in ensuring proper preparation, testing, and aftercare.

Patient preparation

A thorough working knowledge of diagnostic tests will help you prepare patients for them. If you can explain a test with clarity and compassion, you'll help put the patient at ease, gain his trust and cooperation, and thus ensure more accurate results. Helping him understand a procedure based on the doctor's explanations also paves the way for consent that's truly informed.

When preparing a patient, make your explanations clear, straightforward, and complete. For example, before a difficult or painful procedure, such as bone marrow biopsy, you should warn the patient about the type of discomfort he will probably feel. Letting him know exactly what to expect helps him tolerate such a procedure. Preparation should include telling the patient how long the procedure takes and how soon the results will be available.

If you're assisting the doctor with a test, talk to the patient throughout to comfort and encourage him. Prepare him for upcoming sensations, if necessary. Afterward, watch for adverse reactions or complications, and be prepared to implement appropriate care.

Some tests require more detailed instructions to promote cooperation and ensure accurate specimen collection, especially when the patient must modify his behavior before the test or when he will be collecting the specimen himself. For example, you may have to instruct him to observe a special diet, to suspend taking certain medications, or to learn a special collection technique.

Whenever possible, reinforce your verbal explanations with appropriate printed information. Make sure the patient has time to read the information before physical preparation for the test or procedure begins. Many institutions also have videocassettes, telelectures, and films available to augment the patient-teaching process.

Informed consent

Fundamental requirements have been established to protect a patient's rights while he's receiving care. One of the most important rights is informed consent, which states that the patient (or a responsible family member if the patient is legally incompetent) must fully understand what will be done during a test, surgery, or any medical procedure and must understand its risks and implications *before* he can legally consent to it.

Explaining a procedure, how it will be performed, and its potential benefits and risks is primarily the doctor's responsibility. The nurse typically reinforces the doctor's explanation, confirms that the patient comprehends it, and verifies that written consent has been given when necessary. Written consent isn't always necessary for individual tests; informed verbal consent may be adequate. The patient retains the legal right to withdraw consent — verbal or written — at any time and for any reason and to refuse care or treatment.

Safety measures

Keep in mind that proper specimen collection not only helps to ensure accurate results but also protects you and the patient. Use of gloves and other barriers has become routine in many heath care settings. Before you're exposed to a patient's body fluids, be sure you understand and comply with appropriate precautions.

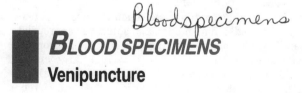

BLOOD SPECIMENS
Venipuncture

Performed to obtain a venous blood sample, venipuncture involves piercing a vein with a needle and collecting blood in a syringe or evacuated tube. Typically, venipuncture is performed using the antecubital fossa. If necessary, however, it can be performed on a vein in the wrist, the dorsum of the hand or foot, or another accessible location. Usually, laboratory personnel carry out the procedure in

Guide to color-top collection tubes

TUBE COLOR	DRAW VOLUME	ADDITIVE	PURPOSE
Red	2 to 20 ml	None	Serum studies
Lavender	2 to 10 ml	EDTA	Whole blood studies
Green	2 to 15 ml	Heparin (sodium, lithium, or ammonium)	Plasma studies
Blue	2.7 or 4.5 ml	Sodium citrate and citric acid	Coagulation studies on plasma
Black	2.7 or 4.5 ml	Sodium oxalate	Coagulation studies on plasma
Gray	3 to 10 ml	Glycolytic inhibitor, such as sodium fluoride, powdered oxalate, or glycolytic-microbial inhibitor	Glucose determinations on serum or plasma
Yellow	12 ml	Acid-citrate-dextrose (ACD)	Whole blood studies

the hospital setting; however, a nurse may perform it occasionally.

Equipment
Tourniquet ■ gloves ■ syringe or evacuated tubes and needle holder ■ 70% ethyl alcohol or povidone-iodine sponges ■ 20G or 21G needle for the forearm or 25G for the wrist, hand, ankle, or for children ■ color-coded tubes containing appropriate additives (see *Guide to color-top collection tubes)* ■ labels ■ laboratory request form ■ 2″ × 2″ gauze pads ■ adhesive bandage.

Preparation of equipment
If you're using evacuated tubes, open the needle packet, attach the needle to its holder, and select the appropriate tubes. If you're using a syringe, attach the appropriate needle to it. Be sure to choose a syringe large enough to hold all the blood required for the test. Label all collection tubes clearly with the patient's name and room number, the doctor's name, and the date and time of collection.

Implementation
● Wash your hands thoroughly and don gloves *to prevent cross-contamination.*
● Tell the patient that you're about to take a blood sample, and explain the procedure *to ease his anxiety and en-*

courage his cooperation. Ask him if he's ever felt faint, sweaty, or nauseated when having blood drawn.
● If the patient is on bed rest, ask him to lie supine, with his head slightly elevated and his arms at his sides. Ask the ambulatory patient to sit in a chair and support his arm securely on an armrest or table.
● Assess the patient's veins *to determine the best puncture site.* (See *Possible venipuncture sites.)* Observe the skin for the vein's blue color, or palpate the vein for a firm rebound sensation.
● Tie a tourniquet 2″ (5 cm) proximal to the area chosen. *By impeding venous return to the heart while still allowing arterial flow, a tourniquet produces venous dilation.* If arterial perfusion remains adequate, you'll be able to feel the radial pulse. (If the tourniquet fails to dilate the vein, have the patient open and close his fist repeatedly. Then ask him to close his fist as you insert the needle and to open it again when the needle is in place.)
● Clean the venipuncture site with a povidone-iodine sponge or with an alcohol sponge. Don't wipe off the povidone-iodine with alcohol *because alcohol cancels the effect of povidone-iodine.* Wipe in a circular motion, spiraling outward from the site *to avoid introducing potentially infectious skin flora into the vessel during the procedure.* If you use alcohol, apply it with friction for 30 seconds, or until the final sponge comes away clean. Allow the skin to dry before performing venipuncture.

• Immobilize the vein by pressing just below the venipuncture site with your thumb and drawing the skin taut.

• Position the needle holder or syringe with the needle bevel up and the shaft parallel to the path of the vein and at a 30-degree angle to the arm. Insert the needle into the vein. If you're using a syringe, venous blood will appear in the hub; withdraw the blood slowly, pulling the plunger of the syringe gently *to create steady suction* until you obtain the required sample. *Pulling the plunger too forcibly may collapse the vein.* If you're using a needle holder and evacuated tube, a drop of blood will appear just inside the needle holder. Grasp the holder securely to stabilize it in the vein, and push down on the collection tube until the needle punctures the rubber stopper. Blood will flow into the tube automatically.

• Remove the tourniquet as soon as blood flows adequately *to prevent stasis and hemoconcentration, which can impair test results.* If the flow is sluggish, leave the tourniquet in place longer, but always remove it before withdrawing the needle.

• After you've drawn the sample, place a gauze pad over the puncture site, and slowly and gently remove the needle from the vein. When using an evacuated tube, remove it from the needle holder *to release the vacuum* before withdrawing the needle from the vein.

• Apply gentle pressure to the puncture site for 2 or 3 minutes or until bleeding stops. *This prevents extravasation into the surrounding tissue, which causes hematoma.*

• After bleeding stops, apply an adhesive bandage.

• If you've used a syringe, transfer the sample to a collection tube. Detach the needle from the syringe, open the collection tube, and gently empty the sample into the tube, being careful to avoid foaming, *which may cause hemolysis.*

• Finally, check the venipuncture site *to make sure a hematoma hasn't developed.* If it has, then apply warm soaks.

• Discard used gloves in the appropriate container.

Special considerations

Never draw a venous sample from an arm or leg already being used for I.V. therapy or blood administration *because this may affect test results.* Don't draw a venous sample from an infection site *because this risks introduction of pathogens into the vascular system.* Likewise, avoid drawing blood from edematous areas, arteriovenous shunts, or sites of previous hematoma or vascular injury.

If you use a blood pressure cuff as a tourniquet, inflate it to a level between the patient's systolic and diastolic pressures *to allow for venous distention without constricting arterial flow.* If the patient has large, distended, highly visible veins, perform venipuncture without a tourniquet *to minimize the risk of hematoma.*

Possible venipuncture sites

The illustrations below show the anatomic locations of veins that can be used for venipuncture. The most commonly used sites are on the forearm, followed by those on the hand. Keep in mind that using the leg veins raises the patient's risk of thrombophlebitis.

If the patient has a clotting disorder or is receiving anticoagulant therapy, maintain firm pressure on the venipuncture site for at least 5 minutes after withdrawing the needle *to prevent possible formation of a hematoma.* Perform venipuncture cautiously in patients who have clotting disorders or who are receiving anticoagulant therapy.

Avoid using veins in the patient's legs for venipuncture, if possible, *because this increases the risk of thrombophlebitis.*

Complications

Hematoma at the needle insertion site is the most common complication of venipuncture. Infection may result from poor technique.

Documentation

Record the date, time, and site of venipuncture; name of the test; the time the sample was sent to the laboratory; and any adverse effects the patient experiences, such as a hematoma or anxiety.

Blood culture

Normally bacteria-free, blood is susceptible to infection through infusion lines, as well as from thrombophlebitis, infected shunts, or bacterial endocarditis from prosthetic heart valve replacements. Bacteria may also invade the vascular system from local tissue infections through the lymphatic system and the thoracic duct.

Blood cultures are performed to detect bacterial invasion (bacteremia) and the systemic spread of such an infection (septicemia) through the bloodstream. In this procedure, a laboratory technician or a nurse collects a venous blood sample by venipuncture at the patient's bedside and then transfers it into two bottles, one containing an anaerobic medium and the other an aerobic medium. The bottles are incubated, encouraging any organisms present in the sample to grow in the media. Blood cultures allow identification of about 67% of pathogens within 24 hours and up to 90% within 72 hours. (See *Isolator blood-culturing system* for a description of another type of culturing procedure.)

Although some authorities consider the timing of culture collections debatable and possibly irrelevant, others advocate drawing three blood samples at least 1 hour apart. The first of these should be collected at the earliest sign of suspected bacteremia or septicemia. To check for suspected bacterial endocarditis, three or four samples may be collected at 5- to 30-minute intervals before starting antibiotic therapy.

Equipment

Tourniquet ■ gloves ■ alcohol sponges ■ povidone-iodine sponges ■ 10-ml syringe for an adult; 6-ml syringe for a child ■ three or four 20G 1½″ needles ■ two or three blood culture bottles (50-ml bottles for adults, 20-ml bottles for infants and children) with sodium polyethanol sulfonate added (one aerobic bottle containing a suitable medium, such as Trypticase soy broth with 10% carbon dioxide atmosphere; one anaerobic bottle with prereduced medium; and, possibly, one hyperosmotic bottle with 10% sucrose medium) ■ laboratory request form ■ small adhesive bandages ■ 2″ × 2″ gauze pads.

Preparation of equipment

Check culture bottle expiration dates and replace outdated bottles.

Implementation

• Tell the patient that you need to collect a series of blood samples to check for infection. Explain the procedure *to ease his anxiety and promote cooperation.* Explain that the procedure usually requires three separate blood samples drawn at different times.
• Wash your hands and put on gloves.
• Tie a tourniquet 2″ (5 cm) proximal to the area chosen. (See "Venipuncture" in this chapter.)
• Clean the venipuncture site with a povidone-iodine sponge or with an alcohol sponge. Don't wipe off the povidone-iodine with alcohol *because alcohol cancels the effect of povidone-iodine.* Start at the site and work outward in a circular motion. Wait 30 to 60 seconds for the solution to dry.
• Perform a venipuncture, drawing 10 ml of blood from an adult or 2 to 6 ml from a child.

Isolator blood-culturing system

A single-tube blood-culturing system, the Isolator uses lysis and centrifugation to help detect septicemia and monitor the effectiveness of antibacterial drug therapy.

The Isolator evacuated tube, used to collect the blood sample, contains a substance that lyses red blood cells. Then, centrifugation concentrates bacteria and other organisms in the sample onto an inert cushioning pad; the concentrate can then be applied directly onto four agar plates.

The Isolator has several advantages over conventional blood-culturing methods. This system:
• eliminates the bottle method's lengthy incubation period, providing faster results
• improves bacterial survival
• results in more valid positive results through direct application onto agar plates, which dilutes any antibiotic present in the sample to a greater degree
• detects more yeast and polymicrobial infections
• improves the laboratory's ability to detect organisms that are difficult to grow
• is easier to use at the patient's bedside and to transport because blood is drawn directly into the Isolator tube.

• Wipe the diaphragm tops of the culture bottles with a povidone-iodine sponge, and change the needle on the syringe used to draw the blood.

• Inject 5 ml of blood into each 50-ml bottle or 2 ml into a 20-ml pediatric culture bottle. (Bottle size may vary with the hospital's protocol, but the sample dilution should always be 1:10.)

• Label the culture bottles with the patient's name and room number, the doctor's name, and the date and time of collection. Indicate the suspected diagnosis and the patient's temperature, and note on the laboratory request form any recent antibiotic therapy. Send the samples to the laboratory immediately.

• Discard the gloves in the appropriate container.

Special considerations

Obtain each set of cultures from a different site. Avoid using existing blood lines for cultures unless the sample is drawn when the line is inserted or unless catheter sepsis is suspected.

Complications

The most common complication of venipuncture is formation of a hematoma. If a hematoma develops, apply warm soaks to the site.

Documentation

In your notes, record the date and time of blood sample collection, the name of the test, the amount of blood collected, the number of bottles used, the patient's temperature, and any adverse reactions to the procedure.

Blood glucose tests

Rapid, easy-to-perform reagent strip tests (such as Glucostix, Chemstrip bG, or Multistix) use a drop of capillary blood obtained by fingerstick, heelstick, or earlobe puncture as a sample. These tests can detect or monitor elevated blood glucose levels in patients with diabetes, screen for diabetes mellitus and neonatal hypoglycemia, and help distinguish diabetic coma from nondiabetic coma. In these tests, a reagent patch on the tip of a hand-held plastic strip changes color in response to the amount of glucose in the blood sample. Comparing the color change with a standardized color chart provides a semiquantitative measurement of blood glucose levels; inserting the strip in a portable blood glucose meter (such as a Glucometer II, Accu-Chek II, or One Touch) provides quantitative measurements that compare in accuracy with other laboratory tests. Some meters store successive

test results electronically to help determine glucose patterns.

These tests can be performed in the hospital, the doctor's office, or the patient's home.

Equipment

Reagent strips ▪ gloves ▪ portable blood glucose meter, if available ▪ gauze pads ▪ alcohol sponges ▪ disposable lancets ▪ small adhesive bandage ▪ watch or clock with a second hand.

Implementation

• Explain the procedure to the patient or to the infant's parents.

• Select the puncture site — usually the fingertip or earlobe for an adult or the heel or great toe for an infant.

• Wash your hands and don gloves.

• If necessary, dilate the capillaries by applying warm, moist compresses to the area for about 10 minutes.

• Wipe the puncture site with an alcohol sponge and dry it thoroughly with a gauze pad.

• To draw a sample from the patient's fingertip with a disposable lancet (smaller than 2 mm), make the puncture on the side of the fingertip and position the lancet perpendicular to the lines of the patient's fingerprints. Pierce the skin sharply and quickly *to minimize the patient's anxiety and pain, and to increase blood flow.* Alternatively, you may want to use a mechanical bloodletting device, such as an Autolet, which uses a spring-loaded lancet.

• After puncturing the finger, wipe away the first drop of blood *to avoid diluting the sample with tissue fluid.* For the same reason, avoid squeezing the puncture site.

• Touch a drop of blood to the reagent patch on the strip; make sure you cover the entire patch.

• After collecting the blood sample, briefly apply pressure to the puncture site *to prevent painful extravasation of blood into subcutaneous tissues.* Ask the adult patient to hold a gauze pad firmly over the puncture site until bleeding stops.

• Leave the blood on the strip for exactly 60 seconds, and then quickly wash it off with a stream of water from a wash bottle. Don't hold the strip under a faucet *because a strong stream of water will wash off too much blood.* Some reagent strips require only that the blood be wiped off, without washing. Follow the manufacturer's instructions exactly *because results will influence insulin dosage.*

• Immediately after washing, compare the color change on the strip with the standardized color chart on the product container. If you're using a blood glucose meter, follow the manufacturer's instructions. Meter designs vary, but they all analyze a drop of blood placed on a

Oral and intravenous glucose tolerance tests

For monitoring trends in glucose metabolism, two tests may offer benefits over testing blood with reagent strips.

Oral glucose tolerance test

The most sensitive test for detecting borderline diabetes mellitus, the oral glucose tolerance test (OGTT) measures carbohydrate metabolism after ingestion of a challenge dose of glucose. The body absorbs this dose rapidly, causing plasma glucose levels to rise and peak within 30 minutes to 1 hour. The pancreas responds by secreting insulin, causing glucose levels to return to normal within 2 to 3 hours. During this period, plasma and urine glucose levels are monitored to assess insulin secretion and the body's ability to metabolize glucose.

Although you may not collect the blood and urine specimens (usually five of each) required for this test, you will be responsible for preparing the patient for the test and monitoring his physical condition during the test.

Begin by explaining the OGTT to the patient. Then, tell him to maintain a high-carbohydrate diet for 3 days and to fast for 10 to 16 hours before the test, as ordered. The patient must not smoke, drink coffee or alcohol, or exercise strenuously for 8 hours before or during the test. Inform him that he will then receive a challenge dose of 100 g of carbohydrate (usually a sweetened carbonated beverage or gelatin).

Tell the patient who will perform the venipunctures and when, and that he may feel slight discomfort from the needle punctures and the pressure of the tourniquet. Reassure him that collecting each blood sample usually takes less than 3 minutes. As ordered, withhold drugs that may affect test results. Remind him not to discard the first voided urine specimen on waking.

During the test period, watch for signs and symptoms of hypoglycemia—weakness, restlessness, nervousness, hunger, and sweating—and report these to the doctor immediately. Encourage the patient to drink plenty of water to promote adequate urine excretion. Provide a bedpan, urinal, or specimen container when necessary.

I.V. glucose tolerance test

This test may be chosen for patients unable to absorb an oral dose of glucose—for example, those with malabsorption disorders, short-bowel syndrome, or those who have had a gastrectomy. The I.V. glucose tolerance test measures blood glucose after an I.V. infusion of 50% glucose over 3 or 4 minutes. Blood samples are then drawn after 30 minutes, 1 hour, 2 hours, and 3 hours. After an immediate glucose peak of 300 to 400 mg/dl (accompanied by glycosuria), the normal glucose curve falls steadily, reaching fasting levels within 1 to 1¼ hours. Failure to achieve fasting glucose levels within 2 to 3 hours typically confirms diabetes.

---

reagent strip that comes with the unit, and they provide a digital display of the resulting glucose level.
• After bleeding has stopped, you may apply a small adhesive bandage to the puncture site.

Special considerations

Before using reagent strips, check the expiration date on the package and replace outdated strips. Also check for special instructions related to the specific reagent. The reagent area of a fresh strip should match the color on the "0" block on the color chart. Protect the strips from light, heat, and moisture.

Before using a blood glucose meter, calibrate it and run it with a control sample *to ensure accurate test results.* Follow the manufacturer's instructions for calibration.

Avoid selecting cold, cyanotic, or swollen puncture sites *to ensure an adequate blood sample.* If you can't obtain a capillary sample, perform venipuncture and place a large drop of venous blood on the reagent strip. If you

want to test blood from a refrigerated sample, allow the blood to return to room temperature before testing it.

To help detect abnormal glucose metabolism and diagnose diabetes mellitus, the doctor may order other blood glucose tests. (See *Oral and intravenous glucose tolerance tests.*)

Home care

If the patient will be using the reagent strip system at home, teach him the proper use of the lancet or Autolet, the reagent strips and color chart, and the portable blood glucose meter, as necessary. Also provide written guidelines.

Documentation

Record the reading from the reagent strip (using a portable blood glucose meter or a color chart) in your notes or on a special flowchart, if available. Also record the time and date of the test.

Arterial puncture for blood gas analysis

Obtaining an arterial blood sample requires percutaneous puncture of the brachial, radial, or femoral artery or withdrawal of a sample from an arterial line. Once drawn, the sample can be analyzed for arterial blood gases.

Arterial blood gas (ABG) analysis evaluates ventilation by measuring blood pH and the partial pressures of oxygen (PaO_2) and carbon dioxide ($PaCO_2$) in arterial blood. Blood pH measurement reveals the blood's acid-base balance. PaO_2 indicates the amount of oxygen that the lungs deliver to the blood, and $PaCO_2$ indicates the lungs' capacity to eliminate carbon dioxide. ABG samples can also be analyzed for oxygen content and saturation and for bicarbonate values.

ABG analysis is ordered commonly for patients who have chronic obstructive pulmonary disease, pulmonary edema, acute respiratory distress syndrome, myocardial infarction, or pneumonia. It's also performed during episodes of shock and after coronary artery bypass surgery, resuscitation from cardiac arrest, changes in respiratory therapy or status, and prolonged anesthesia.

Most ABG samples can be drawn by a respiratory technician or specially trained nurse. Collection from the femoral artery, however, is usually performed by a doctor. Before attempting a radial puncture, Allen's test should be performed to assess the adequacy of the blood supply to the patient's hand. (See *Performing Allen's test.*)

Equipment
10-ml glass syringe or plastic luer-lock syringe specially made for drawing blood gases ■ 1-ml ampule of aqueous heparin (1:1,000) ■ 20G 1¼″ needle ■ 22G 1″ needle ■ alcohol sponge ■ povidone-iodine sponge ■ two 2″ × 2″ gauze pads ■ gloves ■ rubber cap for syringe hub or rubber stopper for needle ■ ice-filled plastic bag ■ label ■ laboratory request form ■ adhesive bandage ■ optional: 1% lidocaine solution.

Many hospitals use a commercial ABG kit that contains all the equipment listed above (except the adhesive bandage and ice). If your hospital doesn't use such a kit, obtain a sterile syringe specially made for drawing blood gases and use a clean emesis basin filled with ice instead of the plastic bag to transport the sample to the laboratory.

Preparation of equipment
Prepare the collection equipment before entering the patient's room. Wash your hands thoroughly; then open the ABG kit and remove the specimen label and the plastic

---

Performing Allen's test

Rest the patient's arm on the mattress or bedside stand, and support his wrist with a rolled towel. Have him clench his fist. Then, using your index and middle fingers, press on the radial and ulnar arteries. Hold this position for a few seconds.

Without removing your fingers from the patient's arteries, ask him to unclench his fist and hold his hand in a relaxed position. The palm will be blanched because pressure from your fingers has impaired the normal blood flow.

Release pressure on the patient's ulnar artery. If the hand becomes flushed, which indicates blood filling the vessels, you can safely proceed with the radial artery puncture. If the hand doesn't flush, perform the test on the other arm.

Arterial puncture technique

The angle of needle penetration in arterial blood gas sampling depends on the artery to be sampled. For the radial artery, which is used most commonly, the needle should enter bevel up at a 30- to 45-degree angle.

bag. Record on the label the patient's name and room number, the date and collection time, and the doctor's name. Fill the plastic bag with ice and set it aside.

To heparinize the syringe, first attach the 20G needle to the syringe. Then open the ampule of heparin. Draw all the heparin into the syringe *to prevent the sample from clotting.* Hold the syringe upright, and pull the plunger back slowly to about the 7-ml mark. Rotate the barrel while pulling the plunger back *to allow the heparin to coat the inside surface of the syringe.* Then, slowly force the heparin toward the hub of the syringe and expel all but about 0.1 ml of heparin.

To heparinize the needle, first replace the 20G needle with the 22G needle. Then, hold the syringe upright, tilt it slightly, and eject the remaining heparin. *Excess heparin in the syringe alters blood pH and PaO_2 values.*

Implementation
● Tell the patient you need to collect an arterial blood sample, and explain the procedure *to help ease anxiety and promote cooperation.* Tell him that the needle stick will cause some discomfort but that he must remain still during the procedure.
● After washing your hands and donning gloves, place a rolled towel under the patient's wrist *for support.* Locate the artery and palpate it for a strong pulse.
● Clean the puncture site with a povidone-iodine sponge or with an alcohol sponge. Don't wipe off the povidone-iodine with alcohol *because alcohol cancels the effect of povidone-iodine.*
● Using a circular motion, clean the area, starting in the center of the site and spiraling outward *to avoid introducing potentially infectious skin flora into the vessel during the procedure.* If you use alcohol, apply it with friction for 30 seconds or until the final sponge comes away clean. Allow the skin to dry.
● Palpate the artery with the index and middle fingers of one hand while holding the syringe over the puncture site with the other hand.
● Hold the needle bevel up at a 30- to 45-degree angle. When puncturing the brachial artery, hold the needle at a 60-degree angle. (See *Arterial puncture technique.*)
● Puncture the skin and the arterial wall in one motion, following the path of the artery.
● Watch for blood backflow in the syringe. Don't pull back on the plunger *because arterial blood should enter the syringe automatically.* Fill the syringe to the 5-ml mark.
● After collecting the sample, press a gauze pad firmly over the puncture site until bleeding stops—at least 5 minutes. If the patient is receiving anticoagulant therapy or has a blood dyscrasia, apply pressure for 10 to 15 minutes; if necessary, ask a co-worker to hold the gauze pad in place while you prepare the sample for transport to the laboratory. Don't ask the patient to hold the pad. *If he fails to apply sufficient pressure, a large, painful hematoma may form, hindering future arterial punctures at that site.*
● Check the syringe for air bubbles *because these can alter PaO_2 values.* If air bubbles appear, remove them by holding the syringe upright and slowly ejecting some of the blood onto a 2″ × 2″ gauze pad.
● Insert the needle into a rubber stopper, or remove the needle and place a rubber cap directly on the needle hub. *This prevents the sample from leaking and keeps air out of the syringe.*
● Put the labeled sample in the ice-filled plastic bag or emesis basin. Attach a properly completed laboratory request form, and send the sample to the laboratory immediately.
● When bleeding stops, apply a small adhesive bandage to the site.
● Monitor the patient's vital signs, and observe for signs of circulatory impairment, such as swelling, discolor-

ation, pain, numbness, or tingling in the bandaged arm or leg. Watch for bleeding at the puncture site.

Special considerations

If the patient is receiving oxygen, make sure that his therapy has been underway for at least 15 minutes before drawing arterial blood.

Unless ordered, don't turn off existing oxygen therapy before drawing arterial blood samples. However, be sure to indicate the amount and type of oxygen therapy the patient is receiving on the laboratory request slip.

If the patient isn't receiving oxygen, indicate that he is breathing room air.

If the patient has just received a breathing treatment or nebulizer treatment, wait about 20 minutes before drawing the sample.

If necessary, you may anesthetize the puncture site with 1% lidocaine solution. Consider such use of lidocaine carefully *because it delays the procedure, the patient may be allergic to the drug, or the resulting vasoconstriction may prevent successful puncture.*

When filling out a laboratory request form for ABG analysis, be sure to include the following information *to help the laboratory staff calibrate the equipment and evaluate results correctly:* the patient's current temperature, most recent hemoglobin level, current respiratory rate, and fraction of inspired oxygen and tidal volume if the patient is on a ventilator.

Complications

If you use too much force when attempting to puncture the artery, the needle may touch the periosteum of the bone, causing the patient considerable pain; or you may advance the needle through the opposite wall of the artery. If this happens, slowly pull the needle back a short distance and check to see if get a blood return. If blood still fails to enter the syringe, withdraw the needle completely and start with a fresh heparinized needle. Do not make more than two attempts to withdraw blood from the same site. *Probing the artery may injure it and the radial nerve. Also, hemolysis will alter test results.*

If arterial spasm occurs, blood will not flow into the syringe and you won't be able to collect the sample. If this happens, replace the needle with a smaller one and attempt the puncture again. *A smaller-bore needle is less likely to cause arterial spasm.*

Documentation

Record the results of Allen's test, the time the sample was drawn, the patient's temperature, the site of the arterial puncture, the length of time pressure was applied to the site to control bleeding, and the type and amount of oxygen therapy the patient was receiving.

URINE SPECIMENS
Urine collection

A random urine specimen, usually collected as part of the physical examination or at various times during hospitalization, permits laboratory screening for urinary and systemic disorders, as well as for drug screening. A clean-catch midstream specimen, once used only to confirm urinary tract infection, is now replacing random collection for many other purposes because it provides a virtually uncontaminated specimen without the need for bladder catheterization.

An indwelling catheter specimen — obtained either by clamping the drainage tube and emptying the accumulated urine into a container or by aspirating a sample with a syringe — requires sterile technique to prevent catheter contamination and urinary tract infection. This method is contraindicated in patients who have recently undergone genitourinary surgery.

Equipment

For a random specimen: bedpan or urinal with cover, if necessary ▪ gloves ▪ graduated container ▪ specimen container with lid ▪ label ▪ laboratory request form.

For a clean-catch midstream specimen: basin ▪ soap and water ▪ towel ▪ gloves ▪ three sterile 2″ × 2″ gauze pads ▪ povidone-iodine solution ▪ sterile specimen container with lid ▪ label ▪ bedpan or urinal, if necessary ▪ laboratory request form. (Commercial clean-catch kits containing antiseptic towelettes, sterile specimen container with lid and label, and instructions for use in several languages are widely used.)

For an indwelling catheter specimen: 10-ml syringe ▪ 21G or 22G 1½″ needle ▪ tube clamp ▪ sterile specimen cup with lid ▪ gloves ▪ alcohol sponge ▪ label ▪ laboratory request form.

Implementation

• Tell the patient that you need a urine specimen for laboratory analysis. Explain the procedure to him and his family, if necessary, *to promote cooperation and prevent accidental disposal of specimens.*

Collecting a random specimen

• Provide privacy. Instruct the patient on bed rest to void into a clean bedpan or urinal, or ask the ambulatory patient to void into either one in the bathroom.

• Don gloves. Then pour at least 120 ml of urine into the specimen container, and cap the container securely. If the patient's urine output must be measured and re-

Aspirating a urine specimen

To aspirate a urine specimen from a rubber indwelling catheter that has no built-in sampling port, insert the syringe needle into the catheter just above where it connects to the drainage tube. This position prevents accidental puncture of the lumen that connects with the catheter balloon. Aspirating the water from this lumen can deflate the balloon and dislodge the catheter.

To aspirate a specimen from a built-in sampling port, wipe the port with an alcohol sponge and insert the needle perpendicular to the catheter.

corded, pour the remaining urine into the graduated container. Otherwise, discard the remaining urine. If you inadvertently spill urine on the outside of the container, clean and dry it *to prevent possible cross-contamination.*
• Label the sample container with the patient's name and room number and the date and time of collection, attach the request form, and send it to the laboratory immediately. *Delaying the sample may alter test results.*
• Clean the graduated container and urinal or bedpan, and return these to their proper storage. Discard disposable items.
• Wash your hands thoroughly *to prevent cross-contamination.* Offer the patient a washcloth and soap and water to wash his hands.

Collecting a clean-catch midstream specimen
• Because the goal of this method is a virtually uncontaminated specimen, explain the procedure to the patient carefully. Provide illustrations to emphasize the correct collection technique, if possible.
• Tell the patient to remove all clothing from the waist down and to stand in front of the toilet as for urination or, if female, to sit far back on the toilet seat and spread her legs. Then have the patient clean the periurethral area (tip of the penis or labial folds, vulva, and urethral meatus) with soap and water and then wipe the area three times, each time with a fresh 2″ × 2″ gauze pad soaked in povidone-iodine solution, or with the wipes provided in a commercial kit. Instruct the female patient to separate her labial folds with the thumb and forefinger. Tell her to wipe down one side with the first pad and discard it, to wipe the other side with the second pad and discard it and, finally, to wipe down the center over the urinary meatus with the third pad and discard it. Stress the importance of cleaning from front to back *to avoid contaminating the genital area with fecal matter.* For the uncircumcised male patient, emphasize the need to retract his foreskin *to effectively clean the meatus* and to keep it retracted during voiding.
• Tell the female patient to straddle the bedpan or toilet *to allow labial spreading.* She should continue to keep her labia separated with her fingers while voiding.
• Instruct the patient to begin voiding into the bedpan, urinal, or toilet *because the urine stream washes bacteria from the urethra and urinary meatus.* Then, without stopping the urine stream, the patient should move the collection container into the stream, collecting about 30 to 50 ml at the midstream portion of the voiding. The patient can then finish voiding into the bedpan, urinal, or toilet.
• Don gloves before discarding the first and last portions of the voiding, and measure the remaining urine in a graduated cylinder for intake and output records, if necessary. Be sure to include the amount in the specimen container when recording the total amount voided.
• Take the sterile container from the patient, and cap it securely. Avoid touching the inside of the container or the lid. If the outside of the container is soiled, clean it and wipe it dry. Remove gloves and discard them properly.

• Wash your hands thoroughly *to prevent cross-contamination.* Tell the patient to wash his hands also.
• Label the container with the patient's name and room number, name of test, type of specimen, collection time, and suspected diagnosis, if known. If a urine culture has been ordered, note any current antibiotic therapy on the laboratory request form. Send the container to the laboratory immediately, or place it on ice *to prevent specimen deterioration and altered test results.*

Collecting an indwelling catheter specimen
• About 30 minutes before collecting the specimen, clamp the drainage tube *to allow urine to accumulate.*
• Put on gloves. If the drainage tube has a built-in sampling port, wipe the port with an alcohol sponge. Uncap the needle on the syringe, and insert the needle into the sampling port at a 90-degree angle to the tubing. Aspirate the specimen into the syringe. (See *Aspirating a urine specimen.)*
• If the drainage tube doesn't have a sampling port and the catheter is made of rubber, obtain the specimen from the catheter. *Other types of catheters will leak after you withdraw the needle.* To withdraw the specimen from a rubber catheter, wipe it with an alcohol sponge just above the point where it connects to the drainage tube. Insert the needle into the rubber catheter at a 45-degree angle and withdraw the specimen. Never insert the needle into the shaft of the catheter *because this may puncture the lumen leading to the catheter balloon.*
• Transfer the specimen to a sterile container, label it, and send it to the laboratory immediately or place it on ice. If a urine culture is to be performed, be sure to list any antibiotic therapy on the laboratory request form.
• If the catheter is not made of rubber or has no sampling port, wipe the area where the catheter joins the drainage tube with an alcohol sponge. Disconnect the catheter, and allow urine to drain into the sterile specimen container. Avoid touching the inside of the sterile container with the catheter, and don't touch anything with the catheter drainage tube *to avoid contamination.* When you have the specimen, wipe both connection sites with an alcohol sponge and join them. Cap the specimen container, label it, and send it to the laboratory immediately or place it on ice.
◆ *Nursing alert.* Make sure you unclamp the drainage tube after collecting the specimen *to prevent urine backflow that may cause bladder distention and infection.* ◆

Home care
Instruct the patient to collect the sample in a clean container with a tight-fitting lid, and to keep it on ice or in the refrigerator (separate from any food items) for up to 24 hours.

Documentation
Record the times of specimen collection and transport to the laboratory. Specify the test, and the appearance, odor, color, and any unusual characteristics of the specimen. If necessary, record the urine volume on the patient's intake and output record.

 ## Timed urine collection

Because hormones, proteins, and electrolytes are excreted in small variable amounts in urine, specimens for measuring these substances must typically be collected over an extended time to yield quantities of diagnostic value.

A 24-hour specimen is used most commonly because it provides an average excretion rate for substances eliminated during this period. Timed specimens may also be collected for shorter periods, such as 2 or 12 hours, depending on the specific information needed.

A timed urine specimen may also be collected after administering a challenge dose of a chemical—inulin, for example—to detect various renal disorders.

Equipment
Large collection bottle with a cap or stopper, or a commercial plastic container ▪ preservative, if necessary ▪ gloves ▪ bedpan or urinal, if patient does not have an indwelling catheter ▪ graduated container, if patient is on intake and output measurement ▪ gloves ▪ ice-filled container, if a refrigerator isn't available ▪ label ▪ laboratory request form ▪ four patient care reminders.

Check with the laboratory to see what preservatives may be needed in the urine specimen, or if a dark collection bottle is required.

Implementation
• Explain the procedure to the patient and his family members, as necessary, *to enlist their cooperation and prevent accidental disposal of urine during the collection period.* Emphasize that loss of even *one* urine specimen during the collection period invalidates the test and requires that it begin again.
• Place patient care reminders over the patient's bed, in his bathroom, on the bedpan hopper in the utility room, and on the urinal or indwelling catheter collection bag. Include the patient's name and room number, the date, and the collection interval.
• Instruct the patient to save all urine during the collection period, to notify you after each voiding, and to avoid contaminating the urine with stool or toilet tissue.

Explain any dietary or drug restrictions and be sure he understands and is willing to comply with them.

For 2-hour collection
● If possible, instruct the patient to drink two to four 8-oz glasses (480 to 960 ml) of water about 30 minutes before collection begins. After 30 minutes, tell him to void. Don gloves and discard this specimen *so the patient starts the collection period with an empty bladder.*
● If ordered, administer a challenge dose of medication (such as glucose solution or corticotropin), and record the time.
● If possible, offer the patient a glass of water at least every hour during the collection period *to stimulate urine production.* After each voiding, don gloves and add the specimen to the collection bottle.
● Instruct the patient to void about 15 minutes before the end of the collection period, if possible, and add this specimen to the collection bottle.
● At the end of the collection period, remove and discard gloves and send the appropriately labeled collection bottle to the laboratory immediately, along with a properly completed laboratory request form.

For 12- and 24-hour collection
● Put on gloves and ask the patient to void. Then discard this urine *so he starts the collection period with an empty bladder.* Record the time.
● After putting on gloves and pouring the first urine specimen into the collection bottle, add the required preservative. Then refrigerate the bottle or keep it on ice until the next voiding, as appropriate.
● Collect all urine voided during the prescribed period. Just before the collection period ends, ask the patient to void again, if possible. Add this last specimen to the collection bottle, pack it in ice *to inhibit deterioration of the specimen,* and remove and discard gloves. Send the specimen to the laboratory. Include a properly completed laboratory request form.

Special considerations
The patient should be hydrated before and during the test *to ensure adequate urine flow.*

Before collection of a timed specimen, make sure the laboratory will be open when the collection period ends *to help ensure prompt, accurate results.* Never store a specimen in a refrigerator containing food or medication *to avoid contamination.* If the patient has an indwelling catheter in place, put the collection bag in an ice-filled container at his bedside.

Instruct the patient to avoid exercise, ingestion of coffee or tea, or any drugs (unless otherwise directed by the doctor) before the test *to avoid altering test results.*

If you accidentally discard a specimen during the collection period, restart the collection. Accidentally discarding a specimen during the test period may result in an additional day of hospitalization, possibly causing the patient personal and financial hardship. Therefore, emphasize the need to save all the patient's urine during the collection period to all persons involved in his care, as well as to family or other visitors.

Home care
If the patient must continue collecting urine at home, provide written instructions for the appropriate method. Tell the patient he can keep the specimens in a brown bag in his refrigerator at home, separate from other refrigerator contents.

Documentation
In the Kardex and in your notes, record the date and interval of collection and that the specimen was sent to the laboratory.

 ## Urine glucose and ketone tests

Reagent tablet and strip tests are used to monitor urine glucose and ketone levels and to screen for diabetes. *Urine ketone tests* monitor fat metabolism, help diagnose carbohydrate deprivation and diabetic ketoacidosis, and help distinguish between diabetic and nondiabetic coma. However, urine glucose tests are less accurate than blood glucose tests, and are now used less frequently because of the increasing convenience of blood self-testing.

The *copper reduction test* (Clinitest) measures the concentration of reducing substances in the urine through the reactions of these substances with a tablet composed of sodium hydroxide, cupric sulfate, and other reagents. When this tablet is added to a test tube containing drops of water and urine, the reaction generates heat. Simultaneously, reduction of cupric ions in the presence of glucose causes a color change. Comparison of this test color with a standardized color chart gives the approximate level of urine glucose. Similarly, the Acetest tablet test produces a color reaction that allows an estimate of urine ketone levels by comparison to a standardized chart.

Glucose oxidase tests (such as Diastix, Tes-Tape, and Chemstrip UG strips) produce color changes when patches of reagents implanted in hand-held plastic strips react with glucose in the patient's urine; *urine ketone strip tests* (such as Chemstrip K and Ketostix) are similar. All test results are read by comparing color changes against a standardized reference chart.

Equipment

For reagent tablet tests: specimen container ▪ 10-ml test tube ▪ medicine dropper ▪ gloves ▪ Clinitest or Acetest tablets ▪ Clinitest or Acetest color chart.

For reagent strip tests: specimen container ▪ gloves ▪ glucose or ketone test strips ▪ reference color chart.

Wear gloves as barrier protection when performing all urine tests.

Implementation

• Explain the test to the patient, and if he's a newly diagnosed diabetic, teach him to perform the test himself. Check his history for medications that may interfere with test results.

• Before each test, instruct the patient not to contaminate the urine specimen with stool or toilet tissue.

• Test the urine specimen immediately after the patient voids.

Clinitest tablet test

• Ask the patient to void, and then ask him to drink a glass of water, if possible. Don gloves and collect a second-voided urine specimen 30 to 45 minutes later.

• Perform the 5-drop test: With the medicine dropper, transfer 5 drops of urine from the specimen container to the test tube. Rinse the dropper and add 10 drops of water to the test tube. Then add one Clinitest tablet to the tube.

• Hold the test tube near the top during the reaction *because the test solution will come to a boil.* Observe the color change that occurs during the reaction.

• Fifteen seconds after effervescence subsides, shake the tube gently. Observe the solution's color and compare it with the Clinitest color chart.

• Remove and discard gloves, and record the test results. Ignore any changes that develop after 15 seconds.

• If the color changes rapidly in the 5-drop test, record the result as "over 2%" glucosuria.

• Alternately, perform the 2-drop test: Transfer 2 drops of urine from the specimen container to the test tube, and then add 10 drops of water and a Clinitest tablet. After the reaction, observe the color of the test solution, and compare it with the Clinitest color chart.

• Remove and discard your gloves, and record the test results.

• Rapid color change in the 2-drop test indicates glycosuria up to 5%.

Acetest tablet test

• Don gloves and collect a second-voided specimen, as for the Clinitest tablet test.

• Place the Acetest tablet on a piece of white paper, and add 1 drop of urine to the tablet.

• After 30 seconds, compare the tablet's color (white, lavender, or purple) with the Acetest color chart. Remove gloves and record the test results.

Glucose oxidase strip tests

• Explain the test to the patient and, if he's diagnosed as diabetic, teach him to perform it himself. Check his history for medications that may interfere with test results. Don gloves before collecting specimens for each of these tests, and remove them to record test results.

• Instruct the patient to void. Ask him to drink a glass of water, if possible, and collect a second-voided specimen after 30 to 45 minutes.

• If you're using Clinistix, dip the reagent end of the strip into the urine for 2 seconds. Remove excess urine by tapping the strip against the container's rim, wait for exactly 10 seconds, and then compare its color with the color chart on the container. Ignore color changes that occur after 10 seconds. Record the result.

• If you're using a Diastix strip, dip the reagent end of the strip into the urine for 2 seconds. Tap off excess urine, wait for exactly 30 seconds, and then compare its color with the standardized color chart on the container. Ignore color changes that occur after 30 seconds. Record the result.

• If you're using a Tes-Tape strip, pull about 1½″ (3.8 cm) of the reagent strip from the dispenser, and dip one end about ¼″ (0.6 cm) into the specimen for 2 seconds. Tap off excess urine, wait exactly 60 seconds, and then compare the darkest part of the tape with the standardized color chart. If the test result exceeds 0.5%, wait an additional 60 seconds and make a final comparison. Record the result.

Ketone strip tests

• Explain the procedure to the patient, and if he's diagnosed as diabetic, teach him to perform the test. Check his medication history. If he's receiving phenazopyridine or levodopa, use Acetest tablets instead *because reagent strips will give inaccurate results.*

• Don gloves and collect a second-voided midstream specimen.

• If you're using Ketostix, dip the reagent end of the strip into the specimen and remove it immediately. Wait exactly 15 seconds, and then compare the color of the strip with the standardized color chart on the container. Ignore color changes that occur after 15 seconds. Record the result.

• If you're using Keto-Diastix, dip the reagent end of the strip into the specimen and remove it immediately. Tap off excess urine, and hold the strip horizontally *to prevent mixing of chemicals between the two reagent squares.* Wait exactly 15 seconds, and then compare the color of the ketone part of the strip with the standardized color chart. After 30 seconds, compare the color of the glucose part of the strip with the chart. Record the results.

Special considerations
Keep reagent strips in a cool, dry place at a temperature below 86° F (30° C), but don't refrigerate them. Keep the containers tightly closed. Don't use discolored or outdated strips.

♦ *Nursing alert.* Because Clinitest tablets contain caustic soda, keep the container tightly closed and in a dry place. If you must handle these tablets, keep your fingers dry *to prevent the tablet from leaving a deposit, which could then be accidentally ingested or brought into contact with eyes, skin, mucous membranes, or clothing, causing caustic burns.* ♦

Documentation
In your notes, record color changes according to the information on the charts on the reagent containers, or use special flowcharts designed to record this information. If you're teaching a patient how to perform the test, keep a record of his progress.

Urine specific gravity

The kidneys maintain homeostasis by varying urine output and its concentration of dissolved salts. Urine specific gravity measures the concentration of urine solutes, which reflects the kidneys' capacity to concentrate urine. The capacity to concentrate urine is among the first functions lost when renal tubular damage occurs.

Urine specific gravity is determined by comparing the weight of a urine specimen with that of an equivalent volume of distilled water, which is 1.000. Because urine contains dissolved salts and other substances, it's heavier than 1.000. Urine specific gravity ranges from 1.003 (very dilute) to 1.035 (highly concentrated); normal values range from 1.010 to 1.025. Specific gravity is commonly measured with a urinometer (a specially calibrated hydrometer designed to float in a cylinder of urine.) The more concentrated the urine, the higher the urinometer floats—and the higher the specific gravity. It may also be measured by a refractometer, which measures the re-

fraction of light as it passes through a urine sample, or by a reagent strip test.

Elevated specific gravity reflects an increased concentration of urine solutes, which occurs in conditions causing renal hypoperfusion, and may indicate congestive heart failure, dehydration, hepatic disorders, or nephrosis. Low specific gravity reflects failure to reabsorb water and concentrate urine; it may indicate hypercalcemia, hypokalemia, alkalosis, acute renal failure, pyelonephritis, glomerulonephritis, or diabetes insipidus.

Although urine specific gravity is commonly measured with a random urine specimen, more accurate measurement is possible with a controlled specimen collected after fluids are withheld for 12 to 24 hours.

Equipment
Calibrated urinometer and cylinder, refractometer, or reagent strips (Multistix) ■ gloves ■ graduated specimen container.

Implementation
• Explain the procedure to the patient, and tell him when you will need the specimen. Explain why you're withholding fluids and for how long *to ensure his cooperation.*

Measuring with a urinometer
• Don gloves and collect a random urine specimen. Allow it to come to room temperature (71.6° F [22° C]) before testing *because this is the temperature at which most urinometers are calibrated.*
• Fill the cylinder about three-fourths full of urine. Then, gently spin the urinometer and drop it into the cylinder.
• When the urinometer stops bobbing, read the specific gravity from the calibrated scale marked directly on the stem of the urinometer. Make sure the instrument floats freely and doesn't touch the sides of the cylinder. Read the scale at the lowest point of the meniscus *to ensure an accurate reading.* (For specific instructions, see *Using a urinometer.*)
• Discard the urine, and rinse the cylinder and urinometer in cool water. *Warm water coagulates proteins in urine, making them stick to the instrument.*
• Remove gloves and wash your hands thoroughly *to prevent cross-contamination.*

Measuring with a refractometer
• Don gloves and collect a random or controlled urine specimen.
• Place a single drop of urine on the refractometer slide.
• Turn on the light and look through the eyepiece, where you will see the specific gravity indicated on a scale. (Some instruments use a digital display.)

Measuring with a reagent strip

• Don gloves and obtain a random or controlled urine specimen.

• Dip the reagent end of the test strip into the specimen for 2 seconds.

• Tap the strip on the rim of the specimen container *to remove excess urine,* and compare the resultant color change with the color chart supplied with the kit.

Special considerations

Test the urinometer in distilled water at room temperature *to check that its calibration is 1.000.* If necessary, correct the urinometer reading for temperature effects; add 0.001 to your observed reading for every 5.4° F (3° C) above the calibration temperature of 71.6° F (22° C); subtract 0.001 for every 5.4° F below 71.6° F.

Documentation

Record the specific gravity, volume, color, odor, and appearance of the collected urine specimen.

Urine pH

The pH of urine—its alkalinity or acidity—reflects the ability of the kidneys to maintain a normal hydrogen ion concentration in plasma and extracellular fluids. The normal hydrogen ion concentration in urine varies, ranging from pH 4.6 to 8.0, but it usually averages around pH 6.0.

The simplest procedure for testing the pH of urine consists of dipping a reagent strip (such as a Combistix) into a fresh specimen of the patient's urine and comparing the resultant color change with a standardized color chart.

An alkaline pH (above 7.0), resulting from a diet low in meat but high in vegetables, dairy products, and citrus fruits, causes turbidity and formation of phosphate, carbonate, and amorphous crystals. Alkaline urine may also result from urinary tract infection and from metabolic or respiratory alkalosis.

An acid pH (below 7.0), resulting from a high-protein diet, also causes turbidity, with formation of oxalate, cystine, amorphous urate, and uric acid crystals. Acid urine may also result from renal tuberculosis, phenylketonuria, alkaptonuria, pyrexia, diarrhea, starvation, and all forms of acidosis.

Measuring urine pH can also help monitor some medications, such as methenamine, that are active only at certain pH levels.

Using a urinometer

With the urinometer floating in a cylinder of urine, position your eye at a level even with the bottom of the meniscus and read the specific gravity from the scale printed on the urinometer.

Meniscus

Reading level

Specific gravity scale

Urine in cylinder

Hydrometer

Mercury bulb

Equipment

Urine specimen container ▪ gloves ▪ reagent strips ▪ color chart. (The reagent strip has a pH indicator as part of a battery of indicators.)

Implementation

• Wash your hands thoroughly and don gloves.
• Provide the patient with a specimen container, and instruct him to collect a clean-catch midstream specimen (see "Urine collection" in this chapter). Dip the reagent strip into the urine, remove it, and tap off the excess urine from the strip.
• Hold the strip horizontally *to avoid mixing reagents from adjacent test areas on the strip.* Then, compare the color on the strip with the standardized color chart on the strip package. This comparison can be made up to 60 seconds after immersing the strip.
• Discard the urine specimen. If you're monitoring the patient's intake and output, measure the amount of urine discarded.
• Discard gloves and wash your hands thoroughly *to prevent cross-contamination.*

Special considerations

Use only a fresh urine specimen *because bacterial growth at room temperature changes urine pH.* Avoid letting a drop of urine run off the pH reagent onto adjacent reagent spots on the strip *because these other reagents will change the pH result.*

Urine collected at night is usually more acidic than urine collected during the day.

Documentation

Record the test results, the time of voiding, and the amount voided.

Straining urine for calculi

Renal calculi, or kidney stones, may develop anywhere in the urinary tract. They may be excreted with the urine or may become lodged in the urinary tract, causing hematuria, urine retention, renal colic and, possibly, hydronephrosis.

Ranging from microscopic to several centimeters in size, calculi are formed in the kidneys when mineral salts—principally calcium oxalate or calcium phosphate—collect around a nucleus of bacterial cells, blood clots, or other particles. Other substances involved in calculus formation may include uric acid, xanthine, and ammonia.

Renal calculi result from many causes, including hypercalcemia, which may occur with hyperparathyroidism, excessive dietary intake, prolonged immobility, abnormal urine pH levels, dehydration, hyperuricemia associated with gout, and some hereditary disorders. Most commonly, calculi form as a result of urine stasis stemming from dehydration (which concentrates urine), benign prostatic hyperplasia, neurologic disorders, or urethral stricture.

Testing for calculi requires careful straining of *all* the patient's urine through a gauze pad or fine-mesh sieve and, at times, quantitative laboratory analysis of questionable specimens. Such testing typically continues until the patient passes the calculi or until after surgery, as ordered.

Equipment

Fine-mesh sieve or 4″ × 4″ gauze pad ▪ graduated container ▪ urinal or bedpan ▪ gloves ▪ laboratory request form ▪ three patient care reminders ▪ specimen container (for use if calculi are found).

Implementation

• Explain the procedure to the patient and his family, if possible, *to ensure cooperation and to stress the importance of straining all his urine.*
• Post a patient care reminder stating STRAIN ALL URINE over his bed, in his bathroom, and on the collection container.
• Tell the patient to notify you after each voiding.
• If a commercial strainer isn't available, unfold a 4″ × 4″ gauze pad, place it over the top of a graduated measuring container, and secure it with a rubber band.
• Don gloves. With the strainer secured over the mouth of the collection container, pour the specimen through the strainer. If the patient has an indwelling catheter, strain all urine from the collection bag before discarding it.
• Examine the strainer for calculi. If you detect any calculi or if the filtrate looks questionable, notify the doctor, place the filtrate in a specimen container, and send it to the laboratory with a laboratory request form.
• If the strainer is intact, rinse it carefully and reuse it. If it has become damaged, discard it and replace it with a new strainer. Remove and discard gloves.

Special considerations

Save and send to the laboratory any small or suspicious-looking residue left in the specimen container *because even tiny calculi can cause hematuria and pain. Calculi may also appear in various colors, each of which has diagnostic value.*

Home care

If the patient will be straining his urine at home, teach him how to use a strainer and emphasize the importance of straining *all* his urine for the prescribed period.

Documentation

Chart the times of specimen collection and transport to the laboratory, if necessary. Describe any filtrate passed, and note any pain or hematuria that occurred during voiding.

STOOL SPECIMENS
Stool collection

Stool is collected to determine the presence of blood, ova and parasites, bile, fat, pathogens, or such substances as ingested drugs. Gross examination of stool characteristics, such as color, consistency, and odor, can reveal such conditions as GI bleeding and steatorrhea. Stool specimens are collected randomly or for specific periods, such as 72 hours. Because stool specimens can't be obtained on demand, their proper collection necessitates careful instructions to the patient to ensure an uncontaminated specimen.

Equipment

Specimen container with lid ■ two tongue blades ■ paper towel or paper bag ■ bedpan or portable commode ■ two patient care reminders (for timed specimens) ■ laboratory request form ■ gloves.

Implementation

• Explain the procedure to the patient and to family members, if possible, *to ensure their cooperation and prevent inadvertent disposal of timed stool specimens.*

Collecting a random specimen

• Tell the patient to notify you when he has the urge to defecate. Have him defecate into a clean, dry bedpan or commode. Instruct him not to contaminate the specimen with urine or toilet tissue *because urine inhibits fecal bacterial growth and toilet tissue contains bismuth, which interferes with test results.*
• Don gloves.
• Using a tongue blade, transfer the most representative stool specimen from the bedpan to the container, and cap the container. If the patient passes blood, mucus, or pus with the stool, be sure to include this with the specimen.

• Wrap the tongue blade in a paper towel and discard it. Remove your gloves, and wash your hands thoroughly *to prevent cross-contamination.*
• Label the specimen container with the patient's name and room number and the date and time of collection. Send it to the laboratory with a laboratory request form immediately *because a fresh specimen provides the most accurate results.* Refrigerate the specimen if it can't be transported to the laboratory immediately. *Note:* Some pathogens are killed by refrigeration. (Do not refrigerate stool collected to confirm the presence of ova and parasites; such a specimen must be examined immediately or discarded.)

Collecting a timed specimen

• Place a patient care reminder stating SAVE ALL STOOL over the patient's bed, in his bathroom, and in the utility room.
• After donning gloves, collect the first defecation, and include this in the total specimen.
• Obtain the timed specimen as you would a random specimen, but remember to transfer all stool to the specimen container.
• If stool must be obtained with an enema, use only tap water or normal saline solution.
• As ordered, send each specimen to the laboratory immediately with a laboratory request form or, if permitted, refrigerate the specimens collected during the test period and send them when collection is complete. Remove and discard gloves.
• Make sure the patient is comfortable after the procedure and that he has the opportunity to thoroughly clean his hands and perianal area. Perineal care may be necessary for some patients.

Special considerations

Never place a stool specimen in a refrigerator that contains food or medication *to prevent contamination.* Notify your nurse manager or the doctor if the stool appears unusual.

Home care

If the patient is to collect a specimen at home, instruct him to collect it in a clean container with a tight-fitting lid, wrap the container in a brown paper bag, and keep it in the refrigerator (separate from any food items) until it can be transported.

Documentation

Record the time of specimen collection and transport to the laboratory. Note stool color, odor, consistency, and any unusual characteristics; also note if the patient had difficulty passing the stool.

Fecal occult blood tests

Fecal occult blood tests are valuable for determining the presence of occult blood (hidden GI bleeding) and for distinguishing between true melena and melena-like stools. Certain medications, such as iron supplements and bismuth compounds, can darken stools so that they resemble melena.

Two common occult blood screening tests are Hematest (an orthotolidin reagent tablet) and the Hemoccult slide (filter paper impregnated with guaiac). Both tests produce a blue reaction in a fecal smear if occult blood loss exceeds 5 ml in 24 hours. A newer test, Colocare, requires no fecal smear.

Occult blood tests are particularly important for early detection of colorectal cancer because 80% of patients with this disorder test positive. However, a single positive test result does not necessarily confirm GI bleeding or indicate colorectal cancer. For a confirmed positive result, the test must be repeated at least three times while the patient follows a meatless, high-residue diet. Still, a confirmed positive test doesn't necessarily indicate colorectal cancer. It does indicate the need for further diagnostic studies; GI bleeding can result from many causes other than cancer, such as ulcers and diverticula. These tests are easily performed on collected specimens or smears from digital rectal examination.

Equipment
Test kit ▪ glass or porcelain plate ▪ tongue blade or other wooden applicator ▪ gloves.

Implementation
● Put on gloves and collect a stool specimen.

Hematest reagent tablet test
● Use a wooden applicator to smear a bit of the stool specimen on the filter paper supplied with the kit. Or, after performing a digital rectal examination, wipe the finger you used for examination on a square of the filter paper.
● Place the filter paper with the stool smear on a glass plate.
● Remove a reagent tablet from the bottle, and immediately replace the cap tightly. Then, place the tablet in the center of the stool smear on the filter paper.
● Add one drop of water to the tablet, and allow it to soak in for 5 to 10 seconds. Add a second drop, letting it run from the tablet onto the specimen and filter paper. If necessary, tap the plate gently to dislodge any water from the top of the tablet.
● After 2 minutes, the filter paper will turn blue if the test is positive. Do not read the color that appears on the tablet itself or develops on the filter paper after the 2-minute period.
● Note the results, and discard the filter paper.
● Remove and discard your gloves, and wash your hands thoroughly.

Hemoccult slide test
● Open the flap on the slide packet, and use a wooden applicator to apply a thin smear of the stool specimen to the guaiac-impregnated filter paper exposed in box A. Or, after performing a digital rectal examination, wipe the finger you used for examination on a square of the filter paper.

Home tests for fecal occult blood

Most fecal occult blood tests require the patient to collect a sample of his stool and smear some of it on a slide. In contrast, some new tests don't require the patient to handle stool, making the procedure safer and simpler. One example is a test called Colocare.

If the patient will perform the Colocare test at home, tell him to avoid red meat and vitamin C supplements for 2 days before the test. He should check with his doctor about discontinuing any medications before the test. Some drugs that may interfere with test results include aspirin, indomethacin, corticosteroids, phenylbutazone, reserpine, dietary supplements, anticancer drugs, and anticoagulants.

Tell the patient to flush the toilet twice just before performing the test to remove any toilet-cleaning chemicals from the tank. Tell him to defecate into the toilet but to throw no toilet paper into the bowl. Within 5 minutes, he should remove the test pad from its pouch and float it printed side up on the surface of the water. Tell him to watch the pad for 15 to 30 seconds for any evidence of blue or green color changes, and have him record the result on the reply card.

Emphasize that he should perform this test with three consecutive bowel movements and then send the completed card to his doctor. However, he should call his doctor immediately if he notes a positive color change in the first test.

• Apply a second smear from another part of the specimen to the filter paper exposed in box B *because some parts of the specimen may not contain blood.*
• Open the flap at the rear of the slide package, and place 2 drops of Hemoccult developing solution on the paper over each smear. A blue reaction will appear in 30 to 60 seconds if the test is positive.
• Record the results of the test and discard the slide package.
• Remove and discard your gloves, and wash your hands thoroughly.

Special considerations

Make sure stool specimens aren't contaminated with urine, soap solution, or toilet tissue, and test them as soon as possible after collection.

Test samples from several different portions of the same specimen *because occult blood from the upper GI tract isn't always evenly dispersed throughout the formed stool; likewise, blood from colorectal bleeding may occur mostly on the outer stool surface.*

Check the condition of the reagent tablets and note their expiration date. Use only fresh tablets and discard outdated ones. Protect Hematest tablets from moisture, heat, and light.

If repeated testing is necessary after a positive screening test, explain the test to the patient. Instruct him to maintain a high-fiber diet and to refrain from eating red meat, poultry, fish, turnips, and horseradish for 48 to 72 hours before the test as well as throughout the collection period *because these substances may alter test results.*

As ordered, have the patient discontinue use of iron preparations, bromides, iodides, rauwolfia derivatives, indomethacin, colchicine, salicylates, potassium, phenylbutazone, oxyphenbutazone, bismuth compounds, steroids, and ascorbic acid for 48 to 72 hours before the test and during it *to ensure accurate test results and to avoid possible bleeding that some of these compounds may cause.*

Home care

If the patient will be using the Hemoccult slide packet at home, advise him to complete the label on the slide packet before specimen collection. If he'll be using a Colocare test packet, advise him that this test is a preliminary screen for occult blood in his stool. Tell him he won't have to obtain a stool specimen to perform the test, but that he should follow your instructions carefully. (See *Home tests for fecal occult blood.*)

Documentation

Record the time and date of the test, the result, and any unusual characteristics of the stool tested. Report positive results to the doctor.

OTHER SPECIMENS
Sputum collection

Secreted by mucous membranes lining the bronchioles, bronchi, and trachea, sputum helps protect the respiratory tract from infection. When expelled from the respiratory tract, sputum carries with it saliva, nasal and sinus secretions, dead cells, and normal oral bacteria. Sputum specimens may be cultured for identification of respiratory pathogens.

The usual method of sputum specimen collection is expectoration, which may require ultrasonic nebulization, hydration, or chest percussion and postural drainage. Less common methods include tracheal suctioning and, rarely, bronchoscopy. Tracheal suctioning is contraindicated within 1 hour of eating and in patients with esophageal varices, nausea, facial or basilar skull fractures, laryngospasm, or bronchospasm. It should be performed cautiously in patients with cardiac disease, because it may precipitate cardiac arrhythmias.

Equipment

For expectoration: sterile specimen container with tight-fitting cap ▪ label ▪ laboratory request form ▪ aerosol (10% sodium chloride, propylene glycol, acetylcysteine, or sterile or distilled water) to induce coughing, as ordered ▪ facial tissues ▪ emesis basin ▪ gloves, if necessary.

For tracheal suctioning: #12 to #14 French sterile suction catheter ▪ water-soluble lubricant ▪ laboratory request form ▪ sterile gloves ▪ sterile in-line specimen trap (Lukens trap) ▪ 3-ml syringe, if necessary ▪ normal saline solution ▪ portable suction machine, if wall unit is unavailable ▪ oxygen therapy equipment. ▪ optional: nasal airway, to obtain a nasotracheal specimen with suctioning, if needed. (Commercial suction kits are available containing all equipment except the suction machine and an in-line specimen container.)

Implementation

• Tell the patient you will collect a specimen of sputum (not saliva), and explain the procedure *to ease his anxiety and promote cooperation.* If possible, collect the specimen early in the morning, before breakfast, *to obtain an overnight accumulation of secretions.*

Attaching a specimen trap to a suction catheter

Wearing gloves, push the suction tubing onto the male adapter of the in-line trap.

Insert the suction catheter into the rubber tubing of the trap.

After suctioning, disconnect the in-line trap from the suction tubing and catheter. To seal the container, connect the rubber tubing to the male adapter of the trap.

Suction tubing

Suction catheter

Collecting sputum by expectoration

• Instruct the patient to sit on a chair or at the edge of the bed. If he can't sit up, place him in high Fowler's position.
• Ask the patient to rinse his mouth with water *to reduce specimen contamination by oral bacteria and food particles.* (Avoid mouthwash or toothpaste *because they may affect the mobility of organisms in the sputum sample.*) Then tell him to cough deeply and expectorate directly into the specimen container. Ask him to produce at least 15 ml of sputum, if possible.
• Put on gloves.
• Cap the container and, if necessary, clean its exterior *to prevent cross-contamination.* Label the container with the patient's name and room number, the doctor's name, ⁀e and time of collection, and initial diagnosis. Also ⁀e on the laboratory request form whether the pa- febrile or was taking antibiotics, and whether ⁀ induced *(because such specimens commonly ⁀d may resemble saliva).* Send the specimen ⁀mmediately.

Collecting sputum by tracheal suctioning

• If the patient can't produce an adequate specimen by coughing, prepare to suction him to obtain the specimen. Explain the suctioning procedure to him and tell him that he may cough, gag, or feel short of breath during the procedure.
• Check the suction machine to be sure it's functioning properly. Then, place the patient in a high or semi-Fowler's position.
• Administer oxygen to the patient before beginning the procedure.
• Wash your hands thoroughly.
• Put on sterile gloves. Consider one hand sterile and the other hand clean *to prevent cross-contamination.*
• Connect the suction tubing to the male adapter of the in-line trap. Attach the sterile suction catheter to the rubber tubing of the trap. (See *Attaching a specimen trap to a suction catheter.*)
• Position a mask over your face *because the patient may cough violently during suctioning.* Tell the patient to tilt his head back slightly. Then lubricate the catheter with

normal saline solution, and gently pass it through the patient's nostril without suction.
• When the catheter reaches the larynx, the patient will cough. As he does, quickly advance the catheter into the trachea. Tell the patient to take several deep breaths through his mouth *to help ease insertion.*
• To obtain the specimen, apply suction for 5 to 10 seconds but never longer than 15 seconds *because prolonged suctioning can cause hypoxia.* If the procedure must be repeated, let the patient rest for four to six breaths. When collection is completed, discontinue the suction, gently remove the catheter, and administer oxygen.
• Detach the catheter from the in-line trap, gather it up in your dominant hand, and pull the glove cuff inside out and down around the used catheter to enclose it for disposal. Remove and discard the other glove and your mask.
• Detach the trap from the tubing connected to the suction machine. Seal the trap tightly by connecting the rubber tubing to the male adapter of the trap. Label the trap's container as an expectorated specimen, and send it to the laboratory immediately with a completed laboratory request form.
• Offer the patient a glass of water or mouthwash.

Special considerations
If you cannot obtain a sputum specimen through tracheal suctioning, perform chest percussion *to loosen and mobilize secretions,* and position the patient for optimal drainage. After 20 to 30 minutes, repeat the tracheal suctioning procedure.

Before sending the specimen to the laboratory, examine it to make sure it is actually sputum, not saliva, *because saliva will produce inaccurate test results.*

Because expectorated sputum is contaminated by normal mouth flora, tracheal suctioning provides a more reliable specimen for diagnosis.

If the patient becomes hypoxic or cyanotic during suctioning, remove the catheter immediately and administer oxygen.

If the patient has asthma or chronic bronchitis, watch for aggravated bronchospasms with use of more than a 10% concentration of sodium chloride or acetylcysteine in an aerosol. If he has suspected tuberculosis, don't use more than 20% propylene glycol with water when inducing a sputum specimen *because a higher concentration inhibits growth of the pathogen and causes erroneous test results.* If propylene glycol isn't available, use 10% to 20% acetylcysteine with water or sodium chloride.

Complications
Patients with cardiac disease may develop arrhythmias during the procedure as a result of coughing, especially when the specimen is obtained by suctioning.

Other complications may include tracheal trauma or bleeding, vomiting, aspiration, and hypoxemia.

Documentation
In your notes, record the method used to obtain the specimen, the time and date of collection, how the patient tolerated the procedure, the color and consistency of the specimen, and its proper disposition.

 # Lumbar puncture

This procedure involves insertion of a sterile needle into the subarachnoid space of the spinal canal, usually between the third and fourth lumbar vertebrae. The procedure may be performed for several reasons: to detect increased intracranial pressure (ICP) or the presence of blood in cerebrospinal fluid (CSF), which indicates cerebral hemorrhage; to obtain CSF specimens for laboratory analysis; or to inject dyes or gases for contrast in radiologic studies of the brain and spinal cord. Lumbar puncture is also used therapeutically to administer drugs or anesthetics and to relieve ICP by removing CSF.

Performed by a doctor with a nurse assisting, lumbar puncture requires sterile technique and careful patient positioning. This procedure is contraindicated in patients with lumbar deformity or infection at the puncture site. It should be performed cautiously in patients with increased ICP, because the rapid reduction in pressure that follows withdrawal of fluid can cause tonsillar herniation and medullary compression.

Equipment
Overbed table ■ one or two pairs of sterile gloves for the doctor ■ sterile gloves for the nurse ■ povidone-iodine solution ■ sterile gauze pads ■ alcohol sponges ■ sterile fenestrated drape ■ 3-ml syringe for local anesthetic ■ 25G ¾″ sterile needle for injecting anesthetic ■ local anesthetic (usually 1% lidocaine) ■ 18G or 20G 3½″ spinal needle with stylet (22G needle for children) ■ three-way stopcock ■ manometer ■ small adhesive bandage ■ three sterile collection tubes with stoppers ■ laboratory request forms ■ labels ■ light source, such as a gooseneck lamp.

Disposable lumbar puncture trays containing most of the needed sterile equipment are generally available.

Implementation
• Explain the procedure to the patient *to ease his anxiety and ensure cooperation.* Be sure a consent form has been signed.

Positioning for lumbar puncture

Have the patient lie on his side at the edge of the bed, with his chin tucked to his chest and his knees drawn up to his abdomen. Make sure the patient's spine is curved and his back is at the edge of the bed, as shown here. This position widens the spaces between the vertebrae, easing insertion of the needle.

To help the patient maintain this position, place one of your hands behind his neck and the other hand behind his knees, and pull gently. Hold the patient firmly in this position throughout the procedure to prevent accidental needle displacement.

Patient positioning

Typically, the doctor inserts the needle between the third and fourth lumbar vertebrae, as shown here.

Needle insertion

Third lumbar vertebra

Fourth lumbar vertebra

Subarachnoid space

• Inform the patient that he may experience headache after lumbar puncture, but reassure him that his cooperation during the procedure minimizes such an effect. (*Note:* Sedatives and analgesics are usually withheld before this test if there is evidence of a central nervous system disorder *because they may mask important symptoms.*)
• Immediately before the procedure, provide privacy and instruct the patient to void.
• Wash your hands thoroughly.
• Open the equipment tray on an overbed table, being careful not to contaminate the sterile field when you open the wrapper.
• Provide adequate lighting at the puncture site, and adjust the height of the patient's bed *to allow the doctor to perform the procedure comfortably.*
• Position the patient (see *Positioning for lumbar puncture*), and reemphasize the importance of remaining as still as possible *to minimize discomfort and trauma.*
• The doctor cleans the puncture site with sterile gauze pads soaked in povidone-iodine solution, wiping in a circular motion away from the puncture site; he uses three different pads *to prevent contamination of spinal tissues by the body's normal skin flora.* After allowing the skin to dry, he may wipe the area in a similar manner with alcohol sponges *to improve his view of the puncture site.* Next, he drapes the area with the fenestrated drape *to provide a sterile field.* (If the doctor uses povidone-iodine sponges instead of sterile gauze pads, he may remove his sterile gloves and put on another pair *to avoid introducing povidone-iodine into the subarachnoid space with the lumbar puncture needle.*)
• If there is no ampule of anesthetic on the equipment tray, clean the injection port of a multidose vial of anesthetic with an alcohol sponge. Then invert the vial 45 degrees so the doctor can insert a 25G needle and syringe and withdraw the anesthetic for injection.
• Before the doctor injects the anesthetic, tell the patient he'll experience a transient burning sensation and local pain. Ask him to report any other persistent pain or sensations *because these may indicate irritation or puncture of a nerve root, requiring repositioning of the needle.*
• When the doctor inserts the sterile spinal needle into the subarachnoid space between the third and fourth lumbar vertebrae, instruct the patient to remain still and breathe normally. If necessary, hold the patient firmly in position *to prevent sudden movement that may displace the needle.*
• If a lumbar puncture is being performed to administer contrast media for radiologic studies or spinal anesthetic, the doctor injects the dye or anesthetic at this time.
• When the needle is in place, the doctor attaches a manometer with a three-way stopcock to the needle hub

to read CSF pressure. If ordered, help the patient extend his legs *to provide a more accurate pressure reading.*

• The doctor then detaches the manometer and allows fluid to drain from the needle hub into the collection tubes. When he has collected approximately 2 or 3 ml in each tube, mark the tubes in sequence, stopper them securely, and label them properly.

• If the doctor suspects an obstruction in the spinal subarachnoid space, he may check for Queckenstedt's sign. He first takes an initial CSF pressure reading. Then, as ordered, compress the patient's jugular vein for 10 seconds. *This temporarily obstructs blood flow from the cranium, increasing ICP and—if no subarachnoid block exists—causes CSF pressure to rise as well.* The doctor then takes pressure readings every 10 seconds until the pressure stabilizes.

• After the doctor collects the specimens and removes the spinal needle, clean the puncture site with povidone-iodine and apply a small adhesive bandage.

• Send the CSF specimens to the laboratory immediately, with properly completed laboratory request forms.

Special considerations

During lumbar puncture, watch closely for signs of adverse reaction: elevated pulse rate, pallor, or clammy skin. Alert the doctor immediately to any significant changes.

The patient may be ordered to lie flat for 8 to 12 hours after the procedure. If necessary, place a patient care reminder on his bed to this effect.

Collected CSF specimens must be sent to the laboratory immediately; they cannot be refrigerated for later transport.

Complications

Headache is the most common adverse effect of lumbar puncture. Others may include a reaction to the anesthetic, meningitis, epidural or subdural abscess, bleeding into the spinal canal, CSF leakage through the dural defect remaining after needle withdrawal, local pain caused by nerve root irritation, edema or hematoma at the puncture site, transient difficulty in voiding, and fever. The most serious complications of lumbar puncture, although rare, are tonsillar herniation and medullary compression.

Documentation

Record the initiation and completion times of the procedure, the patient's response, the administration of drugs, the number of specimen tubes collected, the time of transport to the laboratory, and the color, consistency, and any other characteristics of the collected specimens.

 # Papanicolaou test

Also known as the Pap test or Pap smear, this cytologic test developed in the 1920s by George N. Papanicolaou allows early detection of cervical cancer. The test involves scraping secretions from the cervix, spreading them on a slide, and immediately coating the slide with fixative spray or solution to preserve specimen cells for nuclear staining. Cytologic evaluation then outlines cell maturity, morphology, and metabolic activity. Although cervical scrapings are the most common test specimen, the Pap test also permits cytologic evaluation of the vaginal pool, prostatic secretions, urine, gastric secretions, cavity fluids, bronchial aspirations, and sputum.

Equipment

Bivalve vaginal speculum ▪ gloves ▪ Pap stick (wooden spatula) ▪ long cotton-tipped applicator ▪ three glass microscope slides ▪ fixative (a commercial spray or 95% ethyl alcohol solution) ▪ adjustable lamp ▪ drape ▪ laboratory request forms.

Preparation of equipment

Select a speculum of the appropriate size and gather the equipment in the examining room. Label the glass slides with the patient's name and "E," "C," and "V" *to differentiate endocervical, cervical, and vaginal specimens.*

Implementation

• Explain the procedure to the patient and wash your hands.

• Instruct the patient to void *to relax the perineal muscles and facilitate bimanual examination of the uterus.*

• Provide privacy and instruct the patient to undress below the waist, but to wear her shoes, if desired, *to cushion her feet against the stirrups.* Then instruct her to sit on the examining table and to drape her genital region.

• Place the patient in the lithotomy position, with her feet in the stirrups and her buttocks extended slightly beyond the edge of the table. Adjust the drape.

• Adjust the lamp *to fully illuminate the genital area.* Then, fold back the corner of the drape *to expose the perineum.*

• If you're performing the procedure, first put on gloves. Then take the speculum in your dominant hand and moisten it with warm water *to ease insertion. Avoid using water-soluble lubricants, which can interfere with accurate laboratory testing.*

• Warn the patient that you're about to touch her *to avoid startling her.* Then, gently separate the labia with the thumb and forefinger of your nondominant hand.

• Instruct the patient to take several deep breaths, and insert the speculum into the vagina. Once it's in place, slowly open the blades *to expose the cervix.* Then lock the blades in place.

• Insert a cotton-tipped applicator through the speculum ⅕″ into the cervical os. Rotate it 360 degrees *to obtain an endocervical specimen.* Then remove the cotton-tipped applicator and gently roll it in a circle across the slide marked "E." Refrain from rubbing the applicator on the slide *to prevent cell destruction.* Immediately place the slide in a fixative solution or spray it with a fixative *to prevent drying of the cells, which interferes with nuclear staining and cytologic interpretation.*

• Insert the small curved end of the Pap stick through the speculum and place it directly over the cervical os. Rotate the stick gently but firmly *to scrape cells loose.* Remove the stick, spread the specimen across the slide marked "C," and fix it immediately, as before.

• Insert the opposite end of the Pap stick or a cotton-tipped applicator through the speculum, and scrape the posterior fornix or vaginal pool—an area that collects cells from the endometrium, vagina, and cervix. Remove the stick or applicator, spread the specimen across the slide marked "V," and fix it immediately.

• Unlock the speculum *to ease removal and avoid accidentally pinching the vaginal wall.* Then withdraw the speculum.

• Remove the gloves from your nondominant hand to perform the bimanual exam, which usually follows the Pap test. Then remove and discard your other glove.

• Gently remove the patient's feet from the stirrups and assist her to a sitting position. Provide privacy for her to dress.

• Fill out the appropriate laboratory request forms, including the date of the patient's last menses.

Special considerations

Many preventable factors can interfere with the Pap test's accuracy, so provide appropriate patient teaching beforehand. For example, use of a vaginal douche in the 48-hour period before specimen collection washes away cellular deposits and prevents adequate sampling. Instillation of vaginal medications in the same period makes cytologic interpretation difficult. Collection of a specimen during menstruation prevents adequate sampling because menstrual flow washes away cells; ideally, such collection should take place 5 to 6 days before menses or 1 week after it. Application of topical antibiotics promotes rapid, heavy shedding of cells and requires postponement of the Pap test for at least 1 month.

If the patient has had a complete hysterectomy, collect test specimens from the vaginal pool and cuff.

Complications

Failure to unlock the speculum blades before removal can pinch vaginal tissue.

Although slight cramping normally accompanies this exam, rough handling of the speculum can cause severe cramping.

Scraping an inflamed cervix with the Pap stick can cause slight bleeding.

Documentation

On the patient's chart, record the date and time of specimen collection, any complications, and the nursing action taken.

 # Swab specimens

Correct collection and handling of swab specimens helps the laboratory staff identify pathogens accurately, with a minimum of contamination from normal bacterial flora. Collection normally involves sampling inflamed tissues and exudates from the throat, nasopharynx, wounds, eye, ear, or rectum with sterile swabs of cotton or other absorbent material. Such swabs are immediately placed in a sterile tube containing a transport medium and, in the case of sampling for anaerobes, an inert gas. These specimens are usually collected to identify pathogens and sometimes to identify asymptomatic carriers of certain easily transmitted disease organisms.

Equipment

For a throat specimen: sterile swab ■ tongue blade ■ sterile culture tube with transport medium (or commercial collection kit) ■ penlight ■ gloves ■ label ■ laboratory request form.

For a nasopharyngeal specimen: sterile, flexible cotton-tipped wire swab ■ gloves ■ tongue blade ■ sterile culture tube with transport medium ■ penlight ■ label ■ laboratory request form ■ optional: small open-ended Pyrex tube or nasal speculum.

For a wound specimen: sterile gloves ■ alcohol or povidone-iodine sponges ■ sterile swabs ■ sterile 10-ml syringe ■ sterile 21G needle ■ sterile forceps ■ sterile culture tube with transport medium (or commercial collection kit for aerobic culture) ■ labels ■ special anaerobic culture tube containing carbon dioxide or nitrogen ■ fresh dressings for the wound ■ laboratory request form ■ optional: rubber stopper for needle.

For an ear specimen: gloves ■ sterile swabs ■ sterile culture tube with transport medium ■ normal saline solution ■ two 2″ × 2″ gauze pads ■ label ■ 10-ml syringe and 22G 1″ needle (for tympanocentesis) ▪ label ▪ laboratory request form.

For an eye specimen: sterile gloves ▪ sterile swabs ▪ sterile wire culture loop (for corneal scraping) ▪ sterile culture tube with transport medium ▪ sterile normal saline solution ▪ two 2″ × 2″ gauze pads ▪ label ▪ laboratory request form.

For a rectal specimen: gloves ▪ sterile swab ▪ soap and water ▪ washcloth ▪ normal saline solution ▪ sterile culture tube with transport medium ▪ label ▪ laboratory request form.

Implementation

● Explain the procedure to the patient *to ease his anxiety and ensure cooperation.*

Collecting a throat specimen

● Tell the patient he may gag during the swabbing but that the procedure takes less than a minute.
● Instruct him to sit erect at the edge of the bed or on a chair, facing you. Wash your hands and don gloves.
● Ask the patient to tilt his head back. Depress his tongue with the tongue blade, and illuminate his throat with the penlight *to check for inflamed areas.*
● If the patient starts to gag, withdraw the tongue blade and tell him to breathe deeply. Once he's relaxed, reinsert the tongue blade but not as deeply as before.
● Using the cotton-tipped wire swab, wipe the tonsillar areas from side to side, including any inflamed or purulent sites. Don't touch the tongue, cheeks, or teeth with the swab *to avoid contaminating it with oral bacteria.*
● Withdraw the swab and immediately place it in the culture tube. If you're using a commercial kit, crush the ampule of culture medium at the bottom of the tube and push the swab into the medium *to keep the swab moist.*
● Discard gloves and wash your hands.
● Label the specimen with the patient's name and room number, the doctor's name, and the date, time, and site of collection. On the laboratory request form, indicate if any organism is strongly suspected, especially *Corynebacterium diphtheriae* (requires two swabs and special growth medium), *Bordetella pertussis* (requires a nasopharyngeal culture and special growth medium), and *Neisseria meningitidis* (requires enriched selective media).
● Send the specimen to the laboratory immediately *to prevent growth or deterioration of microbes.*

Collecting a nasopharyngeal specimen

● Tell the patient he may gag or feel the urge to sneeze during the swabbing but that the procedure takes less than 1 minute.
● Instruct him to sit erect at the edge of the bed or on a chair, facing you. Wash your hands and don gloves.

Obtaining a nasopharyngeal specimen

After you've passed the swab into the nasopharynx, *gently* but quickly rotate the swab to collect the specimen. Then remove the swab, taking care not to injure the nasal mucous membrane.

● Ask him to blow his nose *to clear his nasal passages.* Then check his nostrils for patency with a penlight.
● Tell the patient first to occlude one nostril and then the other as he exhales. Listen for the more patent nostril *because you'll insert the swab through it.*
● Ask the patient to cough *to bring organisms to the nasopharynx for a better specimen.*
● Bend the sterile wire swab in a curve and then open the package without contaminating the swab.
● Ask the patient to tilt his head back, and gently pass the swab through the more patent nostril about 3″ to 4″ (8 to 10 cm) into the nasopharynx, keeping the swab near the septum and the floor of the nose. (See *Obtaining a nasopharyngeal specimen.)* Rotate the swab quickly and remove it.
● Alternatively, depress the patient's tongue with a tongue blade, and pass the bent wire swab up behind the uvula. Rotate the swab and withdraw it.
● Remove the cap from the culture tube, insert the swab, and break off the contaminated end. Close the tube tightly, label it for throat culture, fill out laboratory request form, and send the specimen and form to the laboratory im-

Anaerobic specimen collection

Because most anaerobes die when exposed to oxygen, they must be transported in tubes filled with carbon dioxide or nitrogen. The anaerobic specimen collector shown here includes a rubber-stoppered tube filled with carbon dioxide, a small inner tube, and a swab attached to a plastic plunger.

Before specimen collection, the small inner tube containing the swab is held in place with the rubber stopper (as shown on the left). After collecting the specimen, quickly replace the swab in the inner tube and depress the plunger to separate the inner tube from the stopper (right), forcing it into the larger tube and exposing the specimen to a carbon dioxide-rich environment.

Before   **After**

mediately. If you're collecting the specimen to isolate a possible virus, check with the laboratory for the recommended collection technique.
• Discard gloves and wash your hands.

Collecting a wound specimen
• Wash your hands, prepare a sterile field, and put on sterile gloves. With sterile forceps, remove the dressing to expose the wound. Dispose of the soiled dressings properly.

• Clean the area around the wound with an alcohol or povidone-iodine sponge *to reduce the risk of contaminating the specimen with skin bacteria.* Allow the area to dry.
• For an aerobic culture, use a sterile cotton-tipped swab to collect as much exudate as possible, or insert the swab deeply into the wound and gently rotate it. Remove the swab from the wound and immediately place it in the aerobic culture tube. Send the tube to the laboratory immediately with a completed laboratory request form. Never collect exudate from the skin and then insert the same swab into the wound; *this could contaminate the wound with skin bacteria.*
• For an anaerobic culture, insert the sterile cotton-tipped swab deeply into the wound, rotate it gently, remove it, and immediately place it in the anaerobic culture tube (see *Anaerobic specimen collection).* Or, insert a sterile 10-ml syringe, without a needle, into the wound, and aspirate 1 to 5 ml of exudate into the syringe. Then attach the 21G needle to the syringe, and immediately inject the aspirate into the anaerobic culture tube. If an anaerobic culture tube is unavailable, obtain a rubber stopper, attach the needle to the syringe, gently push all the air out of the syringe by pressing on the plunger. Stick the needle tip into the rubber stopper, and send the syringe of aspirate to the laboratory immediately with a completed laboratory request form.
• Apply a new dressing to the wound. (See Chapter 4, Physical treatments.)

Collecting an ear specimen
• Wash your hands and put on gloves.
• Gently clean excess debris from the patient's ear with normal saline solution and gauze pads.
• Insert the swab into the ear canal, and rotate it gently along the walls of the canal.
• Withdraw the swab, being careful not to touch other surfaces *to prevent contaminating the specimen.*
• Place the swab in the culture tube with transport medium.
• Remove the gloves and dispose of them properly. Wash your hands.
• Label the specimen for culture, complete a laboratory request form, and send the sample to the laboratory immediately.

Collecting a middle ear specimen
• Put on gloves and clean the outer ear with normal saline solution and gauze pads. After the doctor punctures the eardrum with a needle and aspirates fluid into the syringe, replace the cap on the needle, label the syringe, complete a laboratory request form, and send the sample to the laboratory immediately.

Collecting an eye specimen
• Wash your hands and put on sterile gloves.
• Gently clean excess debris from the outside of the eye with normal saline solution and gauze pads, wiping from the inner to the outer canthus.
• Retract the lower eyelid *to expose the conjunctival sac.* Gently rub the sterile swab over the conjunctiva, being careful not to touch other surfaces *to avoid contaminating the specimen.* Hold the swab parallel to the eye, rather than pointed directly at it, *to prevent accidental injury caused by sudden movement.* (If a corneal scraping is required, this procedure is performed by a doctor using a wire culture loop.)
• Immediately place the swab or wire loop in the culture tube with transport medium.
• Remove the gloves and dispose of them properly. Wash your hands.
• Label the specimen for culture, complete a laboratory request form, and send the specimen to the laboratory immediately.

Collecting a rectal specimen
• Wash your hands and put on gloves.
• Clean the area around the patient's anus using a washcloth and soap and water.
• Insert the swab, moistened with normal saline solution or sterile broth medium, through the anus and advance it about ⅜″ (1 cm) for infants or 1½″ (4 cm) for adults. While withdrawing the swab, gently rotate it against the walls of the lower rectum to sample a large area of the rectal mucosa.
• Place the swab in a culture tube with transport medium. Then, label the tube for rectal culture, complete a laboratory request form, and send the specimen to the laboratory immediately.
• Remove your gloves and dispose of them properly. Wash your hands.

Special considerations
Note recent antibiotic therapy on the laboratory request form.

For a nasopharyngeal specimen: Because certain organisms, such as *Corynebacterium diphtheriae* and *Bordetella pertussis,* require special growth media, inform the laboratory if you suspect these are present.

For a wound specimen: Although you would normally clean the area around a wound to prevent contamination by normal skin flora, don't clean a perineal wound with alcohol *to avoid irritating sensitive tissues.* Also make sure antiseptic doesn't enter the wound. *Because most anaerobes are destroyed by oxygen,* place the specimen in the culture tube quickly. Ensure that no air enters the tube

and that the double stoppers on the anaerobic collection tube are secure.

For an ear specimen: Insert the swab into the ear gently. Then rotate it carefully *to avoid damaging the eardrum.* Restrain a child or uncooperative patient *to prevent ear trauma from sudden movement.* When sending a specimen in a syringe to the laboratory, secure its cap.

For an eye specimen: Don't use an antiseptic before culturing *to avoid irritating the eye and inhibiting growth of organisms in culture.* Swab the eye carefully *to avoid corneal irritation or trauma.* If the patient is a child or an uncooperative adult, ask a co-worker to restrain the patient's head *to prevent eye trauma from sudden movement.*

Documentation
Record the time, date, and site of specimen collection and recent or current antibiotic therapy. Note any unusual appearance or odor of the specimen.

Bone marrow aspiration and biopsy

A specimen of bone marrow—the major site of blood cell formation—may be obtained by aspiration or needle biopsy. The procedure allows evaluation of overall blood composition by studying blood elements and precursor cells, as well as abnormal or malignant cells. Such aspiration removes cells through a needle inserted into the marrow cavity of the bone; a biopsy removes a small, solid core of marrow tissue through the needle. Both procedures are usually performed by a doctor, but some hospitals authorize specially trained chemotherapy nurses or nurse clinicians to perform them, with the aid of an assistant.

Aspirates are valuable in diagnosing various disorders and cancers, such as oat cell carcinoma, leukemia, and such lymphomas as Hodgkin's disease. Biopsies are often performed simultaneously to stage the disease and to monitor response to treatment.

Equipment
For aspiration: prepackaged bone marrow set, which includes: povidone-iodine sponges ▪ two sterile drapes (one fenestrated, one plain) ▪ ten 4″×4″ gauze pads ▪ ten 2″×2″ gauze pads ▪ two 12-ml syringes ▪ 22G 1″ or 2″ needle ▪ a scalpel ▪ sedative ▪ specimen containers ▪ bone marrow needle ▪ 70% isopropyl alcohol ▪ 1% lidocaine (unopened bottle) ▪ adhesive tape ▪ sterile gloves ▪ glass slides and cover slips ▪ labels.

Common sites for bone marrow aspiration and biopsy

The *posterior superior iliac crest* is the preferred site for aspiration because it's free of nearby vital organs or vessels. For aspiration of bone marrow from this site, the patient is placed either in the lateral position with one leg flexed or in the prone position.

For aspiration or biopsy from the *anterior iliac crest,* the patient is placed in the supine or side-lying position. This site is used with patients who cannot lie prone because of severe abdominal distention. Aspiration from the *sternum* involves the greatest risk but may be used

because this site is near the surface, the cortical bone is thin, and the marrow cavity contains numerous cells and relatively little fat or supporting bone. The sternum is rarely used for biopsy, however, because of its small size and proximity to vital organs.

Posterior superior iliac crest

Anterior iliac crest

Sternum

For biopsy: all equipment listed above ▪ Vim-Silverman, Jamshidi, Illinois sternal, or Westerman-Jensen needle ▪ Zenker's fixative.

Implementation
● Tell the patient the doctor will collect a bone marrow specimen, and explain the procedure *to ease his anxiety and ensure cooperation.* Make sure the patient or a responsible family member understands the procedure and implications of this test and signs a consent form obtained by the doctor.
● Inform the patient that the procedure normally takes 5 to 10 minutes, that test results usually are available in 1 day, and that more than one marrow specimen may be required.
● Check the patient's history for hypersensitivity to the local anesthetic. Tell him which bone — sternum or posterior superior or anterior iliac crest — will be sampled. Inform him that he will receive a local anesthetic and will feel heavy pressure from insertion of the biopsy or aspiration needle, as well as a brief, pulling sensation on removal of the marrow specimen. Tell him the doctor may make a small incision to avoid tearing the skin.

● If the patient has osteoporosis, tell him needle pressure may be minimal; if he has osteopetrosis, inform him a drill may be needed.
● Provide a sedative, as ordered, before the test.
● Position the patient according to the selected puncture site. (See *Common sites for bone marrow aspiration and biopsy.)*
● Using sterile technique, the puncture site is cleaned with povidone-iodine solution and allowed to dry; then the area is draped.
● To anesthetize the site, the doctor infiltrates it with 1% lidocaine, first injecting a small amount intradermally, and then using a larger 22G 1″ to 2″ needle to anesthetize the tissue down to the bone.
● When the needle tip reaches the bone, the doctor anesthetizes the periosteum by injecting a small amount of lidocaine in a circular area about ¾″ (2 cm) in diameter. The needle should be withdrawn from the periosteum after each injection.
● After allowing about 1 minute for the lidocaine to take effect, a scalpel may be used to make a small stab incision in the patient's skin to accommodate the bone marrow needle. *This technique avoids pushing skin into the bone*

marrow and also helps avoid unnecessary skin tearing to help reduce the risk of infection.

Bone marrow aspiration
• The doctor inserts the bone marrow needle at the selected site and lodges it firmly in the bone cortex. If the patient feels sharp pain instead of pressure when the needle first touches bone, the needle was probably inserted outside the anesthetized area. If this happens, the needle should be withdrawn slightly and moved to the anesthetized area.
• The needle is advanced by applying an even, downward force with the heel of the hand or the palm, while twisting it back and forth slightly. A crackling sensation means the needle has entered the marrow cavity.
• Next, the doctor removes the inner cannula, attaches the syringe to the needle, aspirates the required specimen (usually about 1 ml), and withdraws the needle.
• The nurse dons gloves and applies pressure to the aspiration site with a gauze pad for 5 minutes to control bleeding, while an assistant prepares the marrow slides. The area is then cleaned with alcohol to remove the povidone-iodine, the skin dried thoroughly with a 4″ × 4″ gauze pad, and a sterile pressure dressing applied.

Bone marrow biopsy
• The doctor inserts the biopsy needle into the periosteum and advances it steadily until the outer needle passes through the bone cortex into the marrow cavity.
• The biopsy needle is directed into the marrow cavity by alternately rotating the inner needle clockwise and counterclockwise. Then, a plug of tissue is removed, the needle assembly withdrawn, and the marrow specimen expelled into a properly labeled specimen bottle containing Zenker's fixative or formaldehyde.
• The nurse dons gloves and cleans the area around the biopsy site with alcohol to remove the povidone-iodine solution, firmly presses a sterile 2″ × 2″ gauze pad against the incision to control bleeding, and applies a sterile pressure dressing.

Special considerations
Faulty needle placement may yield too little aspirate. If the procedure fails to produce a specimen, the needle must be withdrawn from the bone (but not from the overlying soft tissue), the stylet replaced, and the needle reinserted into a second site within the anesthetized field.

Bone marrow specimens should not be collected from irradiated areas *because radiation may have altered or destroyed the marrow.*

Complications
Bleeding and infection are potentially life-threatening complications of aspiration or biopsy at any site. Complications of sternal needle puncture are uncommon but include puncture of the heart and major vessels, causing severe hemorrhage; puncture of the mediastinum, causing mediastinitis or pneumomediastinum; and puncture of the lung, causing pneumothorax.

If hematoma occurs around the puncture site, apply warm soaks. Give analgesics for site pain or tenderness.

Documentation
Chart the time, date, location, and patient's tolerance of the procedure and the specimen obtained.

Selected references

Clinical Laboratory Tests: Values and Implications. Springhouse, Pa.: Springhouse Corp., 1991.
DeGroot, K.D., and Damato, M.B. *Critical Care Skills.* Norwalk, Conn.: Appleton & Lange, 1987.
Diagnostic Test Implications. Clinical Skillbuilders. Springhouse, Pa.: Springhouse Corp., 1991.
Illustrated Manual of Nursing Practice. Springhouse, Pa.: Springhouse Corp., 1991.
Kee, J.L. *Laboratory and Diagnostic Tests with Nursing Implications,* 3rd ed. Norwalk, Conn.: Appleton & Lange, 1991.
Kinkade, S.L., and Lohrman, J. *Critical Care Nursing Procedures.* Philadelphia: B.C. Decker, Inc., 1990.
Kinney, M.R., et al. *AACN's Clinical Reference for Critical Care Nursing,* 2nd ed. New York: McGraw-Hill Book Co., 1988.
Luckmann, J., and Sorensen, K. *Medical-Surgical Nursing,* 3rd ed. Philadelphia: W.B. Saunders Co., 1987.
Oski, F.A. *Principles and Practices of Pediatrics.* Philadelphia: J.B. Lippincott Co., 1990.
Persons, C. *Critical Care Procedures and Protocols: A Nursing Process Approach.* Philadelphia: J.B. Lippincott Co., 1987.
Ryan, et al. *Kistner's Gynecology,* 5th ed. St. Louis: Mosby-Year Book, Inc., 1990.
Scott, J.R., et al. *Danforth's Obstetrics & Gynecology,* 6th ed. Philadelphia: J.B. Lippincott Co., 1990.
Tietz, N.W. *Clinical Guide to Laboratory Tests,* 2nd ed. Philadelphia: W.B. Saunders Co., 1990.

CHAPTER 4

PHYSICAL TREATMENTS

KATHLEEN MALLOCH, RN, BS, MBA, CNA

Introduction

Used effectively for centuries, many physical treatments have become fundamental nursing procedures. The principles behind such treatments as application of heat and cold—and often the techniques for performing them—remain essentially unchanged. But that doesn't make them any less important than more involved or specialized procedures created by new, high-tech medical treatments. In fact, physical treatments that many nurses might consider routine are those most responsible for maintaining patient comfort, decreasing anxiety, and reducing the risk of infection.

Proven effective

Most physical treatments have endured procedurally intact because of their effectiveness. Some treatments stimulate or support normal physiologic processes. For example, application of heat enhances healing because the warmth causes vasodilation, thereby increasing blood supply to the affected area and making more nutrients available for tissue growth. Antiembolism stockings support blood vessels, increasing venous return and thereby reducing the risk of deep vein thrombosis. Drains allow wound secretions to escape to the surface from underlying tissue, thus assisting the healing process.

Other physical treatments prevent a pathologic response or inhibit a full-blown response. For example, cold application produces vasoconstriction and increases blood viscosity, thereby reducing inflammation, bleeding, and localized tissue edema. Medicated baths relieve itching and reduce the irritation caused by various skin disorders. Wound irrigation performed with an antiseptic solution inhibits bacterial growth. And radiation treatments inhibit or destroy cancerous cells, offering patients palliation, control, or a cure. In all of these instances, nursing assessment and interventions are essential to the success of physical treatments.

Advances in equipment

Improvements in physical treatments have resulted in part from equipment advances. For example, single-use or single-patient disposable products have heightened efficiency and safety. Hot-water bottles and ice collars, sterile gauze dressings, presaturated sterile swabs, and aquamatic K pads are all available for single use. The number and types of disposable items and the variety of prepackaged procedure setup trays available continue to expand. One of the latest such products is the single-patient hyperthermia-hypothermia blanket. This disposable, lightweight vinyl blanket connects to a conventional control module for use both under and over the patient.

A portable fiberglass tub makes it possible to bathe rather than sponge patients on bed rest. The full-sized tub stands as high as the bed, rolls easily on casters, and fills and empties at the bedside through a hose that attaches to any faucet.

Vinyl pressure cuffs improve on the well-known and effective antiembolism stockings. This portable system simulates the normal pumping action of leg muscles by inflating progressively from the ankle to above the calf, assisting venous return and preventing blood backflow.

Nonallergenic adhesive gauze dressings cover an entire wound site with a single sheet of air- and exudate-permeable adhesive gauze. This type of occlusive dressing is particularly well suited for large or curved body areas and holds dressings securely without tape or straps. The gauze can be lifted off easily and painlessly for examination of the wound—even on sensitive or hairy skin—and then can be pressed back into place.

The silicone-foam dressing has improved the care of open, granulating wounds. Poured into the wound in liquid form, this new packing quickly congeals into an absorbent rubber pad with the exact contour of the wound, but it permits air circulation, doesn't cause irritation, and can be reused.

The new portable and disposable equipment saves nursing time because it's easier to use than the equipment it replaces. And nursing time saved means fewer delays in delivering patient care. What's more, disposables reduce the spread of nosocomial infection and—because they're new for each use—enhance patient comfort.

HEAT AND COLD
Direct heat application

Heat applied directly to the patient's body raises tissue temperature and enhances the inflammatory process by causing vasodilation and increasing local circulation. This promotes leukocytosis, suppuration, drainage, and healing. Heat also increases tissue metabolism, reduces pain caused by muscular spasm, and decreases congestion in deep visceral organs.

Direct heat may be dry or moist. Dry heat can be delivered at a higher temperature and for a longer time.

Devices for applying dry heat include the hot water bottle, electric heating pad, K pad, and chemical hot pack.

Moist heat softens crusts and exudates, penetrates deeper than dry heat, doesn't dry the skin, produces less perspiration, and usually is more comfortable for the patient. Devices for applying moist heat include warm compresses for small body areas and warm packs for large areas.

Direct heat treatment can't be used on a patient at risk for hemorrhage. It also is contraindicated if the patient has a sprained limb in the acute stage (because vasodilation would increase pain and swelling), or if he has a condition associated with acute inflammation, such as appendicitis. Direct heat should be applied cautiously to pediatric and elderly patients and to patients with impaired renal, cardiac, or respiratory function; arteriosclerosis or atherosclerosis; and impaired sensation. It should be applied with extreme caution to heat-sensitive areas, such as scar tissue or stomas. Because it raises the risk of burns and possible systemic effects, such as an increased respiratory rate and hypotension, direct heat should be used only when a doctor's order specifies it.

Equipment

Patient thermometer ■ towel ■ adhesive tape or roller gauze ■ gloves, if the patient has an open lesion.

For a hot water bottle: hot tap water ■ pitcher ■ bath (utility) thermometer ■ absorbent, protective cloth covering.

For an electric heating pad: absorbent, protective cloth covering.

For a K pad: distilled water ■ temperature-adjustment key ■ absorbent, protective cloth covering.

For a chemical hot pack (disposable): absorbent, protective cloth covering.

For a warm compress or pack: basin of hot tap water or container of sterile water, normal saline, or other solution, as ordered ■ hot water bottle, K pad, or chemical hot pack ■ linen-saver pad.

The following items may be sterile or nonsterile, depending on the type of procedure required: compress material (flannel, 4" × 4" gauze pads) or pack material (absorbent towels, ABD pads) ■ petroleum jelly ■ cotton-tipped applicators ■ forceps ■ bowl or basin ■ bath (utility) thermometer ■ waterproof covering ■ towel ■ dressing.

Preparation of equipment

Hot water bottle: Fill the bottle with hot tap water *to detect leaks and warm the bottle,* and then empty it. Run hot tap water into a pitcher and measure the water temperature with the bath thermometer. Adjust the temperature as ordered, usually to 115° to 125° F (46.1° to 51.7° C) for adults and 105° to 115° F (40.6° to 46.1° C)

for children under age 2 and elderly patients. Next, pour hot water into the bottle, filling it one-half to two-thirds full. *Partially filling the bottle keeps it lightweight and flexible to mold to the treatment area.* Squeeze the bottle until the water reaches the neck *to expel any air that would make the bottle inflexible and reduce heat conduction.* Fasten the top, and cover the bag with an absorbent, protective cloth *to provide insulation and absorb the patient's perspiration.* Secure the cover with tape or roller gauze.

Electric heating pad: Check the cord for frayed or damaged insulation. Then, plug in the pad and adjust the control switch to the desired setting. Wrap the pad in a protective cloth covering, and secure the cover with tape or roller gauze.

K pad: Check the cord for safety, as above, and fill the control unit two-thirds full with distilled water. Do not use tap water *because it leaves mineral deposits in the unit.* Check for leaks, and then tilt the unit in several directions *to clear the pad's tubing of air, which could interfere with even heat conduction.* Tighten the cap, and then loosen it a quarter turn *to allow heat expansion within the unit.* After making sure the hoses between the control unit and the pad are free of tangles, place the unit on the bedside table, slightly above the patient *so gravity can assist water flow.* If the central supply department has not preset the temperature on the control unit, use the key provided to make this adjustment. The usual temperature is 105° F. Then, place the pad in a protective cloth covering and secure the cover with tape or roller gauze. Plug in the unit, turn it on, and allow the pad to warm for 2 minutes.

Chemical hot pack: Select a pack of the correct size. Then, follow the manufacturer's directions (strike, squeeze, or knead) *to activate the heat-producing chemicals.* Place the pack in a protective cloth covering and secure the cover with tape or roller gauze.

Sterile warm compress or pack: Warm the container of sterile water or solution by setting it in a sink or basin of hot water. Measure the solution's temperature with a sterile bath thermometer. If a sterile thermometer is unavailable, pour some heated sterile solution into a clean container, check the temperature with a regular bath thermometer, and then discard the tested solution. Adjust the temperature of the sterile solution by adding hot or cold water to the sink or basin until the solution reaches 131° F (55° C) for adults or 105° F for children and elderly patients and for an eye compress. Pour the heated solution into a sterile bowl or basin. Then, using sterile technique, soak the compress or pack in the heated solution. If necessary, prepare a hot water bottle, K pad, or chemical hot pack *to keep the compress or pack warm.*

Nonsterile warm compress or pack: Fill a bowl or basin with hot tap water or other solution, and measure the temperature of the fluid with a bath thermometer. Adjust the temperature as ordered, usually to 131° F (55° C) for adults or 105° F (40.6° C) for children and elderly patients and for an eye compress. Then soak the compress or pack in the hot liquid. If necessary, prepare a hot water bottle, K pad, or chemical hot pack *to keep the compress or pack warm.*

Implementation

• Check the doctor's order and assess the patient's condition.
• Explain the procedure to the patient, and tell him not to lean or lie directly on the heating device *because this reduces air space and increases the risk of burns.* Warn the patient against adjusting the temperature of the heating device or adding hot water to a hot water bottle, even if he feels he can tolerate a higher temperature. Advise him to report pain or discomfort immediately and to remove the device himself if necessary.
• Provide privacy and make sure the room is warm and free of drafts. Wash your hands thoroughly.
• Take the patient's temperature, pulse, and respirations *to serve as a baseline.* If heat treatment is being applied to raise the patient's body temperature, monitor temperature, pulse, and respirations throughout the application.
• Expose only the treatment area *because vasodilation will make the patient feel chilly.*

To apply a hot water bottle, an electric heating pad, a K pad, or a chemical hot pack

• Before applying the heating device, press it against the inner aspect of your forearm *to test its temperature and heat distribution.* If it heats unevenly, obtain a new device.
• Apply the device to the treatment area, and if necessary, secure it with tape or roller gauze. Begin timing the application.
• Assess the patient's skin condition frequently, and remove the device if you observe increased swelling or excessive redness, blistering, maceration, or pronounced pallor, or if the patient reports pain or discomfort. Refill the hot water bottle as necessary *to maintain the correct temperature.*
• Remove the device after 20 to 30 minutes, or as ordered.
• Dry the patient's skin with a towel and re-dress the site, if necessary. Take the patient's temperature, pulse, and respirations *for comparison with the baseline.* Position him comfortably in bed.
• If the treatment is to be repeated, store the equipment in the patient's room, out of his reach; otherwise, return the equipment to its proper place.

To apply a warm compress or pack

• Place a linen-saver pad under the treatment area. Spread petroleum jelly (sterile, if necessary) over the affected area. Avoid applying it directly to any areas of skin breakdown or to eye tissues. (You may use sterile cotton-tipped applicators for a sterile procedure.) *The petroleum jelly reduces maceration and the risk of burns by decreasing the rate of heat penetration.*
• Remove the warm compress or pack from the bowl or basin. (Use sterile forceps for a sterile procedure.)
• Wring excess solution from the compress or pack (using sterile forceps for a sterile procedure). *Excess moisture increases the risk of burns.*
• Apply the compress gently to the affected site (using forceps, if warranted). After a few seconds, lift the compress (with forceps, if needed) and check the skin for excessive redness, maceration, or blistering. When you're sure the compress isn't causing a burn, mold it firmly to the skin *to keep out air, which reduces the temperature and effectiveness of the compress.* Work quickly *so the compress retains its heat.*
• Apply a waterproof covering (sterile, if warranted) to the compress. Secure the covering with tape or roller gauze *to prevent it from slipping.*
• Place a hot water bottle, K pad, or chemical hot pack over the compress and waterproof covering *to maintain the correct temperature.* Begin timing the application.
• Check the patient's skin every 5 minutes for signs of tissue intolerance. Remove the device if the skin shows excessive redness, maceration, or blistering or if the patient feels pain or discomfort. Change the compress as necessary to maintain the correct temperature.
• After 15 or 20 minutes or as ordered, remove the compress. (Use forceps, if warranted.) Discard the compress into a waterproof trash bag.
• Dry the patient's skin with a towel (sterile, if necessary). Note the condition of the skin and re-dress the area, if necessary. Take the patient's temperature, pulse, and respiration *for comparison with the baseline.* Then make sure the patient is comfortable.
• Discard liquids and disposable equipment. Return used sterile equipment to the central supply department for sterilization. Clean any remaining equipment and, if the treatment will be repeated, store it in the patient's room, out of his reach; otherwise, return it to storage.

Special considerations

Make sure the patient is positioned in proper alignment *to maintain his comfort during the procedure.* Keep the call button within easy reach, and make sure the patient can remove the heating device if he experiences discomfort.

Unless ordered otherwise, discontinue the heat treatment after 30 minutes *because, by this time, maximum*

Using moist heat to relieve muscle spasm

Tell patients to choose moist heat rather than dry heat when attempting to ease muscle tension or spasm. Moist heat is less drying to the skin, less apt to cause burns, less likely to cause excessive fluid and salt loss through sweating, and more likely to penetrate deeper tissues. Instruct the patient to apply heat for 20 to 30 minutes, as follows:
• Place a moist towel over the painful area.
• Cover the towel with a hot water bottle properly filled and at the correct temperature.
• Remove the hot water bottle and wet pack after 20 to 30 minutes. Don't continue application for longer than 30 minutes because therapeutic value decreases after that time.

vasodilation has probably occurred; vasoconstriction then follows, reversing the effects of the heat treatment. Also, allow at least 1 hour between treatments *to avoid vasoconstriction.*

Because the temperature of a chemical hot pack varies from 101° to 114° F (38.3° to 45.6° C), use a different heating device for treatments requiring a specific or higher temperature.

Don't use an electric heating device near oxygen *because a spark from a frayed wire could cause explosion and fire. Also, to prevent electric shock,* avoid using an electric heating pad near liquid (including on a patient who is incontinent) and avoid handling any electric device with wet hands. When securing a heating device, don't use safety pins *because heated metal can cause burns or electric shock, and accidental puncture of a K pad or chemical hot*

pack can allow fluid to leak, resulting in burns. Avoid crushing or creasing the wires in an electric heating pad *because this may cause portions of the pad to overheat, leading to burns or fire.*

If the patient is unconscious, anesthetized, irrational, neurologically impaired, or insensitive to heat for any reason, stay with him throughout the treatment, and check the site frequently *to avoid such complications as edema, maceration, blotchy redness, and blisters.*

When direct heat is ordered to decrease congestion within internal organs, the application must cover a large enough area *to increase blood volume at the skin's surface.* For relief of pelvic organ congestion, for example, apply heat over the patient's lower abdomen, hips, and thighs. To achieve local relief, you may concentrate heat only over the specified area. (See *Using moist heat to relieve muscle spasm.*)

When applying moist heat to an open wound or to a lesion expected to open during treatment, use sterile technique. When applying moist heat to both eyes, use separate sterile equipment for each eye *to prevent cross-contamination.*

You may use sterile gloves instead of sterile forceps for application of sterile moist compresses or packs. As an alternative method of applying sterile moist compresses, use a bedside sterilizer to sterilize the compresses. Saturate the compress with tap water or other solution and wring it dry. Then place it in the bedside sterilizer at 275° F (135° C) for 15 minutes. Remove the compress with sterile forceps, and wring out the excess solution. Then place the compress in a sterile bowl and measure its temperature with a sterile thermometer. Apply the compress as instructed above when it reaches the correct temperature.

Commercial premoistened sterile compresses may be used as an alternative. Refer to the instructions on the package insert, and follow the same general observations and precautions mentioned above.

Complications
Because tissue damage may result from direct heat application, monitor the temperature of the compress carefully. Assess frequently the condition of the patient's skin under the heat application device.

Documentation
Record the time and date of heat application; the type, temperature or heat setting, duration, and site of application; the patient's temperature, pulse, respirations, and skin condition before, during, and after treatment; signs of complications; and the patient's tolerance of and reaction to treatment.

Radiant heat application

Radiant heat—dry heat shed onto a specific body area rather than applied directly to it—can improve circulation, decrease wound exudation, prevent maceration, and promote healing. Indicated for patients with stasis or slow-healing wounds, this treatment can be delivered during dressing changes and wound debridement.

No specific conditions contraindicate radiant heat treatment, but it must be used judiciously because it can dry the wound excessively; this, in turn, can impair healing. Scar tissue and stomas must be covered during radiant heat treatment, and heat-insensitive patients—such as the very young, elderly, and debilitated—require frequent monitoring to prevent burns.

Radiant heat is delivered by a heat lamp or heat cradle. The heat lamp, called a gooseneck lamp because of its long flexible neck, holds a single light bulb of 25 to 100 watts and conducts heat to a localized treatment site. Bulb wattage and the distance between the lamp and the patient regulate the amount of heat delivered. The heat cradle, a metal frame with one or more sockets for 25-watt bulbs, radiates heat to larger areas, such as the legs or abdomen. The cradle fits over the treatment site. Although its construction permits little control over the distance between the patient and the heat source, you can control the amount of heat delivered by manipulating the number of 25-watt bulbs used and the type and amount of covering tented over the cradle. Some cradles are equipped with thermostats that indicate the temperature and amount of heat projected.

Equipment

Patient thermometer ▪ gloves, if necessary ▪ heat lamp or heat cradle ▪ yardstick or measuring tape ▪ sheet ▪ one or more bath blankets.

Preparation of equipment

Check the doctor's order, and insert the prescribed wattage bulb in the heat lamp or heat cradle. If you're using the heat lamp, place it at the bedside, plug it into an outlet, and turn it on for a few minutes before exposing the patient *to warm the lamp and avoid chilling the patient.* If you're using the heat cradle, position it over the patient before turning it on *to avoid causing burns.*

Implementation

• Assess the patient's condition, explain the procedure to him, and help him into a comfortable position.
• Provide privacy and make sure the room is warm and free of drafts. Wash your hands thoroughly.

• Remove any metal objects from the patient, such as jewelry and orthopedic braces, before starting the treatment. *Metal objects heat rapidly and may cause discomfort or burns.*
• Record the patient's temperature, pulse, and respirations *to serve as a baseline.*
• Expose only the treatment site *to reduce body heat loss and to avoid chilling the patient.*
• Make sure the patient's skin is clean and dry *to reduce the risk of burns.*

Positioning the heat lamp

• Position the prewarmed lamp at the patient's side, not over him, *so if it falls, it won't strike or burn him.*
• Using a yardstick or measuring tape as a guide, adjust the neck of the lamp so the light bulb is the correct distance from the patient's skin. To determine the correct distance, consider the wattage of the bulb and the patient's physical condition, skin pigmentation, and ability to tolerate heat. In most cases, allow 14″ (35.6 cm) between the bulb and the patient's skin for a 25-watt bulb, 18″ (45.7 cm) for a 40-watt bulb, and 24″ to 30″ (61 to 76.2 cm) for a 60-watt or higher bulb.

Positioning the heat cradle

• Place the cradle on the bed, directly over or to the side of the treatment site. Plug in the cord and turn on the device.
• Cover the cradle with a sheet *to prevent drafts and to concentrate the heat on the treatment site. To prevent a fire,* make sure the sheet doesn't touch the bulbs.

Delivering the heat treatment

• With either heating device, time the application carefully.
• Check bulb position and the patient's skin every 5 minutes *to make sure the patient can tolerate the treatment.* If the patient can't tolerate the heat at the prescribed distance, discontinue the treatment and notify the doctor.
• For a cradle equipped with a thermostat, maintain the heat at 86° to 90° F (30° to 32.2° C) or as ordered.
• Turn off the heating device as ordered, usually after 10 to 15 minutes for the first treatment and 20 to 30 minutes for subsequent treatments.
• Dry the patient's skin, re-dress the treatment site if necessary, and obtain temperature, pulse, and respirations *for comparison with the baseline.* Make sure the patient is comfortable.
• If the treatment will be repeated, store the equipment in the patient's room, out of his reach; otherwise, return it to storage.

Special considerations

Avoid application of creams or ointments to the exposed area before the treatment *because they may increase the risk of burns.*

Never enclose a heat lamp and exposed body part under sheets or blankets. *Doing so increases heat intensity and the risk of burns or fire.* The heat cradle can safely support covers only if they don't touch any light bulbs.

To prevent fire or explosion, protect hot light bulbs from paper, cloth, liquids, sprays, and mists.

Caution the patient not to touch the heat lamp or heat cradle *to prevent burns.* If the patient is very young, elderly, unconscious, anesthetized, neurologically impaired, or otherwise insensitive to heat, stay with him during the treatment, and watch for signs of heat intolerance: redness, pain, extreme chills, and changes in vital signs.

Complications

Despite precautions, radiant heat treatment can burn a patient who has extremely sensitive skin.

Documentation

For heat lamp treatment, record the time, date, and duration of treatment; light bulb wattage; distance of the lamp from the patient's skin; the patient's temperature, pulse, and respirations before, during, and after treatment; appearance of the treatment site before and after; and the patient's tolerance for treatment. For heat cradle treatments, also record the number of light bulbs and the number and type of cradle covers used.

Cold application

The application of cold constricts blood vessels; inhibits local circulation, suppuration, and tissue metabolism; relieves vascular congestion; slows bacterial activity in infections; reduces body temperature; and may act as a temporary anesthetic during brief, painful procedures. (See *Reducing pain with ice massage.)* Because treatment with cold also relieves inflammation, reduces edema, and slows bleeding, it may provide effective initial treatment after eye injuries, strains, sprains, bruises, muscle spasms, and burns. Cold does not reduce existing edema, however, because it inhibits reabsorption of excess fluid.

Cold may be applied in dry or moist forms, but ice should not be placed directly on a patient's skin because it may further damage tissue. Moist application is more penetrating than dry because moisture facilitates conduction. Devices for applying dry cold include an ice bag or collar, K pad (which can produce cold or heat), and chemical cold packs and ice packs. Devices for applying moist cold include cold compresses for small body areas and cold packs for large areas.

Apply cold treatments cautiously on patients with impaired circulation, on children, and on elderly or arthritic patients because of the risk of ischemic tissue damage.

Equipment

Patient thermometer ▪ towel ▪ adhesive tape or roller gauze ▪ gloves, if necessary.

For an ice bag or collar: tap water ▪ ice chips ▪ absorbent, protective cloth covering.

For a K pad: distilled water ▪ temperature-adjustment key ▪ absorbent, protective cloth covering.

For a chemical cold pack: Single-use packs are available for applying dry cold. These lightweight plastic packs contain a chemical that turns cold when activated. Reusable, sealed cold packs, filled with an alcohol-based solution, are also available. These packs are stored frozen until use and, after exterior disinfection, may be refrozen and used again.

For a cold compress or pack: basin of ice chips ▪ container of tap water ▪ bath (utility) thermometer ▪ compress material (4″ × 4″ gauze pads or washcloths) or pack material (towels or flannel) ▪ linen-saver pad ▪ waterproof covering.

Preparation of equipment

Ice bag or collar: Select a device of the correct size, fill it with cold tap water, and check for leaks. Then, empty the device and fill it about halfway with crushed ice. *Using small pieces of ice keeps the device flexible for molding to the patient's body.* Squeeze the device *to expel air that might reduce conduction.* Fasten the cap and wipe any moisture from the outside of the device. Wrap the bag or collar in a cloth covering, and secure the cover with tape or roller gauze. *The protective cover prevents tissue trauma and absorbs condensation.*

K pad: Check the cord for frayed or damaged insulation. Then fill the control unit two-thirds full with distilled water. Do not use tap water *because it leaves mineral deposits in the unit.* Check for leaks, and then tilt the unit several times *to clear the pad's tubing of air, which could interfere with conduction.* Tighten the cap. After ensuring that the hoses between the control unit and pad are free of tangles, place the unit on the bedside table, slightly above the patient *so gravity can assist water flow.* If the central supply department has not preset the temperature on the control unit, use the key provided to adjust it to the lowest temperature. Cover the pad with an absorbent, protective cloth and secure the cover with tape or roller gauze. Plug in the unit and turn it on. Allow the pad to cool for 2 minutes before placing it on the patient.

Chemical cold pack: Select a pack of the appropriate size, and follow the manufacturer's directions (strike, squeeze, or knead) *to activate the cold-producing chemicals.* Make certain that the container has not been broken during activation; *such damage may allow the chemicals to leak out.* Wrap the pack in a cloth cover, and secure the cover with tape or roller gauze.

Cold compress or pack: Cool the tap water by placing the container of water in a basin of ice or by adding ice to the water. Using a bath thermometer for guidance, adjust the water temperature to 59° F (15° C) or as ordered. Immerse the compress material or pack material in the water.

Implementation
• Check the doctor's order and assess the patient's condition.
• Explain the procedure to the patient, provide privacy, and make sure the room is warm and free of drafts. Wash your hands thoroughly.
• Record the patient's temperature, pulse, and respirations *to serve as a baseline.*
• Expose only the treatment site *to avoid chilling the patient.*

To apply an ice bag or collar, K pad, or chemical cold pack
• Place the covered cold device on the treatment site and begin timing the application.
• Observe the site frequently for signs of tissue intolerance: blanching, mottling, graying, cyanosis, maceration, or blisters. Also, be alert for shivering and for the patient's complaints of burning or numbness. If any of these signs or symptoms develop, discontinue treatment and notify the doctor.
• Refill or replace the cold device as necessary *to maintain the correct temperature.* Change the protective cover if it becomes wet.
• Remove the device after the prescribed treatment period (usually 30 minutes).

To apply a cold compress or pack
• Place a linen-saver pad under the treatment area.
• Remove the compress or pack from the water, and wring it out *to prevent dripping.* Apply it to the treatment site and begin timing the application.
• Cover the compress or pack with a waterproof covering *to provide insulation and to keep the surrounding area dry.* Secure the covering with tape or roller gauze *to prevent it from slipping.*

Reducing pain with ice massage

Normally, ice should not be applied directly to a patient's skin because it risks damaging the skin surface and underlying tissues. However, when carefully performed, this technique—called ice massage—may help patients tolerate brief, painful procedures, such as biopsy under local anesthesia, bone marrow aspiration, catheterization, chest tube removal, injection into joints, lumbar puncture, and suture removal.

Prepare for ice massage by gathering the ice, a porous covering to hold it in (if desired), and a cloth for wiping water from the patient as the ice melts.

Just before the procedure begins, rub the ice over the appropriate area to numb it. Assess the site frequently; stop rubbing immediately if you detect signs of tissue intolerance.

As the procedure begins, rub the ice over a point near but not at the site. This distracts the patient from the procedure itself and gives him another stimulus on which to concentrate.

If the procedure lasts longer than about 10 minutes, or if you think tissue damage may occur, move the ice to a different site and continue the massage.

If you know in advance that the procedure probably will last longer than 10 minutes, massage the site intermittently—2 minutes of massage alternating with a rest period until the skin regains its normal color. Alternatively, you can divide the area into several sites and apply ice to each one for several minutes at a time.

• Check the application site frequently for signs of tissue intolerance. Also note the patient's complaints of burning or numbness. If these signs or symptoms develop, discontinue treatment and notify the doctor.
• Change the compress or pack as necessary *to maintain the correct temperature.* Remove it after the prescribed treatment period (usually 20 minutes).

To conclude all cold applications
• Dry the patient's skin and re-dress the treatment site according to the doctor's orders. Then, position the patient comfortably, and take his temperature, pulse, and respirations *for comparison with the baseline.*
• Dispose of liquids and soiled materials properly. If treatment will be repeated, clean and store the equipment in

Using cold for a muscle sprain

Cold can help relieve pain and reduce edema during the first 24 to 72 hours after a sprain occurs. Tell the patient to apply cold to the area four times daily for 20 to 30 minutes each time.

For each application, instruct the patient to obtain enough crushed ice to cover the painful area, place it in a plastic bag, and place the bag inside a pillowcase or large piece of cloth, as shown below.

For later applications, the patient may wish to fill a paper cup with water, stand a tongue blade in the cup, and place it in the freezer. After the water freezes, he can peel the paper off the ice and hold it with the protruding handle. If he chooses this method, however, tell him to cover the area with a cloth before applying the ice. Applying ice directly to the skin could cause frostbite or cold shock.

Instruct the patient to rub the ice over the painful area for the specified treatment time. Warn him that, although ice eases pain in a joint that has begun to stiffen, he shouldn't let the analgesic effect encourage overuse of the joint.

After 24 to 72 hours, when heat, redness, and swelling have subsided or when cold no longer helps, the patient should switch to heat application.

the patient's room, out of his reach; otherwise, return it to storage.

Special considerations

Apply cold immediately after an injury *to minimize edema.* (See *Using cold for a muscle sprain.*) Although colder temperatures can be tolerated for a longer time when the treatment site is small, don't continue any application for longer than 1 hour *to prevent reflexive vasodilation.* Application of temperatures below 59° F (15° C) will also cause local reflex vasodilation.

When applying cold to an open wound or to a lesion that may open during treatment, use sterile technique. Also maintain sterile technique during eye treatment, with separate sterile equipment for each eye *to prevent cross-contamination.*

Avoid securing cooling devices with pins *because an accidental puncture may allow extremely cold fluids to leak out and burn the patient's skin.*

If the patient is unconscious, anesthetized, neurologically impaired, irrational, or otherwise insensitive to cold, stay with him throughout the treatment and check the application site frequently for complications. Warn the patient against placing ice directly on his skin *because the extreme cold can cause burns.*

Complications

Thrombi may result from hemoconcentration. Pain, burning, or numbness may result from intense cold.

Documentation

Record the time, date, and duration of cold application; type of device used (ice bag or collar, K pad, or chemical cold pack); site of application; temperature or temperature setting; patient's temperature, pulse, and respirations before and after application; skin appearance before, during, and after application; any signs of complications; and the patient's tolerance for treatment.

 ## Hyperthermia-hypothermia blanket

A blanket-sized aquamatic K pad, the hyperthermia-hypothermia blanket raises, lowers, or maintains body temperature through conductive heat or cold transfer between the blanket and the patient. It can be operated manually or automatically.

In manual operation, the nurse or doctor sets the temperature on the unit. The blanket reaches and maintains this temperature regardless of the patient's temperature. The temperature setting must be manually adjusted to reach a different temperature setting. The nurse monitors the patient's body temperature using a conventional thermometer.

In automatic operation, the unit directly and continually monitors the patient's temperature by means of a thermistor probe (rectal, skin, or esophageal) and alternates heating and cooling cycles as necessary to achieve and maintain the desired body temperature. The thermistor probe also may be used in conjunction with manual operation but is not essential. The unit is equipped with an alarm to warn of abnormal temperature fluctuations, and a circuit breaker that protects against current overload.

The blanket is used most commonly to reduce high fever when more conservative measures — such as baths, ice packs, and antipyretics — are unsuccessful. Its other uses include maintaining normal temperature during surgery or shock; inducing hypothermia during surgery to decrease metabolic activity and thereby reduce oxygen requirements; reducing intracranial pressure; controlling bleeding and intractable pain in patients with amputations, burns, or cancer; and providing warmth in cases of severe hypothermia.

Equipment

Hyperthermia-hypothermia control unit ■ operation manual ■ fluid for the control unit (distilled water or distilled water and 20% ethyl alcohol) ■ thermistor probe (rectal, skin, or esophageal) ■ one or two hyperthermia-hypothermia blankets ■ one or two disposable blanket covers (or one or two sheets or bath blankets) ■ lanolin or a mixture of lanolin and cold cream ■ patient thermometer (for manual mode) ■ adhesive tape ■ towel ■ sphygmomanometer ■ gloves, if necessary ■ optional: protective wraps for the patient's hands and feet.

Disposable hyperthermia-hypothermia blankets are available for single-patient use.

Preparation of equipment

First, read the operation manual. Inspect the unit and each blanket for leaks and the plugs and the connecting wires for broken prongs, kinks, and fraying. If you detect or suspect malfunction, don't use the equipment.

Review the doctor's order, and prepare one or two blankets by covering them with disposable covers (or use a sheet or a bath blanket when positioning the blanket on the patient). *The cover absorbs perspiration and condensation, which could cause tissue breakdown if left on the skin.* Connect the blanket to the control unit, and set the controls for manual or automatic operation and for the desired blanket or body temperature. Make sure the machine is properly grounded before plugging it in. Turn on the machine and add liquid to the unit reservoir, if necessary, as fluid fills the blanket. Allow the blanket to preheat or precool *so the patient receives immediate thermal benefit.* Place the control unit at the foot of the bed.

Implementation

● Assess the patient's condition and explain the procedure to him. Provide privacy and make sure the room is warm and free of drafts. Check hospital policy and, if necessary, make sure the patient or a responsible family member has signed a consent form.

● Wash your hands thoroughly. If the patient is not already wearing a hospital gown, ask him to put one on. Use a gown with cloth ties, not metal snaps or pins *because these could cause heat or cold injury.*

● Take the patient's temperature, pulse, respirations, and blood pressure *to serve as a baseline,* and assess level of consciousness, pupil reaction, limb strength, and skin condition.

● Keeping the bottom sheet in place and the patient recumbent, roll him to one side and slide the blanket halfway under him, so its top edge aligns with his neck. Then roll the patient back, and pull and flatten the blanket across the bed. Place a pillow under the patient's head. Make sure the patient's head doesn't lie directly on the blanket *because the blanket's rigid surface may be uncomfortable and the heat or cold may lead to tissue breakdown.* If necessary, use a sheet or bath blanket as insulation between the patient and the blanket.

● Apply lanolin or a mixture of lanolin and cold cream to the patient's skin where it touches the blanket *to help protect the skin from heat or cold sensation.*

● In automatic operation, insert the thermistor probe in the patient's rectum and tape it in place *to prevent accidental dislodgment.* If rectal insertion is contraindicated, tuck a skin probe deep into the axilla, and secure it with tape. If the patient is comatose or anesthetized, insert an esophageal probe. Plug the other end of the probe into the correct jack on the unit's control panel.

● Place a sheet or, if ordered, the second hyperthermia-hypothermia blanket over the patient. *This increases thermal benefit by trapping cooled or heated air.*

● Wrap the patient's hands and feet, if he wishes, *to minimize chilling and promote comfort.* Monitor vital signs and perform a neurologic assessment every 5 minutes until the desired body temperature is reached; then every 15 minutes until temperature is stable or as ordered.

● Check fluid intake and output hourly or as ordered. Observe the patient regularly for color changes in skin, lips, and nail beds, and for edema, induration, inflammation, pain, or sensory impairment. If these occur, discontinue the procedure and notify the doctor.

● Reposition the patient every 30 minutes to 1 hour, unless contraindicated, *to prevent skin breakdown.* Keep the patient's skin, bedclothes, and blanket cover free of perspiration and condensation, and reapply cream to exposed body parts as needed.

● After turning off the machine, follow the manufacturer's directions. *Some units must remain plugged in for at least 30 minutes to allow the condenser fan to remove water vapor from the mechanism.* Continue to monitor the pa-

tient's temperature until it stabilizes *because body temperature can fall as much as 5° F (2.8° C) after this procedure.*
• Remove all equipment from the bed. Dry the patient and make him comfortable. Supply a fresh hospital gown, if necessary. Cover the patient lightly.
• Continue to perform neurologic checks and monitor vital signs, fluid intake and output, and general condition every 30 minutes for 2 hours and then hourly or as ordered.
• Return the equipment to the central supply department for cleaning, servicing, and storage.

Special considerations
If the patient shivers excessively during hypothermia treatment, discontinue the procedure and notify the doctor immediately. *By increasing metabolism, shivering elevates body temperature.*

Avoid lowering the temperature more than 1 degree every 15 minutes *to prevent premature ventricular contractions.*

Don't use pins to secure catheters, tubes, or blanket covers *because an accidental puncture can result in fluid leakage and burns.*

With hyperthermia or hypothermia therapy, the patient may experience a secondary defense reaction (vasoconstriction or vasodilation, respectively) that causes body temperature to rebound and thus defeat the treatment's purpose.

If the patient requires isolation, place the blanket, blanket cover, and probe in a plastic bag clearly marked with the type of isolation *so the central supply department can give it special handling.* If the blanket is disposable, discard it using appropriate precautions.

To avoid bacterial growth in the reservoir or blankets, always use sterile distilled water and change it monthly. Check to see if hospital policy calls for adding a bacteriostatic agent to the water. Avoid using de-ionized water, *because it may corrode the system.*

Complications
Use of a hyperthermia-hypothermia blanket can cause shivering, marked changes in vital signs, increased intracranial pressure, respiratory distress or arrest, cardiac arrest, oliguria, and anuria.

Documentation
Record the patient's pulse, respirations, blood pressure, neurologic signs, fluid intake and output, skin condition, and position change. Record the patient's temperature and that of the thermal pad every 30 minutes while the pad is in use. Also document the type of hyperthermia-hypothermia unit used; control settings (manual or automatic, and temperature settings); date, time, duration, and patient's tolerance of treatment; and any signs of complications.

Sponge bath

The sponge bath — with tepid water, alcohol, or a mixture of the two — reduces fever by dilating superficial blood vessels, thus releasing heat and lowering body temperature. An alcohol sponge bath effects the fastest temperature reduction because alcohol evaporates faster than water and thus removes heat more rapidly from the skin surface. However, alcohol is also more drying to the skin, and the rapid temperature loss produced by an alcohol bath may cause chilling and a rebound rise in temperature. A tepid-water sponge bath, with or without alcohol, may lower systemic temperature when routine fever treatments fail, particularly for infants and children, whose temperatures tend to rise very high, very quickly.

Equipment
Basin of tepid water, approximately 80° to 93° F (26° to 34° C) ■ 70% isopropyl (rubbing) alcohol, if prescribed ■ bath (utility) thermometer ■ bath blanket ■ linen-saver pad ■ washcloths ■ patient thermometer ■ hot water bottle and cover ■ ice bag and cover ■ towel ■ emesis basin (if using alcohol) ■ clean gown ■ gloves, if the patient has open lesions or has been incontinent.

Preparation of equipment
Prepare a hot water bottle and an ice bag. Then place the bath thermometer in a basin, and run water over it until the temperature reaches the high end of the tepid range (93° F) *because the water will cool during the bath.* Add alcohol, if prescribed, at room temperature in a 1:1 proportion. Immerse the washcloths in the tepid solution until saturated.

Implementation
• Check the doctor's order and assess the patient's condition.
• Check the medication Kardex for recent administration of an antipyretic *because this can affect patient response to the bath.*
• Explain the procedure to the patient, provide privacy, and make sure the room is warm and free of drafts. Wash your hands thoroughly and put on gloves, if necessary.
• Place a linen-saver pad under the patient *to catch any spills* and a bath blanket over him *for privacy.* Then remove his pajamas. Also remove the top bed linen *to avoid wetting it.*

• Take the patient's temperature, pulse, and respiration *to serve as a baseline.*
• Place the hot water bottle with protective covering on the patient's feet *to reduce the sensation of chilliness.* Place the covered ice bag on his head *to prevent headache and nasal congestion that occur as the rest of the body cools.*
• Wring out each washcloth before sponging the patient *so they don't drip and cause discomfort.*
• Place moist washcloths over the major superficial blood vessels in the axillae, groin, and popliteal areas *to accelerate cooling.* Change the washcloths as they warm.
• Bathe each extremity separately for about 5 minutes; then sponge the chest and abdomen for 5 minutes. Turn the patient, and bathe his back and buttocks for 5 to 10 minutes. Keep the patient covered except for the body part you're sponging.
• Add warm water to the basin as necessary *to maintain the desired water temperature.*
• Check the patient's temperature, pulse, and respirations every 10 minutes. Notify the doctor if the patient's temperature doesn't fall within 30 minutes. Stop the bath when the patient's temperature reaches 1° to 2° F above the desired level *because his temperature will continue to fall naturally.* Continue to monitor his temperature until it stabilizes.
• Observe the patient for chills, shivering, pallor, mottling, cyanosis of the lips or nail beds, and changes in vital signs — especially a rapid, weak, or irregular pulse — *because such signs may indicate an emergency.* If any of these signs occur, discontinue the bath, cover the patient lightly, and notify the doctor.
• If no adverse effects occur, bathe the patient for at least 30 minutes *to reduce temperature.*
• Pat each area dry after sponging but avoid rubbing with the towel *because rubbing increases cell metabolism and produces heat.*
• After finishing the bath, make sure the patient is dry and comfortable. Dress him in a fresh gown and cover him lightly.
• Dispose of liquids and soiled materials properly. If the treatment will be repeated, clean and store the equipment in the patient's room, out of his reach; otherwise, return the items to storage.
• Take temperature, pulse, and respirations 30 minutes after the bath *to determine the treatment's effectiveness.*

Special considerations
If ordered, administer an antipyretic 15 to 20 minutes before the sponge bath *to achieve more rapid fever reduction.* If you're giving an alcohol sponge bath, observe the patient's skin for excessive dryness. Also, keep the emesis basin readily available *because alcohol vapors may cause nausea and vomiting.*

Consider covering the patient's trunk with a wet towel for 15 minutes to speed cooling. Resaturate the towel as necessary.

Refrain from bathing the breasts of a postpartum patient *because they could become overly dry or fissures could develop on the nipples.*

Take a rectal temperature, unless contraindicated, *for accuracy.* Axillary temperatures are unreliable *because the cool compresses applied to these areas alter the readings.* If you must take an oral temperature, do so cautiously *because chills may cause the patient to bite down and shatter the thermometer.* If possible, use an electronic thermometer to take an oral temperature *because it gives the temperature reading more quickly and because it isn't covered with glass, which could break in the patient's mouth.*

Home care
Sponge baths to reduce fever are used most commonly in nonhospital settings; febrile hospitalized patients usually receive antibiotics or antipyretics and, if needed, treatment with hypothermia blankets, which lower and maintain body temperature more effectively than sponge baths.

Complications
Accelerated temperature reduction can provoke seizure activity.

Documentation
Record the date, time, and duration of the bath; the type and temperature of the solution; the patient's temperature, pulse, and respirations before, during, and after the procedure; any complications that arise; and the patient's tolerance for treatment.

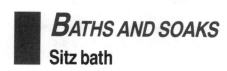

BATHS AND SOAKS
Sitz bath

Also known as a hip bath, a sitz bath involves immersion of the pelvic area in warm or hot water. It is used to relieve discomfort, especially after surgery or childbirth. The bath promotes wound healing by cleaning the perineum and anus, increasing circulation, and reducing inflammation. It also helps relax local muscles.

To be performed correctly, the sitz bath requires frequent checks of water temperature to ensure therapeutic effects, and correct draping of the patient during the bath and prompt dressing after it to prevent vasoconstriction.

Equipment

Sitz tub, portable sitz bath, or regular bathtub ▪ bath mat ▪ rubber mat ▪ bath (utility) thermometer ▪ two bath blankets ▪ towels ▪ hospital gown ▪ gloves, if the patient has an open lesion or has been incontinent ▪ optional: rubber ring, footstool, overbed table, I.V. pole (to hold irrigation bag), wheelchair or cart, dressings.

A disposable sitz bath kit is available for single-patient use. It includes a plastic basin that fits over a commode and an irrigation bag with tubing and clamp.

Preparation of equipment

Make sure the sitz tub, portable sitz bath, or regular bathtub is clean and disinfected. Or, obtain a disposable sitz bath kit from the central supply department.

Position the bath mat next to the bathtub, sitz tub, or commode. If you're using a tub, place the rubber mat on its surface *to prevent falls.* Place the rubber ring on the bottom of the tub *to serve as a seat for the patient,* and cover the ring with a towel *for comfort. Keeping the patient elevated improves water flow over the wound site and avoids unnecessary pressure on tender tissues.*

If you're using a commercial kit, open the package and familiarize yourself with the equipment.

Fill the sitz tub or bathtub one-third to one-half full, so that the water will reach the seated patient's umbilicus. Use warm water (94° to 98° F [34° to 37° C]) for relaxation or wound cleaning and healing, hot water (110° to 115° F [43° to 46° C]) for heat application. Run the water slightly warmer than desired *because it will cool while the patient prepares for the bath.* Measure the temperature of the water using the bath thermometer.

If you're using a commercial kit, fill the basin to the specified line with water at the prescribed temperature. Place the basin under the commode seat, clamp the irrigation tubing to block water flow, and fill the irrigation bag with water of the same temperature as that in the basin. To create flow pressure, hang the bag above the patient's head on a hook, towel rack, or I.V. pole.

Implementation

● Check the doctor's order and assess the patient's condition.
● Explain the procedure to the patient. Wash your hands thoroughly and put on gloves, if necessary.
● Have the patient void.
● Assist the patient to the bath area, provide privacy, and make sure the area is warm and free of drafts. Help the patient undress, as needed.
● Remove and dispose of any soiled dressings. If a dressing adheres to a wound, allow it to soak off in the tub.
● Assist the patient into the tub or onto the commode, as needed. Instruct him to use the safety rail for balance.

Explain that initially the sensation may be unpleasant *because the wound area is already tender.* Assure him that this discomfort will soon be relieved by the warm water.
● For any apparatus except a regular bathtub, if the patient's feet do not reach the floor and the weight of his legs presses against the edge of the equipment, place a small stool under the patient's feet. *This decreases pressure on local blood vessels.* Also place a folded towel against the patient's lower back *to prevent discomfort and promote correct body alignment.*
● Drape the patient's shoulders and knees with bath blankets *to avoid chills that cause vasoconstriction.*
● If you're using the sitz bath kit, open the clamp on the irrigation tubing *to allow a stream of water to flow continuously over the wound site.* Refill the bag with water of the correct temperature as needed, and encourage the patient to regulate the flow himself. Place the patient's overbed table in front of him *to provide support and comfort.*
● If you're using a tub, check the water temperature frequently with the bath thermometer. If the temperature drops significantly, add warm water. For maximum safety, first help the patient stand up slowly *to prevent dizziness and loss of balance.* Then, with the patient holding the safety rail *for support,* run warm water into the tub. Check water temperature. When the water reaches the correct temperature, help the patient sit down again to resume the bath.
● If necessary, stay with the patient during the bath. If you must leave, show him how to use the call button, and ensure his privacy.
● Check the patient's color and general condition frequently. If he complains of feeling weak, faint, or nauseated or shows signs of cardiovascular distress, discontinue the bath, check the patient's pulse and blood pressure, and assist him back to bed. Use a wheelchair or cart to transport the patient to his room if necessary. Notify the doctor.
● When the prescribed bath time has elapsed—usually 15 to 20 minutes—tell the patient to use the safety rail *for balance* and help him to a standing position slowly *to prevent dizziness and to allow him to regain his equilibrium.*
● If necessary, help the patient to dry himself. Re-dress the wound as needed, and assist the patient to dress and to return to bed or back to his room.
● Dispose of soiled materials properly. Empty, clean, and disinfect the sitz tub, bathtub, or portable sitz bath. Return the commercial kit to the patient's bedside for later use.

Special considerations

Use a regular bathtub only if a special sitz tub, portable sitz bath, or commercial sitz bath kit is unavailable. *Because the application of heat to the extremities causes va-*

sodilation and draws blood away from the perineal area, a regular bathtub is less effective for local treatment than a sitz device.

If the patient will be sitting in a bathtub with his extremities immersed in the hot water, check his pulse before, during, and after the bath *to help detect vasodilation that could make him feel faint when he stands up.*

Tell the patient never to touch an open wound *because of the risk of infection.*

Home care
Instruct the patient to adhere to the manufacturer's guidelines for disposable equipment.

Complications
Weakness or faintness can result from heat or the exertion of changing position. Irregular or accelerated pulse may indicate cardiovascular distress.

Documentation
Record the date, time, duration, and temperature of the bath; wound condition before and after treatment, including color, odor, and amount of drainage; any complications; and the patient's response to treatment.

 # Therapeutic bath

Also referred to as balneotherapy, the therapeutic bath combines water and additives to soothe and relax the patient, clean the skin, relieve inflammation and pruritus, and soften and remove crusts, scales, debris, and old medications. Used primarily for their antipruritic and emollient actions, these baths coat irritated skin with a soothing, protective film. Because they constrict surface blood vessels, they also have an anti-inflammatory effect.

Addition of oatmeal powder, soluble cornstarch, or soybean complex to water creates a colloid bath, which has a soothing effect and is used to treat generalized itching. Oil baths are useful for lubricating dry skin and easing eczematous eruptions. Sodium bicarbonate added to water produces an alkaline bath that has a cooling effect and also helps relieve pruritus. A medicated tar bath may be used to treat psoriasis. The film of tar left on the skin works in combination with ultraviolet light to inhibit the rapid cell turnover characteristic of psoriasis. (See *Comparing therapeutic baths,* page 178.)

A bedridden patient may benefit from a local soak with the therapeutic additive instead of a therapeutic tub bath.

Equipment
Bathtub ▪ bath mat ▪ rubber mat ▪ bath (utility) thermometer ▪ therapeutic additive ▪ measuring device ▪ colander or sieve for oatmeal powder ▪ two washcloths ▪ two towels ▪ hospital gown or loose-fitting cotton pajamas ▪ lubricating cream or ointment, if ordered.

Preparation of equipment
Assemble supplies and draw the bath before bringing the patient to the bath area *to prevent chilling him.* Make sure the tub is clean and disinfected *because a patient with skin breakdown is particularly vulnerable to infection.* Place the bath mat next to the tub and the rubber mat on the bottom of the tub *to prevent falls; the therapeutic additive may make the tub exceptionally slippery.* Fill the tub with 6″ to 8″ (15.2 to 20.3 cm) of water at 95° to 100° F (35° to 37.8° C).

The treatment's purpose and the type of additive used will determine the water temperature. Cool to lukewarm water is used for relieving pruritus and when adding tar or starch. Warm baths are soothing, but water warmer than 100° F causes vasodilation, *which could aggravate pruritus.*

Measure the correct amount of therapeutic additive, according to the doctor's order or package instructions. As the tub is filling, thoroughly mix the additive in the water. Add most substances directly to the water, but place oatmeal powder in a sieve or colander under the tub faucet *to help it dissolve.* Begin with two tablespoons of oatmeal powder; then add more powder or water as needed to regulate the thickness of the oatmeal bath.

When giving a tar bath, wear a plastic apron or protective gown *because tar preparations stain clothing.*

Implementation
● Check the doctor's order, and assess the patient's condition.
● Explain the procedure to the patient and have him void. Wash your hands thoroughly and then escort the patient to the bath area. Close the door *to provide privacy and eliminate drafts.*
● Check the water temperature. Assist the patient to undress, and help him into the tub, if necessary. Advise him to use the safety rails *to prevent falls.*
● Tell him the bath may feel unpleasant at first *because his skin is irritated,* but assure him that the medication will soon coat and soothe his skin.
● Ask the patient to stretch out in the tub and submerge his body up to the chin. If he's capable, give him a washcloth to apply the bath solution gently to his face and other body areas not immersed.

Comparing therapeutic baths

TYPE	AGENTS	PURPOSE
Antibacterial	• Acetic acid • Potassium permanganate • Povidone-iodine	Used to treat infected eczema, dirty ulcerations, furunculosis, and pemphigus
Colloidal	• Aveeno colloidal oatmeal • Aveeno colloidal oatmeal, oilated • Starch and baking soda	Used to relieve pruritus and to soothe irritated skin; indicated for any irritated or oozing condition, such as atopic eczema
Emollient	• Bath oils • Mineral oil	Used to clean and hydrate the skin; indicated for any dry skin condition
Tar	• Bath oils with tar • Coal tar concentrate	Used to treat scaly dermatoses, sometimes in combination with ultraviolet light therapy; loosens scales and relieves pruritus

◆ *Nursing alert.* If the patient is taking a tar bath, tell him not to get the bath solution in his eyes *because tar is an eye irritant.* ◆

• Warn the patient against scrubbing his skin *to prevent further irritation.*

• Add warm water to the bath as needed *to maintain a comfortable temperature.*

• Allow the patient to soak for 15 to 30 minutes. If you must stay with him, pull the bath curtain; *this gives him some privacy and protects him from drafts.* If you must leave the room, show the patient how to use the call button, and ensure his privacy.

• After the bath, assist the patient from the tub. Have him use the safety rails *to prevent falls.*

• Help the patient pat his skin dry with towels. Don't rub the skin *because rubbing removes some solutes and oils clinging to the skin and produces friction, which increases pruritus.*

• Apply lubricating cream or ointment, if ordered, *to help hold water in the newly hydrated skin.*

• Provide a fresh hospital gown or loose-fitting cotton pajamas. Advise the patient to avoid wearing pajamas, underwear, or other clothing that isn't cotton and loose-fitting. *Tight clothing and scratchy or synthetic materials can aggravate skin conditions by causing friction and increasing perspiration.*

• Escort the patient to his room and make sure he's comfortable.

• Drain the bath water, clean and disinfect the tub, and dispose of soiled materials properly. *If you have given an oatmeal powder bath, drain and rinse the tub immediately or the powder will cake, making later removal difficult.*

Special considerations

Because pruritus seems worse at night, give a therapeutic bath before bedtime, unless ordered otherwise, *to promote restful sleep. Because the patient with a skin disorder may be self-conscious,* maintain eye contact during conversation and avoid staring at his skin. Also, avoid nonverbal expressions and gestures that show revulsion. If the patient wishes, allow him to talk about his condition and how it affects his self-esteem.

Refrain from using soap during a therapeutic bath *because its drying effect counteracts the bath emollient.*

A patient with skin breakdown chills easily, so protect him from drafts. But after the bath, avoid covering or dressing him too warmly *because perspiration aggravates pruritus.* Instruct the patient not to scratch his skin *to prevent excoriation and infection.*

If the patient is confined to bed, you can place the therapeutic additive in a basin of water at 95° to 100° F (35° to 37.8° C) and apply it with a washcloth, using light, gentle strokes.

Home care

• Instruct the patient to bathe only as often as prescribed. *Excessive bathing can dry the skin.*

• Advise the patient to purchase commercial bath oil. *Salad or cooking oils may give clothes an unpleasant odor, and mineral oil mixes poorly with water.*

• Tell the patient to follow manufacturer's instructions for commercially prepared colloid preparations. Colloid for an oatmeal bath can be made at home by putting one-half cup of raw oatmeal into a blender and blending at medium-high speed until the material has the consistency of flour, then sifting it to remove unground pieces.

Documentation
Record the date, time, and duration of the bath. Note the water temperature, the type and amount of additive, skin appearance before and after the bath, the patient's tolerance of the treatment, and the bath's effectiveness.

 # Soaks

A soak involves the immersion of a body part in warm water or a medicated solution. This treatment helps to soften exudates, facilitate debridement, enhance suppuration, clean wounds or burns, rehydrate wounds, apply medication to infected areas, and increase local blood supply and circulation.

Most soaks are applied with clean tap water and clean technique. Sterile solution and sterile equipment are required for treating wounds, burns, or other breaks in the skin.

Equipment
Basin, or arm or foot tub ▪ bath (utility) thermometer ▪ hot tap water or prescribed solution ▪ cup ▪ pitcher ▪ linen-saver pad ▪ overbed table ▪ footstool ▪ pillows ▪ towels ▪ gauze pads and other dressing materials ▪ gloves, if necessary.

Preparation of equipment
Clean and disinfect the basin or tub. Run hot tap water into a pitcher, or heat the prescribed solution, as applicable. Measure the water or solution temperature with a bath thermometer. If the temperature is not within the prescribed range (usually 105° to 110° F [40.6° to 43.3° C]), add hot or cold water or reheat or cool the solution, as needed. If you're preparing the soak away from the patient's room, heat the liquid slightly above the correct temperature *to allow for cooling during transport.* If the solution for a medicated soak isn't premixed, prepare the dilution and heat it.

Implementation
• Check the doctor's order and assess the patient's condition.

• Explain the procedure to the patient and, if necessary, check his history for previous allergic reaction to the medicated solution. Provide privacy. Wash your hands thoroughly.
• If the soak basin or tub will be placed in bed, make sure the bed is flat beneath it *to prevent spills.* For an arm soak, have the patient sit erect. For a leg or foot soak, ask him to lie down and bend the appropriate knee. For a foot soak in the sitting position, let him sit on the edge of the bed or transfer him to a chair.
• Place a linen-saver pad under the treatment site and, if necessary, cover the pad with a towel *to absorb spillage.*
• Expose the treatment site. Put on gloves before removing any dressing; dispose of the soiled dressing properly. If the dressing is encrusted and stuck to the wound, leave it in place and proceed with the soak. Remove the dressing several minutes later when it has begun to soak free.
• Position the soak basin under the treatment site on the bed, overbed table, footstool, or floor, as appropriate. Pour the heated liquid into the soak basin or tub. Then lower the arm or leg into the basin gradually *to allow adjustment to the temperature change.* Make sure the soak solution covers the treatment site.
• Support other body parts with pillows or towels as needed *to prevent discomfort and muscle strain.* Make the patient comfortable and ensure proper body alignment.
• Check the temperature of the soak solution with the bath thermometer every 5 minutes. If the temperature drops below the prescribed range, remove some of the cooled solution with a cup. Then lift the patient's arm or leg from the basin *to avoid burns,* and add hot water or solution to the basin. Mix the liquid thoroughly and then check its temperature. If the temperature is within the prescribed range, lower the patient's affected part back into the basin.
• Observe the patient for signs of tissue intolerance: extreme redness at the treatment site, excessive drainage, bleeding, or maceration. If such signs develop or the patient complains of pain, discontinue the treatment and notify the doctor.
• After 15 to 20 minutes, or as ordered, lift the patient's arm or leg from the basin and remove the basin.
• Dry the arm or leg thoroughly with a towel. If the patient has a wound, dry the skin around it without touching the wound.
• While the skin is hydrated from the soak, use gauze pads to remove loose scales or crusts.
• Observe the treatment area for general appearance, degree of swelling, debridement, suppuration, and healing. Re-dress the wound, if appropriate.
• Remove the towel and linen-saver pad and make the patient comfortable in bed.

Using intermittent pneumatic compression stockings

For patients with chronic venous disease and sometimes for others at risk for deep venous disease, intermittent pneumatic compression (IPC) stockings may be used during surgery and the postoperative period. These stockings are actually knee- or thigh-length cuffs connected to a pump and hoses. Wrapped from ankle to knee or thigh on each leg, the cuffs imitate normal leg pumping action by sequentially inflating and deflating a series of air cells from the ankle toward the trunk. This milking action propels blood toward the heart, preventing congestion in venous muscle sinuses and valve pockets, and preventing blood backflow. Cuff pressures range from 35 to 55 mm Hg. The cuffs are foam-lined and adjustable to prevent skin irritation.

To operate IPC stockings
Follow the manufacturer's guidelines when operating the IPC unit. The cuffs are marked for placement and positioning. To avoid securing the cuff too tightly, place two fingers between the patient's leg and the cuff before fastening it. If plastic connectors are used, align them on the side of the leg to keep them from pressing against bony prominences when the cuffs are inflated or from pressure against the bed.

Observe cuff filling for at least the first two cycles (approximately 3 or 4 minutes) to ensure correct operation. Only one cuff should fill at a time, from ankle to knee, then thigh. All air cells should then deflate simultaneously. The second cuff follows the same sequence. If the sequence isn't correct and you're sure the cuffs have been properly applied, remove them and have the system checked for malfunction. Also remove the cuffs and check for malfunction if the pump indicator light turns on at any time.

Precautions
Check for proper application, fit, and connections at regular intervals. Assess the patient's skin color, temperature, sensation, and ability to move. If you notice any significant changes, or if the patient experiences numbness, tingling, or leg pain, remove the cuffs and notify the doctor.

• Discard the soak solution, dispose of soiled materials properly, and clean and disinfect the basin. If the treatment is to be repeated, store the equipment in the patient's room, out of his reach; otherwise, return it to the central supply department.

Special considerations
To treat large areas, particularly burns, a soak may be administered in a whirlpool or Hubbard tank.

Documentation
Record the date, time, and duration of the soak; treatment site; solution and its temperature; skin and wound appearance before, during, and after treatment; and the patient's tolerance for treatment.

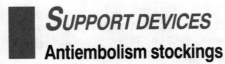

SUPPORT DEVICES
Antiembolism stockings

Elastic antiembolism stockings help prevent deep vein thrombosis (DVT) and pulmonary embolism by compressing superficial leg veins and the soleus muscle. This compression increases venous return by forcing blood into the deep venous system rather than allowing it to pool in the legs and form clots.

Antiembolism stockings can provide equal pressure over the entire leg or a graded pressure that is greatest at the ankle and decreases over the length of the leg. Usually indicated for postoperative, bedridden, elderly, or other patients at risk for DVT, these stockings should not be used on patients with dermatoses or open skin lesions, gangrene, severe arteriosclerosis or other ischemic vascular diseases, pulmonary or any massive edema, recent vein ligation, or vascular or skin grafts. For patients with chronic venous problems, intermittent pneumatic compression stockings may be ordered during surgery and postoperatively. (See *Using intermittent pneumatic compression stockings.)*

Equipment
Tape measure ■ antiembolism stockings of correct size and length ■ talcum powder.

Preparation of equipment
Before applying a knee-length stocking: Measure the circumference of the patient's calf at its widest point and leg length from the bottom of the heel to the back of the knee. (See *Measuring for antiembolism stockings.)*

Measuring for antiembolism stockings

Measure the patient carefully to ensure that his antiembolism stockings provide enough compression for adequate venous return.

To choose a *knee-length* stocking of the correct size, measure the circumference of the calf at its widest point (below) and the leg length from the bottom of the heel to the back of the knee (bottom left).

To choose a *thigh-length* stocking, measure the calf as for a knee-length stocking and the thigh at its widest point (below). Then measure leg length from the bottom of the heel to the gluteal fold (bottom right).

Before applying a thigh-length stocking: Measure the circumference of the calf and thigh at their widest points and the leg length from the bottom of the heel to the gluteal fold.

Before applying a waist-length stocking: Measure the circumference of the calf and thigh at their widest points and the leg length from the bottom of the heel to the waist along the side of the body.

Obtain the correct size stocking according to the manufacturer's specifications. If the patient's measurements are outside the range indicated by the manufacturer, or if his legs are deformed or edematous, ask the doctor if he wants to order custom-made stockings.

Implementation
- Check the doctor's order, and assess the patient's condition. If his legs are cold or cyanotic, notify the doctor before proceeding.
- Explain the procedure to the patient, provide privacy, and wash your hands thoroughly.
- Have the patient lie down. Then dust his ankle with talcum powder *to ease application.*

Applying a knee-length stocking
- Insert your hand into the stocking from the top, and grasp the heel pocket from the inside. Holding the heel, turn the stocking inside out so the foot is inside the

Applying antiembolism stockings: Three key steps

After covering the heel, gather the loose part of the stocking at the toes and pull this portion toward the heel.

Then, gather the loose part of the stocking and bring it over the heel with short, alternating front and back pulls.

Insert index and middle fingers into the gathered part of the stocking at the ankle and ease it upward by rocking it slightly up and down.

stocking leg. *This method allows easier application than gathering the entire stocking and working it up over the foot and ankle.*

• With the heel pocket down, hook the index and middle fingers of both your hands into the foot section. Facing the patient, ease the stocking over the toes, stretching it sideways as you move it up the foot. Ask the patient to point his toes, if possible, *to ease application.*

• Support the patient's ankle with one hand, and use the other hand to pull the heel pocket under the heel. Then center the heel in the pocket.

• Gather the loose portion of the stocking at the toe, and pull only this section over the heel. Gather the loose material at the ankle, and slide the rest of the stocking up over the heel with short pulls, alternating front and back.

• Insert your index and middle fingers into the gathered stocking at the ankle, and ease the fabric up the leg to the knee.

• Supporting the patient's ankle with one hand, use your other hand to stretch the stocking toward the knee, front and back, *to distribute the material evenly.* The stocking top should be 1″ to 2″ (2.5 to 5 cm) below the bottom of the patella.

• Gently snap the fabric around the ankle *to ensure a tight fit and eliminate gaps that could reduce pressure.*

• Adjust the foot section *for fabric smoothness and toe comfort* by tugging on the toe section. If the stocking has a toe window, make sure it's properly positioned.

• Repeat the procedure for the second stocking, if ordered.

Applying a thigh-length stocking

• Follow the procedure for applying a knee-length stocking, taking care to distribute the fabric evenly below the knee before continuing the procedure.

• With the patient's leg extended, stretch the rest of the stocking over the knee.

• Flex the patient's knee, and pull the stocking over the thigh until the top is 1″ to 3″ (2.5 to 7.6 cm) below the gluteal fold.

• Stretch the stocking from the top, front and back, *to distribute the fabric evenly over the thigh.*

• Gently snap the fabric behind the knee *to eliminate gaps that could reduce pressure.*

Applying a waist-length stocking

• Follow the procedure for applying knee-length and thigh-length stockings, and extend the stocking top to the gluteal fold.

• Fit the patient with the adjustable belt that accompanies the stockings. Make sure that neither the waistband nor the fabric interferes with any incision, drainage tube, catheter, or other external device.

Special considerations

Apply the stockings in the morning, if possible, *before edema develops.* If the patient has been ambulating, ask him to lie down and elevate his legs for 15 to 30 minutes before applying the stockings *to facilitate venous return.*

Don't allow the stockings to roll or turn down at the top or toe *because the excess pressure could cause venous strangulation.* Have the patient wear the stockings in bed and during ambulation *to provide continuous protection against thrombosis.*

Check the patient's toes at least once every 4 hours—more often in the patient with a faint pulse or edema. Note skin color and temperature, sensation, swelling, and ability to move. If complications occur, remove the stockings and notify the doctor immediately.

Be alert for an allergic reaction *because some patients cannot tolerate the sizing in new stockings.* Laundering the stockings before applying them reduces this risk. Remove the stockings at least once daily *to bathe the skin and observe for irritation and breakdown.*

Using warm water and mild soap, wash the stockings when soiled. Keep a second pair of stockings handy *for the patient to wear while the other pair is being laundered.*

Home care
If the patient will require antiembolism stockings after discharge, teach him or a family member how to apply them correctly and explain why it's important that he wear them. (See *Applying antiembolism stockings: Three key steps.)* Instruct the patient or family member to care for the stockings properly and to replace them when they lose their elasticity.

Complications
Obstruction of arterial blood flow—characterized by cold and bluish toes, dusky toenail beds, decreased or absent pedal pulses, and leg pain or cramps—can result from application of antiembolism stockings. Less serious complications, such as an allergic reaction and skin irritation, can also occur.

Documentation
Record the date and time of stocking application and removal, stocking length and size, condition of the leg before and after treatment, condition of the toes during treatment, any complications, and the patient's tolerance of the treatment.

 # Elastic bandages

Elastic bandages exert gentle, even pressure on a body part. By supporting blood vessels, these rolled bandages promote venous return and prevent pooling of blood in the legs. They're typically used in place of antiembolism stockings to prevent thrombophlebitis and pulmonary embolism in postoperative or otherwise bedridden patients who can't stimulate venous return by muscle activity.

Elastic bandages also minimize joint swelling after trauma to the musculoskeletal system. Used with a splint, they immobilize a fracture during healing. They can provide hemostatic pressure and anchor dressings over a fresh wound or after surgical procedures, such as vein stripping.

Equipment
Elastic bandage of appropriate width ■ tape or pins ■ gauze pads or absorbent cotton.

Bandages usually come in 2″ to 6″ (5 to 15 cm) widths and 4′ and 6′ (1.2 and 1.8 m) lengths. The 3″ (7.6 cm) width is adaptable to most applications. Also available is an elastic bandage with self-closures that eliminate the need for tape or pins.

Preparation of equipment
Select a bandage that wraps the affected body part completely but isn't excessively long. Generally, use a narrower bandage for wrapping the foot, lower leg, hand, or arm and a wider bandage for the thigh or trunk. The bandage should be clean and rolled before application.

Implementation
• Check the doctor's order, and examine the area to be wrapped for evidence of lesions or skin breakdown. If these conditions are present, consult the doctor before applying the elastic bandage.
• Explain the procedure to the patient, provide privacy, and wash your hands thoroughly. Position the patient comfortably, with the body part to be bandaged in normal functioning position *to promote circulation and prevent deformity and discomfort.*
• Avoid applying a bandage to a dependent extremity. If you're wrapping an extremity, elevate it for 15 to 30 minutes before application *to facilitate venous return.*
• Apply the bandage so that two skin surfaces do not remain in contact when wrapped. Place gauze or absorbent cotton as needed between skin surfaces, such as between toes and fingers or under breasts and arms, *to prevent skin irritation.*
• Hold the bandage with the roll facing upward in one hand and the free end of the bandage in the other hand. Hold the bandage roll close to the part being bandaged *to ensure even tension and pressure.*
• Unroll the bandage as you wrap the body part in a spiral or spiral-reverse method. Never unroll the entire bandage before wrapping *because this could produce uneven*

Bandaging techniques

Circular
Each turn encircles the previous one, covering it completely. Use this technique to anchor a bandage.

Spiral
Each turn partially overlaps the previous one. Use this technique to wrap a long, straight body part or one of increasing circumference.

Spiral-reverse
Anchor the bandage and then reverse direction halfway through each spiral turn. Use this technique to accommodate the increasing circumference of a body part.

Figure eight
Anchor below the joint, and then use alternating ascending and descending turns to form a figure eight. Use this technique around joints.

Recurrent
This technique includes a combination of recurrent and circular turns. Hold the bandage as you make each recurrent turn and then use the circular turns as a final anchor. Use this technique for a stump, a hand, or the scalp.

pressure, *which interferes with blood circulation and cell nourishment.*

• Overlap each layer of bandage by one-half to two-thirds the width of the strip. (See *Bandaging techniques* for specific instructions.)

• Wrap firmly but not too tightly. As you wrap, ask the patient to tell you if the bandage feels comfortable. If he complains of tingling, itching, numbness, or pain, loosen the bandage.

• When wrapping an extremity, anchor the bandage initially by circling the body part twice. *To prevent the bandage from slipping out of place on the foot,* wrap it in a figure eight around the foot, the ankle, and then the foot again before continuing. The same technique works on any joint, such as the knee, wrist, or elbow. Include the heel when wrapping the foot, but never wrap the toes (or fingers) unless absolutely necessary *because the distal extremities are used to detect impaired circulation.*

• When you're finished wrapping, secure the end of the bandage with tape, pins, or self-closures, being careful not to scratch or pinch the patient. Avoid using metal clips *because they typically come loose when the patient moves and may get lost in the bed linens and injure him.*

• Check distal circulation after the bandage is in place *because the elastic may tighten as you wrap.*

• Elevate a wrapped extremity for 15 to 30 minutes *to facilitate venous return.*

• Check distal circulation once or twice every 8 hours *because an elastic bandage that is too tight may result in neurovascular damage.* Lift the distal end of the bandage and assess the skin underneath for color, temperature, and integrity.

• Remove the bandage every 8 hours or whenever it's loose and wrinkled. Roll it up as you unwrap *to ready it for reuse.* Observe the area and provide skin care before rewrapping the bandage.

• Change the bandage at least once daily. Bathe the skin, dry it thoroughly, and observe for irritation and breakdown before applying a fresh bandage.

Special considerations

Wrap an elastic bandage from the distal area to the proximal area *to promote venous return.* Avoid leaving gaps in bandage layers or exposed skin surfaces *because this may result in uneven pressure on the body part.*

Observe the patient for an allergic reaction *because some patients cannot tolerate the sizing in a new bandage.* Laundering it reduces this risk.

Launder the bandage daily or whenever it becomes limp; *laundering restores its elasticity.* Always keep two bandages handy *so one can be applied while the other bandage is being laundered.*

When using an elastic bandage after a surgical procedure on an extremity (such as vein stripping) or with a splint to immobilize a fracture, remove it only as ordered rather than every 8 hours.

Home care

If the patient will be using an elastic bandage at home, teach him or a family member how to apply it correctly and how to assess for restricted circulation. Tell him to keep two bandages available *so he'll always have one to use while the other is being laundered.*

Complications

Arterial obstruction—characterized by a decreased or absent distal pulse, blanching or bluish discoloration of skin, dusky nail beds, numbness and tingling or pain and cramping, and cold skin—can result from elastic bandage application. Edema can occur from obstruction of venous return. Less serious complications include allergic reaction and skin irritation.

Documentation

Record the date and time of bandage application and removal, application site, bandage size, skin condition before application, skin care provided after removal, any complications, the patient's tolerance of the treatment, and any patient teaching.

Binders

Also known as self-closures, binders are lengths of cloth or elasticized material that encircle the chest, abdomen, or groin to provide support, keep dressings in place (especially for patients allergic to tape), reduce tension on wounds and suture lines, and reduce breast engorgement in the non-breast-feeding mother. Typically, cloth binders are fastened with safety pins and elasticized binders are fastened with Velcro. There are no contraindications to their application.

Equipment

Tape measure ■ binder of appropriate size and type ■ safety pins ■ gloves, if necessary.

Commercial elastic binders with Velcro closings are now commonly used instead of standard cotton straight and scultetus binders that require pins. Disposable T-binders are available, and scrotal supports typically replace binders for male patients, except after abdominal-perineal resection. (See *Types of binders,* page 186.) For non-breast-feeding mothers, a snug-fitting support brassiere is usually recommended, but mammary support binders are still available.

Preparation of equipment

Measure the area the binder must fit, and obtain the proper size and type of binder from the central supply department.

Implementation

• Check the doctor's order and assess the patient's condition.

• Explain the procedure to the patient, provide privacy, wash your hands thoroughly, and put on gloves if necessary.

• Raise the patient's bed to its highest position *to avoid muscle strain when applying the binder.*

Types of binders

Breast
Reduces breast engorgement in the non-breast-feeding mother

Scultetus
Keeps suture line intact after abdominal surgery so patient can move more freely, and provides abdominal support after delivery or paracentesis

Straight abdominal
Keeps suture line intact after abdominal surgery so patient can move more freely, and provides abdominal support after delivery or paracentesis

Single T
Keeps perineal dressings in place for the female patient

Double T
Secures perineal dressings for the male patient or for the female patient requiring a bulky dressing

• Change the dressing and inspect the wound or suture line if appropriate.

Applying a straight abdominal binder
• Accordion-fold half of the binder, slip it under the patient, and pull it through from the other side. Make sure the binder is straight, free of wrinkles, and evenly distributed under the patient. Its lower edge should extend well below the hips.
• Overlap one side snugly onto the other. Then insert one finger under the binder's edge *to ensure a snug fit that's still loose enough to avoid impaired circulation and patient discomfort.*
• Starting at the lower edge, pin the binder together with safety pins spaced about 2″ (5 cm) apart. Place pins well

away from a wound, a pressure point, or a tender and inflamed area *to avoid causing undue and uneven pressure.* Slip your fingers under the binder as you insert the pins *to avoid pricking the patient.* Place the pins horizontally *so they don't interfere with body movement.*

• Make darts in the binder as needed *to provide even snugness.* Avoid making the binder too tight around the diaphragm *because it may interfere with breathing.*

Applying a scultetus binder

• Slide the binder under the patient's hips and buttocks so that its top aligns with the waist and its lowest tail crosses the extreme lower abdomen.

• Adjust the binder so that its solid portion is centered under the patient and its tails are evenly distributed on either side. Spread the tails out flat on the bed *so you can pick them up easily.*

• Beginning at the lower edge of the binder, bring one tail straight across the patient's abdomen. If the tail is too long, fold it over flat at the end. Then hold this tail snugly in place as you bring the opposite tail across on top of it, overlapping the first tail's upper half and continuing with succeeding tail pieces. (See *Applying a scultetus binder.*)

• Secure the top strap, using two safety pins placed horizontally *so they won't interfere with body movement.*

Applying a T-binder

• Slip the T-binder under the patient's waist, with its tails extending below the buttocks. Smooth the waistband and tails *to remove twists, which can chafe and create pressure on the patient's skin.*

• Pull the waistband snugly into position at the patient's waistline or lower across the abdomen. Then fasten it with a safety pin. Next, bring the free tail up between the patient's legs over the dressing or perineal pad.

• For a female patient, bring the single tail up to the center of the waist, loop it behind and over the waistband, and secure it to the waistband by pinning through all layers of material. For a male patient, bring the two tails up on either side of the penis *to provide even support for the testicles.* Loop the ends behind and over the waistband on either side of the midline, and fasten them to the waistband by pinning through all layers of material. *Pinning through multiple layers keeps the straps from slipping sideways as the patient moves.*

• Instruct the patient to call you when he wishes to void or defecate *because the binder must be unfastened and then reapplied.*

Applying a scultetus binder

After centering the binder's solid portion under the patient, with tails distributed evenly on each side, bring the lowest tail straight across the patient's abdomen, hold it snugly, and bring the next higher tail across to overlap it. Alternate tails in this manner, with the next higher tail overlapping the one below it by about half its width.

Applying a breast binder

• Slip the binder under the patient's chest so that its lower edge aligns with the waist. Straighten the binder to distribute it evenly on either side of the body.

• Place the binder so that the patient's nipples are centered in the breast tissue. *This ensures proper breast alignment and support and produces faster tissue involution.*

• Pull the binder's edges snugly together and begin pinning upward from the waist. Slip your finger under the binder as you insert the pins *to avoid pricking the patient.* Use at least six pins, and place them horizontally *so they won't interfere with body movement.*

• Make darts in the binder wherever necessary *to provide a snug fit.* Do this by overlapping the material horizontally and pinning it perpendicularly.

• Adjust the shoulder straps to fit properly and secure them with safety pins.

When applying any binder

• Ask the patient if the binder feels comfortable. Tell him that it may feel tight initially but should feel comfortable shortly. Instruct the patient to notify you immediately if the binder feels too tight or too loose or comes apart.

• If the patient can ambulate, ask him to do so *to evaluate the fit of the binder.*

Special considerations

For maximum support, wrap the binder so that it applies even pressure across the body section. Eliminate all wrinkles and avoid placing pressure over bony prominences.

In surgical applications, fasten straight and scultetus binders from the bottom upward *to relieve gravitational pull on the wound.* In obstetric applications, fasten from the top downward *to direct the uterus into the pelvis. Because this places extra pressure on weak abdominal muscles,* observe the patient closely for precipitate delivery. For the obstetric patient, pin the last two straps of the scultetus binder on both sides; for the extremely large patient, pin all straps.

Be careful not to compress any tubes, drains, or catheters and not to position them so that they're working against gravity. Also, don't allow binder placement to interfere with elimination.

Use a double T-binder on a female patient after extensive surgery that requires a large dressing. Use a straight or scultetus binder as a breast binder, if necessary. Pin straps onto the upper front and back for additional support over the shoulders.

Observe the patient and check binder placement every 8 hours. Check the skin for color, palpate it for warmth, check pulses, and assess for tingling or numbness.

Reapply the binder when a dressing needs changing, when the binder becomes loose or too tight, and at other times according to the doctor's orders. When changing the binder, observe the skin for signs of irritation. Provide appropriate skin care before reapplying the binder.

Home care

If the patient will need a binder after discharge from the hospital, teach him and a family member how to remove it, inspect the skin, bathe the area, and reapply it. Tell the patient and family member where binders can be purchased and how to care for them. For a patient with cancer, the American Cancer Society may provide assistance in obtaining binders. If commercially manufactured binders are unavailable, advise the patient and family that a clean towel or discarded sheeting material can be used instead. Periodically reinforce prior teaching and instructions.

Complications

Irritation of the underlying skin can result from perspiration or friction.

Documentation

Record the date and time of binder application, reapplication, and removal; binder type and location; purpose of application; skin condition before and after application; dressing changes or skin care; any complications; and the patient's tolerance of the treatment.

 # Pressure dressings

For effective control of capillary or small-vein bleeding, temporary application of pressure directly over a wound may be achieved with a bulk dressing held by a glove-protected hand, bound into place with a pressure bandage, or held under pressure by an inflated air splint. A pressure dressing requires frequent checks for wound drainage to determine its effectiveness in controlling bleeding. Patients who need a pressure dressing may have such diagnoses as fluid volume deficit, impaired skin integrity, impaired tissue integrity, or altered tissue perfusion.

Equipment

Two or more sterile gauze pads ▪ roller gauze ▪ adhesive tape ▪ clean disposable gloves ▪ metric ruler.

Preparation of equipment

Obtain the pressure dressing quickly *to avoid excessive blood loss.* Use clean cloth for the dressing if sterile gauze pads are unavailable.

Implementation

• Quickly explain the procedure to the patient *to help decrease his anxiety,* and put on gloves.
• Elevate the injured body part *to help reduce bleeding.*
• Place enough gauze pads over the wound to cover it. Don't clean the wound; *you can do this when the bleeding stops.*
• For an extremity or trunk wound, hold the dressing firmly over the wound and wrap the roller gauze tightly across it and around the body part *to provide pressure on the wound.* Secure the bandage with adhesive tape.
• To apply a dressing to the neck, the shoulder, or another location that can't be tightly wrapped, don't use roller gauze. Instead, apply tape directly over the dressings *to provide the necessary pressure at the wound site.*
• Check pulse, temperature, and skin condition distal to the wound site *because excessive pressure can obstruct normal circulation.*
• Check the dressing frequently *to monitor wound drainage.* Use the metric standard of measurement to determine the amount of drainage, and document these serial measurements for later reference. Do not circle a potentially wet dressing with ink *because this provides no per-*

manent documentation in the medical record and also runs *the risk of contaminating the dressing.*
• If the dressing becomes saturated, do not remove it *because this will interfere with the pressure.* Instead, apply an additional dressing over the saturated one and continue to monitor and record drainage.
• Obtain additional medical care as soon as possible.

Special considerations
Apply pressure directly to the wound with your gloved hand if sterile gauze pads and clean cloth are unavailable.

Avoid using an elastic bandage to bind the dressing *because it can't be wrapped tightly enough to create pressure on the wound site.*

Complications
Excessively tight application of a pressure dressing can impair circulation.

Documentation
Once the bleeding is controlled, record the date and time of dressing application, the presence or absence of distal pulses, the integrity of distal skin, the amount of wound drainage, and any complications.

WOUND CARE
Management of surgical wounds

Procedures used to manage surgical wounds have several goals. They help prevent infection by barring pathogens from entering the wound. They protect the skin surface from maceration and excoriation caused by contact with irritating drainage. They allow measurement of wound drainage to monitor fluid and electrolyte balance. And they promote patient comfort.

The two principal methods for managing a draining wound are dressing and pouching. Dressing is the best choice when skin integrity is not compromised by caustic or excessive drainage. Lightly seeping wounds with drains, as well as wounds with minimal purulent drainage, usually can be managed with packing and gauze dressings. (See *Choosing a wound dressing.*) In some cases, such as when a wound becomes chronic, it may require an occlusive dressing. (For more information on dressings, see Chapter 13, Skin care.) Copious, excoriating drainage calls for pouching to protect the skin.

Dressing a wound necessitates sterile technique and sterile supplies to prevent contamination. Such dressings

Choosing a wound dressing

For a wound that requires frequent debriding and dressing changes, usually because of drainage or necrosis, most experts would choose a gauze dressing because it allows air to reach the wound and dry it.

Occlusive dressings
However, some experts believe that moisture at the wound surface promotes reepithelialization in some wounds. Thus, they recommend using occlusive or semiocclusive dressings because these dressings maintain moisture better than gauze dressings do. Occlusive dressings are also more comfortable and less painful, probably because they protect exposed cutaneous nerve endings.

For example, chronic leg ulcers have been treated successfully with occlusive, oxygen-impermeable hydrocolloid dressings. Hydrocolloid dressings are compounds of gelatin, pectin, carboxymethylcellulose sodium, and polyisobutylene. The inner part of such dressings interacts with the wound exudate, forming a hydrated gel over the wound. When you remove the dressing, the gel separates and remains on the wound, preventing damage to the new tissue.

Adhesive semipermeable dressings are not as effective as gauze for draining wounds because they "blister" and then leak.

Other dressings
A dressing containing dextranomer beads has been used successfully for wounds that need frequent cleaning. Burns and large pressure ulcers may benefit from biological dressings made from cadaver skin, pigskin, or human amniotic membranes instead of synthetic ones. These dressings reduce fluid loss, minimize local bacterial growth, and help granulation tissue to form. This ensures that the wound will be in the best possible condition for retaining an autograft. A cotton gauze dressing impregnated with crystallized sodium chloride (Mesalt) may help treat infected wounds.

For more on dressings, see the information on burn care and pressure ulcer treatments in Chapter 13, Skin care.

How to put on sterile gloves

Using your nondominant hand, pick up the opposite glove by grasping the exposed inside of the cuff.

Pull the glove onto your dominant hand. Be sure to keep your thumb folded inward to avoid touching the sterile part of the glove. Allow the glove to come uncuffed as you finish inserting your hand, but don't touch the outside of the glove.

Slip the gloved fingers of your dominant hand under the cuff of the loose glove to pick it up.

should be changed frequently enough to keep the skin dry.

Equipment
Waterproof trash bag ■ clean gloves ■ sterile gloves ■ gown, if indicated ■ sterile 4″ × 4″ gauze pads ■ ABD pads, if needed ■ sterile cotton-tipped applicators ■ topical medication, if ordered ■ adhesive or other tape ■ soap and water ■ optional: skin protectant, nonadherent pads, collodion spray, acetone-free adhesive remover or baby oil, normal saline solution, a graduated container, and Montgomery straps, a fish-net tube elasticized dressing support, or a T-binder.

For a wound with a drain: sterile scissors ■ sterile 4″ × 4″ gauze pads without cotton lining ■ sump drain ■ ostomy pouch or other collection bag ■ precut tracheostomy pads or drain dressings ■ adhesive tape (paper or silk tape if patient is hypersensitive) ■ surgical mask.

For pouching a wound: collection pouch with drainage port ■ sterile gloves ■ skin protectant ■ sterile gauze pads.

Several types of prepared equipment are available, including sterile swabs saturated with povidone-iodine, foam dressing for managing open granulating wounds, adhesive gauze, and complete prepackaged, sterile dressing sets, with or without instruments.

Preparation of equipment
Determine the type of dressing being used. Assemble all equipment in the patient's room. Check the expiration date on each sterile package and inspect for tears. Open the waterproof trash bag and place it near the patient's bed. Position the bag *to avoid reaching across the sterile field or the wound when disposing of soiled articles.* Form a cuff by turning down the top of the trash bag *to provide a wide opening and prevent contamination of instruments or gloves by touching the bag's edge.*

Implementation
• Check the doctor's order for specific wound care and medication instructions. Be sure to note the location of surgical drains *to avoid dislodging them during the procedure.* Assess the patient's condition.

• Identify the patient's allergies, especially to adhesive tape and povidone-iodine or other topical solutions or medications.

• Explain the procedure to the patient, provide privacy, and position the patient as necessary. Expose only the wound site *to avoid chilling the patient.*

Slide your nondominant hand into the glove, holding your dominant thumb as far away as possible to avoid brushing against your arm. Allow the glove to come uncuffed as you finish putting it on, but don't touch the skin side of the cuff with your other gloved hand.

• Wash your hands thoroughly. Put on a gown, if necessary, *to shield your clothing from wound drainage.* Put on clean gloves.

Removing the old dressing

• Loosen the soiled dressing by holding the patient's skin and pulling the tape or dressing toward the wound. *This protects the newly formed tissue and prevents stress on the incision.* Moisten the tape with acetone-free adhesive remover or baby oil, if necessary, *to make removal less painful, particularly from hairy skin.* Don't apply solvents to the incision, *to avoid contaminating the wound.*
• Slowly remove the soiled dressing. If the gauze adheres to the wound, loosen it by moistening with sterile normal saline solution.
• Observe the dressing for the amount, type, color, and odor of drainage.
• Discard the dressing and the gloves in the waterproof trash bag.

Caring for the wound

• Establish a sterile field with all the equipment and supplies you'll need for suture-line care and dressing change, including a sterile dressing set and povidone-iodine swabs. If ointment has been ordered, squeeze the needed amount onto the sterile field. If you're using an antiseptic from an unsterile bottle, pour the antiseptic cleaning agent into a sterile container *so you won't contaminate your gloves.* Then put on sterile gloves. (See *How to put on sterile gloves.*)
• If you won't be using prepackaged sterile povidone-iodine swabs to clean the wound, saturate sterile gauze pads with the prescribed cleaning agent. Avoid using cotton balls *because these may shed particles in the wound, causing irritation, infection, or adhesion.*
• If ordered, obtain a wound culture, then proceed to clean the wound.
• Pick up the moistened gauze pad or swab and squeeze out excess solution.
• Working from the top of the incision, wipe once to the bottom and then discard the gauze pad. With a second moistened pad, wipe from top to bottom in a vertical path next to the incision. (See *Wound-cleaning technique,* page 192.)
• Continue to work outward from the incision in lines running parallel to it. Always wipe from the clean area toward the less clean area, usually top to bottom. Use each gauze pad or swab for only one stroke *to avoid tracking wound exudate and normal body flora from the surrounding skin to the clean areas.* Remember that the suture line is cleaner than the adjacent skin, and the top of the suture line is typically cleaner than the bottom *because more drainage collects at the bottom of the wound.* Avoid cleaning from bottom to top *to prevent further wound contamination.*
• Use sterile cotton-tipped applicators for efficient cleaning of tight-fitting wire sutures, deep and narrow wounds, or wounds with pockets. *Because the cotton on the swab is tightly wrapped, it isn't as likely to leave particles in the wound as a cotton ball.* Remember to wipe only once with each applicator.
• If the patient has a surgical drain, clean the drain's surface last. *Because moist drainage facilitates growth of bacteria,* the drain is considered the most contaminated area. Clean the skin around the drain by wiping in half or full circles from the drain site outward.
• Clean all areas of the wound *to wash away debris, pus, blood, and necrotic material.* Try not to disturb sutures or irritate the incision. Clean to at least 1″ (2.5 cm) beyond the end of the new dressing. If you aren't applying a dressing, clean to at least 2″ (5 cm) beyond the incision.
• Check to see that the incision's edges are lined up properly, and check for signs of infection (heat, redness, swelling, odor), dehiscence, or evisceration. If you observe such signs or the patient reports pain at the wound site, notify the doctor.
• Irrigate the wound, if ordered. (For more information, see "Wound irrigation" in this chapter.)

Wound-cleaning technique

Using a povidone-iodine swab or a sterile gauze pad moistened with the prescribed antiseptic agent, wipe wound areas as shown: Clean a linear wound from top to bottom, and work from the clean area to the less clean area. Use a new swab or pad for each downward stroke. For a puncture wound, wipe the wound area in half or full circles, from the wound site outward, using a new swab or pad for each circular stroke.

• Wash the skin surrounding the wound with soap and water and pat dry. Avoid oil-based soap *because it may interfere with pouch adherence.* Apply any prescribed topical medication.

• Apply a skin protectant if warranted.

• If ordered, pack the wound with gauze pads or strips folded to fit. Avoid using cotton-lined gauze pads *because cotton fibers can adhere to the wound surface and cause complications.* (See *Packing a wound.*) Pack the wound using the wet-to-damp method. *Soaking the packing material in solution and wringing it out so that it is slightly moist provides a moist wound environment which absorbs debris and drainage. But new tissue won't be disrupted when the packing is removed.*

Applying a fresh gauze dressing

• To apply the new dressing, begin by gently placing sterile 4″ × 4″ gauze pads at the wound center and moving progressively outward to the edges of the wound site. Extend the gauze at least 1″ beyond the incision in each direction, and cover the wound evenly with enough sterile dressings (usually two or three layers) to absorb all drainage until the next dressing change. Use ABD pads to form outer layers, if needed, to provide greater absorbency.

• When the dressing is in place, remove and discard your gloves *because the tape may stick to them, making it difficult to apply.*

• Secure the edges of the dressing to the patient's skin with strips of tape *to maintain the sterility of the wound site.* Or secure the dressing with a T-binder or Montgomery straps *to prevent skin excoriation that may be caused*

by the repeated removal of tape necessitated by frequent dressing changes.

• Make sure the patient is comfortable.

• Properly dispose of solutions and trash bag, and clean or dispose of soiled equipment and supplies according to institutional policy. If the patient's wound has purulent drainage, don't return unopened sterile supplies to the sterile supply cabinet *to prevent cross-contamination of other equipment.*

• For the recently postoperative patient or a patient with complications, check the dressing every 30 minutes or as ordered. For the patient with a properly healing wound, check it at least once every 8 hours.

Dressing a wound with a drain

• Prepare a drain dressing by using sterile scissors to cut a slit in a sterile 4″ × 4″ gauze pad. Fold the pad in half, and cut inward from the center of the folded edge. Don't use a cotton-lined gauze pad *because cutting the gauze opens the lining and releases cotton fibers into the wound.* Prepare a second pad the same way.

• Gently press one folded pad close to the skin around the drain so that the tubing fits into the slit. Press the second folded pad around the drain from the opposite direction so that the two pads encircle the tubing.

• Layer as many uncut sterile 4″ × 4″ gauze pads or ABD pads around the tubing as needed *to absorb expected drainage.* Tape the dressing in place or use a T-binder or Montgomery straps. (See *How to make Montgomery straps,* page 194.)

Pouching a wound

• If the patient's wound is draining heavily or if drainage may damage surrounding skin, you'll need to create a pouch.

• Measure the wound, and cut an opening ⅛″ (0.3 cm) larger than the wound in the collection pouch's facing.

• Apply a skin protectant, as needed. Some protectants are incorporated within the collection pouch and also provide adhesion.

• Make sure the drainage port at the bottom of the pouch is firmly closed *to prevent leaks.* Then gently press the contoured pouch opening around the wound, beginning at its lower edge, *to catch any drainage.*

• To empty the pouch, put on gloves, insert its bottom half into a graduated collection container, and open the drainage port. Note the color, consistency, odor, and amount of fluid. Obtain a culture specimen, if ordered, and send it to the laboratory immediately. Remember to follow isolation precautions when handling infectious drainage.

• Wipe the bottom of the pouch and the drainage port with a gauze pad *to remove any drainage that could irritate the patient's skin or cause an odor.* Then reseal the port. Change the pouch only if it leaks or fails to adhere to the skin. *More frequent changes are unnecessary and only irritate the patient's skin.*

Special considerations

Because many doctors prefer to change the first postoperative dressing themselves *to check the incision,* avoid changing the first dressing unless you have specific instructions to do so. If you have no such order and drainage comes through the dressing, reinforce the dressing with fresh sterile gauze. Request an order to change the dressing, or ask the doctor to change it as soon as possible. A reinforced dressing shouldn't remain in place longer than 24 hours *because it's an excellent medium for bacterial growth.* Replace any dressing that becomes wet from the outside—from spilled drinking water, bath water, or urine, for example—as soon as possible *to prevent wound contamination.*

Consider all dressings and drains infectious.

Use acetone-free adhesive remover to remove any adhesive tape residue. If the doctor wants to avoid debriding the wound, place nonadherent pads directly over the incision before applying gauze pads *because gauze adheres to the wound and debrides it.*

If the patient has two wounds in the same area, cover each separately with layers of sterile 4″ × 4″ gauze pads. Then cover both sites with an ABD pad secured to the patient's skin with tape. Don't eliminate the gauze pads and use only an ABD pad to cover both sites *because*

Packing a wound

Pack the wound cavity carefully with moist gauze pads folded to fit. Make sure that all wound surfaces are covered and kept moist so that complete debridement can take place.

Pack the wound only until all wound surfaces and edges are covered. Packing that overlaps the edge can cause maceration of surrounding tissues.

drainage quickly saturates a single pad, promoting cross-contamination.

When packing a wound, don't pack it too tightly *because this may prevent wound edges from contracting and also compresses adjacent capillaries.* Avoid using overly damp packing *because it retards wound closure from within and increases the risk of infection.*

To save time when dressing a wound with a drain, use precut tracheostomy pads or drain dressings instead of custom-cutting gauze pads to fit around the drain. If the patient is sensitive to adhesive tape, use paper or silk tape *because these cause less skin reaction and will peel off*

How to make Montgomery straps

An abdominal dressing requiring frequent changes can be secured with Montgomery straps to promote the patient's comfort. If ready-made straps aren't available, follow these steps to make your own:

• Cut four to six strips of 2″ or 3″ (5 cm to 7.6 cm) wide nonallergenic tape of sufficient length to allow the tape to extend about 6″ (15.2 cm) beyond the wound on each side. (The length of the tape varies, depending on the patient's size and the type and amount of dressing.)

• Fold one end of each strip 2″ or 3″ back on itself (sticky sides together) to form a nonadhesive tab. Then cut a small hole in the folded tab's center, close to its top edge. Make as many pairs of straps as you'll need to snugly secure the dressing.

• Clean the patient's skin to prevent irritation. After the skin dries, apply a skin protectant. Then apply the sticky side of each tape to a skin barrier sheet composed of opaque hydrocolloidal or nonhydrocolloidal materials, and apply the sheet directly to the skin near the dressing. Next, thread a separate piece of gauze ties, umbilical tape, or twill tape (about 12″ [30.5 cm]) through each pair of holes in the straps and fasten each tie as you would a shoelace. Don't stress the surrounding skin by securing the ties too tightly.

• Repeat this procedure according to the number of Montgomery straps needed.

• Replace Montgomery straps whenever they become soiled (every 2 or 3 days). If skin maceration occurs, place new tapes about 1″ (2.5 cm) away from any irritation.

more easily than adhesive tape. Use a surgical mask to cradle a chin or jawline dressing; *this provides a secure dressing and avoids the need for shaving the patient's hair.*

If ordered, use a collodion spray or other similar topical protectant instead of a gauze dressing; *this moisture- and contaminant-proof covering dries in a clear impermeable film that leaves the wound visible for observation and avoids the friction caused by a dressing.*

If a sump drain isn't adequately collecting wound secretions, reinforce it with an ostomy pouch or other collection bag. Use waterproof tape to strengthen a spot on the front of the pouch near the adhesive opening; then cut a small "X" in the tape. Feed the drain catheter into the pouch through the "X" cut. Seal the cut around the tubing with more waterproof tape, and then connect the tubing to the suction pump. *This method frees the drainage port at the bottom of the pouch so you don't have to remove the tubing to empty the pouch.* If you use more than one collection pouch for a wound or wounds, be sure to record the volume of drainage separately for each pouch. Avoid using waterproof material over the dressing *because it*

reduces air circulation and predisposes the wound to infection from accumulated heat and moisture.

Home care

Include the patient in all aspects of wound management as early as possible *to allay anxiety and promote self-care.* Teach the importance of aseptic techniques, how to examine the wound for signs of infection and other healing problems, and how to change the dressing. Teach proper positioning, lighting, and use of mirrors so the patient or family members can view the wound clearly. Provide written instructions for all procedures to be performed at home. Urge the patient to call his doctor if he detects signs of infection.

Complications

Allergy to an antiseptic cleaning agent, prescribed topical medication, or adhesive tape may result in skin redness, rash, excoriation, or infection.

Documentation

Record the date, time, and type of wound management procedure; amount of soiled dressing and packing removed; wound appearance (size, condition of margins, presence of necrotic tissue) and odor, if present; type, color, consistency, and amount of drainage for each wound; presence and location of drains; any additional procedures, such as irrigation, packing, or application of a topical medication; type and amount of new dressing or pouch applied; and the patient's tolerance of the procedure.

Record special or detailed wound care instructions and pain management steps on the nursing care plan. Record the color and amount of measurable drainage on the intake and output sheet.

Suture removal

The goal of this procedure is to remove skin sutures from a healed wound without damaging newly formed tissue. The timing of suture removal depends on the shape, size, and location of the sutured incision; the absence of inflammation, drainage, and infection; and the patient's general condition. Usually, for a sufficiently healed wound, sutures are removed 7 to 10 days after insertion. Techniques for removal depend on the method of suturing, but all require sterile procedure to prevent contamination. Although sutures usually are removed by a doctor, in many institutions a nurse may remove them on the doctor's order.

Equipment

Waterproof trash bag ▪ adjustable light ▪ clean gloves, if the wound is dressed ▪ sterile gloves ▪ sterile forceps or sterile hemostat ▪ normal saline solution ▪ sterile gauze pads ▪ antiseptic cleaning agent ▪ sterile curve-tipped suture scissors ▪ povidone-iodine sponges ▪ optional: adhesive butterfly strips or Steri-Strips and compound benzoin tincture or other skin protectant.

Prepackaged, sterile suture-removal trays are available.

Preparation of equipment

Assemble all equipment in the patient's room. Check the expiration date on each sterile package and inspect for tears. Open the waterproof trash bag and place it near the patient's bed. Position the bag properly *to avoid reaching across the sterile field or the suture line when disposing of soiled articles.* Form a cuff by turning down the top of the trash bag *to provide a wide opening and prevent con-*

tamination of instruments or gloves by touching the bag's edge.

Implementation

- If your institution allows you to remove sutures, check the doctor's order *to confirm the exact time and details of this procedure.*
- Check for patient allergies, especially to adhesive tape and povidone-iodine or other topical solutions or medications.
- Tell the patient that you're going to remove the stitches from his wound. Assure him that this procedure typically is painless, but that he may feel a tickling sensation as the stitches come out. Reassure him that because his wound is healing properly, removing the stitches won't weaken the incision.
- Provide privacy, and position the patient so he's comfortable without placing undue tension on the suture line. *Because some patients experience nausea or dizziness during the procedure,* have the patient recline if possible. Adjust the light to have it shine directly on the suture line.
- Wash your hands thoroughly. If the patient's wound has a dressing, put on clean gloves and carefully remove it. Discard the dressing and the gloves in the waterproof trash bag.
- Observe the patient's wound for possible gaping, drainage, inflammation, signs of infection, or embedded sutures. Notify the doctor if the wound has failed to heal properly. The absence of a healing ridge under the suture line 5 to 7 days postinsertion indicates that the line needs continued support and protection during the healing process.
- Establish a sterile work area with all the equipment and supplies you'll need for suture removal and wound care. Put on sterile gloves and open the sterile suture removal tray if you're using one.
- Observing sterile technique, clean the suture line *to decrease the number of microorganisms present and reduce the risk of infection.* The cleaning process should also moisten the sutures sufficiently *to facilitate removal.* You can soften them further, if necessary, with normal saline solution.
- Then proceed according to the type of suture you're removing. (See *Methods for removing sutures,* page 196.) *Because the visible part of a suture is exposed to skin bacteria and is considered contaminated,* be sure to cut sutures at the skin surface on one side of the visible part of the suture. Remove the suture by lifting and pulling the visible end off the skin *to avoid drawing this contaminated portion back through subcutaneous tissue.*
- If ordered, remove only every other suture *to maintain some support for the incision.* Then go back and remove the remaining sutures.

Methods for removing sutures

Removal techniques depend in large part on the type of sutures you must remove. The illustrations below show removal steps for four common suture types. Keep in mind that, for all suture types, it's important to grasp and cut sutures in the correct place to avoid pulling the exposed (thus contaminated) suture material through subcutaneous tissue.

Plain interrupted sutures
Using sterile forceps, grasp the knot of the first suture and raise it off the skin. This will expose a small portion of the suture that was below skin level. Place the rounded tip of sterile curved-tip suture scissors against the skin and cut through the exposed portion of the suture. Then, still holding the knot with the forceps, pull the cut suture up and out of the skin in a smooth continuous motion to avoid causing the patient pain. Discard the suture. Repeat the process for every other suture, initially; if the wound doesn't gape, you can then remove the remaining sutures as ordered.

Mattress interrupted sutures
If possible, remove the small visible portion of the suture opposite the knot by cutting it at each visible end and lifting the small piece away from the skin *to prevent pulling it through and contaminating subcutaneous tissue.* Then remove the rest of the suture by pulling it out in the direction of the knot, as shown in the illustration at the top of the next column. If the visible portion is too small to cut twice, cut it once and pull the entire suture out in the opposite direction. Repeat for the remaining sutures and monitor the incision carefully for infection.

Plain continuous sutures
Cut the first suture on the side opposite the knot. Next, cut the same side of the next suture in line. Then lift the first suture out in the direction of the knot. Proceed along the suture line, grasping each suture where you grasped the knot on the first one.

Mattress continuous sutures
Follow the procedure for removing mattress interrupted sutures, first removing the small visible portion of the suture, if possible, *to prevent pulling it through and contaminating subcutaneous tissue.* Then extract the rest of the suture in the direction of the knot.

• After removing sutures, wipe the incision gently with gauze pads soaked in an antiseptic cleaning agent or with a povidone-iodine sponge. Apply a light sterile gauze dressing, if needed, *to prevent infection and irritation from clothing.* Then discard your gloves.

• Make sure the patient is comfortable. According to the doctor's preference, inform the patient that he may shower in 1 or 2 days if the incision is dry and heals well.

• Properly dispose of solutions and trash bag, and clean or dispose of soiled equipment and supplies according to institutional policy.

Special considerations
Be sure to check the doctor's order for the time of suture removal. Usually, you'll remove sutures on the head and neck 3 to 5 days after insertion; on the chest and abdomen, 5 to 7 days after insertion; and on the lower extremities, 7 to 10 days after insertion.

However, if the patient has interrupted sutures or an incompletely healed suture line, remove only those sutures specified by the doctor. He may want to leave some sutures in place for an additional day or two *to support the suture line.*

If the patient has both retention and regular sutures in place, check the doctor's order for the sequence in which they are to be removed. *Because retention sutures link underlying fat and muscle tissue and give added support to the obese or slow-healing patient,* these usually remain in place for 14 to 21 days.

Be particularly careful to clean the suture line before attempting to remove mattress sutures. *This decreases the risk of infection when the visible, contaminated part of the stitch is too small to cut twice for sterile removal and must be pulled through the tissue.* After you have removed mattress sutures this way, monitor the suture line carefully *for subsequent infection.*

If the wound dehisces during suture removal, apply butterfly adhesive strips or Steri-Strips to support and approximate the edges and call the doctor immediately to repair the wound.

Apply butterfly adhesive strips or Steri-Strips after any suture removal, if desired, *to give added support to the incision line and prevent lateral tension on the wound from forming a wide scar.* Use a small amount of compound benzoin tincture or other skin protectant *to ensure adherence.* Leave the strips in place for 3 to 5 days, or as ordered.

Home care
If the patient is being discharged, teach him how to remove the dressing and care for the wound. Instruct him to call the doctor immediately if he observes wound discharge or any other abnormal change. Tell him that

the redness surrounding the incision should gradually disappear and only a thin line should show after a few weeks.

Documentation
Record the date and time of suture removal, type and number of sutures, appearance of the suture line, any signs of wound complications, any dressings or butterfly strips applied, and the patient's tolerance for the procedure.

Removal of skin staples and clips

Skin staples or clips may be used instead of standard sutures to close lacerations or surgical wounds. Because they can secure a wound more quickly than sutures, they may substitute for surface sutures where cosmetic results are not a prime consideration, such as in abdominal closure. When properly placed, staples and clips distribute tension evenly along the suture line with minimal tissue trauma and compression, facilitating healing and minimizing scarring. Because staples and clips are made from surgical stainless steel, tissue reaction to them is minimal. Usually, doctors remove skin staples and clips, but some institutions permit qualified nurses to perform this procedure.

Skin staples and clips are contraindicated when wound location requires cosmetically superior results or when the incision site makes it impossible to maintain at least a 5 mm distance between the staple and underlying bones, vessels, or internal organs.

Equipment
Waterproof trash bag ▪ adjustable light ▪ clean gloves, if needed ▪ sterile gloves ▪ sterile gauze pads ▪ sterile staple or clip extractor ▪ povidone-iodine solution or other antiseptic cleaning agent ▪ sterile cotton-tipped applicators ▪ optional: butterfly adhesive strips or Steri-Strips, compound benzoin tincture or other skin protectant.

Prepackaged, sterile, disposable staple or clip extractors are available.

Preparation of equipment
Assemble all equipment in the patient's room. Check the expiration date on each sterile package and inspect for tears. Open the waterproof trash bag and place it near the patient's bed. Position the bag *to avoid reaching across the sterile field or the wound when disposing of soiled articles.* Form a cuff by turning down the top of the bag *to provide*

Removing a staple

Position the extractor's lower jaws beneath the span of the first staple, as shown in the first illustration. Squeeze the handles until they're completely closed; then lift the staple away from the skin, as shown in the second illustration. The extractor changes the shape of the staple and pulls the prongs out of the intradermal tissue.

a wide opening and prevent contamination of instruments or gloves by touching the bag's edge.

Implementation
• If your institution allows you to remove skin staples and clips, check the doctor's order *to confirm the exact timing and details of this procedure.*
• Check for patient allergies, especially to adhesive tape and povidone-iodine or other topical solutions or medications.
• Explain the procedure to the patient. Tell him that he may feel a slight pulling or tickling sensation, but little discomfort, during staple removal. Reassure him that because his incision is healing properly, removing the supporting staples or clips won't weaken the incision line.

• Provide privacy, and place the patient in a comfortable position that doesn't place undue tension on the incision. *Because some patients experience nausea or dizziness during the procedure,* have the patient recline if possible. Adjust the light to shine directly on the incision.
• Wash your hands thoroughly.
• If the patient's wound has a dressing, put on clean gloves and carefully remove it. Discard the dressing and the gloves in the waterproof trash bag.
• Assess the patient's incision and notify the doctor of gaping, drainage, inflammation, or other signs of infection.
• Establish a sterile work area with all the equipment and supplies you'll need for removing staples or clips and for cleaning and dressing the incision. Open the package containing the sterile staple or clip extractor, maintaining asepsis. Put on sterile gloves.
• Wipe the incision gently with sterile gauze pads soaked in an antiseptic cleaning agent, or with sterile cotton-tipped applicators, *to remove surface encrustations.*
• Pick up the sterile staple or clip extractor. Then, starting at one end of the incision, remove the first staple or clip. (See *Removing a staple.*) Hold the extractor over the trash bag, and release the handle to discard the staple or clip.
• Repeat the procedure for each staple or clip until all are removed.
• Apply a sterile gauze dressing, if needed, *to prevent infection and irritation from clothing.* Then discard your gloves.
• Make sure the patient is comfortable. According to the doctor's preference, inform the patient that he may shower in 1 or 2 days if the incision is dry and healing well.
• Properly dispose of solutions and the trash bag, and clean or dispose of soiled equipment and supplies according to institutional policy.

Special considerations
Carefully check the doctor's order for the time and extent of staple or clip removal. The doctor may want you to remove only alternate staples or clips initially and to leave the others in place for an additional day or two *to support the incision.*

When removing a staple or clip, place the extractor's jaws carefully between the patient's skin and the staple or clip *to avoid patient discomfort.* If extraction is difficult, notify the doctor; *staples or clips placed too deeply within the skin or left in place too long may resist removal.*

If the wound dehisces after staples or clips are removed, apply butterfly adhesive strips or Steri-Strips to approximate and support the edges, and call the doctor immediately to repair the wound. (See *Types of adhesive skin closures.)*

You may also apply butterfly adhesive strips or Steri-Strips after removing staples or clips even if the wound is healing normally *to give added support to the incision and prevent lateral tension from forming a wide scar.* Use a small amount of compound benzoin tincture or other skin protectant *to ensure adherence.* Leave the strips in place for 3 to 5 days.

Home care
If the patient is being discharged, teach him how to remove the dressing and care for the wound. Instruct him to call the doctor immediately if he observes wound discharge or any other abnormal change. Tell him the redness surrounding the incision should gradually disappear, and that after a few weeks only a thin line should show.

Documentation
Record the date and time of staple or clip removal, the number of staples or clips removed, appearance of the incision, any dressings or butterfly strips applied, any signs of wound complications, and the patient's tolerance for the procedure.

Management of wound dehiscence and evisceration

Although the typical surgical wound heals without incident, occasionally the edges of a wound may fail to join, or may separate even after they seem to be healing normally. This development, called wound dehiscence, may lead to an even more serious complication: evisceraton, where a portion of the viscera (usually a bowel loop) protrudes through the incision. Evisceration, in turn, can lead to peritonitis and septic shock. (See *Recognizing dehiscence and evisceration,* page 200.) Dehiscence and evisceration are most likely to occur 6 or 7 days after surgery. By then, sutures may have been removed and the patient can cough easily and breathe deeply—both of which strain the incision.

Several factors can contribute to these complications. Poor nutrition—whether from inadequate intake or a condition such as diabetes mellitus—may hinder wound healing. Chronic pulmonary or cardiac disease can also slow healing because the injured tissue doesn't get needed nutrients and oxygen. Localized wound infection may limit closure, delay healing, and weaken the incision. And stress on the incision from coughing or vomiting may cause abdominal distention or severe stretching. A

Types of adhesive skin closures

Steri-Strips are used as a primary means of keeping a wound closed after suture removal. They're made of thin strips of sterile, nonwoven, porous fabric tape.

Butterfly closures consist of sterile, waterproof adhesive strips. A narrow, nonadhesive "bridge" connects the two expanded adhesive portions. These strips are used to close small wounds and to assist healing after suture removal.

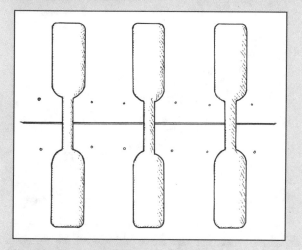

midline abdominal incision, for instance, has a high risk of wound dehiscence.

Equipment
Two sterile towels ■ 1 liter of normal sterile saline solution ■ sterile irrigation set, including a basin, a solution

Recognizing dehiscence and evisceration

In wound dehiscence, the layers of the surgical wound separate. With evisceration, the viscera (in this case, a bowel loop) protrude through the surgical incision.

Wound dehiscence

Evisceration of bowel loop

container, and a 50-ml catheter-tip syringe ■ several large abdominal dressings ■ sterile, waterproof drape ■ linen-saver pads ■ sterile gloves.

If the patient will return to the operating room, make sure you also gather the following equipment: I.V. administration set and I.V. fluids ■ equipment for nasogastric intubation ■ sedative, as ordered ■ suction apparatus.

Implementation

● Provide reassurance and support *to ease the patient's anxiety.* Tell him to stay in bed. If possible, stay with him while someone else notifies the doctor and collects the necessary equipment.

● Place a linen-saver pad under the patient *to keep the sheets dry when you moisten the exposed viscera.*

● Using sterile technique, unfold a sterile towel *to create a sterile field.* Open the package containing the irrigation set, and place the basin, solution container, and 50-ml syringe on the sterile field.

● Open the bottle of normal saline solution and pour about 400 ml into the solution container. Also pour about 200 ml into the sterile basin.

● Open several large abdominal dressings and place them on the sterile field.

● Put on the sterile gloves and place one or two of the large abdominal dressings into the basin *to saturate them with saline solution.*

● Place the moistened dressings over the exposed viscera. Then place a sterile, waterproof drape over the dressings *to prevent the sheets from getting wet.*

● Moisten the dressings every hour by withdrawing saline solution from the container through the syringe and then gently squirting the solution on the dressings.

● When you moisten the dressings, inspect the color of the viscera. If it appears dusky or black, notify a doctor immediately. *With its blood supply interrupted, a protruding organ may become ischemic and necrotic.*

● Keep the patient on absolute bed rest in low Fowler's position (no more than 20 degrees elevation) with his knees flexed. *This prevents injury and reduces stress on an abdominal incision.*

● Monitor the patient's pulse, respirations, blood pressure, and temperature every 15 minutes *to detect shock.*

● If necessary, prepare the patient to return to the operating room. Gather the equipment and start an I.V. infusion, as ordered.

● Insert a nasogastric tube and connect it to continuous or intermittent low suction, as ordered.

● Also administer preoperative medications to the patient as ordered.

● Depending on the circumstances, some of these procedures may not be done at the bedside. For instance, nasogastric intubation may make the patient gag or vomit, causing further evisceration. For this reason, the doctor may choose to have the tube inserted in the operating room with the patient under anesthesia.

● Continue to reassure the patient while you prepare him for surgery. Be sure he has signed a consent form and the operating room staff has been informed about the procedure.

Special considerations

As always, the best treatment is prevention. If you're caring for a postoperative patient who's at risk for poor healing, be sure he gets an adequate supply of protein, vitamins, and calories. Monitor his dietary deficiencies, and discuss any problems with a doctor and a dietitian.

When changing wound dressings, always use sterile technique. Inspect the incision with each dressing change and, if you recognize the early signs of infection, start treatment before dehiscence or evisceration can occur. If local infection develops, clean the wound as necessary to eliminate a buildup of purulent drainage. Always make sure bandages aren't so tight that they limit blood supply to the wound.

After surgery on obese or elderly patients with weak or pendulous abdominal walls, apply an abdominal binder. *You'll do this because large amounts of fatty tissue make approximating the wound edges more difficult and because fatty tissue heals slowly.* A large abdomen can also cause excessive stretching and abdominal wall tension.

Encourage the high-risk patient to splint his abdomen with a pillow during straining, coughing, or sneezing.

If a postoperative patient detects a sudden gush of pinkish serous drainage on his dressing, inspect the incision for dehiscence. If the wound seems to be separating slowly and evisceration hasn't developed, place the patient in the supine position. Apply a butterfly bandage to the wound edges and call the doctor.

Complications

Infection, which can lead to peritonitis and possibly septic shock, is the most severe and most common complication of wound dehiscence and evisceration. Caused by bacterial contamination or by drying of normally moist abdominal contents, infection can impair circulation and lead to necrosis of the affected organ. Immediately covering the wound with sterile, moist dressings reduces the risk of contamination and drying.

Assess for local infection by observing the wound for drainage, purulence, or odor. Inspect the incision for redness, swelling, or local inflammation. Suspect infection with a poorly approximated wound. Also look for signs of systemic infection, such as an increased white blood cell count, fever, and tachycardia.

Documentation

Note when the problem occurred, the patient's activity preceding the problem, his condition, and the time the doctor was notified. Describe the appearance of the wound or eviscerated organ; the amount, color, consistency, and odor of any drainage; and any nursing actions taken. Record the patient's vital signs, his response to the incident, and the doctor's actions.

Finally, be sure you change the patient care plan to reflect nursing actions needed to promote proper healing.

Management of traumatic wounds

Because most traumatic wounds are caused by accidental injury in unsterile conditions, they carry a high risk of local infection that can delay healing, increase scar formation, and lead to a systemic infection such as septicemia. Care of such wounds aims to remove bacteria, prevent infection, promote healing, and minimize scarring.

While caring for a traumatic wound, the nurse can also assess its condition. The type of wound and degree of contamination usually determine which cleaning technique and cleaning agent are most appropriate. Large, deep, or obviously dirty wounds may require analgesic medication and such special procedures as debridement and irrigation.

Equipment

Two sterile basins ▪ ordered antiseptic cleaning agent ▪ normal saline solution ▪ sterile 4″ × 4″ gauze pads ▪ sterile gloves and clean gloves ▪ sterile cotton-tipped applicators ▪ dry sterile dressing, nonadherent pad, or petroleum gauze ▪ linen-saver pad ▪ optional: scissors, towel, goggles, mask, gown, 50-ml catheter-tip syringe, surgical scrub brush, oral irrigating device, antibiotic ointment, porous tape, sterile forceps, sutures and suture set.

Preparation of equipment

Assemble needed equipment at the patient's bedside. Fill one basin with the ordered cleaning agent and the other with normal saline solution. Make sure the treatment area has enough light to allow careful observation of the wound. Depending on the nature and location of the wound, wear sterile or clean gloves *to avoid spreading infection.*

Implementation

• Wash your hands.

• Explain the procedure to the patient and provide privacy.

• Assess the patient's pain. Administer pain medication, if ordered, except intradermally injected local anesthetics, which are administered by the doctor.

• Place a linen-saver pad under the area to be cleaned.

• If necessary, cut the hair around the wound with scissors *to facilitate cleaning and treatment.*

• Wet a sterile 4″ × 4″ gauze pad with the ordered cleaning agent. Never clean a wound with cotton balls or cotton-filled gauze pads *because cotton fibers may be pulled off and left in the wound, causing contamination.* Clean the wound gently using a circular motion, working outward from the center of the wound to approximately 2″ (5 cm) past its edge. *This motion removes nearby sources of contamination and stimulates circulation to the wound site.* Discard the soiled gauze pad and use fresh ones as necessary.

• Continue cleaning for approximately 5 minutes or until the wound appears clean.

• Wet several 4″ × 4″ gauze pads with the normal saline and rinse the wound with the same circular motion used in cleaning.

• Extremely dirty wounds that require additional cleaning may be scrubbed with a surgical brush or irrigated with jet lavage (such as a 50-ml catheter-tip syringe or an oral irrigating device, such as a Water Pik). Don't use a bulb syringe or I.V. tubing *because these can't provide enough force to remove embedded debris.* Wear goggles, mask, gown, and sterile gloves when you're manually removing embedded debris *to avoid contaminating yourself with aerosolized particles.*

• After the wound has been cleaned, the doctor may debride it *to remove dead tissue and to reduce the risk of infection and scarring.*

• If necessary, the doctor may suture the wound edges using the suture kit provided, or apply sterile strips of porous tape, depending on the wound's depth.

• Apply the ordered antibacterial ointment *to help prevent infection.*

• Apply a dry sterile dressing over the wound *to absorb drainage and to protect the site from bacterial contamination.* Apply a nonadherent pad or petroleum gauze to abrasions *to keep the dressing from sticking to the wound.*

Special considerations

Do not clean a wound with alcohol *because it causes pain and dehydrates tissue.*

The doctor may perform extensive debriding and suturing in the operating room, using the suture kit provided. If this is necessary, pack the wound with gauze pads soaked in normal saline solution before moving the patient to the operating room. Recognize that a wound in an area subjected to repeated traumatic injury may require splinting *to promote complete healing.*

Check the patient's medical history for previous tetanus immunization and, if ordered, arrange for current immunization.

Teach the patient how to care for his wound, and, if necessary, inform him when to return to have his sutures removed.

Complications

The most common complication of traumatic wounds is infection.

Documentation

Record the date and time of the procedure, the size and condition of the wound, the administration of medications, and specific wound care measures.

 # Wound irrigation

Irrigation cleans tissues and flushes cell debris and drainage from an open wound. Irrigation with an antiseptic or antibiotic solution helps the wound heal properly from the inside tissue layers outward to the skin surface; it also helps prevent premature surface healing over an abscess pocket or infected tract. Performed properly, wound irrigation requires strict sterile technique. After irrigation, open wounds usually are packed to absorb additional drainage.

Equipment

Waterproof trash bag ■ linen-saver pad ■ emesis basin ■ clean gloves ■ sterile gloves ■ gown, if indicated ■ prescribed irrigant, such as sterile normal saline solution, hydrogen peroxide, or antibiotic solutions ■ sterile water or normal saline solution ■ soft rubber catheter ■ 50- to 60-ml piston syringe ■ sterile container ■ antiseptic cleaning agent ■ materials as needed for wound care ■ sterile irrigation and dressing set ■ povidone-iodine sponges ■ sterile petroleum jelly.

Preparation of equipment

Assemble all equipment in the patient's room. Check the expiration date on each sterile package and inspect for tears. Check the sterilization date and the date that each bottle of irrigating solution was opened; don't use any solution that's been open longer than 24 hours.

Using aseptic technique, dilute the prescribed irrigant to the correct proportions with sterile water or normal saline solution, if necessary. Let the solution stand until it reaches room temperature, or warm it to 90° to 95° F (32.2° to 35° C).

Open the waterproof trash bag and place it near the patient's bed *to avoid reaching across the sterile field or the wound when disposing of soiled articles.* Form a cuff by turning down the top of the trash bag *to provide a wide opening and prevent contamination by touching the bag's edge.*

Implementation

• Check the doctor's order, and assess the patient's condition. Identify the patient's allergies, especially to povidone-iodine or other topical solutions or medications.

• Explain the procedure to the patient, provide privacy, and position the patient correctly for the procedure. Place the linen-saver pad under the patient *to catch any spills and avoid linen changes.* Place the emesis basin below the wound *so the irrigating solution flows from the wound into the basin.*

• Wash your hands thoroughly. If necessary, put on a gown *to protect your clothing from wound drainage and contamination.* Put on clean gloves.

• Remove the soiled dressing; then discard the dressing and gloves in the trash bag.

• Establish a sterile field with all the equipment and supplies you'll need for irrigation and wound care. Pour the prescribed amount of irrigating solution into a sterile container *so you won't contaminate your sterile gloves later by picking up unsterile containers.* Put on sterile gloves.

• Fill the syringe with the irrigating solution; then connect the rubber catheter to the syringe. Gently instill a slow, steady stream of irrigating solution into the wound until the syringe empties. (See *Irrigating a deep wound.*) Make sure the solution flows from the clean to the dirty area of the wound *to prevent contamination of clean tissue by exudate.* Be sure the solution reaches all areas of the wound.

• Pinch the catheter closed before you withdraw the syringe *to prevent aspirating drainage and contaminating the equipment.*

• Refill the syringe, reconnect it to the catheter, and repeat the irrigation.

• Continue to irrigate the wound until you've administered the prescribed amount of solution or until the solution returns clear. Note the amount of solution administered. Then remove and discard the catheter and syringe in the waterproof trash bag.

• Keep the patient positioned *to allow further wound drainage into the basin.*

• Clean the area around the wound with povidone-iodine sponges or an antiseptic cleaning agent *to help prevent skin breakdown and infection.*

• Pack the wound, if ordered, and apply a sterile dressing. Remove and discard your gloves and gown.

• Make sure the patient is comfortable.

• Properly dispose of drainage, solutions, and trash bag, and clean or dispose of soiled equipment and supplies according to institutional policy. *To prevent contamination of other equipment,* don't return unopened sterile supplies to the sterile supply cabinet.

Irrigating a deep wound

When preparing to irrigate a deep wound, attach a soft rubber catheter to a piston-type syringe. Soft rubber minimizes tissue trauma, irritation, and bleeding. Then gently insert the catheter into the recesses of the wound until you feel resistance. Avoid forcing the catheter into the wound to prevent tissue damage or, in an abdominal wound, intestinal perforation.

Irrigate the wound with gentle pressure until the solution returns clean. Then position the emesis basin under the wound to collect any remaining drainage.

Special considerations

Try to coordinate wound irrigation with the doctor's visit *so he can inspect the wound.* Use only the irrigant specified by the doctor *because others may be erosive or otherwise harmful.* When using an irritating irrigant, such as Dakin's solution, spread sterile petroleum jelly around the wound site *to protect the patient's skin.* Remember to follow your institution's policy concerning wound and skin precautions when appropriate. Irrigate with a bulb syringe only if a piston syringe is unavailable; *the piston syringe reduces the risk of aspirating drainage.* If the wound is small or not particularly deep, you may want to use just the syringe for irrigation.

Home care

If the wound must be irrigated at home, teach the patient or a family member how to perform it using strict aseptic technique. Ask for a return demonstration of the proper technique. Provide written instructions. Arrange for home health supplies and nursing visits, as appropriate. Urge the patient to call his doctor if he detects signs of infection.

Complications

Wound irrigation increases the risk of infection. Excoriation and increased pain may also occur.

Documentation

Record the date and time of irrigation, amount and type of irrigant, appearance of the wound, any sloughing tissue or exudate, amount of solution returned, any skin care performed around the wound, any dressings applied, and the patient's tolerance of the treatment.

Closed-wound drain management

Typically inserted during surgery in anticipation of substantial postoperative drainage, a closed-wound drain promotes healing and prevents swelling by suctioning the serosanguineous fluid that accumulates at the wound site. By removing this fluid, the closed-wound drain helps reduce the risk of infection and skin breakdown as well as the number of dressing changes. Hemovac and Jackson-Pratt closed drainage systems are used most commonly.

A closed-wound drain consists of perforated tubing connected to a portable vacuum unit. The distal end of the tubing lies within the wound and usually leaves the body from a site other than the primary suture line to preserve the integrity of the surgical wound. The tubing exit site is treated as an additional surgical wound; the drain is usually sutured to the skin.

If the wound produces heavy drainage, the closed-wound drain may be left in place for longer than 1 week. Drainage must be emptied and measured frequently to maintain maximum suction and prevent strain on the suture line.

Equipment

Graduated cylinder ■ sterile laboratory container, if needed ■ alcohol sponges ■ gloves ■ trash bag ■ sterile gauze pads ■ antiseptic cleaning agent ■ prepackaged povidone-iodine swabs.

Implementation

● Check the doctor's order and assess the patient's condition.

● Explain the procedure to the patient, provide privacy, and wash your hands.

● Unclip the vacuum unit from the patient's bed or gown.

● Using aseptic technique, release the vacuum by removing the spout plug on the collection chamber. The container expands completely as it draws in air.

● Empty the unit's contents into a graduated cylinder, and note the amount and appearance of the drainage. If diagnostic tests will be performed on the fluid specimen, pour the drainage directly into a sterile laboratory container, note the amount and appearance, and send it to the laboratory.

● Maintaining aseptic technique, use an alcohol sponge to clean the unit's spout and plug.

● *To reestablish the vacuum that creates the drain's suction power,* fully compress the vacuum unit. With one hand holding the unit compressed *to maintain the vacuum,* replace the spout plug with your other hand. (See *Using a closed-wound drainage system.)*

● Check the patency of the equipment. Make sure the tubing is free of twists, kinks, and leaks *because the drainage system must be airtight to work properly.* The vacuum unit should remain compressed when you release manual pressure; rapid reinflation indicates an air leak. If this occurs, recompress the unit and make sure the spout plug is secure.

● Secure the vacuum unit to the patient's bedding or, if he is ambulatory, to his gown. Fasten it below wound level *to promote drainage.* Do not apply tension on drainage tubing when fastening the unit *to prevent possible dislodgement.* Remove and discard your gloves and wash your hands thoroughly.

● Observe the sutures that secure the drain to the patient's skin; look for signs of pulling or tearing, and for swelling or infection of surrounding skin. Gently clean

Using a closed-wound drainage system

The portable closed-wound drainage system draws drainage from a wound site, such as the chest wall postmastectomy shown at left, by means of a Y tube. To empty the drainage, remove the plug and empty it into a graduated cylinder. To reestablish suction, compress the drainage unit against a firm surface to expel air and, while holding it down, replace the plug with your other hand, as shown at right.

the sutures with sterile gauze pads soaked in an antiseptic cleaning agent or with a povidone-iodine swab.
• Properly dispose of drainage, solutions, and trash bag, and clean or dispose of soiled equipment and supplies according to institutional policy.

Special considerations
Empty the system and measure its contents once during each shift if drainage has accumulated, more often if drainage is excessive. *Removing excess drainage maintains maximum suction and avoids straining the drain's suture line.*

   If the patient has more than one closed drain, number the drains *so you can record drainage from each site.*
◆ *Nursing alert.* Be careful not to mistake chest tubes for closed-wound drains *because the vacuum of a chest tube should never be released.* ◆

Complications
Occlusion of the tubing by fibrin, clots, or other particles can reduce or obstruct drainage.

Documentation
Record the date and time you empty the system, the appearance of the drain site and presence of swelling or signs of infection, any equipment malfunction and consequent nursing action, and the patient's tolerance of the treatment. On the intake and output sheet, record drainage color, consistency, type, and amount. If the patient has more than one closed-wound drain, number the drains and record the above information separately for each drainage site.

RADIATION THERAPY
External radiation therapy

About 60% of all cancer patients are treated with some form of external radiation therapy. Also called radiotherapy, this treatment delivers radiation—X-rays or gamma rays—directly to the cancer site. Its effects are local, since only the area being treated experiences direct effects.

   Radiation doses are based on the type, stage, and location of the tumor, as well as on the patient's size, condition, and overall treatment goals. Doses are given in increments, usually 3 to 5 times a week, until the total dose is reached.

The goals of radiation therapy include *cure,* in which the cancer is completely destroyed and not expected to recur; *control,* in which the cancer does not progress or regress, but is expected to progress at some later time; or *palliation,* in which radiation is given to relieve symptoms (such as bone pain, seizures, bleeding, headache) caused by the cancer.

Radiation therapy may be augmented by chemotherapy, brachytherapy (radiation implant therapy), or surgery, as needed. (For information on chemotherapy, see Chapter 5, Drug Administration.)

External beam radiation therapy is delivered by machines that aim a concentrated beam of high-energy particles (photons and gamma rays) at the target site. Two types of machines are commonly used: units containing cobalt or cesium as radioactive sources for gamma rays, and linear accelerators that use electricity to produce X-rays. Linear accelerators produce high energy with great penetrating ability. Some (known as orthovoltage machines) produce less powerful electron beams that may be used for superficial tumors.

Equipment
Radiation therapy machine ▪ film badge or pocket dosimeter.

Implementation
• Explain the treatment to the patient and his family. Review the treatment goals, and discuss the range of potential adverse effects and interventions to minimize them. Also discuss possible long-term complications and treatment issues. Educate the patient and his family about local cancer services.
• Check to see that the radiation oncology department has obtained informed consent.
• Review the patient's clinical record for recent laboratory and imaging results, and alert the radiation oncology staff to any abnormalities or pertinent results (such as myelosuppression, paraneoplastic syndromes, oncologic emergencies, and tumor progression).
• Transport the patient to the radiology department.
• The patient begins by undergoing simulation (treatment planning), in which the target area is mapped out on his body using a machine similar to the radiotherapy machine. Then the target area is tattooed or marked in ink on his body *to ensure accurate treatments.*
• The doctor and radiation oncologist determine the duration and frequency of treatments, depending on the patient's body size, size of portal, extent and location of cancer, and treatment goals.

• The patient is positioned on the treatment table beneath the machine. Treatments last from a few seconds to a few minutes. Reassure the patient that he won't feel anything and that he will not be radioactive. After treatment is complete, the patient may return home or to his room.

Special considerations
Explain to the patient that the full benefit of radiation treatments may not occur until several weeks or months after treatments begin. Instruct him to report any long-term adverse effects.

Emphasize the importance of keeping follow-up appointments with the doctor.

Refer the patient to a support group, such as a local chapter of the American Cancer Society.

Home care
Instruct the patient and his family on proper skin care and management of the adverse effects of treatment.

Complications
Adverse effects arise gradually and diminish gradually after treatments. They may be acute, subacute (accumulating as treatment progresses), chronic (following treatment), and long-term (arising months to years after treatment). Adverse effects are localized to the area of treatment, and their severity depends on the total radiation dosage, underlying organ sensitivity, and the patient's overall condition.

Common acute and subacute adverse effects can include altered skin integrity, altered GI and genitourinary function, altered fertility and sexual function, altered bone marrow production, fatigue, and alopecia.

Long-term complications or adverse effects may include radiation pneumonitis, neuropathy, skin and muscle atrophy, telangiectasia, fistulas, altered endocrine function, and secondary malignancies.

Other complications of treatment include headache, alopecia, xerostomia, dysphagia, stomatitis, altered skin integrity (wet or dry desquamation), nausea, vomiting, heartburn, diarrhea, cystitis, and fatigue.

Documentation
Record radiation precautions taken during treatment; interventions used, and evaluation of the interventions; grading of adverse effects; teaching given to the patient and family and their responses to it; the patient's tolerance of isolation procedures and the family's compliance with procedures; discharge plans and teaching; and referrals to local cancer services, if any.

Radiation implant therapy

In this treatment, also called brachytherapy, the doctor uses implants of radioactive isotopes (encapsulated in seeds, needles, or sutures) to deliver ionizing radiation within a body cavity or interstitially to a tumor site. Implants can deliver a continuous radiation dose over several hours or days to a specific site while minimizing exposure to adjacent tissues. The implants may be permanent or temporary. Isotopes such as cesium 137 (^{137}Cs), gold 198 (^{198}Au), iodine 125 (^{125}I), iridium 192 (^{192}Ir), palladium 103 (^{103}Pd), and phosphorus 32 (^{32}P) are used to treat cancers. (See *Radioisotopes and their uses,* page 208.)

Common implant sites include the brain, breast, cervix, endometrium, lung, neck, oral cavity, prostate, and vagina.

Brachytherapy is commonly combined with external radiation therapy (teletherapy) for increased effectiveness.

For treatment, the patient is usually placed in a private room (with its own bathroom) located as far away from high-traffic areas as practical. If monitoring shows an increased radiation hazard, adjacent rooms and hallways may also need to be restricted. Consult your hospital's radiation safety policy for specific guidelines.

Equipment
Film badge or pocket dosimeter ▪ RADIATION PRECAUTION sign for door ▪ radiation precaution warning labels ▪ masking tape ▪ lead-lined container ▪ long-handled forceps ▪ male T-binder and two sanitary napkins with safety pin (if Burnett applicator is being used) ▪ optional: lead shield and lead strip.

Preparation of equipment
Place the lead-lined container and long-handled forceps in a corner of the patient's room. Mark a "safe line" on the floor with masking tape 6 feet (180 cm) from the patient's bed *to warn visitors to keep clear of the patient to minimize their radiation exposure.* If desired, place a portable lead shield in the back of the room *to use when providing care.*

Place an emergency tracheotomy tray in the room if an implant will be inserted in the oral cavity or neck.

Implementation
• Explain the treatment and its goals to the patient. Before treatment begins, review radiation safety procedures, visitation policies, potential adverse effects, and inter-

ventions for those effects. Also review long-term concerns and home care issues.

• Place the RADIATION PRECAUTION sign on the door.

• Check to see that informed consent has been obtained.

• Ensure that all laboratory tests are performed before beginning treatment. If laboratory work is required during treatment, the badged technician obtains the specimen, labels the collection tube with a radioactive precaution label, and alerts the laboratory personnel before bringing it. If urine tests are needed for ^{32}P therapy, ask the radiation oncology department or laboratory technician how to transport these specimens safely.

• Affix a radiation precaution warning label to the patient's identification wristband.

• Affix warning labels to the patient's chart and Kardex *to ensure staff awareness of the patient's radioactive status.*

• Wear a film badge or dosimeter at waist level during the entire shift. Turn in the radiation badge monthly or according to your hospital's protocol. Pocket dosimeters measure immediate exposures. In many centers, these measurements aren't part of the permanent exposure record but are used to ensure that nurses receive the lowest possible exposure.

• Each nurse must have a personal, nontransferable film badge or ring badge. *Badges document each person's cumulative lifetime radiation exposure.* Only primary caregivers are badged and allowed into the patient's room.

• To minimize exposure to radiation, use the three principles of time, distance, and shielding: Time — plan to give care in the shortest time possible. *Less time equals less exposure.* Distance — work as far away from the radiation source as possible. Give care from the side opposite the implant or from a position allowing the greatest working distance possible. *The intensity of radiation exposure varies inversely as the square of the distance from the source.* Shielding — use a portable shield, if needed and desired.

• Give essential nursing care only; omit bed baths. If ordered, provide perineal care, making sure that wipes, sanitary pads, and similar items are bagged correctly and monitored. (Refer to your hospital's radiation policy.)

• Dressing changes over an implanted area must be supervised by the radiation technician or another designated caregiver.

• Before discharge, a patient's temporary implant must be removed and properly stored by the radiation oncology department. A patient with a permanent implant may not be released until his radioactivity level is less than 5 millirems (mrem) per hour at one meter's distance.

Special considerations
Nurses and visitors who are pregnant or trying to conceive or father a child must not attend patients receiving

Radioisotopes and their uses

Unstable elements, radioisotopes emit three kinds of energy particles as they "decay" to a stable state. These particles are ranked by their penetrating power. *Alpha particles* possess the lowest energy level and are easily stopped by a sheet of paper. More powerful *beta particles* can be stopped by the skin's surface. *Gamma rays*, the most powerful, can only be stopped by dense shielding, such as lead. Some isotopes commonly used in cancer treatments are listed below.

ISOTOPE AND INDICATIONS	DESCRIPTION	NURSING CONSIDERATIONS
Cesium 137 (^{137}Cs) Gynecologic cancers	• 30-year half-life • Emits gamma particles • Encased in steel capsules which are placed temporarily in the patient in the operating room	• Elevate the head of the bed no more than 45 degrees. • Encourage fluids and implement a low-residue diet. • Encourage quiet activities; enforce strict bed rest, as ordered.
Iodine 125 (^{125}I) Localized or unresectable tumors; slow-growing tumors; recurrent disease	• 60-day half-life • Emits gamma particles • Permanently implanted as tiny seeds or sutures directly into the tumor or tumor bed	• Because seeds may become dislodged, no linens, body fluids, instruments, or utensils may leave the patient's room until they're monitored. • If a seed is dislodged and found, call the radiation department; use long-handled forceps to put it in a lead-lined container in the room. • Monitor body fluids to detect displaced seeds. Give the patient a 24-hour urine container that can be closed.
Iridium 192 (^{192}Ir) Localized or unresectable tumors	• 74-day half-life • Emits gamma particles • Temporarily implanted as seeds strung inside special catheters that are implanted around the tumor	• If a catheter is dislodged, call the radiation department; use long-handled forceps to put the implant in a lead-lined container in the room.
Palladium 103 (^{103}Pd) Superficial, localized or unresectable intrathoracic or intra-abdominal tumors	• 17-day half-life • Emits gamma particles • Permanently implanted as seeds in the tumor or tumor bed	• See Iodine 125.
Phosphorus 32 (^{32}P) Polycythemia, leukemia, bone metastasis, and malignant ascites	• 14-day half-life • Emits beta particles • Used as an I.V. solution rather than an implant because of its low energy level	• No shielding is required other than a lucite syringe shield. • Patients receiving ^{32}P are placed in a private room with a separate bathroom.
Gold 198 (^{198}Au) Localized male genitourinary tumors	• 3-day half-life • Emits gamma particles • Permanently implanted as tiny seeds directly into the tumor or tumor bed	• If a seed is dislodged and found, call the radiation oncology department for disposal.

radiation implant therapy *because the gonads and developing embryo and fetus are highly susceptible to the damaging effects of ionizing radiation.*

If the patient must be moved out of his room, notify the appropriate department of the patient's status *to give receiving personnel time to make appropriate preparations to receive the patient.* When moving the patient, ensure that the route is clear of equipment and other persons, and that the elevator, if there is one, is keyed and ready to receive the patient. Move the patient in a bed or wheelchair, accompanied by two badged caregivers. If the patient is delayed along the way, stand as far away from the bed as possible until you can continue.

The patient's room must be monitored daily by the radiation oncology department, and disposables must be monitored and removed according to hospital guidelines.

If a code is called on a patient with an implant, follow your hospital's code procedures as well as these steps: Notify the code team of the patient's radioactive status *to exclude any team member who is pregnant or trying to conceive or father a child.* Also notify the radiation oncology department. Cover the implant site with a strip of lead shielding if possible. Don't allow anything to leave the patient's room until it's monitored for radiation. The primary care nurse must remain in the room (as far away from the patient as possible) *to act as a resource person for the patient and to provide film badges or dosimeters to code team members.*

If an implant becomes dislodged, notify the radiation oncology department staff and follow their instructions. Typically, the dislodged implant is collected with long-handled forceps and placed in a lead-shielded canister.

Tell the patient who has had a cervical implant to expect slight to moderate vaginal bleeding after being discharged from the hospital. This flow normally changes color from pink to brown to white. Instruct her to notify the doctor if bleeding increases, persists for more than 48 hours, or has a foul odor. Explain to the patient that she may resume most normal activities but should avoid sexual intercourse and the use of tampons until after her follow-up visit to the doctor (about 6 weeks after discharge). Instruct her to take showers rather than baths for 2 weeks, to avoid douching unless allowed by the doctor, and to avoid activities that cause abdominal strain for 6 weeks.

Refer the patient for sexual or psychological counseling if needed.

If a patient with an implant dies on the unit, notify the radiation oncology department *so they can remove a temporary implant and store it properly.* If the implant was permanent, radiation oncology staff members will determine which precautions to follow before postmortem

care can be provided and before the body can be moved to the morgue.

Complications

Depending on the implant site and total radiation dosage, complications of implant therapy may include dislodgment of the radiation source or applicator, tissue fibrosis, xerostomia, radiation pneumonitis, muscle atrophy, sterility, vaginal dryness or stenosis, fistulas, hypothyroidism, altered bowel habits, infection, airway obstruction, diarrhea, cystitis, myelosuppression, neurotoxicity, and secondary cancers. Encourage the patient and family members to keep in contact with the radiation oncology department and to call them if concerns or physical changes occur.

Documentation

Record radiation precautions taken during treatment; adverse effects of therapy; teaching given to the patient and family and their responses to it; the patient's tolerance of isolation procedures and the family's compliance with procedures; and referrals to local cancer services.

 ## Radioactive iodine therapy

Because the thyroid gland concentrates iodine, radioactive iodine 131 (^{131}I) can be used to treat thyroid cancer. This isotope emits beta and gamma radiation, and its half-life (the time required for it to decay to 50% of its original activity) is 8 days. Usually administered orally, ^{131}I is used to treat postoperative residual cancer, recurrent disease, inoperable primary thyroid tumors, invasion of the thyroid capsule, or thyroid ablation as well as cancers that have metastasized to cervical or mediastinal lymph nodes or other distant sites.

Because ^{131}I is absorbed systemically, all body secretions, especially urine, must be considered radioactive. For ^{131}I treatments, the patient usually is placed in a private room (with its own bathroom) located as far away from high-traffic areas as practical. If monitoring shows increased radiation hazard, adjacent rooms and hallways may also need to be restricted. Consult your hospital's radiation safety policy for specific guidelines.

In lower doses, radioactive ^{131}I also may be used to treat hyperthyroidism. Most patients receive this treatment on an outpatient basis and are sent home with appropriate home care instructions.

HOME CARE

What to do after ¹³¹I treatment

- Instruct the patient to report any long-term adverse reactions. In particular, review signs and symptoms of hypothyroidism and hyperthyroidism. Also ask him to report any signs and symptoms of thyroid cancer, such as enlarged lymph nodes, dyspnea, bone pain, nausea, vomiting, and abdominal discomfort.
- Although the patient's radiation level at discharge will be safe, suggest that he take extra precautions during the first week, such as using separate eating utensils, sleeping in a separate bedroom, and avoiding bodily contact.
- Sexual intercourse may be resumed 1 week after ¹³¹I treatment. However, urge a female patient to avoid pregnancy for 6 months after treatment, and tell a male patient to avoid impregnating his partner for 3 months after treatment.

Equipment

Film badges, pocket dosimeters, or ring badges ■ RADIATION PRECAUTION sign for door ■ radiation precaution warning labels ■ waterproof gowns ■ clear and red plastic bags for contaminated articles ■ plastic wrap ■ absorbent plastic-lined pads ■ masking tape ■ radioresistant gloves ■ trash cans ■ optional: portable lead shield.

Preparation of equipment

Assemble all necessary equipment in the patient's room. Keep an emergency tracheotomy tray just outside the room or in a handy place at the nurses' station. Place the RADIATION PRECAUTION sign on the door. Affix warning labels to the patient's chart and Kardex *to ensure staff awareness of the patient's radioactive status.*

Place an absorbent plastic back pad on the bathroom floor and under the sink; if the patient's room is carpeted, cover it with such a pad as well. Place an additional pad over the bedside table. Secure plastic wrap over the telephone, television controls, bed controls, mattress, call button, and toilet. *These measures prevent radioactive contamination of working surfaces.*

Keep large trash cans in the room lined with plastic bags (two clear bags inserted inside an outer red bag). Monitor all objects before they leave the room.

Notify the dietitian to supply foods and beverages only in disposable containers and with disposable utensils.

Implementation

- Explain the procedure and review treatment goals with the patient and his family. Before treatment begins, review radiation safety procedures, visitation policies, potential adverse effects, interventions, and home care procedures. (See *What to do after ¹³¹I treatment.*)
- Verify that the doctor has obtained informed consent.
- Check for allergies to iodine-containing substances such as contrast media or shellfish. Review the medication history for thyroid-containing or thyroid-altering drugs and for lithium carbonate, *which may increase ¹³¹I uptake.*
- Review the patient's health history for vomiting, diarrhea, productive cough, and sinus drainage, *which could increase the risk of radioactive secretions.*
- If necessary, remove the patient's dentures *to avoid contaminating them and to reduce radioactive secretions.* Tell him they'll be replaced 48 hours after treatment.
- Affix a RADIATION PRECAUTION label to the patient's identification wristband.
- Encourage the patient to use the toilet rather than a bedpan or urinal, and to flush it three times after each use *to reduce radiation levels.*
- Instruct the patient to remain in his room except for tests or other special reasons. Allow him to ambulate.
- Unless contraindicated, instruct the patient to increase his fluid intake to 3 quarts daily.
- Encourage the patient to chew or suck on hard candy *to keep salivary glands stimulated and to prevent them from becoming inflamed (which may develop in the first 24 hours.)*
- Ensure that all laboratory tests are performed before beginning treatment. If laboratory work is required, the badged laboratory technician obtains the specimen, labels the collection tube with a RADIOACTIVE PRECAUTION label, and alerts the laboratory personnel before transporting it. If urine tests are needed, ask the radiation oncology department or laboratory technician how to transport these specimens safely.
- Wear a film badge or dosimeter at waist level during the entire shift. Turn in the radiation badge monthly or according to your hospital's protocol, and be sure to record your exposures accurately. *Pocket dosimeters measure immediate exposures. These measurements may not be part of the permanent exposure record but help to ensure that nurses receive the lowest possible exposure.*
- Each nurse must have a personal, nontransferable film badge or ring badge. *Badges document each person's cumulative lifetime radiation exposure.* Only primary caregivers are badged and allowed into the patient's room.
- Wear gloves to touch the patient or objects in his room.
- Allow visitors to spend no more than 30 minutes every 24 hours with the patient. Stress that no visitors will be allowed who are under age 18 or who are pregnant or trying to conceive or father a child.

• Restrict direct contact to no more than 30 minutes or 20 millirems (mrem) per day. If the patient is receiving 200 millicuries (mCi) of ^{131}I, remain with him only 2 to 4 minutes and stand no closer than 1' (30 cm) away. If standing 3' (1 m) away, the time limit is 20 minutes; if standing 5' (1.5 m) away, the limit is 30 minutes.

• Give essential nursing care only; omit bed baths. If ordered, provide perineal care, making sure that wipes, sanitary pads, and similar items are bagged correctly and monitored.

• If the patient vomits or urinates on the floor, notify the nuclear medicine department and use nondisposable radioresistant gloves when cleaning the spill. After cleanup, wash your gloved hands, remove the gloves and leave them in the room, then rewash your hands.

• If the patient must be moved from his room, notify the appropriate department of the patient's status *so that receiving personnel can make appropriate arrangements to receive him.* When moving the patient, ensure that the route is clear of equipment and other persons and that the elevator, if there is one, is keyed and ready to receive the patient. Move the patient in a bed or wheelchair, accompanied by two badged caregivers. If the patient is delayed along the way, stand as far away from him as possible until you can continue.

• The patient's room must be cleaned by the radiation oncology department, not by housekeeping. The room must be monitored daily, and disposables must be monitored and removed according to hospital guidelines.

• At discharge, schedule the patient for a follow-up examination. Also arrange for a whole-body scan approximately 7 to 10 days after ^{131}I treatment.

• Inform the patient and his family of community support services for cancer patients.

Special considerations

Nurses and visitors who are pregnant or trying to conceive or father a child must not attend or visit patients receiving ^{131}I therapy *because the gonads and developing embryo and fetus are highly susceptible to the damaging effects of ionizing radiation.*

If a code is called on a patient undergoing ^{131}I therapy, follow your hospital's code procedures as well as these steps. Notify the code team of the patient's radioactive status *to exclude any team member who is pregnant or trying to conceive or father a child.* Also notify the radiation oncology department. Don't allow anything out of the patient's room until it's monitored. The primary care nurse must remain in the room (as far as possible from the patient) *to act as a resource person for the patient and to provide film badges or dosimeters to code team members.*

If the patient dies on the unit, notify the radiology safety officer who will determine which precautions to follow before postmortem care is provided and before the body can be moved to the morgue.

Complications

Myelosuppression is common in patients who have extensive disease or who undergo repeated ^{131}I treatments.

Radiation pulmonary fibrosis may develop if extensive lung metastasis was present when ^{131}I was administered.

Other complications may include nausea, vomiting, headache, radiation thyroiditis, fever, sialadenitis, or pain and swelling at metastatic sites.

Documentation

Record radiation precautions taken during treatment, teaching given to the patient and family and their responses to it, the patient's tolerance of isolation procedures and the family's compliance with procedures, and referrals to local cancer counseling services.

Selected references

Bucholtz, J. "Radiation Therapy," in *Core Curriculum for Oncology Nursing.* Philadelphia: W.B. Saunders Co., 1987.

Campbell, A.D. "Pneumatic Compression Stockings: Preventing Deep Vein Thrombosis and Pulmonary Embolus," *Today's O.R. Nurse* 12(7):4-9, July 1990.

Cooper, D.M. "Optimizing Wound Healing: A Practice Within Nursing's Domain," *Nursing Clinics of North America* 25(1):165-80, March 1990.

Eriksson, J.H. *Oncologic Nursing: A Study and Learning Tool.* Springhouse Notes. Springhouse, Pa.: Springhouse Corp., 1989.

Fahey, V. "An In-depth Look at Deep Vein Thrombosis," *Nursing89* 19(1):86-93, January 1989.

Greenfield, L. "Thyroid Tumors," in *Principles and Practice of Radiation Oncology.* Edited by Perez, C., and Brady, L. Philadelphia: J.B. Lippincott Co., 1987.

Hassey, K.M. "Principles of Radiation Safety and Protection," *Seminars in Oncology Nursing* 3(1):23-29, February 1987.

Jones, P., and Millman, A. "Wound Healing and the Aged Patient," *Nursing Clinics of North America* 25(1):263-77, March 1990.

McCaffery, M., and Beebe, A. *Pain: Clinical Manual for Nursing Practice.* St. Louis: Mosby-Year Book, Inc., 1989.

Porteous, M.J., et al. "Thigh-length Versus Knee-length Stockings in the Prevention of Deep Vein Thrombosis," *British Journal of Surgery* 76(3):296-97, March 1989.

Scurr, J.H., et al. "Regimen for Improved Effectiveness of Intermittent Pneumatic Compression in Deep Venous Thrombosis Prophylaxis," *Surgery* 102(5):816-20, November 1987.

Taylor, C., et al. *Fundamentals of Nursing: The Art and Science of Nursing Care.* Philadelphia: J.B. Lippincott Co., 1989.

Timby, B.K., et al. *Clinical Nursing Procedures.* Philadelphia: J.B. Lippincott Co., 1989.

CHAPTER **5**

DRUG ADMINISTRATION

SUSAN J. HART, RN,C, MSN, CCRN

Introduction

Administering drugs is one of your most crucial nursing responsibilities. To ensure safe and effective drug therapy for your patients, you need to be familiar with the indications, customary dosages, and intended effects of prescribed drugs. And you need to assess each patient before administering a drug, delaying or withholding it if necessary. Just as important, you need the skills to be able to administer a drug capably, minimizing your patient's anxiety and maximizing the drug's effectiveness. This chapter will help you perform this task by providing the information you need to give drugs by injection, instillation, inhalation, topical application, and intravascular route. You'll also learn how to add drugs to an I.V. solution, give I.V. bolus injections, and prepare and administer chemotherapeutic drugs.

Selecting the appropriate route

Drugs may be administered by many routes. The *topical*, or dermatomucosal, route includes aural, ocular, nasal, and vaginal administration, oropharyngeal inhalation, and transdermal absorption. The *enteral* route, the most commonly used one, involves drug absorption through the GI tract. The *parenteral* route includes intradermal, subcutaneous, intramuscular, I.V., intrathecal, and intraosseous infusions or injections. The *epidural* route involves giving a drug (usually an anesthetic or narcotic analgesic) through a catheter inserted near the spinal cord by a lumbar puncture.

More than any other factor, the administration route determines the onset of drug effect. For example, drugs administered I.V. act almost instantly because they're immediately available in the bloodstream. Antibiotics, for instance, are commonly given I.V. to provoke a quick, continuous response. Other drugs must be given I.V. because they're ineffective or even dangerous when given by other routes.

Conversely, some drugs—such as NPH insulin or penicillin G procaine—can't be given I.V. because they obstruct blood flow. Drugs administered intrathecally, such as spinal anesthetics, also act rapidly. However, drugs administered orally must be absorbed into the bloodstream before they can take effect. Because their peak effects are therefore delayed, oral drugs are used most often when the patient's condition doesn't require an immediate drug effect.

Avoiding medication errors

Before you administer any medication, always compare the doctor's order with the order on the patient's medication record. Then mentally check off the first five "rights" of drug administration: *right patient, right drug, right dose, right route, and right time*. If the doctor's order and the patient's medication record match, then compare the label on the medication to the medication record. If you find any discrepancies, withhold the drug and verify the order with the doctor or the pharmacist. If a patient questions any of his drugs, always double-check the orders and the dose before administration. Also check the drug's expiration date.

Before giving any drug, you need to be aware of two more "rights": the patient's *right to know why he's getting the drug and what adverse effects to expect, if any;* and his *right to refuse medication*.

Some drugs—such as narcotics, barbiturates, and other controlled substances—have automatic stop dates, mandated by law. Other medications, such as antibiotics, have stop dates set by hospital policy. Check your hospital's policy on how to handle outdated orders, and check drug expiration dates. Also learn your hospital's policies on acceptance and documentation of verbal orders and correct use of p.r.n. (as needed) orders.

Understanding patient response and drug interactions

Assessing a patient's response to medication requires a thorough understanding of his condition and the drug's desired or expected effect. If a patient is receiving an antiarrhythmic, for example, but continues to have premature ventricular contractions, you should tell the doctor that the drug isn't producing the desired effect.

When assessing the patient's response to therapy, also consider the results of laboratory tests, which can indicate a therapeutic effect, adverse effect, or toxic level. For example, prothrombin times help to evaluate the therapeutic effect of warfarin sodium, and low serum potassium levels may signal an adverse effect of certain diuretics. Be aware that some drugs may affect diagnostic test results, causing "false positives." (For example, codeine may elevate cerebrospinal fluid pressure.)

Monitor the patient's condition carefully; such changes as weight loss or gain can affect the action of some drugs. Other factors—such as the patient's age, body build, sex, and emotional state—also may affect the patient's response to drug therapy.

Because many patients receive more than one drug, you should also understand drug *interactions*. A drug interaction is a change in drug absorption, distribution, metabolism, and excretion that may occur with or shortly after administration of another drug. A desirable interaction is the basis for combination therapy, which may be used for additive effect, for helping to maintain an effective blood level, and for minimizing or preventing adverse effects. Some interactions, however, can have undesirable results, such as weakening a drug's desired effects or exaggerating its toxic ones. For example, patients who smoke require larger doses of theophylline than nonsmokers because cigarette smoke activates oxidative enzymes in the liver, increasing drug metabolism.

Watching for adverse effects

When you administer drugs, you also need to recognize and identify adverse effects, toxic reactions, and drug allergies. Some *adverse effects* are transient and subside as the patient develops a tolerance for the drug. Other adverse effects may require a change in therapy.

Toxic reactions to a drug can be acute, resulting from excessive doses, as in acetaminophen overdose, or chronic, resulting from progressive accumulation of the drug in the body. Toxic reactions can also result from impaired metabolism or excretion that can cause elevated blood levels of a drug.

Drug allergy (hypersensitivity) results from an antigen-antibody reaction in susceptible patients. Such a reaction can range from mild urticaria to potentially fatal anaphylaxis. Therefore, always be sure to check for allergies before administering medications. In some instances, sensitivity tests may be done before giving the first dose. Be aware that a negative history does not rule out a future allergic reaction.

Other undesirable effects to watch for when administering drugs include idiosyncratic reactions and dependence.

Document carefully

Documentation aims to preserve an accurate record of patient assessment and interventions as well as your reasons for giving the care specified. Documenting a patient's medications provides a legal record of drugs he received during his hospital stay. Medication administration involves documenting on a medication administration record as well as in the nurses' notes. Many hospitals also require documentation of narcotic administration in a central record.

After administering a drug, document the following on the patient's Kardex or computer file: drug name, dosage, route and time of administration, and your signature and title. In the nurses' notes, include any assessment data that refer to the patient's response to the medication or any adverse effects of the medication.

If your hospital documents medications by computer, be sure to enter each drug immediately after you give it. This gives all health care team members access to current medication information and is especially important if the system has no hard-copy backup. If a patient refuses or is unable to take medication, or if—in your judgment—the patient shouldn't receive the medication, document this on the medication administration record and in the nurses' notes.

Many hospitals use a medication administration record to document medication orders and administration. Usually contained in a Kardex file, the medication administration record serves as the central source for recording the doctor's medication orders and documenting administration. It becomes part of the patient's permanent medical record. When using the medication administration record, know and follow your hospital's policy and procedure for recording medication orders and charting medication administration. Make sure medication orders include the patient's full name, date ordered, drug dose, administration route or method, frequency, and time ordered for the first dose. Some drugs may be ordered with a specific number of doses or a stop date. If that's so, be sure to note this on the medication administration record. Always write legibly. Use only acceptable abbreviations and use them correctly. When in doubt as to how to abbreviate a term, spell it out. When documenting parenteral medications, be sure to include the injection site and the route you used. After administering the first dose, sign your full name, licensure status, and identifying initials in the appropriate place on the medication administration record.

If all medications have been given according to the care plan, no further documentation is needed. However, if your hospital's medication administration record does not include a place to document parenteral administration sites, patient's response to p.r.n. medications, or any deviation from the medication order, further narrative documentation is necessary. Document any patient teaching given, as well as the patient's response and knowledge level.

TOPICAL ADMINISTRATION
Application of topical skin medications

Topical drugs are applied directly to the skin surface. They include lotions, pastes, ointments, creams, powders, shampoos, and aerosol sprays. The medication is absorbed through the epidermal layer into the dermis. The extent of absorption depends on the vascularity of the region. Except for nitroglycerin and certain supplemental hormone replacements, topical medications are commonly used for local, rather than systemic, effects. Ointments have a fatty base, which is an ideal vehicle for such drugs as antimicrobials and antiseptics. Typically, topical medications should be applied two or three times a day to achieve their therapeutic effect.

Equipment
Patient's medication record and chart ▪ prescribed medication ▪ sterile tongue blades ▪ gloves ▪ 4″ × 4″ sterile gauze pads ▪ transparent semipermeable dressing ▪ adhesive tape ▪ solvent (such as cottonseed oil).

Implementation
• Verify the order on the patient's medication record by checking it against the doctor's order on the chart.
• Make sure the label on the medication agrees with the medication order. Read the label again before you open the container and as you remove the medication from the container.
• Confirm the patient's identity by asking his name and checking the name, room number, and bed number on his wristband.
• Provide privacy.
• Explain the procedure thoroughly to the patient *because, after discharge, he may have to apply the medication by himself.*
• Wash your hands *to prevent cross-contamination*, and glove your dominant hand.
• Help the patient assume a comfortable position that provides access to the area to be treated.
• Expose the area to be treated. Make sure the skin or mucous membrane is intact (unless the medication has been ordered to treat a skin lesion, such as an ulcer). *Application of medication to broken or abraded skin may cause unwanted systemic absorption and result in further irritation.*
• If necessary, clean the skin of debris, including crusts, epidermal scales, and old medication. You may have to change the glove if it becomes soiled.

Applying a paste, a cream, or an ointment
• Open the container. Place the lid or cap upside down *to prevent contamination of the inside surface.*
• Remove a tongue blade from its sterile wrapper and cover one end with medication from the tube or jar. Then, transfer the medication from the tongue blade to your gloved hand.
• Apply the medication to the affected area with long, smooth strokes that follow the direction of hair growth. *This technique avoids forcing medication into hair follicles, which can cause irritation and lead to folliculitis.* Avoid excessive pressure when applying the medication *because it could abrade the skin.*

• *To prevent contamination of the medication,* use a new tongue blade each time you remove medication from the container.

Removing an ointment
• To remove ointment, wash your hands; then rub solvent on them and apply it liberally to the treated area in the direction of hair growth. Alternatively, saturate a sterile gauze pad with the solvent and use this pad to gently remove the ointment. Remove excess oil by gently wiping the area with the sterile gauze pad. Don't rub too hard to remove the medication *because you could irritate the skin.*

Applying other topical medications
• To apply *shampoos,* follow package directions. (See *Using medicated shampoos,* page 216.)
• To apply *aerosol sprays,* shake the container, if indicated, *to completely mix the medication.* Hold the container 6″ to 12″ (15 to 30 cm) from the skin or follow the manufacturer's recommendation. Spray the medication evenly over the treatment area *to apply a thin film.*
• To apply *powders,* dry the skin surface, making sure to spread skin folds where moisture collects. Then apply a thin layer of powder over the treatment area.
• *To protect applied medications and prevent them from soiling the patient's clothes,* tape an appropriate amount of sterile gauze pad or a transparent semipermeable dressing over the treated area. If you're applying topical medication to the patient's hands or feet, cover the site with white cotton gloves for the hands or terry cloth scuffs for the feet.
• Assess the patient's skin for signs of irritation, allergic reaction, or breakdown.

Special considerations
Never apply medication without first removing previous applications *to prevent skin irritation from an accumulation of medication.*

Be sure to wear gloves *to prevent absorption by your own skin.* If the patient has an infectious skin condition, use sterile gloves and dispose of old dressings according to your hospital's policy.

Don't apply ointments to mucous membranes as liberally as you would to skin *because mucous membranes are usually moist and absorb ointment more quickly than skin does.* Also, don't apply too much ointment to any skin area. *It may cause irritation and discomfort, stain clothing and bedding, and make removal difficult.*

Never apply ointment to the eyelids or ear canal unless ordered. *The ointment may congeal and occlude the tear duct or ear canal.*

Using medicated shampoos

Medicated shampoos include keratolytic and cytostatic agents, coal tar preparations, and lindane (gamma benzene hexachloride) solutions. They can be used to treat such conditions as dandruff, psoriasis, and head lice. However, they're contraindicated in patients with broken or abraded skin.

Since application instructions may vary among brands, check the label on the shampoo before starting the procedure *to ensure use of the correct amount.* Keep the shampoo away from the patient's eyes. If any shampoo should accidentally get in his eyes, irrigate promptly with water. Selenium sulfide, used in cytostatic agents, is extremely toxic if ingested.

To apply a medicated shampoo, follow these steps:
• Prepare the patient for shampoo treatment. (See "Hair care" in Chapter 1.)
• Shake the bottle of shampoo well *to mix the solution evenly.*
• Wet the patient's hair thoroughly and wring out excess water.
• Apply the proper amount of shampoo, as directed on the label.
• Work the shampoo into a lather, adding water as necessary. Part the hair and work the shampoo into the scalp, taking care not to use your fingernails.
• Leave the shampoo on the scalp and hair for as long as instructed (usually 5 to 10 minutes). Then rinse the hair thoroughly.
• Towel-dry the patient's hair.
• After the hair is dry, comb or brush it. Use a fine-tooth comb to remove nits if necessary.

Inspect the treated area frequently for adverse effects, such as signs of an allergic reaction.

Complications
Skin irritation, a rash, or an allergic reaction may occur.

Documentation
Record the medication applied, the time, date and site of application, and the condition of the patient's skin at the time of application. Note subsequent effects of the medication, if any.

Transdermal drug administration

Through an adhesive disk or measured dose of ointment applied to the skin, transdermal drugs deliver constant, controlled medication directly into the bloodstream for prolonged systemic effect. Medications currently available in transdermal form include nitroglycerin, used to control angina; scopolamine, used to treat motion sickness; estradiol for postmenopausal hormone replacement; clonidine, used to treat hypertension; and fentanyl, a narcotic analgesic used to control chronic pain. Nitroglycerin ointment dilates coronary vessels for up to 4 hours; a nitroglycerin disk can produce the same effect for as long as 24 hours. The scopolamine disk can relieve motion sickness for as long as 72 hours; transdermal estradiol lasts for up to 1 week; clonidine lasts for 24 hours; and fentanyl lasts up to 72 hours.

Contraindications for transdermal application include skin allergies or skin reactions to the drug. Transdermal drugs should not be applied to broken or irritated skin because they would increase irritation, or to scarred or calloused skin, which may impair absorption.

Equipment
Patient's medication record and chart ■ prescribed medication (disk or ointment) ■ application strip or measuring paper (for nitroglycerin ointment) ■ adhesive tape ■ plastic wrap (optional for nitroglycerin ointment) or semipermeable dressing ■ optional: gloves.

Implementation
• Verify the order on the patient's medication record by checking it against the doctor's order.
• Wash your hands and, if necessary, don gloves.
• Check the label on the medication *to make sure you'll be administering the correct drug in the correct dose.*
• Confirm the patient's identity by asking his name and checking the name, room number, and bed number on his wristband.
• Explain the procedure to the patient and provide privacy.
• As needed, remove any previously applied medication.

Applying transdermal ointment
• Place the prescribed amount of ointment on the application strip or measuring paper, taking care not to get any on your skin. (See *Applying nitroglycerin ointment.*)
• Apply the strip to any dry, hairless area of the body. Don't rub the ointment into the skin.
• Tape the application strip and ointment to the skin.
• If desired, cover the application strip with the plastic wrap, and tape the wrap in place.

Applying nitroglycerin ointment

Unlike most topical medications, nitroglycerin ointment is used for its transdermal *systemic* effect. It's used to dilate the veins and arteries, thus improving cardiac perfusion in a patient with cardiac ischemia or angina pectoris.

To apply nitroglycerin ointment, start by taking the patient's baseline blood pressure *so that you can compare it with later readings.* Gather your equipment. Nitroglycerin ointment, which is prescribed by the inch, comes with a rectangular piece of ruled paper, to be used in applying the medication. Squeeze the prescribed amount of ointment onto the ruled paper, as shown below. Put on gloves, if desired, *to avoid contact with the medication.*

After measuring the correct amount of ointment, tape the paper—drug side down—directly to the skin, as

shown below. (Some hospitals require you to use the paper to apply the medication to the patient's skin, usually on the chest or arm. Spread a thin layer of the ointment over a 3″ [7.6 cm] area.) For increased absorption, the doctor may request that you cover the site with plastic wrap or a transparent semipermeable dressing.

After 5 minutes, record the patient's blood pressure. If it has dropped significantly and he has a headache (from vasodilation of blood vessels in his head), notify the doctor immediately. He may reduce the dose. If the patient's blood pressure has dropped, but he has no symptoms, instruct him to lie still until it returns to normal.

Applying a transdermal disk
- Open the package and remove the disk.
- Without touching the adhesive surface, remove the clear plastic backing.
- Apply the disk to a dry, hairless area—behind the ear, for example, as with scopolamine. (See *Applying a transdermal medication disk,* page 218.)

After applying transdermal medications
- Store the medication as ordered.
- Instruct the patient to keep the area around the disk or ointment as dry as possible.
- If you didn't wear gloves, wash your hands immediately after applying the disk or ointment *to avoid absorbing the drug yourself.*

Special considerations
Reapply daily transdermal medications at the same time every day *to ensure a continuous effect,* but alternate the application sites *to avoid skin irritation.* Before reapplying nitroglycerin ointment, remove the plastic wrap, application strip, and any remaining ointment from the patient's skin at the previous site.

When applying a scopolamine disk, instruct the patient not to drive or operate machinery until his response to the drug has been determined.

Warn a patient using clonidine disks to check with his doctor before using any over-the-counter cough preparations *because these may counteract the effects of the drug.*

Applying a transdermal medication disk

If the patient will be receiving medication by transdermal disk, instruct him in its proper use, as described below:
• Explain to the patient that the disk consists of several layers. The layer closest to his skin contains a small amount of the drug and allows prompt introduction of the drug into the bloodstream (as indicated by the dots). The next layer controls release of the drug from the main portion of the patch. The third layer contains the main dose of the drug. The outermost layer comprises an aluminized polyester barrier.
• Teach the patient to apply the disk to appropriate skin areas, such as on the upper arm or chest, or behind the ear. Warn him to avoid touching the gel or surrounding tape. Tell him to use a different site for each application to avoid skin irritation. If necessary, he can shave the site. Tell him to avoid any area that may cause uneven absorption, such as skin folds, scars, and calluses, or any irritated or damaged skin areas. Also, tell him not to apply the disk below the elbow or knee.
• Instruct the patient to wash his hands after application to remove any medication that may have rubbed off.
• Warn the patient not to get the disk wet. Tell him to discard the disk if it leaks or falls off, and then to clean the site and apply a new disk at a different site.
• Instruct the patient to apply the disk at the same time at the prescribed interval to ensure continuous drug delivery. Bedtime application is ideal because body movement is reduced during the night. Finally, tell him to apply a new disk about 30 minutes before removing the old one.

Complications

Skin irritation, such as pruritus or a rash, may occur. The patient may also suffer adverse effects of the drug administered. For example, transdermal nitroglycerin medications may cause headaches and, in elderly patients, postural hypotension. Scopolamine has various adverse effects; dry mouth and drowsiness are the most common. Transdermal estradiol carries an increased risk of endometrial cancer, thromboembolic disease, and birth defects. Clonidine may cause severe rebound hypertension, especially if withdrawn suddenly.

Documentation

Record the type of medication, the date, time, and site of application, and the dose. Also note any adverse effects and the patient's response.

Application of eye medications

Eye medications—drops, ointments, and disks—serve diagnostic and therapeutic purposes. During an eye examination, eyedrops can be used to anesthetize the eye, dilate the pupil to facilitate examination, and stain the cornea to identify corneal abrasions, scars, or other anomalies. Eye medications can also be used to lubricate the eye, treat certain eye conditions (such as glaucoma and infections), protect the vision of neonates, and lubricate the eye socket for insertion of a prosthetic eye.

Understanding the ocular effects of medications is important because certain drugs may cause eye disorders or have serious ocular effects. For example, anticholinergics, which are often used during eye examinations, can precipitate acute glaucoma in patients with a predisposition to the disorder.

Equipment
Prescribed eye medication ■ patient's medication record and chart ■ sterile cotton balls ■ gloves ■ warm water or normal saline solution ■ sterile gauze pads ■ facial tissues ■ optional: ocular dressing.

Preparation of equipment
Make sure the medication is labeled for ophthalmic use. Then check the expiration date. Remember to date the container the first time you use the medication. After it's opened, an eye medication may be used for a maximum of 2 weeks *to avoid contamination.*

Inspect ocular solutions for cloudiness, discoloration, and precipitation, but remember that some eye medications are suspensions and normally appear cloudy. Don't use any solution that appears abnormal. If the tip of an eye ointment tube has crusted, turn the tip on a sterile gauze pad *to remove the crust.*

Implementation
• Verify the order on the patient's medication record by checking it against the doctor's order on his chart.
• Wash your hands.
• Check the medication label against the medication record.
• Make sure you know which eye to treat *because different medications or doses may be ordered for each eye.*
• Confirm the patient's identity by asking his name and checking the name, room number, and bed number on his wristband.
• Explain the procedure to the patient and provide privacy. Don gloves.
• If the patient is wearing an eye dressing, remove it by gently pulling it down and away from his forehead. Take care not to contaminate your hands.
• Remove any discharge by cleaning around the eye with sterile cotton balls or sterile gauze pads moistened with warm water or normal saline solution. With the patient's eye closed, clean from the inner canthus to the outer canthus, using a fresh sterile cotton ball or sterile gauze pad for each stroke.

• *To remove crusted secretions around the eye,* moisten a gauze pad with warm water or normal saline solution. Ask the patient to close the eye, and then place the gauze pad over it for a minute or two. Remove the pad, and then reapply moist sterile gauze pads, as necessary, until the secretions are soft enough to be removed without traumatizing the mucosa.
• Have the patient sit or lie in the supine position. Instruct him to tilt his head back and toward the side of the affected eye *so excess medication can flow away from the tear duct, minimizing systemic absorption through the nasal mucosa.*
• Remove the dropper cap from the medication container, if necessary, and draw the medication into it. Be careful to avoid contaminating the dropper tip or bottle top.
• Before instilling the eyedrops, instruct the patient to look up and away. *This moves the cornea away from the lower lid and minimizes the risk of touching the cornea with the dropper if the patient blinks.*

Instilling eyedrops
• You may steady the hand in which you're holding the dropper by resting it against the patient's forehead. Then, with your other hand, gently pull down the lower lid of the affected eye and instill the drops in the conjunctival sac. Try to avoid placing the drops directly on the eyeball. (See *Instilling eye medications,* page 220.)

Applying eye ointment
• Squeeze a small ribbon of medication on the edge of the conjunctival sac from the inner to the outer canthus. Cut off the ribbon by turning the tube. If you wish, you can steady the hand holding the medication tube by bracing it against the patient's forehead or cheek.

Using a medication disk
• A medication disk can release medication in the eye for up to 1 week. Pilocarpine, for example, can be administered this way to treat glaucoma. (For specific instructions, refer to *How to insert and remove an eye medication disk,* page 221.)

After instilling eyedrops or eye ointment
• Instruct the patient to close his eyes gently, without squeezing the lids shut. If you instilled drops, tell the patient to blink. If you applied ointment, tell him to roll his eyes behind closed lids *to help distribute the medication over the surface of the eyeball.*
• Use a clean tissue to remove any excess solution or ointment leaking from the eye. Use a fresh tissue for each eye *to prevent cross-contamination.*
• Apply a new eye dressing if necessary. (See "Hot and cold eye compresses" in Chapter 14.)

Instilling eye medications

To instill eyedrops, pull the lower lid down to expose the conjunctival sac. Have the patient look up and away, and squeeze the prescribed number of drops into the sac. Release the patient's eyelid and have him blink to distribute the medication.

To apply an ointment, gently lay a thin strip of the medication along the conjunctival sac from the inner canthus to the outer canthus. Avoid touching the tip of the tube to the patient's eye. Then, release the eyelid and have the patient roll his eye behind closed lids to distribute the medication.

• Return the medication to the storage area. Make sure you store it according to the label's instructions.
• Wash your hands.

Special considerations

When administering an eye medication that may be absorbed systemically (such as atropine), gently press your thumb on the inner canthus for 1 to 2 minutes after instilling drops while the patient closes his eyes. *This helps prevent medication from flowing into the tear duct.*

To maintain the drug container's sterility, never touch the tip of the bottle or dropper to the patient's eyeball, lids, or lashes. Discard any solution remaining in the dropper before returning the dropper to the bottle. If the dropper or bottle tip has become contaminated, discard it and obtain another sterile dropper. *To avoid cross-contamination,* never use a container of eye medication for more than one patient.

Teach the patient to instill eye medications *so that he can continue treatment at home, if necessary.* Review the procedure and ask for a return demonstration.

Complications

Instillation of some eye medications may cause transient burning, itching, and redness. Rarely, systemic effects may also occur.

Documentation

Record the medication instilled or applied, the eye or eyes treated, and the date, time, and dose. Note any adverse effects and the patient's response.

Instillation of eardrops

Eardrops may be instilled to treat infection and inflammation, to soften cerumen for later removal, to produce local anesthesia, or to facilitate removal of an insect trapped in the ear by immobilizing and smothering it. Instillation of ear drops is usually contraindicated if the patient has a perforated eardrum; however, it may be permitted with certain medications and adherence to sterile technique. Other conditions may also prohibit instillation of certain medications into the ear. For instance, instillation of drops containing hydrocortisone is contraindicated if the patient has herpes, another viral infection, or a fungal infection.

Equipment

Prescribed eardrops ▪ patient's medication record and chart ▪ light source ▪ facial tissue or cotton-tipped applicator ▪ optional: cotton ball, bowl of warm water.

How to insert and remove an eye medication disk

Small and flexible, the oval eye medication disk consists of three layers: two soft outer layers and a middle layer containing the medication. Floating between the eyelids and the sclera, the disk stays in the eye while the patient sleeps and even during swimming and athletic activities. The disk frees the patient from having to remember to instill his eyedrops. Once the disk is in place, ocular fluid moistens it, releasing the medication. Eye moisture or contact lenses don't adversely affect the disk. The disk can release medication for up to 1 week before needing replacement. Pilocarpine, for example, can be administered this way to treat glaucoma.

Contraindications include conjunctivitis, keratitis, retinal detachment, and any condition where constriction of the pupil should be avoided.

To insert an eye medication disk

Arrange to insert the disk before the patient goes to bed. *This minimizes the blurring that usually occurs immediately after disk insertion.*
• Wash your hands and don gloves.
• Press your fingertip against the oval disk so it lies lengthwise across your fingertip. It should stick to your finger. Lift the disk out of its packet.
• Gently pull the patient's lower eyelid away from the eye and place the disk in the conjunctival sac. It should lie horizontally, not vertically. The disk will adhere to the eye naturally.

• Pull the lower eyelid out, up, and over the disk. Tell the patient to blink several times. If the disk is still visible, pull the lower lid out and over the disk again. Tell the patient that once the disk is in place, he can adjust its position by *gently* pressing his finger against his closed lid. Caution him against rubbing his eye or moving the disk across the cornea.
• If the disk falls out, wash your hands, rinse the disk in cool water, and reinsert it. If the disk appears bent, replace it.
• If both of the patient's eyes are being treated with medication disks, replace both disks at the same time *so that both eyes receive medication at the same rate.*
• If the disk repeatedly slips out of position, reinsert it under the upper eyelid. To do this, gently lift and evert the upper eyelid and insert the disk in the conjunctival sac. Then, gently pull the lid back into position and tell the patient to blink several times. Again, the patient may press gently on the closed eyelid to reposition the disk. The more the patient uses the disk, the easier it should be for him to retain it. If he can't, notify the doctor.
• If the patient will continue therapy with an eye medication disk after discharge, teach him to insert and remove it himself. To check his mastery of these skills, have him demonstrate insertion and removal techniques for you.
• Also, teach the patient about possible adverse reactions. Foreign-body sensation in the eye, mild tearing or redness, increased mucous discharge, eyelid redness, and itchiness can occur with the use of disks. Blurred vision, stinging, swelling, and headaches can occur with pilocarpine, specifically. Mild symptoms are common but should subside within the first 6 weeks of use. Tell the patient to report persistent or severe symptoms to his doctor.

To remove an eye medication disk

• You can remove an eye medication disk with one or two fingers. To use one finger, put on gloves and evert the lower eyelid to expose the disk. Then use the forefinger of your other hand to slide the disk onto the lid and out of the patient's eye. To use two fingers, evert the lower lid with one hand to expose the disk. Then pinch the disk with the thumb and forefinger of your other hand and remove it from the eye.
• If the disk is located in the upper eyelid, apply long circular strokes to the patient's closed eyelid with your finger until you can see the disk in the corner of the patient's eye. Once the disk is visible, you can place your finger directly on the disk and move it to the lower sclera. Then remove it as you would a disk located in the lower lid.

Positioning the patient for eardrop instillation

Before instilling eardrops, have the patient lie on his side. Then straighten the patient's ear canal to help the medication reach the eardrum. In an adult, gently pull the auricle *up and back;* in an infant or young child, gently pull *down and back,* as shown here.

Adult

Child

Preparation of equipment
Verify the order on the patient's medication record by checking it against the doctor's order.

To avoid adverse effects (such as vertigo, nausea, and pain) resulting from instillation of eardrops that are too cold, warm the medication to body temperature in the bowl of warm water or carry it in your pocket for 30 minutes before administration. If necessary, test the temperature of the medication by placing a drop on your wrist. *(If the medication is too hot, it may burn the patient's eardrum.)* Before using a glass dropper, make sure it's not chipped *to avoid injuring the ear canal.*

Implementation
• Wash your hands.
• Confirm the patient's identity by asking his name and checking the name, room number, and bed number on his wristband.
• Provide privacy if possible. Explain the procedure to the patient.
• Have the patient lie on the side opposite the affected ear.
• Straighten the patient's ear canal. For an adult, pull the auricle of the ear up and back. For an infant or child under age 3, gently pull the auricle down and back *because the ear canal is straighter at this age.* (See *Positioning the patient for eardrop instillation.)*
• Using a light source, examine the ear canal for drainage. If you find any, clean the canal with the tissue or cotton-tipped applicator *because drainage can reduce the medication's effectiveness.*
• Compare the label on the eardrops to the order on the patient's medication record. Check the label again while drawing the medication into the dropper. Check the label for the final time before returning the eardrops to the shelf or drawer.
• *To avoid damaging the ear canal with the dropper,* gently support the hand holding the dropper against the patient's head. Straighten the patient's ear canal once again and instill the ordered number of drops. *To avoid patient discomfort,* aim the dropper so that the drops fall against the sides of the ear canal, not on the eardrum. Hold the ear canal in position until you see the medication disappear down the canal. Then release the ear.
• Instruct the patient to remain on his side for 5 to 10 minutes *to allow the medication to run down into the ear canal.*
• If ordered, tuck the cotton ball loosely into the opening of the ear canal *to prevent the medication from leaking out.* Be careful not to insert it too deeply into the canal *because this would prevent drainage of secretions and increase pressure on the eardrum.*
• Clean and dry the outer ear.
• If ordered, repeat the procedure in the other ear after 5 to 10 minutes.
• Assist the patient into a comfortable position.
• Wash your hands.

Special considerations

Remember that some conditions make the normally tender ear canal even more sensitive, so be especially gentle when performing this procedure. Wash your hands before and after caring for the patient's ear and between caring for each ear.

To prevent injury to the eardrum, never insert a cotton-tipped applicator into the ear canal past the point where you can see the tip. After applying eardrops to soften cerumen, irrigate the ear as ordered *to facilitate its removal.*

If the patient has vertigo, keep the side rails of his bed up and assist him during the procedure, as necessary. Also, move slowly and unhurriedly *to avoid exacerbating his vertigo.*

Teach the patient to instill the eardrops correctly so that he can continue treatment at home, if necessary. Review the procedure and let the patient try it himself while you observe.

Documentation

Record the medication, the ear treated, and the date, time, and number of eardrops instilled. Also note any signs or symptoms that arise during the procedure, such as drainage, redness, vertigo, nausea, or pain.

Hand-held oropharyngeal inhalers

Hand-held inhalers include the metered-dose inhaler or nebulizer, the turbo-inhaler, and the nasal inhaler. These devices deliver topical medications to the respiratory tract, producing local and systemic effects. The mucosal lining of the respiratory tract absorbs the inhalant almost immediately. Examples of common inhalants are bronchodilators, used to improve airway patency and facilitate mucous drainage, and mucolytics, which attain a high local concentration to liquefy tenacious bronchial secretions.

These inhalers may be contraindicated in patients who can't form an airtight seal around the device, and in patients who lack the coordination or clear vision necessary to assemble a turbo-inhaler. Contraindications for specific inhalant drugs are also possible. For example, bronchodilators are contraindicated if the patient has tachycardia or a history of cardiac arrhythmias associated with tachycardia.

Equipment

Patient's medication record and chart ▪ metered-dose inhaler, turbo-inhaler, or nasal inhaler (see *Types of hand-held inhalers,* page 224) ▪ prescribed medication ▪ normal saline solution (or another appropriate solution) for gargling ▪ optional: emesis basin.

Implementation

• Verify the order on the patient's medication record by checking it against the doctor's order.
• Wash your hands.
• Check the label on the inhaler against the order on the medication record.
• Confirm the patient's identity by asking his name and by checking his name, room number, and bed number on his wristband.
• Explain the procedure to the patient.

Using a metered-dose inhaler

• Shake the inhaler bottle *to mix the medication and aerosol propellant.*
• Remove the mouthpiece and cap from the bottle.
• Insert the metal stem on the bottle into the small hole on the flattened portion of the mouthpiece. Then turn the bottle upside down.
• Have the patient exhale; then place the mouthpiece in his mouth and close his lips around it.
• As you firmly push the bottle down against the mouthpiece, instruct the patient to inhale slowly and to continue inhaling until his lungs feel full. *This action draws the medication into his lungs.* Compress the bottle against the mouthpiece only once.
• Remove the mouthpiece from the patient's mouth, and tell him to hold his breath for several seconds *to allow the medication to reach the alveoli.* Then instruct him to exhale slowly through pursed lips *to keep the distal bronchioles open, allowing increased absorption and diffusion of the drug and better gas exchange.*
• Have the patient gargle with normal saline solution, if desired, *to remove medication from the mouth and back of the throat.* (The lungs retain only about 10% of the inhalant; most of the remainder is exhaled, but substantial amounts may remain in the oropharynx.)
• Rinse the mouthpiece thoroughly with warm water *to prevent accumulation of residue.*

Using a turbo-inhaler

• Hold the mouthpiece in one hand, and with the other hand, slide the sleeve away from the mouthpiece as far as possible.
• Unscrew the tip of the mouthpiece by turning it counterclockwise.
• Firmly press the colored portion of the medication capsule into the propeller stem of the mouthpiece.
• Screw the inhaler together again securely.

Types of hand-held inhalers

These devices use air under pressure to produce a mist containing tiny droplets of medication. Drugs delivered in this form (such as mucolytics or bronchodilators) can travel deep into the lungs.

Nasal inhaler	**Metered-dose inhaler**	**Turbo-inhaler with capsules**

• Holding the inhaler with the mouthpiece at the bottom, slide the sleeve all the way down and then up again *to puncture the capsule and release the medication.* Do this only once.

• Have the patient exhale completely and tilt his head back. Then instruct him to place the mouthpiece in his mouth, close his lips around it, and inhale once — quickly and deeply — through the mouthpiece.

• Tell the patient to hold his breath for several seconds *to allow the medication to reach the alveoli.* (Instruct him not to exhale through the mouthpiece.)

• Remove the inhaler from the patient's mouth, and tell him to exhale as much air as possible.

• Repeat the procedure until all the medication in the device is inhaled.

• Have the patient gargle with normal saline solution, if desired, *to remove medication from the mouth and back of the throat.* Be sure to provide an emesis basin if the patient needs one.

• Discard the empty medication capsule, put the inhaler in its can, and secure the lid. Rinse the inhaler with warm water at least once a week.

Using a nasal inhaler

• Have the patient blow his nose *to clear his nostrils.*

• Shake the medication cartridge and then insert it in the adapter. (When inserting a refill cartridge, first remove the protective cap from the stem.)

• Remove the protective cap from the adapter tip.

• Hold the inhaler with your index finger on top of the cartridge and your thumb under the nasal adapter. The adapter tip should be pointing toward the patient.

• Have the patient tilt his head back. Then tell him to place the adapter tip into one nostril while occluding the other nostril with his finger.

• Instruct the patient to inhale gently as he presses the adapter and the cartridge together firmly *to release a measured dose of medication.* Be sure to follow the manufacturer's instructions. With some medications, such as dexamethasone sodium phosphate (Turbinaire), inhaling during administration is not desirable.

• Tell the patient to remove the inhaler from his nostril and to exhale through his mouth.

• Shake the inhaler, and have the patient repeat the procedure in the other nostril.

• Have the patient gargle with normal saline solution *to remove medication from the mouth and throat.*

• Remove the medication cartridge from the nasal inhaler, and wash the nasal adapter in lukewarm water.

Let the adapter dry thoroughly before reinserting the cartridge.

Special considerations

When using a turbo-inhaler or a nasal inhaler, make sure the pressurized cartridge isn't punctured or incinerated. Store the medication cartridge below 120° F (48.9° C).

Spacer inhalers may be recommended to provide greater therapeutic benefit for children or patients who have difficulty with coordination. A spacer attachment is an extension to the inhaler's mouthpiece that provides more dead-air space for mixing the medication. Some inhalers have built-in spacers.

If you're using a turbo-inhaler, keep the medication capsules wrapped until needed *to keep them from deteriorating.*

Teach the patient how to use the inhaler *so that he can continue treatments himself after discharge,* if necessary. Explain that overdosage — which is common — can cause the medication to lose its effectiveness. Tell him to record the date and time of each inhalation and his response *to prevent overdosage and to help the doctor determine the drug's effectiveness.* Also, note if the patient uses an unusual amount of medication — for example, more than one cartridge for a metered-dose nebulizer every 3 weeks. Inform the patient of possible adverse reactions.

Documentation

Record the inhalant administered, the dose, and the time. Note any significant change in the patient's heart rate after bronchodilation, and any other adverse reactions.

Instillation of nasal medications

Nasal medications may be instilled by means of drops, a spray (using an atomizer), or an aerosol (using a nebulizer). Most drugs instilled by these methods produce local rather than systemic effects. Drops can be directed at a specific area; sprays and aerosols diffuse medication throughout the nasal passages.

Most nasal medications, such as phenylephrine, are vasoconstrictors, which relieve nasal congestion by coating and shrinking swollen mucous membranes. Because vasoconstrictors may be absorbed systemically, they are usually contraindicated in hypertensive patients. Other types of nasal medications include antiseptics, anesthetics, and corticosteroids. Local anesthetics may be administered to promote patient comfort during rhinolaryngologic examination, laryngoscopy, bronchoscopy, and endotracheal intubation. Corticosteroids reduce inflammation in allergic or inflammatory conditions and in nasal polyps.

Equipment

Prescribed medication ▪ patient's medication record and chart ▪ emesis basin (with nose drops only) ▪ facial tissues ▪ optional: pillow, small piece of soft rubber or plastic tubing, gloves.

Implementation

• Verify the order on the patient's medication record by checking it against the doctor's order. Note the concentration of the medication. Phenylephrine, for example, is available in various concentrations from 0.125% to 1%.
• Confirm the patient's identity by asking his name and checking the name, room number, and bed number on his wristband.
• Explain the procedure to the patient and provide privacy.
• Wash your hands. Don gloves if you notice any drainage from the nares.

Instilling nose drops

• When possible, position the patient so the drops flow back into the nostrils, toward the affected area. (See *Positioning the patient for nose drop instillation,* page 226.)
• Draw up some medication into the dropper.
• Push up the tip of the patient's nose slightly. Position the dropper just above the nostril, and direct its tip toward the midline of the nose *so the drops flow toward the back of the nasal cavity rather than down the throat.*
• Insert the dropper about ⅜″ (1 cm) into the nostril. Make sure the dropper doesn't touch the sides of the nostril because *this would contaminate the dropper or could cause the patient to sneeze.*
• Instill the prescribed number of drops, observing the patient carefully for any signs of discomfort.
• *To prevent the drops from leaking out of the nostrils,* ask the patient to keep his head tilted back for at least 5 minutes and to breathe through his mouth. *This also allows sufficient time for the medication to constrict mucous membranes.*
• Keep an emesis basin handy *so the patient can expectorate any medication that flows into the oropharynx and mouth.* Use a facial tissue to wipe any excess medication from the patient's nostrils and face.
• Clean the dropper by separating the plunger and pipette and flushing them with warm water. Allow them to air-dry.

Using a nasal spray

• Have the patient sit upright with his head tilted back slightly. If this position is uncomfortable, have the patient

Positioning the patient for nose drop instillation

To reach the ethmoidal and sphenoidal sinuses, have the patient lie on his back with his neck hyperextended and his head tilted back over the edge of the bed. Support his head with one hand to prevent neck strain.

To reach the maxillary and frontal sinuses, have the patient lie on his back with his head toward the affected side and hanging slightly over the edge of the bed. Ask him to rotate his head laterally after hyperextension, and support his head with one hand to prevent neck strain.

Ethmoidal sinuses

Sphenoidal sinus

Maxillary sinuses

Frontal sinuses

lie on his back with his shoulders elevated, neck hyperextended, and head tilted back over the edge of the bed. Support his head with one hand *to prevent neck strain.*
• Remove the protective cap from the atomizer.
• *To prevent air from entering the nasal cavity and to allow the medication to flow in properly,* occlude one of the patient's nostrils with your finger. Insert the atomizer tip into the open nostril.
• Instruct the patient to inhale, and as he does so, squeeze the atomizer once, quickly and firmly. Use just enough force to coat the inside of the patient's nose with medication. Then tell the patient to exhale through his mouth.
• If ordered, spray the nostril again. Then repeat the procedure in the other nostril.
• Instruct the patient to keep his head tilted back for several minutes and to breathe slowly through his nose *so the medication has time to work.* Tell him not to blow his nose for several minutes.

Using a nasal aerosol
• Instruct the patient to blow his nose gently *to clear his nostrils.*

• Insert the medication cartridge according to the manufacturer's directions. With some models, you'll fit the medication cartridge over a small hole in the adapter. When inserting a refill cartridge, first remove the protective cap from the stem. Spacer inhalers may be recommended. (See "Hand-held oropharyngeal inhalers" in this chapter.)
• Shake the aerosol well immediately before each use, and remove the protective cap from the adapter tip.
• Hold the aerosol between your thumb and index finger with your index finger positioned on top of the medication cartridge.
• Tilt the patient's head back, and carefully insert the adapter tip in one nostril while sealing the other nostril with your finger.
• Press the adapter and cartridge together firmly *to release one measured dose of medication.*
• Shake the aerosol and repeat the procedure to instill medication into the other nostril.
• Remove the medication cartridge and wash the nasal adapter in lukewarm water daily. Allow the adapter to dry thoroughly before reinserting the cartridge.

To administer drops to relieve ordinary nasal congestion, help the patient to a reclining or supine position with his head tilted slightly toward the affected side. Aim the dropper upward, toward the patient's eye, rather than downward, toward his ear.

Special considerations
Before instilling nose drops in a young child or an uncooperative patient, attach a small piece of tubing to the end of the dropper *to avoid damaging mucous membranes.*

When using an aerosol, be careful not to puncture or incinerate the pressurized cartridge. Store it at temperatures below 120° F (48.9° C).

To prevent the spread of infection, label the medication bottle so that it will be used only for that patient.

Ideally, a nasal spray should be self-administered by the patient. Teach the patient how to instill nasal medications correctly *so he can continue treatment after discharge,* if necessary. Caution him against using nasal medications longer than prescribed *because they may cause a rebound effect that worsens the condition.* A rebound effect occurs when the medication loses its effectiveness and relaxes the vessels in the nasal turbinates, producing a stuffiness that can be relieved only by discontinuing the medication.

Inform the patient of possible adverse reactions. For example, explain that when receiving corticosteroids by aerosol therapy, therapeutic effects may not appear for 2 days to 2 weeks.

Complications
Some nasal medications may cause restlessness, palpitations, nervousness, and other systemic effects. For example, excessive use of corticosteroid aerosols may cause hyperadrenocorticism and adrenal suppression.

Documentation
Record the medication instilled and its concentration, the number of drops or instillations administered, and whether the medication was instilled in one or both nostrils. Also note the time, date, and any resulting adverse effects.

Insertion of vaginal medications

Vaginal medications include suppositories, creams, gels, and ointments. These medications can be inserted as topical treatment for infection (particularly *Trichomonas vaginalis* and monilial vaginitis) or inflammation, or as a contraceptive. Suppositories melt when they contact the vaginal mucosa, and their medication diffuses topically — as effectively as creams, gels, and ointments.

Vaginal medications usually come with a disposable applicator that enables placement of medication in the anterior and posterior fornices. Vaginal administration is most effective when the patient can remain lying down afterward to retain the medication.

Equipment
Patient's medication record and chart ■ prescribed medication and applicator, if necessary ■ gloves ■ water-soluble lubricant ■ small sanitary pad.

Implementation
● If possible, plan to give vaginal medications at bedtime, when the patient is recumbent.
● Verify the order on the patient's medication record by checking it against the doctor's order.
● Confirm the patient's identity by asking her name and checking the name, room number, and bed number on her wristband.
● Wash your hands, explain the procedure to the patient, and provide privacy.
● Ask the patient to void.
● Ask the patient if she would rather insert the medication herself. If so, provide appropriate instructions. If not, proceed with the following steps.
● Help her into the lithotomy position.
● Expose only the perineum.

How to insert a vaginal suppository

If the suppository is small, place it in the tip of an applicator. Then, lubricate the applicator, hold it by the cylinder, and insert it into the vagina. To ensure the patient's comfort, direct the applicator down initially (toward the spine), and then up and back (toward the cervix), as shown here. When the suppository reaches the distal end of the vagina, depress the plunger.

Remove the applicator while the plunger is still depressed.

Inserting a suppository
• Remove the suppository from the wrapper and lubricate it with water-soluble lubricant.
• Put on gloves and expose the vagina.
• With an applicator or the forefinger of your free hand, insert the suppository about 2" (5 cm) into the vagina. (See *How to insert a vaginal suppository.*)

Inserting ointments, creams, or gels
• Insert the plunger into the applicator. Then fit the applicator to the tube of medication.
• Gently squeeze the tube to fill the applicator with the prescribed amount of medication. Lubricate the applicator.
• Put on gloves and expose the vagina.
• Insert the applicator as you would a small suppository and administer the medication by depressing the plunger on the applicator.

After vaginal insertion
• Remove and discard your gloves.
• Wash the applicator with soap and warm water and store it, unless it is disposable. If the applicator can be used again, label it *so it will be used only for the same patient.*
• *To prevent the medication from soiling the patient's clothing and bedding,* provide a sanitary pad.
• Help the patient return to a comfortable position, and advise her to remain in bed as much as possible for the next several hours.
• Wash your hands thoroughly.

Special considerations
Refrigerate vaginal suppositories that melt at room temperature. If possible, teach the patient how to insert vaginal medication. *She may have to administer it herself after discharge.* Give her a patient-teaching sheet if one is available. Instruct the patient not to wear a tampon after inserting vaginal medication *because it would absorb the medication and decrease its effectiveness.*

Complications
Vaginal medications may cause local irritation.

Documentation
Record the medication administered, the time, and the date. Note adverse effects and any other pertinent information.

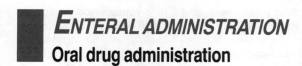

ENTERAL ADMINISTRATION
Oral drug administration

Because oral administration of drugs is usually safest, most convenient, and least expensive, most drugs are commonly administered by this route. Drugs for oral administration are available in many forms: tablets, enteric-coated tablets, capsules, syrups, elixirs, oils, liquids, suspensions, powders, and granules. Some require special preparation before administration, such as mixing with juice to make them more palatable; oils, powders, and granules most often require such preparation.

   Oral drugs are sometimes prescribed in higher dosages than their parenteral equivalents because, after absorption through the GI system, they are immediately broken down by the liver before they reach the systemic circulation. Oral administration is contraindicated for unconscious patients; it may also be contraindicated in patients with nausea and vomiting, and in those unable to swallow.

Equipment

Patient's medication record and chart ▪ prescribed medication ▪ medication cup ▪ optional: appropriate vehicle, such as jelly or applesauce, for crushed pills commonly used with children or elderly patients and juice, water, or milk for liquid medications; drinking straw; mortar and pestle for crushing pills.

Implementation

• Verify the order on the patient's medication record by checking it against the doctor's order.
• Wash your hands.
• Check the label on the medication three times before administering it *to make sure you'll be giving the prescribed medication.* Check when you take the container from the shelf or drawer, again before you pour the medication into the medication cup, and again before returning the container to the shelf or drawer. If you're administering a unit-dose medication, check the label for the final time at the patient's bedside immediately after pouring the medication and before discarding the wrapper.
• Confirm the patient's identity by asking his name and checking the name, room number, and bed number on his wristband.
• Assess the patient's condition, including level of consciousness and vital signs, as needed. *Changes in the patient's condition may warrant withholding medication.* For example, you may need to withhold a medication that will slow the patient's heart rate if his apical pulse rate is below 60.
• Give the patient his medication and, as needed, an appropriate vehicle or liquid *to aid swallowing, minimize adverse effects, or promote absorption.* For example, cyclophosphamide is given with fluids to minimize adverse effects; antitussive cough syrup is given without a fluid to avoid diluting its soothing effect on the throat. If appropriate, crush the medication *to facilitate swallowing.*
• Stay with the patient until he has swallowed the drug. If he seems confused or disoriented, check his mouth *to make sure he has swallowed it.* Return and reassess the patient's response within 1 hour after giving the medication.

Special considerations

Make sure you have a written order for every medication given. Verbal orders should be signed by the doctor within the specified time period. (Hospitals usually require a signature within 24 hours; long-term care facilities, within 48 hours.)

Measuring liquid medications

To pour liquids, hold the medication cup at eye level. Use your thumb to mark off the correct level on the cup.

Then set the cup down and read the bottom of the meniscus at eye level *to ensure accuracy.* If you've poured too much medication into the cup, discard the excess. Don't return it to the bottle. Here are a few additional tips:
• Hold the container so that the medication flows from the side opposite the label *so it won't run down the container and stain or obscure the label.* Remove drips from the lip of the bottle first, then from the sides, using a clean, damp paper towel.
• For a liquid measured in drops, use only the dropper supplied with the medication.

Use care in measuring out the prescribed dose of liquid oral medication. (See *Measuring liquid medications.*)

Don't give medication from a poorly labeled or unlabeled container. Don't attempt to label or reinforce drug labels yourself. *This must be done by a pharmacist.*

Never give a medication poured by someone else. Never allow your medication cart or tray out of your sight. *This prevents anyone from rearranging the medications or taking one without your knowledge.* Never return unwrapped or prepared medications to stock containers. Instead, dispose of them and notify the pharmacy. Keep in mind that the disposal of any narcotic drug must be cosigned by another nurse, as mandated by law.

If the patient questions you about his medication or the dosage, check his medication record again. If the medication is correct, reassure him. Make sure you tell him about any changes in his medication or dosage. Instruct him, as appropriate, about possible adverse effects. Ask him to report anything that he feels may be an adverse effect.

To avoid damaging or staining the patient's teeth, give acid or iron preparations through a straw. An unpleasant-tasting liquid can usually be made more palatable if taken through a straw *because the liquid contacts fewer taste buds.*

Oral medications are relatively easy to give to infants *because of their natural sucking instinct and, in infants under 4 months, their undeveloped sense of taste.*

If the patient can't swallow a whole tablet or capsule, ask the pharmacist if the drug is available in liquid form or if it can be administered by another route. If not, ask him if you can crush the tablet or open the capsule and mix it with food. Keep in mind that many enteric-coated or time-release medications and gelatin capsules should not be crushed. Remember to contact the doctor for an order to change the route of administration when necessary.

Documentation

Note the drug administered, the dose, the date and time, and the patient's reaction, if any. If the patient refuses a drug, document the refusal and notify the charge nurse and the patient's doctor, as needed. Also note if a drug was omitted or withheld for other reasons, such as radiology or laboratory tests, or if, in your judgment, the drug was contraindicated at the ordered time. Sign out all narcotics given on the appropriate narcotics central record.

Instillation of drugs through a nasogastric tube

Besides providing an alternate means of nourishment, the nasogastric (NG) tube allows direct instillation of medication into the GI system of patients who can't ingest it orally. Before instillation, the patency and positioning of the tube must be carefully checked because this procedure is contraindicated if the tube is obstructed or improperly positioned or if the patient is vomiting around the tube or his bowel sounds are absent.

Oily medications and enteric-coated or sustained-release tablets are contraindicated for instillation through an NG tube. Oily medications cling to the sides of the tube and resist mixing with the irrigating solution. And crushing enteric-coated or sustained-release tablets to facilitate transport through the tube destroys their intended effect.

Equipment

Patient's medication record and chart ■ prescribed medication ■ towel or linen-saver pad ■ 50- or 60-ml piston type catheter-tip syringe ■ feeding tubing ■ two 4″ × 4″ gauze pads ■ stethoscope ■ gloves ■ diluent ■ cup for mixing medication and fluid ■ spoon ■ 50 ml of water ■ rubber band ■ gastrostomy tube and funnel, if needed ■ optional: pill-crushing equipment (mortar and pestle, for example), clamp (if not already attached to tube).

For maximum control of suction, use a piston syringe instead of a bulb syringe. The liquid for diluting the medication can be juice, water, or a nutritional supplement.

Preparation of equipment

Gather necessary equipment for use at the patient's bedside. Liquids should be at room temperature. *Administering cold liquid through the NG tube can cause abdominal cramping.* Although this is not a sterile procedure, make sure the cup, syringe, spoon, and gauze are clean.

Implementation

• Verify the order on the patient's medication record by checking it against the doctor's order.
• Wash your hands and don gloves.
• Check the label on the medication three times before preparing it for administration *to make sure you'll be giving the medication correctly.*
• If the prescribed medication is in tablet form, crush the tablets *to ready them for mixing in a cup with the diluting liquid.* Bring the medication and equipment to the patient's bedside.
• Explain the procedure to the patient, if necessary, and provide privacy.
• Confirm the patient's identity by asking his name and checking the name, room number, and bed number on his wristband.
• Unpin the tube from the patient's gown. *To avoid soiling the sheets during the procedure,* fold back the bed linens to the patient's waist and drape his chest with a towel or linen-saver pad.
• Elevate the head of the bed so the patient is in Fowler's position, as tolerated.
• After unclamping the tube, take the 50- or 60-ml syringe and create a 10-cc air space in its chamber. Then attach the syringe to the end of the tube.
• Auscultate the patient's abdomen about 3″ (7.6 cm) below the sternum with the stethoscope. Then, gently insert the 10 cc of air into the tube. You should hear the air bubble entering the stomach. If you hear this sound, gently draw back on the piston of the syringe. *The appearance of gastric contents implies that the tube is patent and in the stomach.* (However, only an X-ray positively

confirms the tube's position.) If no gastric contents appear when you draw back on the piston of the syringe, the tube may have risen into the patient's esophagus, in which case you'll have to advance it before proceeding.

• If you meet resistance when aspirating for stomach contents, stop the procedure. *Resistance may indicate a nonpatent tube or improper tube placement.* (Keep in mind that some smaller NG tubes may collapse when aspiration is tried.) If the tube seems to be in the stomach, resistance probably means the tube is lying against the stomach wall. *To relieve resistance,* withdraw the tube slightly or turn the patient.

• After you have established that the tube is patent and in the correct position, clamp the tube, detach the syringe, and lay the end of the tube on the 4″ × 4″ gauze pad.

• Mix the crushed tablets with the diluent. If the medication is in capsule form, open the capsules and empty their contents into the liquid. Pour liquid medications directly into the diluting liquid. Stir well with the spoon. (If the medication was in tablet form, make sure the particles are small enough to pass through the eyes at the distal end of the tube.)

• Reattach the syringe, without the piston, to the end of the tube and open the clamp.

• Deliver the medication slowly and steadily. (See *Giving medications through an NG tube.*)

• If the medication flows smoothly, slowly add more until the entire dose has been given. If the medication doesn't flow properly, don't force it. It may be too thick to flow through the tube. If so, dilute it with water. If you suspect tube placement is inhibiting flow, stop the procedure and reevaluate the placement.

• Watch the patient's reaction throughout the instillation. If he shows any sign of discomfort, stop the procedure immediately.

• As the last of the medication flows out of the syringe, start to irrigate the tube by adding 30 to 50 ml of water. (If your patient is a child, use only 15 to 30 ml of water.) *Irrigation clears medication from the sides of the tube and from the distal end, reducing the risk of clogging.*

• When the water stops flowing, quickly clamp the tube. Detach the syringe and dispose of it properly.

• Fasten the NG tube to the patient's gown.

• Remove the towel or linen-saver pad and replace bed linens.

• Leave the patient in Fowler's position, or have him lie on his right side with the head of the bed partially elevated. Have him maintain this position for at least 30 minutes after the procedure *to facilitate the downward flow of medication into his stomach and prevent esophageal reflux.*

Giving medications through an NG tube

Holding the nasogastric (NG) tube at a level somewhat above the patient's nose, pour up to 30 ml of diluted medication into the syringe barrel. *To prevent air from entering the patient's stomach,* hold the tube at a slight angle and add more medication before the syringe empties. If necessary, raise the tube slightly higher to increase the flow rate.

After you've delivered the whole dose, position the patient on her right side, head slightly elevated, *to minimize esophageal reflux.*

• You may be asked to deliver medications through a gastrostomy tube. (See *Giving medications through a gastrostomy tube,* page 232.) If medication is prescribed for a patient with a gastrostomy feeding button, ask the doctor to order the liquid form of the drug, if possible. If not, you may administer a tablet or capsule if it is dissolved in 30 to 50 ml of warm water (15 to 30 ml for children). To administer medication this way, use the

Giving medications through a gastrostomy tube

Surgically inserted into the stomach, a gastrostomy tube reduces the risk of fluid aspiration into the lungs, a constant danger with a nasogastric (NG) tube.

To administer medication by this route, prepare the patient and medication as you would for an NG tube. Then, gently lift the dressing around the tube *to assess the skin for irritation caused by gastric secretions*. Report any redness or irritation to the doctor. If no irritation appears, follow these steps:

• Remove the dressing that covers the tube. Then remove the dressing or plug at the tip of the tube and attach the syringe or funnel to the tip.

• Release the clamp and instill about 10 ml of water into the tube through the syringe *to check for patency*. If the water flows in easily, the tube is patent. If it flows in slowly, raise the funnel to increase pressure. If the water still doesn't flow properly, stop the procedure and notify the doctor.

• Pour up to 30 ml of medication into the syringe or funnel. Tilt the tube *to allow air to escape as the fluid flows downward*. Just before the syringe empties, add medication as needed.

• After giving the medication, pour in about 30 ml of water *to irrigate the tube*.

• Tighten the clamp, place a 4″ × 4″ gauze pad on the end of the tube, and secure it with a rubber band.

• Cover the tube with two more 4″ × 4″ gauze pads, and secure them firmly with tape.

• Keep the head of the bed elevated for at least 30 minutes after the procedure *to aid digestion*.

---

same procedure as for feeding the patient through the button (see Chapter 10, Gastrointestinal care). Then draw up the dissolved medication into a syringe and inject it into the feeding tube.

• Next, withdraw the medication syringe and flush the tube with 50 ml of warm water. (For children, flush the tube with 30 ml.)

• Then replace the safety plug, and keep the patient upright at a 30-degree angle for 30 minutes after giving the medication.

Special considerations

To prevent instillation of too much fluid (more than 400 ml of liquid at one time for an adult), plan the drug instillation so that it doesn't coincide with the patient's regular tube feeding, if possible.

When you must schedule a tube feeding and medication instillation simultaneously, administer the medication first *to ensure that the patient receives the prescribed drug therapy even if he can't tolerate an entire feeding*. Remember to avoid giving the patient foods that interact adversely with the medication.

If the patient receives continuous tube feedings, stop the feeding and check the quantity of residual stomach contents. If it's greater than 150 ml, withhold the medication and feeding and notify the doctor. *An excessive amount of residual contents may indicate intestinal obstruction or paralytic ileus*.

If the NG tube is attached to suction, be sure to turn off the suction for 20 to 30 minutes after administering medication.

If possible, teach the patient who requires long-term treatment to instill his medication himself through the NG tube. Have him observe you as you perform the procedure several times before you allow him to try it himself.

Be sure to remain with the patient when he performs the procedure for the first few times *so you can provide assistance and answer any questions*. As the patient performs the procedure, give him positive reinforcement and correct any errors in his technique, as necessary.

Documentation

Record the instillation of medication, the date and time of instillation, the dose, and the patient's tolerance of the procedure. On his intake and output sheet, note the amount of fluid instilled.

Buccal and sublingual drug administration

Certain drugs are given buccally or sublingually to prevent their destruction or transformation in the stomach or small intestine. These drugs act quickly because the oral mucosa's thin epithelium and abundant vasculature allow direct absorption into the bloodstream. Drugs given buccally include erythrityl tetranitrate and methyltestosterone; drugs given sublingually include ergotamine tartrate, erythrityl tetranitrate, isoproterenol hydrochloride, isosorbide dinitrate, and nitroglycerin. With this method, the patient must be observed carefully to ensure he doesn't swallow the drug or suffer mucosal irritation.

Equipment
Patient's medication record and chart ■ prescribed medication ■ medication cup.

Implementation
● Verify the order on the patient's medication record by checking it against the doctor's order on his chart.
● Wash your hands with warm water and soap. Explain the procedure to the patient if he's never taken a drug buccally or sublingually before.
● Check the label on the medication three times before administering it *to make sure you'll be giving the prescribed medication.* Check when you take the container from the shelf or drawer, right before pouring the medication into the medication cup, and before returning the container to the shelf or drawer. If you're administering a unit-dose medication, check the label for the third time immediately after pouring the medication and again before discarding the wrapper. (Remember: Don't open a unit-dose medication until you're at the patient's bedside.)
● Confirm the patient's identity by asking his name and checking the name and room and bed number on his wristband.
● For buccal administration, place the tablet in the buccal pouch, between the cheek and gum. For sublingual administration, place the tablet under the patient's tongue. (See *Placing drugs in the oral mucosa.*)
● Instruct the patient to keep the medication in place until it dissolves completely *to ensure absorption.*
● Caution him against chewing the tablet or touching it with his tongue *to prevent accidental swallowing.*
● Tell him not to smoke before the drug has dissolved *because nicotine's vasoconstrictive effects slow absorption.*

Placing drugs in the oral mucosa

Buccal and sublingual administration routes allow some drugs, such as nitroglycerin or methyltestosterone, to enter the bloodstream rapidly without being degraded in the GI tract. To give a drug sublingually, place it under the patient's tongue, as shown below, and ask him to leave it there until it's dissolved.

To give a drug buccally, insert it between the patient's cheek and teeth, as shown below. Ask him to close his mouth and hold the tablet against his cheek until the tablet is absorbed.

Special considerations
Don't give liquids *because some buccal tablets may take up to 1 hour to be absorbed.* In that case, the patient should rinse his mouth with water *between* doses. Tell the angina patient to wet the nitroglycerin tablet with saliva and keep it under the tongue until fully absorbed.

Complications

Some buccal medications may irritate the mucosa. Alternate sides of the mouth for repeat doses *to prevent continuous irritation of the same site.* Sublingual medications — erythrityl tetranitrate, for example — may cause a tingling sensation under the tongue. If the patient finds this annoying, try placing the drug in the buccal pouch instead.

Documentation

Record the medication administered, the dose, the date and time, and the patient's reaction, if any.

Administration of rectal suppositories or ointments

A rectal suppository is a small, solid, medicated mass, usually cone-shaped, with a cocoa butter or glycerin base. It may be inserted to stimulate peristalsis and defecation or to relieve pain, vomiting, and local irritation. Rectal suppositories commonly contain drugs that reduce fever, induce relaxation, interact poorly with digestive enzymes, or have a taste too offensive for oral use. Rectal suppositories melt at body temperature and are absorbed slowly.

Because insertion of a rectal suppository may stimulate the vagus nerve, this procedure is contraindicated in patients with potential cardiac arrhythmias. It may have to be avoided in patients with recent rectal or prostate surgery because of the risk of local trauma or discomfort during insertion.

An ointment is a semisolid medication used to produce local effects. It may be applied externally to the anus or internally to the rectum. Rectal ointments commonly contain drugs that reduce inflammation or relieve pain and itching.

Equipment

Rectal suppository or tube of ointment and ointment applicator ▪ patient's medication record and chart ▪ 4″ × 4″ gauze pads ▪ gloves ▪ water-soluble lubricant ▪ optional: bedpan.

Preparation of equipment

Store rectal suppositories in the refrigerator until needed *to prevent softening and possible decreased effectiveness of the medication.* A softened suppository is also difficult to handle and insert. To harden it again, hold the suppository (in its wrapper) under cold running water.

Implementation

● Verify the order on the patient's medication record by checking it against the doctor's order.
● Wash your hands with warm soap and water.
● Confirm the patient's identity by asking his name and checking the name, room number, and bed number on his wristband.
● Explain the procedure and the purpose of the medication to the patient.
● Provide privacy.

Inserting a rectal suppository

● Place the patient on his left side in Sims' position. Drape him with the bedcovers *to expose only the buttocks.*
● Put on gloves. Remove the suppository from its wrapper, and lubricate it with water-soluble lubricant.
● Lift the patient's upper buttock with your nondominant hand *to expose the anus.*
● Instruct the patient to take several deep breaths through his mouth *to help relax the anal sphincters and reduce anxiety or discomfort during insertion.*
● Using the index finger of your dominant hand, insert the suppository — tapered end first — about 3″ (7.6 cm), until you feel it pass the internal anal sphincter. Try to direct the tapered end toward the side of the rectum *so it contacts the membranes.* (See *How to administer a rectal suppository or ointment.)*
● Ensure the patient's comfort. Encourage him to lie quietly and, if applicable, to retain the suppository for the appropriate length of time. A suppository administered to relieve constipation should be retained as long as possible (at least 20 minutes) to be effective. Press on the anus with a gauze pad if necessary until the urge to defecate passes.
● Discard the used equipment.

Applying an ointment

● *To apply externally,* wear gloves or use a gauze pad to spread medication over the anal area.
● *To apply internally,* attach the applicator to the tube of ointment and coat the applicator with water-soluble lubricant.
● Expect to use approximately 1″ (2.5 cm) of ointment. *To gauge how much pressure to use during application,* try squeezing a small amount from the tube before you attach the applicator.
● Lift the patient's upper buttock with your nondominant hand *to expose the anus.*
● Instruct the patient to take several deep breaths through his mouth *to relax the anal sphincters and reduce anxiety or discomfort during insertion.*
● Gently insert the applicator, directing it toward the umbilicus.

- Slowly squeeze the tube *to eject the medication.*
- Remove the applicator and place a folded 4″ × 4″ gauze pad between the patient's buttocks to absorb excess ointment.
- Disassemble the tube and applicator. Recap the tube, and clean the applicator thoroughly with soap and warm water.

Special considerations

Because the intake of food and fluid stimulates peristalsis, a suppository for relieving constipation should be inserted about 30 minutes before mealtime *to help soften the feces in the rectum and facilitate defecation.* A medicated retention suppository should be inserted between meals.

Instruct the patient to avoid expelling the suppository. However, if he has difficulty retaining it, place him on a bedpan.

Make sure the patient's call button is handy and watch for his signal *because he may be unable to suppress the urge to defecate.* For example, a patient with proctitis has a highly sensitive rectum and may not be able to retain a suppository for long.

Be sure to inform the patient that the suppository may discolor his next bowel movement. Anusol suppositories, for example, can give feces a silver-gray pasty appearance.

Documentation

Record the administration time, the dose, and the patient's response.

PARENTERAL ADMINISTRATION
Cartridge-injection system

A cartridge-injection system, such as the Tubex or Carpuject, is a convenient, easy-to-use method of injection that facilitates accuracy and sterility. The device consists of a plastic cartridge-holder syringe and a prefilled medication cartridge with needle attached.

The medication is premixed and premeasured, which saves time and helps ensure an exact dose. The medication remains sealed in the cartridge and sterile until the injection is administered

The disadvantage of this system is that not all drugs are available in cartridge form. However, compatible drugs can be added to partially filled cartridges.

How to administer a rectal suppository or ointment

When applying a suppository, direct its tapered end toward the side of the rectum so it contacts the membranes, encouraging absorption of the medication.

When applying an ointment, be sure to lubricate the applicator to minimize pain on insertion. Direct the applicator tip toward the patient's umbilicus.

Equipment

Patient's medication record and chart ▪ plastic cartridge-holder syringe ▪ medication-filled cartridge-needle unit ▪ alcohol sponge ▪ additional medication, if prescribed.

The 2-ml Carpuject-type syringe can be adapted to fit a 1-ml cartridge. Plastic syringes can be used with cartridges of any size.

Implementation

• Verify the order on the patient's medication record by checking it against the doctor's order.
• Wash your hands.

Using a Tubex system

• Hold the base of the unit and pull the plunger back. Place the medication cartridge inside the barrel of the unit. Then secure the cartridge by turning the plunger clockwise while holding the barrel. Finally, lock the barrel in place by turning it clockwise.
• Explain the procedure to the patient and provide privacy.
• Remove the needle guard just before the injection. A popping sound indicates that the seal was secure. Expel any air bubbles from the syringe cartridge and administer the medication, as prescribed.
• After the injection, don't resheath the needle *to avoid needle-stick injuries*. Remove the medication cartridge by unscrewing the plunger and barrel and removing the cartridge from the barrel. Discard the cartridge in an appropriate sharps container.

Using a plastic syringe (Carpuject)

• Make sure the medication and dose are correct before loading the syringe.
• Grasp the barrel of the syringe with the open side facing you and pull back the plunger as far as possible.
• Disengage the locking screw by turning it counterclockwise.
• Insert the cartridge-needle unit — needle end first — into the open side of the syringe. Advance and engage the locking screw, and turn it clockwise beyond its initial resistance until it will no longer rotate.
• Advance the plunger rod and screw it clockwise onto the threaded insert in the rubber plunger.
• Remove the needle guard, expel excess air from the cartridge, and administer the injection.
• After the injection, don't resheath the needle *to avoid needle-stick injuries*. Disengage the plunger rod from the plunger by rotating it counterclockwise and pulling it back as far as possible, taking care not to touch the needle.
• Disengage the locking screw by rotating it counterclockwise. Turn the syringe over, and allow the cartridge

to drop out of the holder. Discard the unit in an appropriate sharps container.

Adding a compatible medication to a partially filled cartridge

• Hold the cartridge with the needle end up. Remove the sheath and pull back the plunger rod so the surface of the rubber piston in contact with the medication is set at the mark equal to the combined medication volume.
• Wipe the diaphragm of the vial containing the compatible medication with an alcohol sponge.
• Insert the needle into the single-dose vial. Depress the plunger rod to inject into the vial an amount of air equal to the prescribed amount of medication to be withdrawn from the vial. Pull the rod back *to withdraw the medication.*
• Remove the needle from the vial, expel excess air, and replace the needle guard.
• Proceed to the patient's room to give the injection. Discard the equipment in an appropriate sharps container.

Special considerations

To use a 2-ml syringe holder with a 1-ml cartridge-needle unit, insert a 1-ml cartridge-needle unit into the syringe, engage it in the usual manner, and proceed with the injection. Disengage the cartridge-needle unit and discard it.

Before combining drugs in a cartridge, check appropriate sources for incompatibilities and contraindications. After mixing the drugs, check again for signs of incompatibility, such as discoloration and precipitation. If combining drugs involves the use of a multidose vial, you may want to use a separate needle and syringe to inject air *to prevent contaminating the vial with the cartridge medication.* If combining drugs involves the use of an ampule, you don't have to inject air into it *because an ampule doesn't contain a vacuum.*

Empty cartridges can be obtained and used for medications not readily available in the prefilled cartridge form.

Never use a cartridge-needle unit for successive injections or as a multidose container. Discard the unit after one injection.

To maintain sterility, keep the rubber sheath or needle guard in place until just before the injection.

For patients in isolation, disposable syringes are recommended instead of the cartridge-injection system. If the cartridge-injection system is used under such circumstances, the syringe holder should be kept in the patient's room and must be cleaned properly before it's removed from the room. Once removed from the room, it should be sterilized before being used for other patients or discarded.

248

Documentation
Record the medications administered, the injection site, and the time of administration. Describe any subsequent effects of the medications.

Admixture of drugs in a syringe

Combining two drugs in one syringe avoids the discomfort of two separate injections. Usually, drugs can be mixed in a syringe in one of four ways. They may be combined from two multidose vials (as, for example, regular and long-acting insulin), from one multidose vial and one ampule, from two ampules, or from a cartridge-injection system combined with either a multidose vial or ampule.

Such combinations are contraindicated when the drugs aren't compatible, and when the combined doses exceed the amount of solution that can be absorbed from a single injection site.

Equipment
Prescribed medications ■ patient's medication record and chart ■ alcohol sponges ■ syringe and needle ■ optional: cartridge-injection system and filter needle.

The type and size of the syringe and needle depend on the prescribed medications, the patient's body build, and the route of administration.

Medications that come in prefilled cartridges require a cartridge-injection system. (See "Cartridge-injection system" in this chapter.)

Implementation
• Verify that the drugs to be administered agree with the patient's medication record and the doctor's orders.
• Calculate the dose to be given.
• Wash your hands.

To mix drugs from two multidose vials
• Using an alcohol sponge, wipe the rubber stopper on the first vial. _This decreases the risk of contaminating the medication as you insert the needle into the vial._
• Pull back the syringe plunger until the volume of air drawn into the syringe equals the volume to be withdrawn from the drug vial.
• Without inverting the vial, insert the needle into the top of the vial, making sure that the needle's bevel tip doesn't touch the solution. Inject the air into the vial and withdraw the needle. _This replaces air in the vial to prevent creation of a partial vacuum when the drug is withdrawn._

• Repeat the above steps for the second vial. Then, after injecting the air into the second vial, invert the vial, withdraw the prescribed dose, and then withdraw the needle.
• Wipe the rubber stopper of the first vial again and insert the needle, taking care not to depress the plunger. Invert the vial, withdraw the prescribed dose, and then withdraw the needle.

To mix drugs from a multidose vial and an ampule
• Using an alcohol sponge, clean the vial's rubber stopper.
• Pull back on the syringe plunger until the volume of air drawn into the syringe equals the volume to be withdrawn from the drug vial.
• Insert the needle into the top of the vial and inject the air. Then invert the vial and withdraw the prescribed dose. Put the sterile needle cover over the needle.
• Wrap the ampule's neck with a piece of sterile gauze or an alcohol sponge _to protect yourself from injury in case the glass splinters._ Break open the ampule, directing the force away from you.
• If desired, switch to the filter needle at this point _to filter out any glass splinters._
• Insert the needle into the ampule. Be careful not to touch the outside of the ampule with the needle. Draw the correct dose into the syringe.
• If you switched to the filter needle, change back to a regular needle to administer the injection.

To mix drugs from two ampules
• An opened ampule doesn't contain a vacuum. To mix drugs from two ampules in a syringe, calculate the prescribed doses and open both ampules, using aseptic technique. If desired, use a filter needle to draw up the drugs. Then change to a regular needle to administer them.

Special considerations
Insert a needle through the vial's rubber stopper at a slight angle, bevel up, and exert slight lateral pressure. _This way you won't cut a piece of rubber out of the stopper, which can then be pushed into the vial._

When mixing drugs from multidose vials, be careful not to contaminate one drug with the other. Ideally, the needle should be changed after drawing the first medication into the syringe. This isn't always possible _because many disposable syringes do not have removable needles._
♦ _Nursing alert._ Never combine drugs if you are unsure of their compatibility, and never combine more than two drugs. (See _Combining drugs in a syringe: A compatibility guide,_ page 238.) Although drug incompatibility usually causes a visible reaction, such as clouding, bubbling, or precipitation, some incompatible combinations produce no visible reaction even though they alter the chemical na-

Combining drugs in a syringe: A compatibility guide

	atropine	butorphanol	chlorpromazine	codeine	diazepam	glycopyrrolate	hydromorphone	hydroxyzine	meperidine	morphine	nalbuphine	pentobarbital	phenobarbital	promethazine	scopolamine	secobarbital	sodium bicarbonate	thiopental	
atropine	■	Y	Y		N	Y	Y	Y	Y	P	Y	P		P	P				atropine
butorphanol	Y	■	Y		N			Y	P	Y		N		Y	Y				butorphanol
chlorpromazine	Y	Y	■		N	Y	Y	P	P	P		N		P	P			N	chlorpromazine
codeine				■	N	Y		Y											codeine
diazepam	N	N	N	N	■	N	N	N	N	N	N	N	N	N	N	N	N	N	diazepam
glycopyrrolate	Y		Y	Y	N	■	Y	Y	Y	Y		N		Y	Y	N	N	N	glycopyrrolate
hydromorphone	Y		Y		N	Y	■	Y				Y		Y	Y				hydromorphone
hydroxyzine	Y	Y	P	Y	N	Y	Y	■	P	Y	Y	N		P	Y				hydroxyzine
meperidine	Y	P	P		N	Y		P	■	N		N		Y	P			N	meperidine
morphine	P	Y	P		N	Y		Y	N	■		N?		P?	P			N	morphine
nalbuphine	Y				N			Y			■	N		Y	Y				nalbuphine
pentobarbital	P	N	N		N	N	Y	N	N	N?	N	■		N	Y		Y	Y	pentobarbital
phenobarbital					N								■						phenobarbital
promethazine	P	Y	P		N	Y	Y	P	Y	P?	Y	N		■	P			N	promethazine
scopolamine	P	Y	P		N	Y	Y	Y	P	P	Y	Y		P	■			Y	scopolamine
secobarbital					N	N										■			secobarbital
sodium bicarbonate					N	N						Y					■	N	sodium bicarbonate
thiopental			N		N	N			N	N		Y		N	Y		N	■	thiopental

KEY

Y Compatible

N Not compatible

P Provisionally compatible: use within 15 minutes of preparation

? Conflicting reports on compatibility; mixing not recommended

(A blank space indicates no available data on compatibility.)

ture and action of the drugs. Check appropriate references and a pharmacist when you are unsure about specific compatibility. When in doubt, administer two separate injections. ◆

Some medications are compatible for only a brief time after being combined and should be administered within 10 minutes after mixing. After this time, environmental factors—such as temperature, exposure to light, and humidity—may alter compatibility.

To reduce the risk of contamination, most hospitals dispense parenteral medications in single-dose vials. Insulin is one of the few drugs still packaged in multidose vials. Be careful when mixing regular and long-acting insulin. Draw up the regular insulin first *to avoid contamination by the long-acting suspension. (If a minute amount of the regular insulin is accidentally mixed with the long-acting insulin, it won't appreciably change the effect of the long-acting insulin.)* Check your hospital's policy before mixing insulins.

When you combine a cartridge-injection system and a multidose vial, use a separate needle and syringe to inject air into the multidose vial. *This prevents possible contamination of the multidose vial by the cartridge-injection system.*

Documentation
Record the drugs administered, the injection site, and the time of administration. Document adverse drug effects or other pertinent information.

Heparin insulin

Subcutaneous injection

When injected into the adipose (fatty) tissues beneath the skin, a drug moves into the bloodstream more rapidly than if given by mouth. Subcutaneous injection allows slower, more sustained drug administration than intramuscular injection; it also causes minimal tissue trauma and carries little risk of striking large blood vessels and nerves.

Absorbed mainly through the capillaries, drugs recommended for subcutaneous injection include nonirritating aqueous solutions and suspensions contained in 0.5 to 2.0 ml of fluid. Heparin and insulin, for example, are usually administered subcutaneously.

Drugs and solutions for subcutaneous injection are injected through a relatively short needle, using meticulous sterile technique. The most common subcutaneous injection sites are the outer aspect of the upper arm, anterior thigh, loose tissue of the lower abdomen, buttocks, and upper back. Injection is contraindicated in sites that are inflamed, edematous, scarred, or covered by a mole, birthmark, or other lesion. It may also be contraindicated in patients with impaired coagulation mechanisms.

Equipment
Prescribed medication ■ patient's medication record and chart ■ needle of appropriate gauge and length ■ gloves ■ 1- to 3-ml syringe ■ alcohol sponges ■ optional: antiseptic cleaning agent, filter needle, insulin syringe, insulin pump.

Preparation of equipment
Verify the order on the patient's medication record by checking it against the doctor's order.

Inspect the medication *to make sure it's not abnormally discolored or cloudy and that it doesn't contain precipitates.*

Wash your hands. Select a needle of the proper gauge and length. An average adult patient requires a 25G ⅝″ needle; an infant, a child, or an elderly or thin patient, a 25G to 27G ½″ needle.

Remember to check the label on the medication against the medication record. Read the label again as you draw up the medication for injection.

For single-dose ampules: Wrap the ampule's neck in an alcohol sponge and snap off the top, directing the force away from your body. If desired, attach a filter needle to the needle and withdraw the medication. Tap the syringe *to clear air from it.* Cover the needle with the needle sheath.

Before discarding the ampule, check the label against the patient's medication record.

Discard the filter needle and the ampule. Attach the appropriate needle to the syringe.

For single-dose or multidose vials: Reconstitute powdered drugs according to the label's instructions. Make sure that all crystals have dissolved in the solution. Warming the vial by holding it and rolling it between your palms may help to dissolve the drug more quickly.

Clean the vial's rubber stopper with an alcohol sponge. Pull the syringe plunger back until the volume of air in the syringe equals the volume of drug to be withdrawn from the vial.

Insert the needle into the vial. Inject the air, invert the vial, and keep the needle's bevel tip below the level of the solution as you withdraw the prescribed amount of medication. Cover the needle with the needle sheath. Tap the syringe *to clear any air from it.*

Check the drug label against the patient's medication record before returning the multidose vial to the shelf or drawer or before discarding the single-dose vial.

insulin = arms, abdomen, thighs, buttocks

Locating subcutaneous injection sites

Subcutaneous injection sites (shown by dotted areas) include the fat pads on the abdomen, upper hips, upper back, and lateral upper arms and thighs. For subcutaneous injections administered repeatedly, such as insulin, rotate sites. Choose one injection site in one area, move to a corresponding injection site in the next area, and so on. When returning to an area, choose a new site in that area. Preferred injection sites for insulin are the arms, abdomen, thighs and buttocks. Preferred injection sites for heparin injections are in the lower abdominal fat pad just below the umbilicus.

Implementation

● Confirm the patient's identity by asking his name and checking the name, room number, and bed number on his wristband.
● Explain the procedure to the patient and provide privacy.
● Select an appropriate injection site. (See *Locating subcutaneous injection sites.*) Rotate sites according to a schedule for patients who require repeated injections. Use different areas of the body unless contraindicated by the specific drug. (Heparin, for example, should be injected only in certain sites.)

● Put on gloves.
● Position and drape the patient if necessary.
● Clean the injection site with an alcohol sponge, beginning at the center of the site and moving outward in a circular motion. Allow the skin to dry before injecting the drug *to avoid a stinging sensation from introducing alcohol into subcutaneous tissues.*
● Loosen the protective needle sheath.
● With your nondominant hand, grasp the skin around the injection site firmly to elevate the subcutaneous tissue, forming a 1″ (2.5-cm) fat fold.
● Holding the syringe in your dominant hand, insert the loosened needle sheath between the fourth and fifth fingers of your other hand while still pinching the skin around the injection site. Pull back the syringe with your dominant hand *to uncover the needle by grasping the syringe like a pencil.* Don't touch the needle.
● Position the needle with its bevel up.
● Tell the patient he'll feel a prick as the needle is inserted.
● Insert the needle quickly in one motion. (See *Technique for subcutaneous injections.*) Release the patient's skin *to avoid injecting the drug into compressed tissue and irritating nerve fibers.*
● Pull back the plunger slightly *to check for blood return.* If none appears, begin injecting the drug slowly. If blood appears upon aspiration, withdraw the needle, prepare another syringe, and repeat the procedure.
● Don't aspirate for blood return when giving insulin or heparin. *It's not necessary with insulin and may cause a hematoma with heparin.*
● After injection, remove the needle gently but quickly at the same angle used for insertion.
● Cover the site with an alcohol sponge, and massage the site gently (unless you have injected a drug that contraindicates massage, such as heparin or insulin) *to distribute the drug and facilitate absorption.*
● Remove the alcohol sponge and check the injection site for bleeding or bruising.
● Dispose of injection equipment according to hospital policy. *To avoid needle-stick injuries,* don't resheath the needle.

Special considerations

If the medication is available in prefilled syringes, adjust the angle and depth of insertion according to needle length.

For insulin injections

To establish more consistent blood insulin levels, rotate insulin injection sites within anatomic regions. Absorption varies from one region to another. Preferred insulin injection sites are the arms, abdomen, thighs, and buttocks.

Make sure the type of insulin, unit dosage, and syringe are correct.

When combining insulins in a syringe, make sure they are compatible. Regular insulin can be mixed with all other types. Prompt insulin zinc suspension (Semilente insulin) cannot be mixed with NPH insulin. Follow hospital policy regarding which insulin to draw up first.

Before drawing up insulin suspension, gently roll and invert the bottle to ensure even drug particle distribution. Don't shake the bottle *because this can cause foam or bubbles to develop in the syringe.*

Some patients may benefit from an insulin infusion pump. (See *Types of insulin infusion pumps,* page 242.)

For heparin injections

The preferred site for heparin injection is the lower abdominal fat pad, 2″ (5 cm) beneath the umbilicus, between the right and the left iliac crests. *Injecting heparin into this area, which isn't involved in muscular activity, reduces the risk of local capillary bleeding.* Always rotate the sites from one side to the other.

Don't administer any injections within 2″ of a scar, a bruise, or the umbilicus.

Don't aspirate to check for blood return *because this may cause bleeding into the tissues at the site.*

Don't rub or massage the site after the injection. *Rubbing can cause localized minute hemorrhages or bruises.*

If the patient bruises easily, apply ice to the site for the first 5 minutes after the injection *to minimize local hemorrhage,* then apply pressure.

Complications

Concentrated or irritating solutions may cause formation of sterile abscesses. Repeated injections in the same site can cause lipodystrophy. A natural immune response, this complication can be minimized by rotating injection sites.

Documentation

Record the time and date of the injection, the medication administered and the dose, the injection site and route, and the patient's reaction to the medication.

Intradermal injection

Used primarily for diagnostic purposes, as in allergy or tuberculin testing, intradermal injections are administered in small amounts, usually 0.5 ml or less, into the

Technique for subcutaneous injections

Before giving the injection, elevate the subcutaneous tissue at the site by grasping it firmly.

Insert the needle at a 45- or 90-degree angle to the skin surface, depending upon needle length and the amount of subcutaneous tissue at the site. Some medications, such as heparin, should always be injected at a 90-degree angle.

outer layers of the skin. Because little systemic absorption of intradermally injected agents takes place, this type of injection is used primarily to produce a local effect.

The ventral forearm is the most commonly used site for intradermal injection because of its easy accessibility and lack of hair. In extensive allergy testing, the outer aspect of the upper arms may be used, as well as the area of the back located between the scapulae (see *Intradermal injection sites,* page 243.)

Types of insulin infusion pumps

A continuous subcutaneous insulin infusion pump provides long-term insulin therapy for patients with insulin-dependent diabetes mellitus. Complications include infection at the injection site, catheter clogging, and insulin loss from loose reservoir-catheter connections. Insulin pumps work on either a closed-loop or an open-loop system.

Open-loop system
The open-loop pump is used most commonly. It infuses insulin but can't respond to blood glucose changes. These portable, self-contained, programmable insulin pumps are smaller and less obtrusive than ever—about the size of a credit card—and have fewer buttons.

The pump delivers insulin in small (basal) doses every few minutes and large (bolus) doses that the patient sets manually. The system consists of a reservoir containing the insulin syringe, a small pump, an infusion-rate selector that allows insulin release adjustments, a battery, and a plastic catheter with an attached needle leading from the syringe to the subcutaneous injection site. The needle is typically held in place with waterproof tape. The patient can wear the pump on his belt

or in his pocket—practically anywhere as long as the infusion line has a clear path to the injection site.

The infusion-rate selector automatically releases about half the total daily insulin requirement. The patient releases the remainder in bolus amounts before meals and snacks. The patient must change the syringe daily; he must change the needle, catheter, and injection site every other day.

Closed-loop system
The self-contained closed-loop system detects and responds to changing blood glucose levels. The typical closed-loop system includes a glucose sensor, a programmable computer, a power supply, a pump, and an insulin reservoir. The computer triggers continuous insulin delivery in appropriate amounts from the reservoir.

Nonneedle catheter system
In an alternate, nonneedle delivery system, a tiny plastic catheter is inserted into the skin over a needle. The needle is then withdrawn, leaving the catheter in place. This pump can be placed in the abdomen, thigh, or flank and should be changed every 2 or 3 days.

Open-loop infusion pump

Close-up of the pump

Equipment

Patient's medication record and chart ■ tuberculin syringe with a 26G or 27G ½" to ⅝" needle ■ prescribed medication ■ gloves ■ alcohol sponges.

Implementation

• Verify the patient's identity by checking his name, room number, and bed number on his wristband against his medical record.
• Tell him where you will be giving the injection.
• Instruct the patient to sit up and to extend his arm and support it on a flat surface, with the ventral forearm exposed.
• Put on gloves.
• With an alcohol sponge, clean the surface of the ventral forearm about two or three fingerbreadths distal to the antecubital space. Be sure the test site you have chosen is free of hair or blemishes. Allow the skin to dry completely before administering the injection.
• While holding the patient's forearm in your hand, stretch the skin taut with your thumb.
• With your free hand, hold the needle at a 15-degree angle to the patient's arm, with its bevel up.
• Insert the needle about ⅛" below the epidermis at sites 2" (5 cm) apart. Stop when the needle's bevel tip is under the skin, and inject the antigen slowly. You should feel some resistance as you do this, and a wheal should form as you inject the antigen. (See *Giving an intradermal injection,* page 244.) If no wheal forms, you have injected the antigen too deeply; withdraw the needle and administer another test dose at least 2" (5 cm) from the first site.
• Withdraw the needle at the same angle at which it was inserted. Do not rub the site. *This could irritate the underlying tissue, which may affect test results.*
• Circle each test site with a marking pen, and label each site according to the recall antigen given. Instruct the patient to refrain from washing off the circles until the test is completed.
• Dispose of needles and syringes according to hospital policy.
• Remove and discard your gloves.
• Assess the patient's response to the skin testing in 24 to 48 hours.

Special considerations

In patients hypersensitive to the test antigens, a severe anaphylactic response can result. This requires immediate epinephrine injection and other emergency resuscitation procedures. Be especially alert after giving a test dose of penicillin or tetanus antitoxin.

Intradermal injection sites

The most common intradermal injection site is the ventral forearm. Other sites (indicated by dotted areas) include the upper chest, upper arm, and shoulder blades. Skin in these areas is usually lightly pigmented, thinly keratinized, and relatively hairless, facilitating detection of adverse reactions.

Documentation

Record the type and amount of medication given on the patient's medication record. Also record the time given and the location of the injection site. Note any skin reactions as well as any other adverse reactions.

Intramuscular injection

[handwritten: Stretch skin site taut]

[handwritten: Draw 0.2cc air into syringe p you have drawn medicine in]

Intramuscular (I.M.) injections deposit medication deep into muscle tissue, which is well-vascularized and can absorb it quickly. This route of administration provides rapid systemic action and absorption of relatively large doses (up to 5 ml in appropriate sites). I.M. injections are recommended for patients who are uncooperative or can't take medication orally and for drugs that are altered by digestive juices. Because muscle tissue has few sensory nerves, I.M. injection allows less painful administration of irritating drugs.

The site for an I.M. injection must be chosen carefully, taking into account the patient's general physical status and the purpose of the injection. I.M. injections should not be administered at inflamed, edematous, or irritated

Giving an intradermal injection

Secure the forearm. Insert the needle at a 10- to 15-degree angle so it just punctures skin surface. When injected, the drug should raise a small wheal.

sites or at those containing moles, birthmarks, scar tissue, or other lesions. I.M. injections may also be contraindicated in patients with impaired coagulation mechanisms, and in patients with occlusive peripheral vascular disease, edema, and shock, because these conditions impair peripheral absorption. I.M. injections require sterile technique to maintain the integrity of muscle tissue.

Oral or I.V. routes are preferred for administration of drugs that are poorly absorbed by muscle tissue, such as phenytoin, digoxin, chlordiazepoxide, diazepam, and haloperidol.

Equipment
Patient's medication record and chart ▪ prescribed medication ▪ diluent or filter needle, if needed ▪ 3- to 5-ml syringe ▪ 20G to 25G 1″ to 3″ needle ▪ gloves ▪ alcohol sponges.

The prescribed medication must be sterile. The needle may be packaged separately or already attached to the syringe. Needles used for I.M. injections are longer than subcutaneous needles *because they must reach deep into the muscle.* Needle length also depends on the injection site, the patient's size, and the amount of subcutaneous fat covering the muscle. The needle gauge for I.M. injections should be larger to accommodate viscous solutions and suspensions.

Preparation of equipment
Verify the order on the patient's medication record by checking it against the doctor's order. Also note if the patient has any allergies, especially before the first dose.

Check the prescribed medication for color and clarity. Also note the expiration date. Never use medication that is cloudy or discolored or that contains a precipitate unless the manufacturer's instructions allow it. Remember also that for some drugs (such as suspensions) the presence of drug particles is normal. Observe for any abnormal changes. If in doubt, check with the pharmacist.

Choose equipment appropriate to the prescribed medication and injection site and make sure it works properly. The needle should be straight, smooth, and free of burrs.

Wipe the stopper of the medication vial with an alcohol sponge, and then draw up the prescribed amount of medication using the three-label check system — read the label as you select the medication, as you draw up the medication, and after you have completed drawing up the medication *to verify the correct dosage.*

Then draw about 0.2 cc of air into the syringe according to hospital policy. When the syringe is inverted during the injection, the air bubble rises to the plunger end of the syringe and follows the medication into the injection site. *The air clears the needle of medication and helps prevent leakage into the subcutaneous tissue following injection by creating an air block that reduces reflux (tracking) along the needle path.*

Gather all necessary equipment and proceed to the patient's room.

Implementation
• Confirm the patient's identity by asking his name and checking his wristband for name, room number, and bed number.
• Provide privacy and explain the procedure to the patient.
• Wash your hands.
• Select an appropriate injection site. The gluteal muscles (gluteus medius and minimus and the upper outer corner of the gluteus maximus) are used most commonly for healthy adults, although the deltoid muscle may be used for a small-volume injection (2 ml or less). For infants and children, the vastus lateralis muscle of the thigh is used most often *because it's usually the best developed and contains no large nerves or blood vessels, minimizing the risk of serious injury.* The rectus femoris muscle may also be used in infants but is usually contraindicated in adults. Remember to always rotate injection sites for patients who require repeated injections.
• Position and drape the patient appropriately, making sure the site is well-exposed and that lighting is adequate.
• Loosen the protective needle sheath, but don't remove it.

• After selecting the injection site, gently tap it *to stimulate nerve endings and minimize pain when the needle is inserted.* (See *Locating I.M. injection sites,* page 246.) Then clean the skin at the site with an alcohol sponge. Move the sponge outward in a circular motion to a circumference of about 2″ (5 cm) from the injection site. Then allow the skin to dry *to avoid introducing alcohol into the needle puncture, which causes pain.* Keep the alcohol sponge for later use.

• Don gloves. With the thumb and index finger of your nondominant hand, gently stretch the skin of the injection site taut.

• Holding the syringe in your dominant hand, remove the needle sheath by slipping it between the free fingers of your nondominant hand and then drawing back the syringe.

• Position the syringe at a 90-degree angle to the skin surface, with the needle a couple of inches from the skin. Tell the patient that he will feel a prick as you insert the needle. Then quickly and firmly thrust the needle through the skin and subcutaneous tissue, deep into the muscle.

• Support the syringe with your nondominant hand, if desired. Pull back slightly on the plunger with your dominant hand to aspirate for blood. If no blood appears, place your thumb on the plunger rod and *slowly* inject the medication into the muscle. *A slow, steady injection rate allows the muscle to distend gradually and accept the medication under minimal pressure.* You should feel little or no resistance against the force of the injection. The air bubble in the syringe should follow the medication into the injection site.

♦ *Nursing alert.* If blood appears in the syringe on aspiration, the needle is in a blood vessel. If this occurs, stop the injection, withdraw the needle, prepare another injection with new equipment, and inject another site. Don't inject the bloody solution. ♦

• After the injection, gently but quickly remove the needle at a 90-degree angle.

• Using a gloved hand, cover the injection site immediately with the used alcohol sponge, apply gentle pressure, and unless contraindicated, massage the relaxed muscle *to help distribute the drug and promote absorption.*

• Remove the alcohol sponge and inspect the injection site for signs of active bleeding or bruising. If bleeding continues, apply pressure to the site; if bruising occurs, you may apply ice.

• Watch for adverse reactions at the site for 30 minutes after the injection.

• Discard all equipment according to universal precautions and your hospital's policy. Don't attempt to recap needles; dispose of them in an appropriate sharps container *to avoid needle-stick injuries.*

Special considerations

To slow absorption, some drugs for I.M. administration are dissolved in oil or other special solutions. Mix these preparations well before drawing them into the syringe.

Never use the gluteal muscles (which develop from repeated walking) as the injection site for a child under age 3 or who has been walking for less than a year. Never inject into sensitive muscles, especially those that twitch or tremble when you assess site landmarks and tissue depth with your fingertips. *Injections in these trigger areas may cause sharp or referred pain, such as the pain caused by nerve trauma.*

Keep a rotation record that lists all available injection sites, divided into various body areas, for patients who require repeated injections. Rotate from a site in the first area to a site in each of the other areas. Then return to a site in the first area that is at least 1″ (2.5 cm) away from the previous injection site in that area.

If the patient has experienced pain or emotional trauma from repeated injections, consider numbing the area before cleaning it by holding ice on it for several seconds. If you must inject more than 5 ml of solution, divide the solution and inject it at two separate sites.

Always encourage the patient to relax the muscle you'll be injecting *because injections into tense muscles are more painful than usual and may bleed more readily.*

I.M. injections can damage local muscle cells, causing elevated serum enzyme levels (creatine phosphokinase, [CPK]) that can be confused with the elevated enzymes resulting from damage to cardiac muscle, as in myocardial infarction. To distinguish between skeletal and cardiac muscle damage, diagnostic tests for suspected myocardial infarction must identify the isoenzyme of CPK specific to cardiac muscle (CPK-MB [CPK_2]) and include tests for lactate dehydrogenase (LDH) and aspartate aminotransferase (AST), formerly SGOT. If it's important to measure these enzyme levels, suggest that the doctor switch to I.V. administration, with dosages adjusted accordingly.

Complications

Accidental injection of concentrated or irritating medications into subcutaneous tissue, or into other areas where it can't be fully absorbed, can cause sterile abscesses to develop. Such abscesses result from a natural immune response in which phagocytes attempt to remove the foreign matter.

Failure to rotate sites in patients who require repeated injections can lead to deposits of unabsorbed medications. Such deposits can reduce the desired pharmacologic effect and may lead to abscess formation or tissue fibrosis.

Locating I.M. injection sites

Deltoid *2ml or less*

First find the lower edge of the acromial process and the point on the lateral arm in line with the axilla. Insert the needle 1″ to 2″ (2.5 to 5 cm) below the acromial process, usually two to three fingerbreadths, at a 90-degree angle or angled slightly toward the process. Typical injection: 0.5 ml (range: 0.5 to 2 ml).

Dorsogluteal

Inject above and outside a line drawn from the posterior superior iliac spine to the greater trochanter of the femur. Or divide the buttock into quadrants and inject in the upper outer quadrant, about 2″ to 3″ (5 to 7.6 cm) below the iliac crest. Insert the needle at a 90-degree angle. Typical injection: 1 to 4 ml (range: 1 to 5 ml).

Ventrogluteal *1-5ml*

First, locate the greater trochanter of the femur with the heel of your hand. Then, spread your index and middle fingers from the anterior superior iliac spine to as far along the iliac crest as you can reach. Insert the needle between the two fingers at a 90-degree angle to the muscle. (Remove your hand before inserting the needle.) Typical injection: 1 to 4 ml (range: 1 to 5 ml).

Vastus lateralis

Use the lateral muscle of the quadriceps group, from a handbreadth below the greater trochanter to a handbreadth above the knee. Insert the needle into the middle third of the muscle parallel to the surface on which the patient is lying. You may have to bunch the muscle before insertion. Typical injection: 1 to 4 ml (range: 1 to 5 ml; 1 to 3 ml for infants).

Documentation
Chart the drug administered, dose, date, time, route of administration, and injection site. Also, note the patient's tolerance of injection and its effects, including any adverse effects.

Z-track injection

This method of intramuscular injection prevents leakage, or tracking, into the subcutaneous tissue. Typically, it's used to administer drugs that irritate and discolor subcutaneous tissue, primarily iron preparations, such as iron dextran. It may also be used in elderly patients who have decreased muscle mass. Lateral displacement of the skin during the injection helps to seal the drug in the muscle.

This procedure requires careful attention to technique because leakage into subcutaneous tissue can cause patient discomfort and may permanently stain some tissues.

Equipment
Patient's medication record and chart ▪ two 20G 1¼" to 2" needles ▪ prescribed medication ▪ gloves ▪ 3- to 5-ml syringe ▪ two alcohol sponges.

Preparation of equipment
Verify the order on the patient's medication record by checking it against the doctor's order. Wash your hands. Make sure the needle you're using is long enough to reach the muscle. As a rule of thumb, a 200-pound patient requires a 2" needle; a 100-pound patient, a 1¼" to 1½" needle. Attach one needle to the syringe and draw up the prescribed medication. Then draw 0.2 to 0.5 cc of air (depending on hospital policy) into the syringe. Remove the first needle and attach the second *to prevent tracking the medication through the subcutaneous tissue as the needle is inserted.*

Implementation
• Confirm the patient's identity, explain the procedure, and provide privacy.
• Place the patient in the lateral position, exposing the gluteal muscle to be used as the injection site. The patient may also be placed in the prone position.
• Clean an area on the upper outer quadrant of the patient's buttock with an alcohol sponge.
• Don gloves. Then displace the skin laterally by pulling it away from the injection site. (See *Displacing the skin for Z-track injection*, page 248.)

• Insert the needle into the muscle at a 90-degree angle.
• Aspirate for blood return; if none appears, inject the drug slowly, followed by the air. *Injecting air after the drug helps clear the needle and prevents tracking the medication through subcutaneous tissues as the needle is withdrawn.*
• Wait 10 seconds before withdrawing the needle *to ensure dispersion of the medication.*
• Withdraw the needle slowly. Then release the displaced skin and subcutaneous tissue *to seal the needle track.* Don't massage the injection site or allow the patient to wear a tight-fitting garment over the site *because it could force the medication into subcutaneous tissue.*
• Encourage the patient to walk or to move about in bed *to facilitate absorption of the drug from the injection site.*
• Discard the needles and syringe in an appropriate sharps container. Do not recap needles *to avoid needlestick injuries.*
• Remove and discard your gloves.

Special considerations
Never inject more than 5 ml of solution into a single site using the Z-track method. Alternate gluteal sites for repeat injections.

If the patient is on bed rest, encourage active range-of-motion (ROM) exercises or perform passive ROM exercises *to facilitate absorption from the injection site.*

Complications
Discomfort and tissue irritation may result from drug leakage into subcutaneous tissue.

Documentation
Record the medication, dosage, date, time, and site of injection on the patient's medication record. Include the patient's response to the injected drug.

Intraosseous infusion

When rapid venous infusion is difficult or impossible, intraosseous infusion allows delivery of fluids, medications, or whole blood into the bone marrow. Performed on infants and children, this technique is used in such emergencies as cardiopulmonary arrest or circulatory collapse, hypokalemia from traumatic injury or dehydration, status epilepticus, status asthmaticus, burns, near-drowning, and overwhelming sepsis.

Any drug that can be given I.V. can be given by intraosseous infusion; drug absorption and effectiveness are comparable to the I.V. route. Intraosseous infusion

Displacing the skin for Z-track injection

By blocking the needle pathway after injection, this technique allows I.M. injection while minimizing the risk of subcutaneous irritation and staining from such drugs as iron dextran. The illustrations below show how to perform a Z-track injection.

Before the procedure begins, the skin, subcutaneous fat, and muscle lie in their normal positions.

To begin, place your finger on the skin surface, and pull the skin and subcutaneous layers out of alignment with the underlying muscle. You should move the skin about ½″ (1 cm).

Insert the needle at a 90-degree angle in the site where you initially placed your finger. Inject the drug and withdraw the needle.

Finally, remove your finger from the skin surface, allowing the layers to return to their normal positions. The needle track (shown by the dotted line) is now broken at the junction of each tissue layer, trapping the drug in the muscle.

has been used as an acceptable alternative for infants and children.

Intraosseous infusion is commonly undertaken at the anterior surface of the tibia. Alternate sites include the iliac crest, spinous process, or (rarely) the upper anterior portion of the sternum. Only personnel trained in this procedure should perform it. Usually, a nurse will assist. (See *Understanding intraosseous infusion.*)

This procedure is contraindicated in osteogenesis imperfecta, osteopetrosis, and ipsilateral fracture, because of the potential for subcutaneous extravasation. Infusion through an area with cellulitis or an infected burn increases the risk of infection.

Equipment
Bone marrow biopsy needle or specially designed intraosseous infusion needle (cannula and obturator) ▪ povidone-iodine sponges ▪ sterile gauze pads ▪ sterile gloves ▪ sterile drape ▪ bone marrow set ▪ heparinized saline

flush solution ■ I.V. fluids and tubing ■ 1% lidocaine ■ 3-
to 5-ml syringe.

Preparation of equipment
Prepare I.V. fluids and tubing, as ordered.

Implementation
• If the patient is conscious, explain the procedure *to
allay his fears and promote his cooperation.* Ensure that
the patient or a responsible family member understands
the procedure and signs a consent form.
• Check the patient's history for hypersensitivity to the
local anesthetic. If the patient isn't an infant, tell him
which bone site will be infused. Inform him that he will
receive a local anesthetic and will feel pressure from
needle insertion.
• Provide a sedative, if ordered, before the procedure.
• Position the patient based on the selected puncture site.
• Using sterile technique, clean the puncture site with
a povidone-iodine sponge and allow it to dry. Then cover
the area with a sterile drape.
• Using sterile technique, hand the doctor the 3- to 5-ml
syringe with 1% lidocaine *so that he may anesthetize the
infusion site.*
• The doctor inserts the cannula and obturator through
the skin and into the bone at an angle of 10 to 15 degrees
from vertical. He advances it with a to-and-fro rotary
motion through the periosteum until the needle penetrates the marrow cavity. The needle should "give" suddenly as it enters the marrow and should stand erect
when released.
• Then the doctor removes the obturator from the needle
and attaches a 5-ml syringe. He aspirates some bone
marrow *to confirm needle placement.*
• The doctor replaces this syringe with a syringe containing 5 ml of heparinized saline flush solution and
flushes the cannula *to confirm needle placement and clear
the cannula of clots or bone particles.*
• Next, the doctor removes the syringe of flush solution
and attaches I.V. tubing to the cannula *to allow infusion
of medications and I.V. fluids.*
• Put on sterile gloves.
• Clean the infusion site with povidone-iodine sponges,
and then secure the site with tape and a sterile gauze
dressing.
• Monitor vital signs and check the infusion site for bleeding, extravasation, and postinfusion infection.

Special considerations
Intraosseous infusion should be discontinued as soon as
conventional vascular access is established (within 2 to
4 hours, if possible). *Prolonged infusion significantly increases the risk of infection.*

Understanding intraosseous infusion

During intraosseous infusion, the bone marrow
serves as a noncollapsible vein; thus, fluid infused
into the marrow cavity rapidly enters the circulation
via an extensive network of venous sinusoids.
Here, the needle is shown positioned in the patient's tibia.

After needle removal, place a sterile dressing over
the injection site, and apply firm pressure to the site for
5 minutes.

Intraosseous flow rates are determined by needle size
and flow through the bone marrow. Fluids should flow
freely if needle placement is correct. Normal saline solution has been administered intraosseously at a rate of
600 ml/minute and up to 2,500 ml/hour when delivered
under pressure of 300 mm Hg through a 13G needle.

Complications
Common complications of intraosseous infusion include
extravasation of fluid into subcutaneous tissue, resulting
from incorrect needle placement; subperiosteal effusion,
resulting from failure of fluid to enter the marrow space;
and clotting in the needle, resulting from delayed infusion
or failure to flush the needle after placement. Other complications include subcutaneous abscess, osteomyelitis,
and epiphyseal injury.

Documentation
Record the time, date, location, and the patient's tolerance of the procedure. Document the amount of fluid
infused on the input and output record.

Intra-articular injection

An intra-articular injection delivers drugs directly to the synovial cavity of a joint to relieve pain, help preserve function, prevent contractures, and delay muscle atrophy. Drugs commonly administered intra-articularly include corticosteroids, anesthetics, and lubricants. Rarely, antiseptics, analgesics, and counterirritants may be injected by this route. Before intra-articular injection, synovial fluid may be withdrawn to relieve pressure or to be tested in the laboratory.

Usually performed by a doctor with a nurse assisting, intra-articular injection requires sterile technique. It's contraindicated in patients with joint infection, joint instability or fracture, or systemic fungal infection.

Equipment
Patient's medication record and chart ■ 3-ml and 5- or 10-ml syringes ■ labels ■ prescribed medication ■ sterile towel, gloves, cotton balls, and gauze pads ■ pillows ■ sterile emesis basin ■ antiseptic cleaning agent ■ sterile fenestrated drape ■ local anesthetic ■ 25G ⅝" needle ■ 18G 1½" needle ■ adhesive bandage ■ optional: sterile test tubes for synovial fluid aspiration, with appropriate additives and specimen labels, and 10- or 20-ml syringe for aspirating synovial fluid specimen.

Sterile povidone-iodine sponges may be used instead of the antiseptic cleaning agent and the sterile cotton balls or gauze pads.

Preparation of equipment
Verify the order on the patient's medication record by checking it against the doctor's order. Wash your hands. Draw the prescribed amount of medication into the 5- or 10-ml syringe before entering the patient's room. Label the syringe with the name of the medication and the amount. Take the container from which you drew the medication with you *so the doctor can verify the syringe contents.*

Implementation
• Confirm the patient's identity, explain the procedure to him, and provide privacy.
• Position the patient comfortably. The joint to be injected should be stabilized, supported (with pillows, if necessary), and fully exposed. (See *Locating intra-articular injection sites.)*
• Using aseptic technique, open the sterile towel and place it on the bedside stand *to create a sterile field.*
• Using aseptic technique, open the syringes, needles, and cotton balls or gauze pads and drop them onto the sterile field.
• After putting on sterile gloves, the doctor picks up sterile cotton balls or gauze pads and holds them over the emesis basin.
• Pour the antiseptic cleaning agent over the cotton balls or gauze pads.
• The doctor cleans the injection site with the saturated cotton balls or gauze pads. After draping the site, he checks the label on the local anesthetic as you hold the bottle. Then turn it upside down so the doctor can fill the 3-ml syringe.
• The doctor anesthetizes the skin and subcutaneous tissue at the injection site using the 25G ⅝" needle.

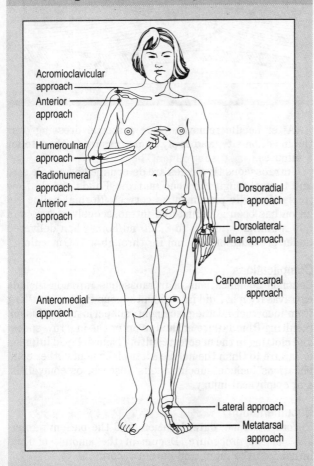

Locating intra-articular injection sites

Acromioclavicular approach
Anterior approach
Humeroulnar approach
Radiohumeral approach
Anterior approach
Anteromedial approach
Dorsoradial approach
Dorsolateral-ulnar approach
Carpometacarpal approach
Lateral approach
Metatarsal approach

To aspirate synovial fluid

• Position the sterile test tubes in the correct order.
• The doctor withdraws synovial fluid with the 18G 1½" needle using the 10-ml syringe. He leaves the needle in the joint *for the subsequent injection of medication.* The syringe containing the specimen can be set aside until after the procedure.
• After completing the intra-articular injection, the doctor will attach a needle to the specimen syringe and insert appropriate specimens into the test tubes. Label the test tubes appropriately and send them to the laboratory.

To perform intra-articular injection

• Hand the 5- or 10-ml medication syringe—with an 18G 1½" needle attached—to the doctor, who then injects the medication into the synovial cavity. (If synovial fluid was aspirated, remove the needle and hand the doctor the medication syringe. He attaches the syringe to the needle already in the joint and injects the medication.)
• After the injection, apply pressure to the site and (if appropriate) massage the area gently for 1 or 2 minutes *to facilitate absorption.*
• Apply an adhesive bandage to the site.

Special considerations

Advise the patient to avoid excessive use of the affected joint *because the injected medications may mask pain.*

Complications

Because the medication may infiltrate and initially irritate surrounding tissue, local joint pain may actually increase for 24 to 48 hours after an intra-articular injection. However, fever, persistent increased pain, redness, and swelling may indicate septic arthritis, a serious complication caused by contamination.

Documentation

Record the injected medication, dose, date, time and site of injection, and the doctor's name in your notes. Also note the amount of synovial fluid aspirated, any laboratory studies requested, and the patient's tolerance of the injection.

 # Addition of drugs to an I.V. solution

Various transfer devices can be used to add drugs to an I.V. solution. The common syringe and needle are used to draw up medications, reconstitute powdered drugs, and make transfers. A single- or double-headed needle is used to transfer dissolved medication in a vial to an I.V. bottle while keeping the vacuum intact. A syringe with a filter needle or filter straw can be used to transfer medication from an ampule to a bottle or bag.

Before adding any drug to an I.V. solution, it's necessary to verify the compatibility of the solution with the drug. Adding drugs to blood is contraindicated because it complicates identifying the source of an adverse reaction.

Equipment

Patient's medication record and chart ▪ compatibility and stability guide ▪ drug to be added ▪ I.V. solution ▪ diluent, if necessary ▪ I.V. administration set or sterile I.V. cap ▪ syringe with filter needle ▪ double-headed needle ▪ medication-added labels ▪ alcohol sponges ▪ optional: ampule transfer device, 100-, 250-, or 500-ml container.

You'll also need a needle when using a syringe with a filter needle or filter straw and an ampule transfer device. A 4" × 4" gauze pad helps prevent cuts when you break open an ampule. Always use a small, thin needle (such as a 25G 1") for multiple punctures of a vial or bag. *A small puncture reseals better.*

Preparation of equipment

Verify the order on the patient's medication record by checking it against the doctor's order. Check hospital policy *to see if you're permitted to add the drug to the I.V. solution.* If so, find out how the drug to be added is packaged, and then obtain the appropriate transfer device and any necessary diluent. Inspect the I.V. container for cracks or leaks. Check the compatibility and dosage of the drug, diluent, and I.V. solution. If the drug's stability is limited, mix it in a 100-, 250-, or 500-ml container *to avoid waste and loss of potency.*

Implementation

• Wash your hands.
• Confirm the patient's identity by asking his name and checking the name, room number, and bed number on his wristband.
• Verify that you have the correct drug by comparing its label with the order on the medication record. Read the label as you prepare the drug additive and again after you've added it to the solution.

To use a syringe and needle

• Remove the protective cap from the drug vial and wipe the top of the vial with a sterile alcohol sponge.
• If the drug to be added is a powder, aspirate the correct amount of diluent into the syringe and inject it into the drug vial. Roll the vial between your hands *to dissolve all particles.*

• Wipe the injection port on the I.V. container with an alcohol sponge.
• Inject the drug and gently rotate the vial or invert or rotate the bag *to mix the solution.*

To use a single-headed needle or pin
• Remove the protective cap from the needle or pin on top of the drug vial.
• Invert the drug vial and insert the pin into the I.V. container's main port *so the vacuum draws the drug into the container.* Remove the vial and gently rotate the container *to mix the solution.*

To use a double-headed needle or pin
• Remove the protective cap from the drug vial and wipe the rubber seal with an alcohol sponge, if desired. If you're adding medication to an I.V. bag, remove the protective outer wrapping.
• If the drug to be added is a powder, add the appropriate diluent with a needle and syringe and roll the vial between your hands *to dissolve all particles.*
• Remove the outside cover of the double-headed needle *to expose the shorter needle.* Insert this needle into the drug vial and remove the other half of the needle cover *to expose the longer needle.*
• Wipe the injection port on the I.V. container with an alcohol sponge. Invert the medication vial, and insert the longer needle into the center hole of the appropriate seal. The vacuum then draws the drug into the I.V. container. Remove the vial and gently rotate the container *to mix the solution.*

To use a syringe with a filter needle or straw
• Place the filter needle or straw on the syringe. Then wipe the ampule's neck with an alcohol sponge, wrap it in a 4″ × 4″ gauze pad, and snap off the top, directing the force away from your body.
• Aspirate the ampule's contents with the syringe. Then replace the filter needle or straw with a 25G 1″ needle.
• Inject the drug into the I.V. container and rotate the container *to mix the solution.*

After preparing the solution
• Recheck the drug dose and I.V. solution *to prevent error.*
• Connect the I.V. administration set or sterile protective cap (provided by the manufacturer) to the I.V. container *to prevent contamination.*
• Fill out the medication-added label and place it on the I.V. container. The label should include the date, drug dose, your initials, time the drug was added to the I.V. container, and patient's name, room number, and bed number.

Special considerations
Maintain sterile technique throughout this procedure.

When making multiple drug transfers, add only one drug at a time. Always add the most concentrated drug first and any colored drugs last. Mix the solution thoroughly and examine it for precipitation, discoloration, or cloudiness after adding each drug.

To add a drug to an I.V. solution that has already been hung, always close the flow clamp *to prevent delivering a bolus of the drug to the patient.* Insert a syringe and needle into the injection port of the I.V. container after wiping it with an alcohol sponge. Always rotate the container gently *to mix the solution.* Then open the flow clamp and adjust the flow rate.

When administering an I.V. solution with drugs or other additives, watch for signs of drug sensitivity or intolerance.

Complications
Excessively high drug concentrations in the I.V. solution can cause complications such as sclerosis, thrombosis, hemolysis, or phlebitis. Extravasation of some drugs into subcutaneous tissues can cause tissue necrosis.

Documentation
Record the date and time of administration, your initials or name, the drug name and dosage, the amount and type of I.V. solution infused, and the duration of infusion.

Drug infusion through a secondary I.V. line

A secondary I.V. line is a complete I.V. set — container, tubing, and microdrip or macrodrip system — connected to the lower Y port (secondary port) of a primary line instead of to the I.V. catheter or needle. It can be used for continuous or intermittent drug infusion. When used continuously, a secondary I.V. line permits drug infusion and titration while the primary line maintains a constant total infusion rate.

When used intermittently, a secondary I.V. line is commonly called a *piggyback set.* In this case, the primary line maintains venous access between drug doses. Typically, a piggyback set includes a small I.V. container, short tubing, and a macrodrip system. This set connects to the primary line's upper Y port, also known as a piggyback port. (See *Needle-free piggyback system* for more information.) Antibiotics and histamine$_2$ receptor antagonists are most commonly administered by intermittent (piggyback) infusion. To make this set work, the primary I.V. container must be positioned below the piggyback container. (The manufacturer provides an extension hook for that purpose.)

I.V. pumps may be used to maintain constant infusion rates, especially with a drug such as lidocaine. A pump allows more accurate titration of drug dosage and helps maintain venous access because the drug is delivered under sufficient pressure to prevent clot formation in the I.V. cannula.

Equipment

Patient's medication record and chart ▪ prescribed I.V. medication ▪ prescribed I.V. solution ▪ administration set with secondary injection port ▪ 22G 1″ needle ▪ alcohol sponges ▪ 1″ adhesive tape ▪ time tape ▪ labels ▪ infusion pump ▪ extension hook and appropriate solution for intermittent piggyback infusion ▪ optional: normal saline solution for infusion with incompatible solutions.

For intermittent infusion, the primary line typically has a piggyback port with a backcheck valve that stops the flow from the primary line during drug infusion and returns to the primary flow after infusion. A volume-control set can also be used with an intermittent infusion line. (For more information, refer to "Use of a volume-control set" in Chapter 6.)

Preparation of equipment

Verify the order on the patient's medication record by checking it against the doctor's order. Wash your hands. Inspect the I.V. container for cracks, leaks, or contamination, and check drug compatibility with the primary solution. See if the primary line has a secondary injection port. If it doesn't, and the medication will be given regularly, replace the I.V. set with a new one that has a secondary injection port.

If necessary, add the drug to the secondary I.V. solution. To do so, remove any seals from the secondary container and wipe the main port with an alcohol sponge. Inject the prescribed medication and gently agitate the solution *to mix the medication thoroughly.* Properly label the I.V. mixture. Insert the administration set spike and attach the needle. Open the flow clamp and prime the line. Then close the flow clamp.

Some medications now come in vials suitable for hanging directly on an I.V. pole. Instead of preparing medication and injecting it into a container, you can inject diluent directly into the medication vial. Then you can spike the vial, prime the tubing, and hang the set as directed.

Needle-free piggyback system

Some drugs can be piggybacked with a needle-free system, which consists of a blunt-tipped plastic insertion device and a rubber injection port. The port may be part of a special administration set or an adaptor for existing administration sets. This rubber injection port has a preestablished slit that can open and reseal immediately.

The needle-free system aims to reduce the risk of accidental needle-stick injuries.

Blunt-tipped syringe

Self-sealing injection port

Implementation

● Confirm the patient's identity by asking his name and checking the name, room number, and bed number on his wristband.

● If the drug is incompatible with the primary I.V. solution, replace the primary solution with a fluid that's compatible with both solutions, such as normal saline, and flush the line before starting the drug infusion. Many hospital protocols require removing the primary I.V. solution and inserting a sterile I.V. plug into the container until you're ready to rehang it. *This will maintain sterility of the solution* and prevent someone else from inadvertently restarting the incompatible solution before the line is flushed with normal saline solution.

● Hang the secondary set's container and wipe the injection port of the primary line with an alcohol sponge.

● Insert the needle from the secondary line into the injection port and tape it securely to the primary line.

● To run the secondary set's container by itself, lower the primary set's container with an extension hook. To run both containers simultaneously, place them at the same height. (See *Assembling a piggyback set,* page 254.)

● Open the clamp and adjust the drip rate. For continuous infusion, set the secondary solution to the desired drip rate; then adjust the primary solution *to achieve the desired total infusion rate.*

Assembling a piggyback set

A piggyback set is useful for intermittent drug infusion. To work properly, its drug container must be positioned higher than the primary set's container.

Extension hook

Piggyback set

Slide clamp

Primary set

Piggyback Y port
(with backcheck valve)

Flow control clamp

Secondary Y port
(to serve secondary set)

• For intermittent infusion, adjust the primary drip rate as required upon completion of the secondary solution. If the secondary solution tubing is being reused, close the clamp on the tubing and follow the hospital's policy: Either remove the needle and replace it with a new one, or leave it securely taped in the injection port and label it with the time it was first used. In this case, also leave the empty container in place until you replace it with a new dose of medication at the prescribed time. If the tubing won't be reused, discard it appropriately with the I.V. container.

Special considerations

If hospital policy allows, use a pump for drug infusion. Put a time tape on the secondary container *to help prevent an inaccurate administration rate.*

When reusing secondary tubing, change it according to hospital policy, usually every 48 to 72 hours. Similarly, inspect the injection port for leakage with each use, and change it more often if needed.

Unless you're piggybacking lipids, don't piggyback a secondary I.V. line to a total parenteral nutrition line *because of the risk of contamination.* Check your hospital's policy for possible exceptions.

Complications

Adverse effects and reactions to the infused drug can occur. Repeated punctures of the secondary injection port can damage the seal, possibly allowing leakage or contamination.

Documentation

Record the amount and type of drug and the amount of I.V. solution on the intake and output and medication records. Note the date, duration, and rate of infusion, and the patient's response, where applicable.

Drug administration through a heparin lock

An intermittent infusion injection device—or heparin lock—eliminates the need for multiple venipunctures or for maintaining venous access with a continuous I.V. infusion. This device allows intermittent administration by infusion or by the I.V. bolus or I.V. push injection methods.

Dilute heparin or saline solutions are often injected as the final step in this procedure to prevent clotting in the device. When heparin is used, the device must be flushed with normal saline solution before and after the prescribed medication is administered in case the heparin and the medication are incompatible. The device may then be reflushed with the heparin flush solution.

Equipment

Patient's medication record and chart ■ three 3-ml syringes with 22G or 25G 1″ needles ■ normal saline solution ■ alcohol sponges ■ extra heparin lock ■ prescribed medication in an I.V. container with administration set and needle (for infusion) or in a syringe with needle (for I.V. bolus or push) ■ tourniquet ■ tape ■ gloves ■ optional:

T connector, dilute heparin solution, sterile bacteriostatic water.

The concentration of dilute heparin solution ranges from 10 to 100 units/ml. The solution is available in a cartridge-injection system in doses of 10 to 100 units/ml. If this system is used, substitute its syringe for the 3-ml syringe and the heparin cartridge for the heparin solution. Normal saline solution is available in a similar cartridge system.

Preparation of equipment
Verify the order on the patient's medication record by checking it against the doctor's order. Wash your hands, don gloves, and then wipe the tops of the normal saline solution, heparin flush solution, and medication containers with alcohol sponges. Fill two of the 3-ml syringes (bearing 22G needles) with normal saline solution; if required by hospital policy, draw 1 ml of heparin flush solution into the third syringe. If you'll be infusing medication, insert the administration set spike into the I.V. container, attach the appropriate-sized needle, and prime the line. If you'll be giving an I.V. injection, fill a syringe with the prescribed drug.

Implementation
• Confirm the patient's identity by asking his name and checking the name, room number, and bed number on his wristband. Explain the procedure.
• Don gloves. Wipe the injection port of the intermittent infusion device with an alcohol sponge and insert the needle of a saline-filled syringe.
• Aspirate the syringe and observe for blood *to verify the patency of the device.* If none appears, apply a tourniquet slightly above the site, keep it in place for about 1 minute, and then aspirate again. If blood still doesn't appear, remove the tourniquet and inject the normal saline solution slowly.
♦ *Nursing alert.* Stop the injection immediately if you feel any resistance *because resistance indicates that the device is occluded.* If this occurs, insert a new heparin lock. ♦
• If you feel no resistance, watch for signs of infiltration (puffiness or pain at the site) as you slowly inject the saline solution. If these signs occur, insert a new heparin lock.
• If blood is aspirated, slowly inject the saline and observe for signs of infiltration. *The saline solution flushes out any residual heparin solution that might be incompatible with the medication.*
• Withdraw the saline syringe and needle.

To administer I.V. bolus or push injections
• Insert the needle and syringe with the medication for the I.V. bolus or push injection into the injection port of the device.
• Inject the medication at the required rate. Then remove the needle from the injection port.
• Insert the needle of the remaining saline-filled syringe into the injection port and slowly inject the saline solution *to flush all medication through the device.*
• Remove the needle and syringe, and insert and inject the heparin (or saline) flush solution *to prevent clotting in the device.*

To administer an infusion
• Insert and tape the needle attached to the administration set.
• Open the infusion line and adjust the flow rate as necessary.
• Infuse medication for the prescribed length of time; then flush the device with normal saline solution and heparin flush solution, as you would after a bolus or push injection, according to your hospital's policy.
• To administer fluids and drugs simultaneously or to administer a medication incompatible with the primary I.V. solution, you may want to use a T connector. (See *Using a T connector,* page 256.)

Special considerations
If you're giving a bolus injection of a drug that's incompatible with saline, such as diazepam (Valium), flush the device with bacteriostatic water.

Some hospitals use diluted heparin solution (100 units/ml or 10 units/ml) *to prevent clotting in the cannula.* Other hospitals use 2 to 3 ml of normal saline solution instead. A few hospitals use other solutions or dilutions. Check your hospital's policy.

Intermittent infusion devices should be changed regularly (usually every 48 to 72 hours), according to universal precautions guidelines and hospital policy.

If you're unable to rotate injection sites because the patient has fragile veins, document this fact in your notes.

Complications
Infiltration and a specific reaction to the infused drug are the most common complications.

Documentation
Record the type and amount of drug administered and the times of administration. Include all I.V. solutions used to dilute the medication and flush the line on the intake record. Also document the use of dilute heparin solution.

Using a T connector

The T connector is a piece of small-bore extension tubing 3″ to 6″ (7.6 to 15.2 cm) long. It's fitted with an injection port near the luer-lock connection. This additional injection site allows simultaneous administration of drugs and fluids or of primary I.V. solution and a drug incompatible with it.

To add the T connector, wash your hands and don gloves to minimize exposure to body fluids. Then, explain to the patient what you are about to do, to reduce his anxiety at seeing another piece of I.V. equipment.

Prime the tubing with I.V. fluid, then attach one end of the T connector to the I.V. tubing. Open the slide clamp. Now you're ready to connect the luer-lock tip to the injection cap. Remove the leur-lock tip-protector cap and carefully insert this tip into the injection cap.

Secure this connector in place with tape. Another I.V. needle can be inserted into the latex injection cap. Finally, document your actions.

I.V. bolus injection

This bolus injection method allows rapid I.V. drug administration. It may be used in an emergency to provide an immediate drug effect. Alternately, it may be used to achieve peak drug levels in the bloodstream or to deliver drugs that can't be diluted, such as diazepam, digoxin, and phenytoin. It may also be used to administer drugs that can't be given I.M. because they're toxic to muscle tissue or because the patient's ability to absorb them is impaired.

The term *bolus* usually refers to the concentration or amount of a drug. I.V. push is a technique for rapid intravenous injection.

Bolus doses of medication may be injected directly into a vein or through an existing I.V. line, or through an implanted vascular access port (VAP). The medication administered by these methods usually takes effect rapidly, so the patient must be monitored for an adverse reaction, such as cardiac arrhythmia. I.V. bolus injections

are contraindicated when rapid drug administration could cause life-threatening complications. For certain drugs, the safe rate of injection is specified by the manufacturer.

Some hospital policies specify that only nurses trained in this technique (such as emergency department, critical care, or chemotherapy nurses) can give bolus injections.

Equipment
Patient's medication record and chart ■ prescribed medication ■ 20G needle and syringe ■ diluent, if needed ■ tourniquet ■ povidone-iodine sponge ■ alcohol sponge ■ sterile 2″ × 2″ gauze pad ■ gloves ■ adhesive bandage ■ tape ■ optional: winged-tip needle with catheter and second syringe (and needle) filled with normal saline solution; non-coring needle if used with a vascular access port; heparin flush solution.

Winged-tip needles are frequently used for this purpose largely because they can be quickly and easily inserted. This makes them ideal for repeated drug administration, as in weekly or monthly chemotherapy. Another useful dosage form is the ready injectable. (See *Using a ready injectable.)*

Preparation of equipment

Verify the order on the patient's medication record by checking it against the doctor's order. Know the actions, adverse effects, and administration rate of the drug to be injected. Draw up the prescribed medication in the syringe and dilute it if necessary.

Implementation

• Confirm the patient's identity, wash your hands, put on gloves, and explain the procedure.

To give direct injections

• Select the largest vein suitable for an injection. *The larger the vein, the more diluted the drug will become, minimizing vascular irritation.*
• Apply a tourniquet above the injection site *to distend the vein.*
• Clean the injection site with an alcohol sponge or a povidone-iodine sponge, working outward from the puncture site in a circular motion *to prevent recontamination with skin bacteria.*
• If you're using the drug syringe's needle, insert it into the vein at a 30-degree angle with the bevel up. The bevel should reach ¼" (0.6 cm) into the vein. If you're using a winged-tip needle, insert the needle (bevel up), tape the butterfly wings in place when you see blood return in the tubing, and attach the syringe containing the drug.
• Pull back on the plunger of the syringe and check for blood backflow, *which indicates that the needle is in the vein.*
• Remove the tourniquet and inject the drug at the appropriate rate.
• Pull back slightly on the plunger of the syringe and check for blood backflow again. *If blood appears, it indicates that the needle remained in place and all of the injected medication entered the vein.*
• If you're using a winged-tip needle, flush the line with the normal saline solution from the second syringe *to ensure delivery of all the medication into the vein.*
• Withdraw the needle and apply pressure to the injection site with the sterile gauze pad for at least 3 minutes *to prevent hematoma formation.*
• Apply the adhesive bandage to the site after bleeding has stopped.

To give injections through an existing I.V. line

• Check the compatibility of the medication with the I.V. solution.
• Close the flow clamp, wipe the injection port with an alcohol sponge, and inject the drug as you would a direct injection. (Some I.V. lines have a secondary injection port or a T connector; others have a latex cap at the end of the I.V. tubing where the needle is attached.)

Using a ready injectable

A ready injectable — commercially premeasured medication packaged with a syringe and needle — allows for rapid drug administration in an emergency. Usually, preparing a ready injectable takes only 15 to 20 seconds. Other advantages include the reduced risk of breaking sterile technique during administration and the easy identification of medication and dose.

When using a commercially prefilled syringe, make sure to administer precisely the dose prescribed. For example, if a 50 mg/ml cartridge is supplied but the patient's prescribed dose is 25 mg, you must administer only 0.5 ml — half of the volume contained in the cartridge. Be alert for potential medication errors whenever dispensing medications in premeasured dosage forms.

• Open the flow clamp and readjust the flow rate.
• If the drug isn't compatible with the I.V. solution, flush the line with normal saline solution before and after the injection. (For additional information, see "Drug administration through a heparin lock" in this chapter.)

To give a bolus injection through a vascular access port

• Wash your hands, don gloves, and clean the injection site with an alcohol sponge or a povidone-iodine sponge, starting at the center of the port and working outward with a circular motion over a 4" to 5" (10 to 12.7 cm) diameter. Do this three times.
• Palpate the area over the port *to locate the port septum.*
• Anchor the port between your thumb and the first two fingers of your nondominant hand. Then using your dominant hand, insert the needle into the appropriate area of the device and deliver the injection. (See "Implanted vascular access devices" in Chapter 6.)

Special considerations

Because drugs administered by I.V. bolus or push injection are delivered directly into the circulatory system and can produce an immediate effect, signs of an acute allergic reaction or anaphylaxis can develop rapidly. If any signs of anaphylaxis occur (dyspnea, cyanosis, convulsions, or increasing respiratory distress), notify the doctor immediately and begin emergency procedures, as necessary. Also watch for signs of extravasation, such as swelling, the absence of blood backflow, and a sluggish flow rate. If extravasation occurs, stop the injection,

Antidotes for vesicant extravasation

Substances commonly used as antidotes for vesicant extravasation are listed below, along with the extravasated drugs for which they may be given. Antidotes may be instilled through the existing I.V. line or injected subcutaneously with a 1-ml tuberculin syringe in a circle around the infiltrated area. The needle should be changed before each injection of antidote. Some antidotes may be used in combination.

Hyaluronidase (15 units/ml)
This drug may be given as an antidote to aminophylline, calcium solutions, contrast media, dextrose solutions (concentrations of 10% or more), total parenteral nutrition solutions, nafcillin, potassium solutions, vinblastine, vincristine, or vindesine.

Sodium bicarbonate 8.4%
This drug may be given as an antidote to carmustine, daunorubicin, doxorubicin, vinblastine, or vincristine.

Phentolamine
This drug may be given as an antidote to dobutamine, dopamine, epinephrine, metaraminol, or norepinephrine.

Sodium thiosulfate 10%
This drug may be given as an antidote to dactinomycin, mechlorethamine, or mitomycin.

Hydrocortisone sodium succinate (100 mg/ml)
This drug, usually followed by topical application of 1% hydrocortisone cream, may be given as an antidote to doxorubicin or vincristine.

Ascorbic acid
This drug may be injected as an antidote to dactinomycin.

Sodium edetate
This drug may be administered as an antidote to plicamycin.

estimate the amount of infiltration, and notify the doctor. If you're giving diazepam or chlordiazepoxide hydrochloride through a winged-tip needle or I.V. line, flush with bacteriostatic water instead of normal saline solution *to prevent drug precipitation caused by incompatibility.*

Complications
Excessively rapid drug administration may cause adverse effects, depending on the drug administered.

Documentation
Record the amount and type of drug administered, time of injection, appearance of the site, duration of administration, and patient's tolerance of the procedure. Also note the drug's effect and any adverse reactions.

Management of intravenous extravasation

Extravasation is the leakage of infused solution from a vein into surrounding tissue. The result of a needle puncturing the vessel wall or leakage around a venipuncture site, extravasation causes local pain and itching, edema, blanching, and decreased skin temperature in the affected extremity. Extravasation of I.V. solution is often referred to as infiltration, because the fluid infiltrates the tissues.

Extravasation of a small amount of isotonic fluid or a nonirritating drug usually causes only minor discomfort. Treatment involves routine comfort measures, such as the application of warm compresses. However, extravasation of some drugs can severely damage tissue through irritative, sclerotic, vesicant, corrosive, or vasoconstrictive action. (See *Antidotes for vesicant extravasation.*) In these cases, emergency measures must be taken to minimize tissue damage and necrosis, prevent the need for skin grafts or, rarely, avoid possible amputation.

Equipment
Three 25G ⅝″ needles ■ antidote for extravasated drug in appropriate syringe ■ 5-ml syringe ■ three tuberculin syringes ■ alcohol sponge or gauze pad soaked in antiseptic cleaning agent ■ 4″ × 4″ gauze pad ■ cold and warm compresses ■ optional: anti-inflammatory drug ■ 8.4% sodium bicarbonate ■ normal saline solution.

Preparation of equipment
Attach one 25G ⅝″ needle to the syringe containing the antidote. Connect the two remaining 25G ⅝″ needles to two tuberculin syringes. Then fill the remaining tuberculin syringe with the anti-inflammatory drug, if needed.

Implementation

Opinions differ on the preferred treatment for extravasation; hospital policy will dictate specific actions. They may include some or all of the following steps.

• Stop the infusion immediately and remove the I.V. needle unless you need the route to infiltrate the antidote. Carefully estimate the amount of extravasated solution and notify the doctor.

• Disconnect the tubing from the I.V. needle. Attach the 5-ml syringe to the needle and try to withdraw 3 to 5 ml of blood *to remove any medication or blood in the tubing or needle and provide a path to the infiltrated tissues.*

• Clean the area around the extravasation site with an alcohol sponge or 4″ × 4″ gauze pad soaked in an antiseptic cleaning agent. Then insert the needle of the empty tuberculin syringe into the subcutaneous tissue around the site, and gently aspirate as much of the solution as possible from the tissue.

• Instill the prescribed antidote into the subcutaneous tissue around the site. Then, if ordered, slowly instill an anti-inflammatory drug subcutaneously *to help reduce inflammation and edema.*

• If ordered, instill the prescribed antidote through the I.V. needle.

• Apply cold compresses to the affected area for 24 hours, or apply an ice pack for 20 minutes every 4 hours *to cause vasoconstriction that may localize the drug and slow cell metabolism.* After 24 hours, apply warm compresses and elevate the affected extremity *to reduce discomfort and promote fluid reabsorption.* If the extravasated drug is a vasoconstrictor, such as norepinephrine or metaraminol bitartrate, apply warm compresses only.

• Continuously monitor the I.V. site for signs of abscess or necrosis.

Special considerations

If you're administering a potentially tissue-damaging drug by I.V. bolus or push, first start an I.V. infusion, preferably with normal saline solution. Infuse a small amount of the saline solution, and check for signs of infiltration before injecting the drug.

Know the antidote (if any) for an I.V. drug that can cause tissue necrosis if extravasation occurs. Make sure you're familiar with your hospital's policy regarding the administration of such drugs and their antidotes.

Tell the patient to report any discomfort at the I.V. site. During infusion, frequently check the site for signs of infiltration.

Documentation

Record the site of the extravasation, the patient's symptoms, the estimated amount of infiltrated solution, nursing treatment, the time, and the name of the doctor notified.

Continue to document the appearance of the infiltrated site and any associated symptoms.

Preparation and handling of chemotherapeutic drugs

Administration of chemotherapeutic drugs may cause teratogenic, mutagenic, or carcinogenic effects in patients. However, the risks associated with the caregiver's preparation and handling of these drugs haven't been fully determined. Nor has a preferential technique for handling these drugs been found. Despite these uncertainties, nurses who give chemotherapeutic drugs should follow guidelines from the Occupational Safety and Health Administration (OSHA). What's more, they should keep current with the latest safety guidelines and protocols.

Typically, chemotherapeutic drugs are prepared by a pharmaceutical company or in the hospital pharmacy using a laminar airflow hood and procedures to ensure minimal exposure to potential hazards. Only nurses, doctors, or pharmacists with specialized training should prepare chemotherapeutic drugs.

Equipment

Chemotherapeutic drug ▪ I.V. solution ▪ diluent, if necessary ▪ patient's medication record and chart ▪ compatibility and stability reference source ▪ medication labels ▪ Class II biological safety cabinet (if available) ▪ 18G or 19G needle and hydrophobic filter or dispensing pin ▪ syringes, needles and I.V. tubing with luer-lock fittings ▪ long-sleeved gown ▪ gloves ▪ face shield or goggles ▪ eyewash ▪ plastic absorbent pad ▪ alcohol sponges or sterile gauze pads ▪ impervious containers labeled CAUTION: CHEMOTHERAPY or BIOHAZARD for disposal of unused drug or equipment.

Preparation of equipment

Verify the drug, dosage, and route of administration by checking the medication record against the doctor's order. Check the expiration dates of drugs, solutions, and diluents.

Select syringes, needles, and I.V. tubing with luer-lock fittings *to prevent contamination by leakage.*

Use an 18G or 19G needle and a hydrophobic filter or dispensing pin *to prevent aerosol release from vials.*

Label all syringes, bottles, or bags containing chemotherapeutic drugs with the following information:

• patient's name, identification, and room number

• drug name and dose

- route of administration
- date and time of preparation
- expiration date and time
- vesicant
- storage requirements, if applicable.

Implementation
• Prepare the prescribed drugs in accordance with current product instructions regarding compatibility, stability, and reconstitution technique.

To avoid unnecessary or excessive drug exposure
• Prepare drugs in a Class II biological safety cabinet *for maximum protection.* The blower on the hood should be left on 24 hours a day, 7 days a week. Alternatively, prepare drugs in a quiet work space, away from heating or cooling vents and other personnel.
• Use protective garments (long-sleeved gown, gloves, face shield or goggles) as indicated by institutional policy. Do not wear equipment outside of the preparation area.
• Do not eat, drink, smoke, or apply cosmetics in the drug preparation area.
• Cover the work surface with a clean plastic absorbent pad *to minimize contamination by droplets or spills.* Change the pad when completing each shift or after a spill.
• Consider all equipment used in drug preparation and any unused drug as hazardous waste and dispose according to hospital policy.

To manage accidental exposure
• If skin contact occurs, wash the involved area thoroughly with soap (not a germicidal agent) and water.
• If eye contact occurs, flood the involved eye with water or an isotonic eyewash for at least 5 minutes while holding the eyelid open.
• Obtain a medical evaluation as soon as possible after accidental exposure.

Special considerations
Exercise precautions to avoid skin contact if the medication leaks. Clean all spills immediately according to hospital policy.

Dispose of waste (unused drug and preparation equipment) in impervious containers labeled CAUTION: CHEMOTHERAPY or BIOHAZARD. These must be incinerated or handled as toxic waste.

Complications
Chromosomal damage or liver damage may result from chronic exposure to chemotherapeutic drugs.

Documentation
Document exposure incidents according to established hospital policies.

Administration of chemotherapeutic drugs

Chemotherapeutic drugs may be administered by many routes. These include oral, subcutaneous, I.M., I.V. (using peripheral or central veins), intra-arterial, intracavitary, intrathecal, and intraperitoneal routes. (See *An alternate approach to intraperitoneal chemotherapy.)* The route chosen by the oncologist reflects the drug's pharmacology and the patient's condition. However, most chemotherapeutic drugs are given intravenously.

Chemotherapeutic drugs are hazardous and errors in dosage or administration can cause severe effects or even death. Therefore, these drugs should be reconstituted in a laminar airflow hood by trained personnel. (See "Preparation and handling of chemotherapeutic drugs" in this chapter.) In addition, the patient requires a comprehensive assessment before treatment so that adverse reactions can be prevented or managed effectively.

Equipment
Chemotherapeutic drug ▪ patient's medication record and chart ▪ brown paper bag or aluminum foil if the drug is photosensitive ▪ normal saline solution ▪ syringes and needles ▪ infusion pump or control device (if I.V. infusion is ordered) ▪ gloves ▪ impervious containers labeled CAUTION: CHEMOTHERAPY or BIOHAZARD for disposal of unused drug or equipment.

Preparation of equipment
Verify the drug, dosage, and route of administration by checking the medication record against the doctor's order. Be sure you know the immediate and delayed adverse reactions of the drug being administered. Follow administration guidelines for appropriate procedures in this chapter.

Implementation
• Obtain baseline data, including the patient's history relevant to planned chemotherapy and related medications, the patient's and family's understanding of chemotherapy, and the results of laboratory studies (such as complete blood count, blood urea nitrogen, platelets, creatinine level, and liver function studies).

An alternate approach to intraperitoneal chemotherapy

Administering chemotherapeutic drugs into the peritoneal cavity has several benefits for patients with malignant ascites or ovarian cancer that has spread to the peritoneum. This technique passes drugs directly to the tumor area in the peritoneal cavity, exposing malignant cells to very high concentrations of chemotherapy—up to 1,000 times what could be safely given systemically. What's more, the semipermeable peritoneal membrane permits prolonged exposure of malignant cells to the drug.

Typically, this therapy is performed using a peritoneal dialysis kit, but drugs can also be administered to the peritoneal cavity directly, via the Tenckhoff catheter, shown at right. This method can be performed on an outpatient basis if necessary, and uses equipment that is readily available on most units with oncology patients.

In this technique, the chemotherapy bag is connected directly to the Tenckhoff catheter with a length of I.V. tubing, the solution is infused, and the catheter and I.V. tubing are clamped. Then the patient is asked to change positions every 10 to 15 minutes for 1 hour to move the solution around in the peritoneal cavity. After the prescribed "dwell time," the chemotherapy is al-

lowed to drain into an I.V. bag. The patient is encouraged to change positions to facilitate drainage. Then the I.V. tubing and catheter are clamped, the I.V. tubing is removed, and a new p.r.n. adapter is fitted to the catheter. Finally, the catheter is flushed with a syringe of heparinized saline.

• Check the patient's chart for the complete chemotherapy protocol order, including the patient's name, the drug's name and dosage, and the route, rate, and frequency of administration. Also check the doctor's order for laboratory values for administration. *The order may specify a reduced drug dosage based on laboratory values.*

• Check to see if antiemetics, fluids, diuretics, or electrolyte supplements have been ordered before, during, or after drug administration.

• Ensure that the patient or a responsible family member has signed the consent form.

• Don gloves when priming I.V. tubing, when purging air bubbles from syringes or I.V. tubing, and when administering chemotherapeutic drugs. *Gloves prevent direct skin contact with drugs.*

• Examine the patient's veins *to determine an administration site,* starting with his hand and proceeding to his forearm. (Remember, the use of veins in the dorsum of the hand or wrist is controversial if you're giving a vesicant drug.)

• Avoid using an existing I.V. line to administer these drugs. Perform a new venipuncture proximal to the old site *to ensure proper needle placement and vein patency.*

Never use a chemotherapeutic drug to test vein patency. Infuse 10 to 20 ml of normal saline solution *to maintain patency.* Administer nonvesicant agents by I.V. push or admixed in a bag of I.V. fluid. Give vesicant agents by I.V. push through a piggyback set connected to a rapidly infusing I.V.

• During administration, watch closely for signs of a hypersensitivity reaction or extravasation. Check for blood return after each 5 ml of medication is injected or according to established guidelines.

• If you suspect extravasation, stop the infusion immediately, leave the needle in place, and notify the doctor. Know the applicable policy for treating extravasation.

• Infuse 20 ml of normal saline solution between all chemotherapeutic medications and before discontinuing the I.V. line.

• Dispose of used needles and syringes carefully. *To prevent aerosol dispersion of chemotherapeutic drugs,* don't clip needles. Place them intact in an impervious container for incineration.

• Dispose of I.V. bags, bottles, gloves, and tubing in a covered trash container. Chemotherapy trash should be incinerated.

• Even though you've used gloves, wash your hands thoroughly with warm soap and water after giving any chemotherapeutic drug.

Special considerations
Evaluate the patient's and family's desire for information and their level of understanding. Instruct them about the chemotherapy, treatment protocol, and schedule of administration. Teach them to recognize the signs and symptoms of extravasation or any other unusual sensations. Instruct them about posttreatment care.

Observe the I.V. administration site frequently for signs of extravasation or allergic reaction (swelling, redness, urticaria). If the patient reports pain, stop the drug immediately and evaluate the site.

During infusion, some drugs need protection from direct sunlight to avoid possible drug breakdown. Cover the vial with a brown paper bag or aluminum foil.

When administering vesicants, avoid sites where damage to underlying tendons or nerves may occur (such as veins in the antecubital fossa, near the wrist, or in the dorsal surface of the hand).

Flush with normal saline solution between drugs *to avoid incompatibility* and after treatment *to clear the line.*

Observe the patient at regular intervals and after treatment for adverse reactions.

If you're unable to remain with the patient during the entire infusion, use a control device or infusion pump *to ensure delivery of the drug within the prescribed time and rate.*

Complications
Adverse effects of chemotherapeutic drugs include extravasation, causing inflammation, ulceration, and possibly necrosis; and loss of vein patency, caused by fibrosis. Other effects include alopecia, anemia, neutropenia, thrombocytopenia, photosensitivity, urticaria, hyperpigmentation, telangiectasis, hyperkeratosis, radiation recall (if drugs are given with or soon after radiotherapy), nausea, vomiting, anorexia, esophagitis, diarrhea, constipation, and stomatitis. Keep in mind that adverse effects vary depending on the drug, dosage, and route of administration.

Anaphylactic reactions may occur with any chemotherapeutic drug. Stop the infusion immediately if the patient displays a local or generalized reaction. Maintain venous access and institute emergency measures as appropriate.

Documentation
Record the location and description of the I.V. site before treatment (and presence of blood return during bolus administration); drugs and dosages administered; sequence of drug administration; needle type and size used; amount and type of flushing solution; and the site's condition after treatment. Also record any adverse reactions, the patient's tolerance of treatment, and the topics you've taught the patient and his family.

SPECIAL ADMINISTRATION TECHNIQUES
Epidural administration of analgesics

In this procedure, the doctor injects or infuses medication into the epidural space, which lies just outside the subarachnoid space where cerebrospinal fluid (CSF) flows. The drug diffuses slowly into the subarachnoid space of the spinal canal and then into the CSF, which carries it directly into the spinal area—bypassing the blood-brain barrier. In some cases, the doctor injects drugs directly into the subarachnoid space. (See *Understanding intrathecal injections.)*

Epidural analgesia helps manage acute or chronic pain, including moderate to severe postoperative pain. It's especially useful in patients with cancer or degenerative joint disease. This procedure works well because opiate receptors are located along the entire spinal cord. Narcotic drugs act directly on the receptors of the dorsal horn to produce localized analgesia without motor blockade. Narcotics such as morphine, fentanyl, and hydromorphone are administered as either an I.V. bolus dose or by continuous infusion, either alone or in combination with bupivacaine (a local anesthetic). The infusion, given via an epidural catheter, is preferable because it allows a smaller drug dosage to be given continuously. The epidural catheter, inserted near the spinal cord, eliminates the risks of multiple I.M. injections, minimizes adverse cerebral and systemic effects, and eliminates the analgesic peaks and valleys that usually occur with intermittent I.M. injections. (See *Placement of a permanent epidural catheter,* page 264.)

Typically, epidural catheter insertion is performed by an anesthesiologist using aseptic technique. Once the catheter has been inserted, the nurse is responsible for monitoring the infusion and assessing the patient.

Epidural analgesia is contraindicated in patients who have local or systemic infection, neurologic disease, anticoagulant therapy, coagulopathy, spinal arthritis or deformity, hypotension, marked hypertension, or allergy to the prescribed drug.

Equipment

Volume infusion device and epidural infusion tubing (depending on hospital policy) ▪ patient's medication record and chart ▪ prescribed epidural solutions ▪ transparent dressing or sterile gauze pads ▪ epidural tray ▪ labels for epidural infusion line ▪ silk tape ▪ optional: monitoring equipment for blood pressure and pulse, apnea monitor.

Have on hand the following drugs and equipment for emergency use: naloxone 0.4 mg I.V.; ephedrine 50 mg I.V.; oxygen; intubation set; hand-held resuscitation bag.

Preparation of equipment

Prepare the infusion device according to the manufacturer's instructions and hospital policy. Obtain an epidural tray. Be sure the pharmacy has been notified ahead of time regarding the medication order *because epidural solutions require special preparation.* Check the medication concentration and infusion rate against the doctor's order.

Implementation

• Explain the procedure and its possible complications to the patient. Tell him he'll feel some pain as the catheter is inserted. Answer any questions he has. Make sure that a consent form has been properly signed and witnessed.
• Position the patient on his side in the knee-chest position, or have him sit on the edge of the bed and lean over a bedside table.
• After the catheter is in place, prime the infusion device, confirm the appropriate medication and infusion rate, and then adjust the device for the correct rate.
• Help the anesthesiologist connect the infusion tubing to the epidural catheter. Then connect the tubing to the infusion pump.
• Bridge-tape all connection sites and label the catheter, infusion tubing, and infusion pump with EPIDURAL INFUSION *to prevent accidental infusion of other drugs into the epidural lines.* Then start the infusion.
• Tell the patient to report immediately any feeling of pain. Instruct him to use a pain scale from 0 to 10, with 0 denoting no pain and 10 denoting the worst pain imaginable. A response of 3 or less typically indicates tolerable pain. If the patient reports a higher pain score, the infusion rate may need to be increased. Call the doctor or change the rate within prescribed limits.
• If ordered, place the patient on an apnea monitor for the first 24 hours after beginning the infusion.
• Change the dressing over the catheter's exit site every 24 to 48 hours, or as needed. The dressing is usually transparent *to allow inspection of drainage* and commonly appears moist or slightly blood-tinged.
• Change the infusion tubing every 48 hours, or as specified by hospital policy.

Understanding intrathecal injections

An intrathecal injection allows the doctor to inject medication into the subarachnoid space of the spinal canal. Certain drugs — such as anti-infectives, or antineoplastics used to treat meningeal leukemia — are administered by this route because they can't readily penetrate the blood-brain barrier through the bloodstream. Intrathecal injection may also be used to deliver anesthetics, such as lidocaine hydrochloride, to achieve regional anesthesia (as in spinal anesthesia or epidural block).

An invasive procedure performed by a doctor under sterile conditions with the nurse assisting, intrathecal injection requires informed patient consent. The injection site is usually between the third and fourth (or fourth and fifth) lumbar vertebrae, well below the spinal cord, to avoid the risk of paralysis. This procedure may be preceded by aspiration of spinal fluid for laboratory analysis.

Contraindications to intrathecal injection include inflammation or infection at the puncture site, septicemia, and spinal deformities (especially when considered as an anesthesia route).

To remove an epidural catheter

• Typically, the anesthesiologist orders analgesics and removes the catheter. However, hospital policy may allow a specially trained nurse to remove the catheter.
• If you feel resistance when removing the catheter, stop and call the doctor for further orders.
• The doctor will want to examine the catheter tip *to rule out any damage during removal,* so be sure to save the catheter.

Special considerations

Assess the patient's respiratory rate and blood pressure every 2 hours for 8 hours, then every 4 hours for 8 hours, during the first 24 hours after starting the infusion. Then assess the patient once per shift, depending on his condition or unless ordered otherwise. Notify the doctor if the patient's respiratory rate is less than 10 breaths/minute or if his systolic blood pressure is less than 90 mm Hg.

Assess the patient's sedation level, mental status, and pain relief status every hour initially, then every 2 to 4 hours, until adequate pain control is achieved. Notify the doctor if the patient appears drowsy or experiences nausea and vomiting, refractory itching, or inability to void,

Placement of a permanent epidural catheter

An epidural catheter is implanted beneath the patient's skin and inserted near the spinal cord at the first lumbar (L1) interspace.

For temporary analgesic therapy (less than 1 week), the catheter may exit directly over the spine and be taped up the patient's back to the shoulder. However, for prolonged therapy, the catheter may be tunneled subcutaneously to an exit site on the patient's side or abdomen, or over his shoulder.

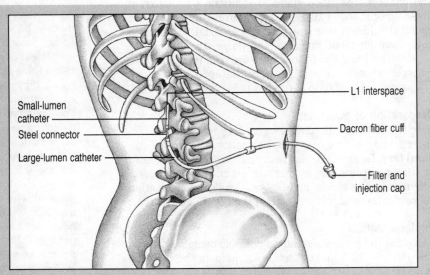

which are adverse effects of certain narcotic analgesics, or if he complains of unrelieved pain.

Assess lower-extremity motor strength every 2 to 4 hours. *If sensory and motor loss occurs, large motor nerve fibers have been affected and dosage may need to be decreased.*

Keep in mind that drugs given epidurally diffuse slowly and may cause adverse effects, including excessive sedation, up to 12 hours after epidural infusion has been discontinued.

The patient should always have a peripheral I.V. line (either continuous infusion or heparin lock) open *to allow immediate administration of emergency drugs.*

If CSF leaks into the dura mater during removal of an epidural catheter, the patient usually experiences headache. This postanalgesia headache worsens with postural changes, such as standing or sitting. The headache can be treated with a " blood patch," in which the patient's own blood (about 10 ml) is withdrawn from a peripheral vein and then injected into the epidural space. When the epidural needle is withdrawn, the patient is instructed to sit up. Because the blood clots seal off the leaking area, the blood patch should relieve the patient's headache immediately. The patient need not restrict his activity after this procedure.

Home care

Home use of epidural analgesia is possible only if the patient or his family is willing and able to learn the care needed. The patient also must be willing and able to abstain from alcohol and street drugs *because these substances potentiate opiate action.*

Complications

The most common complication of epidural infusion is numbness and leg weakness, which may occur after the first 24 hours and is drug- and concentration-dependent. Identifying the dosage level that provides adequate pain control without causing excessive numbness and weakness requires that the doctor titrate the dosage.

Other complications include respiratory depression, which usually occurs during the first 24 hours (treated with naloxone, 0.2 to 0.4 mg I.V.), pruritus (treated with nalbuphine, 5 mg I.V., or diphenhydramine, 25 mg I.V.), and nausea and vomiting (treated with prochlorperazine, 5 to 10 mg I.V., or metoclopramide, 10 mg I.V.).

Documentation

Record the patient's response to treatment, catheter patency, condition of the dressing and insertion site, vital signs, and assessment results. Also document the labeling of the epidural catheter, changing of the infusion bags, ordered analgesics, if any, and the patient's response.

Selected references

Akahoshi, M.P., et al. "Patient Controlled Analgesia via Intrathecal Catheter in Outpatient Oncology Patients," *Journal of Intravenous Nursing* 11(5):289-92, September-October 1988.

Bigelow-Kemp, B., et al. *Fundamentals of Nursing,* 2nd ed. Glenview, Ill.: Scott, Foresman & Co., 1989.

Brown, J.M. "Innovative Antibiotic Therapy at Home," *Journal of Intravenous Nursing* 11(6):397-401, November-December 1988.

Clayton, B., and Stock, Y. *Basic Pharmacology for Nurses,* 9th ed. St. Louis: C.V. Mosby Co., 1989.

Cohen, M.S. "Continuous Epidural Infusions for Acute Postoperative Pain," Part 1. *Current Reviews for Postanesthesia Care Nurses* 11(12):90-96, August 1989.

Crisis Drugs. Clinical SkillBuilders Series. Springhouse, Pa.: Springhouse Corp., 1991.

Drug Information for the Health Care Professional, 2 vols., 11th ed. Rockville, Md.: United States Pharmacopeial Convention, Inc., 1991.

Earnest, V. *Clinical Skills and Assessment Techniques in Nursing Practice.* Glenview, Ill.: Scott, Foresman & Co., 1989.

Endocrine Problems. NurseReview Series. Springhouse, Pa.: Springhouse Corp., 1991.

Facts and Comparisons. St. Louis, Mo.: Facts and Comparisons, Inc. Updated monthly.

Fiser, D.H. "Intraosseous Infusion," *New England Journal of Medicine* 322(22):1579-81, May 31, 1990.

Handy, C.M. "Vascular Access Devices: Hospital to Home Care," *Journal of Intravenous Nursing* (Supp.) 12(1):10S-18S, January-February 1989.

Illustrated Manual of Nursing Practice, 2nd ed. Springhouse, Pa.: Springhouse Corp., 1994.

I.V. Therapy. Clinical SkillBuilders Series. Springhouse, Pa.: Springhouse Corp., 1991.

Keen, M.F. "Get on the Right Track with Z-track Injections," *Nursing90* 20(8):59, August 1990.

Malloy, Janice. "Administering Intraperitoneal Chemotherapy: A New Approach," *Nursing91* 21(1):58-62, January 1991.

Masoorli, S., and Angeles, T. "PICC Lines: The Latest Home Care Challenge," *RN* 53(1):44-51, January 1990.

Medication Administration and I.V. Therapy Manual, 2nd ed. Springhouse, Pa.: Springhouse Corp., 1993.

Millam, D. "Avoiding Needle-stick Injuries," *Nursing90* 20(1):61-64, January 1990.

Nursing94 Drug Handbook. Springhouse, Pa.: Springhouse Corp., 1994.

Perry, A.G., and Potter, P.A. *Clinical Nursing Skills and Techniques,* 2nd ed. St. Louis: Mosby-Year Book, Inc., 1990.

Photoguide to Drug Administration. Springhouse, Pa.: Springhouse Corp., 1991.

Physicians' Desk Reference, 47th ed. Oradell, N.J.: Medical Economics Co., Inc., 1993.

Tenenbaum, L. *Cancer Chemotherapy: A Reference Guide.* Philadelphia: W.B. Saunders Co., 1989.

Trissel, L.A. *Handbook on Injectable Drugs,* 5th ed. Bethesda, Md.: American Society of Hospital Pharmacists, 1988.

Wheeler, C.A. "Pediatric Intraosseous Infusion: An Old Technique in Modern Health Care Technology," *Journal of Intravenous Nursing* 12(6):371-76, November-December 1989.

Ziegfeld, C.R. *Core Curriculum for Oncology Nursing.* Philadelphia: W.B. Saunders Co., 1987.

INTRAVASCULAR THERAPY

CHARLES KROZEK, RN, BA, MN

Introduction

Currently, more than 80% of hospitalized patients receive some form of I.V. therapy. Although you may not be called upon to insert all types of I.V. lines, you will be responsible for maintaining these lines and preventing complications throughout therapy.

This chapter will explain the administration methods and primary uses of I.V. therapy. You'll review how to prepare for I.V. therapy; how to insert, maintain, and remove specific I.V. lines and devices; how to control infection and maintain flow rates; and how to monitor the patient's response to therapy. What's more, you'll find out about patient-teaching responsibilities and home care issues.

I.V. delivery methods

Selection of an I.V. delivery method depends upon the therapy's purpose and duration; the patient's diagnosis, age, and health history; and the condition of his veins. For example, in peripheral I.V. therapy, you'll administer I.V. solutions through a vein in the arm, the hand or, less frequently, the leg or foot. Typically, this method is used for short-term or intermittent therapy.

Uses of I.V. therapy

The most common uses of I.V. therapy are maintaining and restoring fluid and electrolyte balance, administering drugs, transfusing blood, and delivering parenteral nutrition.

The I.V. route allows rapid, effective drug administration. Commonly infused drugs include antibiotics, thrombolytics, histamine$_2$-receptor antagonists, antineoplastic agents, cardiovascular drugs, anticonvulsants and, most recently, patient-controlled analgesics. Usually, you'll give an I.V drug over a short period—in some cases by direct injection, called I.V. push. (See Chapter 5, Drug administration.)

With blood transfusion, your nursing responsibilities include administering blood and blood components as well as monitoring patients receiving therapy. Transfusion aims to maintain adequate blood volume, prevent cardiogenic shock, increase the blood's oxygen carrying capacity, and maintain hemostasis.

Parenteral nutrition refers to the administration of nutrients by the I.V. route. Low-concentration parenteral nutrition solutions are administered through a peripheral vein; more highly concentrated ones through a central vein. If you're caring for a patient receiving parenteral nutrition, you'll need to know how to recognize changes in fluid and electrolyte status and in glucose, amino acid, mineral, and vitamin levels. You'll also need to judge your patient's response to the nutrient solution and to detect early signs of complications.

Patient teaching

Many patients are apprehensive about I.V. therapy. To allay their fears, you can provide information that explains and clarifies this therapy. Use pamphlets and videotapes if available. If possible, show the patient the actual equipment and explain how it will be used during therapy.

Allow the patient to express fears and concerns, and convey reassurance by answering his questions fully. You may wish to involve a family member or caregiver in these discussions to further reassure the patient.

Home I.V. therapy

More and more patients are receiving I.V. therapy at home. Home therapy benefits patients by making them feel more comfortable and allowing them to perform many of their normal activities. Its lower cost benefits both patients and hospitals.

Home care patients may receive fluids or such medications as antibiotics, antifungals, chemotherapeutic agents, insulin, chelating agents, or analgesics. More recently, some blood products have been given at home following an initial transfusion in the hospital.

Candidates for home I.V. therapy should be selected carefully. Such patients must be willing and able to administer therapy safely, learn the potential complications and interventions, understand the basics of asepsis, and obtain the necessary supplies. Patients who need help must enlist a home caregiver, such as a family member or friend, to assist them in administering I.V. therapy.

When teaching the home care patient, demonstrate procedures and answer any questions. Have the patient or family members give return demonstrations whenever possible. Teaching should begin in the hospital and should be completed before the patient is discharged. You may wish to include a family member or caregiver in your patient teaching.

Documentation

You need to document I.V. therapy for many reasons. First, an accurate description of your care provides legal protection for you and the hospital. Furthermore, thorough documentation furnishes health care insurers with the records they need of the equipment and supplies used. You may document I.V. therapy on progress notes, a special I.V. therapy sheet or flowchart, or a nursing care plan on the patient's chart. You also must document it on the intake and output sheet.

PERIPHERAL LINES
Preparation for I.V. therapy

Proper selection and preparation of equipment is essential to accurate delivery of an I.V. solution. Selection of an I.V. administration set depends on the rate and type of infusion desired and the type of I.V. solution container used. Two types of drip system are available: the macrodrip and the microdrip set. The macrodrip set can deliver a solution in large quantities and at rapid rates because it delivers a larger amount of solution with each drop than the microdrip set. The microdrip set, used for pediatric and certain adult patients requiring small or closely regulated amounts of I.V. solution, delivers a smaller quantity of solution with each drop.

Administration tubing with a secondary injection port permits separate or simultaneous infusion of two solutions; tubing with a piggyback port and a backcheck valve permits intermittent infusion of a secondary solution and, on its completion, a return to infusion of the primary solution. Vented I.V. tubing is selected for solutions in nonvented bottles; nonvented tubing for solutions in bags or vented bottles. Assembly of I.V. equipment requires aseptic technique to prevent contamination, which can cause local or systemic infection.

Equipment
I.V. solution ▪ I.V. administration set ▪ in-line filter, if needed ▪ I.V. pole ▪ alcohol sponges ▪ medication and label, if necessary.

Preparation of equipment
Verify the type, volume, and expiration date of the I.V. solution. Discard any outdated solution. If the solution is contained in a glass bottle, inspect for chips or cracks; if it is in a plastic bag, squeeze to detect leaks. Examine the I.V. solution for particles, abnormal discoloration, and cloudiness. If present, discard the solution and notify the pharmacy or dispensing department. If ordered, add medication to the solution, and place a completed medication-added label on the container. (For instructions, see "Addition of drugs to an I.V. solution" in Chapter 5.) Remove the administration set from its box and observe for cracks, holes, and missing clamps.

Implementation
● Wash your hands thoroughly *to prevent introducing contaminants during preparation.*
● Slide the flow clamp of the administration set tubing down to the drip chamber or injection port, and close the clamp.

Preparing a bag
● Place the bag on a flat, stable surface or hang it on an I.V. pole. Then remove the protective cap or tear the tab from the tubing insertion port.
● Remove the protective cap from the administration set spike.
● Holding the port carefully and firmly with one hand, insert the spike with your other hand.

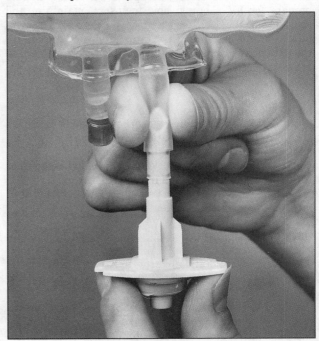

● Hang the bag on the I.V. pole, if you haven't already, and squeeze the drip chamber until it is half full.

Preparing a nonvented bottle
● Remove the bottle's metal cap and inner disk, if present.
● Place the bottle on a stable surface and wipe the rubber stopper with an alcohol sponge.
● Remove the protective cap from the administration set spike, and push the spike through the center of the bottle's rubber stopper. Avoid twisting or angling the spike *to prevent pieces of the stopper from breaking off and falling into the solution.*

• Invert the bottle. If its vacuum is intact, you'll hear a hissing sound and see air bubbles rise (this may not occur if you've already added medication). If the vacuum is not intact, discard the bottle and begin again.
• Hang the bottle on the I.V. pole and squeeze the drip chamber until it is half full.

Preparing a vented bottle
• Remove the bottle's metal cap and latex diaphragm *to release the vacuum.* If the vacuum is not intact (except after medication has been added), discard the bottle and begin again.
• Place the bottle on a stable surface and wipe the rubber stopper with an alcohol sponge.
• Remove the protective cap from the administration set spike, and push the spike through the insertion port next to the air vent tube opening.
• Hang the bottle on the I.V. pole and squeeze the drip chamber until it is half full.

Priming the I.V. tubing
• If necessary, attach a filter to the opposite end of the I.V. tubing, and follow the manufacturer's instructions for filling and priming it. Purge the tubing before attaching the filter *to avoid forcing air into the filter and possibly clogging some filter channels.* Most filters are positioned with the distal end of the tubing facing upward *so that the solution will completely wet the filter membrane and all air bubbles will be eliminated from the line.* (See *When to use an in-line filter,* page 270.)
• If you're not using a filter, aim the distal end of the tubing over a wastebasket or sink and slowly open the flow clamp. (Most distal tube coverings allow the solution to flow without having to remove the protective cover.)
• Leave the clamp open until I.V. solution flows through the entire length of tubing, forcing out all air.
• Invert all Y injection sites and backcheck valves and tap them, if necessary, *to fill them with solution.*

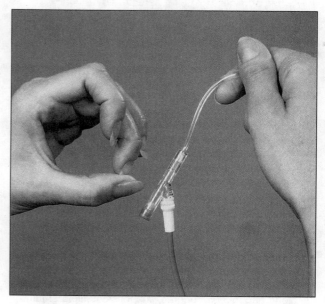

• After priming the tubing, close the clamp. Then loop the tubing over the I.V. pole.
• Label the container with the patient's name and room number, the date and time, the container number, the ordered rate and duration of infusion, and your initials.

Special considerations
Before initiation of I.V. therapy, the patient should be instructed in what to expect. (See *Teaching your patient about I.V. therapy,* page 271.)

When to use an in-line filter

An in-line filter removes pathogens and particles from I.V. solutions, helping to reduce the risk of infusion phlebitis. But because in-line filters are expensive and their installation cumbersome and time-consuming, they're not used routinely. Many institutions require use of a filter only when administering an admixture. If you're unsure of whether to use a filter, check hospital policy or follow this list of do's and don'ts.

Do's
Use an in-line filter:
• when administering solutions to an immunodeficient patient.
• when administering total parenteral nutrition.
• when using additives comprising many separate particles, such as antibiotics requiring reconstitution, or when administering several additives.
• when using rubber injection sites or plastic diaphragms repeatedly.
• when phlebitis is likely to occur.

 Be sure to change the in-line filter according to the manufacturer's recommendations (typically every 24 to 96 hours). *If you don't, bacteria trapped in the filter release endotoxin, a pyrogen small enough to pass through the filter into the bloodstream.*

 Use an add-on filter of larger pore size (1.2 microns) when infusing lipid emulsions and albumin mixed with nutritional solutions.

Don'ts
Don't use an in-line filter:
• when administering solutions with large particles *that will clog a filter and stop I.V. flow,* such as blood and its components, suspensions, lipid emulsions, and high-molecular-volume plasma expanders.
• when administering a drug dose of 5 mg or less *(because the filter may absorb it).*

 Always use aseptic technique when preparing I.V. solutions. If you contaminate the administration set or container, replace it with a new one *to prevent introducing contaminants into the system.*

 If necessary, you can use vented tubing with a vented bottle. To do this, don't remove the latex diaphragm.

Instead, insert the spike into the larger indentation in the diaphragm.

 Change I.V. tubing every 48 or 72 hours according to hospital policy or more frequently if you suspect contamination. Change the filter according to manufacturer's recommendations or sooner if it becomes clogged.

Documentation
Document the type of solution used and any additives to the solution.

Use of a volume-control set

A volume-control set — an I.V. line with a graduated chamber — delivers precise amounts of fluid and shuts off when the fluid is exhausted, preventing air from entering the I.V. line. This device is used as a primary line in children for continuous infusion of fluids or medication. It also may be used as a secondary line in adults for intermittent infusion of medication.

Equipment
Volume-control set ■ I.V. pole (for setting up a primary I.V. line) ■ I.V. solution ■ 20G to 22G 1″ needle ■ alcohol sponges ■ medication in labeled syringe and 20G to 22G 1″ needle ■ tape ■ label.

 Although various models of volume-control sets are available, each one consists of a graduated fluid chamber (120 to 250 ml) with a spike and a filtered air line on top and administration tubing underneath. Floating-valve sets have a valve at the bottom that closes when the chamber empties; membrane-filter sets have a rigid filter at the bottom that, when wet, prevents the passage of air.

Preparation of equipment
Ensure the sterility of all equipment and inspect it carefully *to ensure the absence of flaws.* Take the equipment to the patient's bedside.

Implementation
• Wash your hands, and explain the procedure to the patient. If an I.V. line is already in place, observe its insertion site for signs of infiltration or infection.
• Remove the volume-control set from its box and close all the clamps.
• Remove the protective cap from the volume-control set spike, insert the spike into the I.V. solution container, and hang the container on the I.V. pole.

Teaching your patient about I.V. therapy

Many patients feel apprehensive about peripheral I.V. therapy. So before you begin therapy, teach your patient what to expect before, during, and after the procedure. Thorough patient teaching can reduce anxiety, making therapy easier. Follow these guidelines.

Before insertion
• Describe the procedure. Tell him that "intravenous" means inside the vein and that a plastic catheter or needle will be placed in his vein. Explain that fluids containing certain nutrients or medications will flow from a bag or bottle, through a length of tubing, then through the plastic catheter or needle into his vein.
• Tell him approximately how long the catheter or needle will stay in place. Explain that the doctor will decide how much and what type of fluid the patient needs.
• If the patient will receive a local anesthetic at the insertion site, ask him if he's allergic to lidocaine. If in doubt, use another anesthetic. Tell him this injection will numb the site to reduce the pain of I.V. device insertion.
• If no anesthetic will be used, tell the patient that he may feel transient pain at the insertion site but that the discomfort will stop once the catheter or needle is in place.

• Tell him that I.V. fluid may feel cold at first, but that this sensation should last only a few minutes.

During therapy
• Instruct the patient to report any discomfort after the catheter or needle has been inserted and the fluid has begun to flow.
• Explain any restrictions, as ordered. As appropriate, tell the patient that he may be able to walk while receiving I.V. therapy and, depending on the insertion site and the device, he also may be able to shower or take a tub bath during therapy.
• Teach him how to care for the I.V. line. Tell him not to pull at the insertion site or tubing, not to remove the container from the I.V. pole, and not to kink the tubing or lie on it. Instruct him to call a nurse if the flow rate suddenly slows down or speeds up.

At removal
• Explain that removing a peripheral I.V. line is a simple procedure. Tell the patient that pressure will be applied to the site until the bleeding stops. Reassure him that once the device is out and the bleeding stops, he'll be able to use the affected arm or leg as before therapy.

• Open the air vent clamp and close the upper slide clamp. Then open the lower clamp on the I.V. tubing, slide it upward until it's slightly below the drip chamber, and close the clamp.

• If you're using a valve set, open the upper clamp until the fluid chamber fills with about 30 ml of solution. Then close the clamp and carefully squeeze the drip chamber until it is half full.
• If you're using a volume-control set with a membrane filter, open the upper clamp until the fluid chamber fills with about 30 ml of solution, and then close the clamp.
• Open the lower clamp and squeeze the drip chamber flat with two fingers of your opposite hand. *If you squeeze the drip chamber with the lower clamp closed, you'll damage the membrane filter.*

• Keeping the drip chamber flat, close the lower clamp. Now release and reshape the drip chamber so it fills halfway.

• Open the lower clamp, prime the tubing, and close the clamp. To use as a primary line, insert an adapter into the catheter or needle hub. To use as a secondary line, attach a needle to the adapter on the volume-control set. Wipe the Y port of the primary tubing with an alcohol sponge, and insert the needle. Then tape the connection.

• To add medication, wipe the injection port on the volume-control set with an alcohol sponge, and inject the medication. Place a label on the chamber, indicating the drug, the dose, and the date. Don't write directly on the chamber *because the plastic absorbs ink.*

• Open the upper clamp, fill the fluid chamber with the prescribed amount of solution, and close the clamp. Gently rotate the chamber *to mix the medication.*

• Turn off the primary solution (if present) or lower the drip rate *to maintain an open line.*

• Open the lower clamp on the volume-control set, and adjust the drip rate as ordered. After completion of the infusion, open the upper clamp and let 10 ml of I.V. solution flow into the chamber and through the tubing *to flush them.*

• If you're using the volume-control set as a secondary I.V. line, close the lower clamp and reset the flow rate of the primary line. If you're using the set as a primary I.V. line, close the lower clamp, refill the chamber to the prescribed amount, and begin the infusion again.

Special considerations

Always check compatibility of the medication and the I.V. solution. If you're using a membrane-filter set, avoid administering suspensions, lipid emulsions, blood, or blood components through it.

If you're using a floating-valve set, the diaphragm may stick after repeated use. If it does, close the air vent and upper clamp, invert the drip chamber, and squeeze it. If the diaphragm opens, reopen the clamp and continue to use the set. If the drip chamber of a floating-valve diaphragm set overfills, immediately close the upper clamp and air vent, invert the chamber, and squeeze the excess fluid from the drip chamber back into the graduated fluid chamber.

Documentation

If you add a drug to the volume-control set, record the amount and type of medication, the amount of fluid used to dilute it, and the date and time of infusion.

■ Insertion of a peripheral I.V. line

This procedure involves selection of a venipuncture device and insertion site, application of a tourniquet, preparation of the site, and venipuncture. Selection of a venipuncture device and site depends on the type of solution to be used; the frequency and duration of infusion; the patient's age, size, and condition; the patency and location of accessible veins; and, when possible, the patient's preference. Typically, selection focuses on a vein in the nondominant arm or hand. The most favorable venipuncture sites are the cephalic and basilic veins in the lower arm and the veins in the dorsum of the hand; least favorable are the leg and foot veins because of the increased risk of thrombophlebitis.

Antecubital veins can be used if no other venous access is available; to accommodate a large-bore needle; or to administer drugs requiring large volume dilution.

Use of a peripheral line allows administration of fluids, medication, blood, and blood components, and maintains I.V. access to the patient. Insertion is contraindicated in a sclerotic vein, in an edematous or impaired arm or hand, and in the presence of burns or an arteriovenous fistula. Subsequent venipunctures should be performed proximal to a previously used or injured vein.

Equipment

Alcohol sponges ■ povidone-iodine sponges ■ antimicrobial ointment, according to hospital policy ■ gloves ■ tourniquet (rubber tubing or a blood pressure cuff) ■ two I.V. needles or I.V. catheter devices ■ sterile 2″ × 2″ gauze pads or a transparent semipermeable dressing ■ 1″ non-allergenic tape ■ I.V. solution with attached and primed administration set ■ I.V. pole ■ sharps container ■ optional: armboard, roller gauze, tube gauze, warm packs,

EQUIPMENT

Comparing venipuncture devices

Most I.V. infusions are delivered through one of three basic types of venipuncture devices: an over-the-needle catheter, a through-the-needle catheter, or a winged infusion set.

Over-the-needle catheter
Purpose: long-term therapy for the active or agitated patient.
Advantages: accidental puncture of the vein is less likely than with a needle; more comfortable for the patient once it's in place; contains radiopaque thread for easy location; some units come with a syringe attached that permits easy check of blood return; some units are equipped with wings.
Disadvantage: more difficult to insert than other devices.

Through-the-needle catheter
Purpose: long-term therapy for the active or agitated patient.
Advantages: accidental puncture of the vein is less likely than with a needle; more comfortable for the patient once it's in place; available in many lengths; most plastic catheters contain radiopaque thread, permitting easy location; one variant, the peripherally inserted central catheter, is inserted in the antecubital vein by

a specially prepared nurse.
Disadvantages: leaking at the site may occur, especially in an elderly patient; if a needle guard isn't used, the catheter may be severed.

Winged infusion set
Purpose: short-term therapy for any cooperative adult patient; therapy of any duration for an infant or child or for an elderly patient with fragile or sclerotic veins.
Advantages: easiest intravascular device to insert; ideal for I.V. push drugs.
Disadvantage: may easily cause infiltration if a rigid-needle winged infusion device is used.

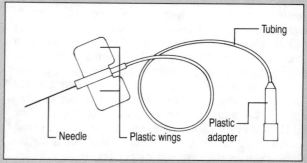

antimicrobial solution (such as 70% alcohol, tincture of iodine, povidone-iodine, or chlorhexidine), local anesthetic (such as 1% lidocaine without epinephrine), U-100 insulin syringe with a 27G needle.

Commercial venipuncture kits are available with or without an I.V. needle or I.V. catheter device (see *Comparing venipuncture devices*). In many hospitals, venipuncture equipment is kept on a tray or cart, allowing

choice of the correct needle or catheter and easy replacement of contaminated items.

Preparation of equipment
Check the information on the label of the I.V. solution container, including the patient's name and room number, the type of solution, the time and date of its preparation, the preparer's name, and the ordered infusion rate. Com-

Locating hard-to-find veins

You can locate hard-to-find peripheral veins more easily by using a transillumination device such as the Landry Vein Light. This device uses bright light from a pair of adjustable fiber-optic arms to reveal the blood vessels. Secure the light to the patient's limb with tape. Dim the room lights. With the device on its brightest setting, scan the limb below the tourniquet for a vein. The vein appears as a dark line between the fiber-optic arms.

Fiber-optic arms

Peripheral vein

Needle

Fastener tape

Interior spotlight

pare the doctor's orders with the solution label *to verify that the infusion is the correct one.* Then select the smallest gauge needle or catheter device available for the infusion unless subsequent therapy will require a larger one. *Smaller gauges cause less trauma to veins, allow greater blood flow around their tips, and reduce the clotting risk.*

If you're using a winged infusion set, connect the adapter to the administration set, and unclamp the line until fluid flows from the open end of the needle cover. Then close the clamp and place the needle on a sterile surface, such as the inside of its packaging.

If you're using a catheter device, open its package *to allow easy access.*

Implementation

• Place the I.V. pole in the proper slot in the patient's bed frame. If you're using a portable I.V. pole, position it close to the patient.

• Hang the I.V. solution with attached primed administration set on the I.V. pole.

• Verify the patient's identity by comparing the information on the solution container with the patient's wristband.

• Wash your hands thoroughly *to avoid spreading microorganisms.* Then explain the procedure to the patient *to ensure his cooperation and reduce anxiety. Anxiety can cause a vasomotor response resulting in venous constriction.*

Selecting the site

• Select the puncture site—preferably a vein in the nondominant arm. For fluid replacement, choose a small vein unless a large vein will be needed for subsequent therapy; *this leaves the large veins available for emergency infusion.* If long-term therapy is anticipated, start with a vein at the most distal site *so you can move proximally as needed for subsequent I.V. insertion sites.* For infusion of an irritating medication, choose a large vein (with plenty of subcutaneous tissue) distal to any nearby joint. Be sure the vein can accommodate the cannula if used.

• Place the patient's arm in a dependent position *to increase capillary fill of the lower arms and hands.* If the patient's skin is cold, warm it by rubbing and stroking the arm, or cover the entire arm with warm packs for 5 to 10 minutes.

Applying the tourniquet

• Apply a tourniquet about 6″ (15.2 cm) above the intended puncture site *to dilate the vein.* Check for a distal pulse. If it is not present, release the tourniquet and reapply it with less tension *to prevent arterial occlusion.*

• Lightly palpate the vein with your index and middle fingers, while stretching it to prevent rolling. If the vein feels hard or ropelike, select another.

• If the vein is easily palpable but not sufficiently dilated, one or more of the following techniques may help raise the vein. Flick the skin over the vein with one or two sharp snaps of your finger, place the extremity in a dependent position for several seconds, rub or stroke the skin upward toward the tourniquet or, if you have selected a vein in the arm or hand, tell the patient to open and close his fist several times. If necessary, you may be able to locate a vein using transillumination. (See *Locating hard-to-find veins.*)

• Leave the tourniquet in place for no more than 2 minutes. If you cannot find a suitable vein and prepare the site in that time, release the tourniquet for a few minutes. Then reapply it and continue the procedure.

Preparing the site

• Put on gloves. Clip the hair around the insertion site, if necessary, and clean the site with one of the following antimicrobials: 70% alcohol solution, povidone-iodine, tincture of iodine, or chlorhexidine. Do not apply alcohol after an iodophor prep *because alcohol negates the effect of the iodophor.* Work in a circular motion outward from the site to a diameter of 2″ to 4″ (5 to 10 cm) *to remove flora that would otherwise be introduced into the vascular system with the venipuncture.* Allow the antimicrobial solution to dry.

• If ordered, administer a local anesthetic. Make sure the patient is not sensitive to lidocaine. (See *Administering a local anesthetic,* page 276.)
• Hold the skin taut below the site *to stabilize the selected vein.*
• Grasp the needle or catheter. If you're using a *winged infusion set,* hold the short edges of the wings (with the needle's bevel facing upward) between the thumb and forefinger of your dominant hand. Then squeeze the wings together. If you're using an *over-the-needle catheter,* grasp the plastic hub with your dominant hand, remove the

cover, and examine the catheter tip. If the edge isn't smooth, discard and replace the device. If you're using a *through-the-needle catheter,* grasp the needle hub with one hand, and unsnap the needle cover. Then rotate the catheter device until the bevel faces upward.
• Using the thumb of your opposite hand, stretch the skin taut below the puncture site *to stabilize the vein.*

• Lightly press the vein with your thumb about 1½″ (3.8 cm) from the intended insertion site. The vein should feel round, firm, fully engorged, and resilient.
• Tell the patient that you are about to insert the device.
• For the direct approach, hold the needle bevel up and enter the skin directly over the vein at a 30- to 45-degree angle. For the indirect approach, enter the skin slightly adjacent to the vein. Direct the device into the side of the vein wall *to avoid perforating the vein's opposite wall.*
• Advance the device steadily until you meet resistance. Don't penetrate the vein. Lower the needle to a 15- to 20-degree angle, and slowly pierce the vein. You may not always feel a "pop" or a sensation of release when the device enters the vein.

Administering a local anesthetic

Many doctors order a local anesthetic when starting peripheral I.V. therapy. (However, the Intravenous Nurses Society doesn't recommend the practice.) If you'll be giving a local anesthetic, follow these guidelines:
• Using a U-100 insulin syringe with a 27G needle, draw up 0.1 ml of 1% lidocaine without epinephrine.
• Clean the venipuncture site.
• Put on gloves. Insert the needle next to the vein, introducing about one-third of it into the skin subcutaneously at a 30-degree angle (as shown). The lateral approach

poses less risk of accidental vein puncture (indicated by blood appearing in the syringe). If the vein is deep, however, inject the lidocaine over the top of it. Just be careful not to inject the anesthetic into the vein.

• Hold your thumb on the plunger of the syringe during insertion to avoid unnecessary movement once the needle is under the skin.
• Without aspirating, quickly inject the lidocaine until a small wheal appears, as shown below. You may not have to administer the entire amount in the syringe.

• Quickly withdraw the syringe and massage the wheal with an alcohol swab. This will make the wheal disappear so the vein won't be hidden. However, you'll see a small pinprick of blood. The skin will be numb for about 30 minutes.
• Once the skin is numb, insert the venipuncture device into the vein.

• When you observe blood flashback behind the hub, tilt the needle slightly upward and advance it farther into the vein *to prevent puncture of the posterior vein wall.* (You may not see blood return with a small vein.)
• If you're using a *winged infusion set,* advance the needle fully, if possible, and hold it in place. Release the tourniquet, open the administration set clamp slightly, and check for free flow or infiltration.
• If you're using an *over-the-needle catheter,* advance the device to at least half of its length *to ensure that the catheter itself, not just the introducer needle, has entered the vein.* Then remove the tourniquet.
• Grasp the catheter hub to hold it in place in the vein, and withdraw the needle. As you withdraw it, press lightly on the catheter tip *to prevent bleeding.* (See photograph at right.)
• Advance the catheter up to the hub or until you meet resistance.

• To advance the catheter while infusing I.V. solution, release the tourniquet and remove the inner needle. Using aseptic technique, attach the I.V. tubing and begin the infusion. While stabilizing the vein with one hand, use the other to advance the catheter into the vein. When the catheter is advanced, decrease the I.V. flow rate. *This method reduces the risk of puncturing the vein's opposite wall because the catheter is advanced without the steel needle and because the rapid flow dilates the vein.*

• To advance the catheter before starting the infusion, first release the tourniquet. While stabilizing the vein with one hand, use the other to advance the catheter up to the hub. Next, remove the inner needle and, using aseptic technique, quickly attach the I.V. tubing. *This method often results in less blood being spilled.*

• If you're using a *through-the-needle catheter*, remove the tourniquet, hold the needle in place with one hand and, with your opposite hand, grasp the catheter through the protective sleeve. Then, slowly thread the catheter through the needle until the hub is within the needle collar. Never pull back on the catheter without pulling back on the needle *to avoid severing and releasing the catheter into the circulation, causing an embolus.* If you feel resistance from a valve, withdraw the catheter and needle slightly and reinsert them, rotating the catheter as you pass the valve. Then withdraw the metal needle, and cover it with the protector. Remove the stylet and protective sleeve, and attach the administration set to the catheter hub. Open the administration set clamp slightly, and check for free flow or infiltration.

Dressing the site

• After the venipuncture device has been inserted, clean the skin completely. If necessary, dispose of the inner needle in a needle receptacle. Then regulate the flow rate.

How to apply a transparent semipermeable dressing

Instead of using tape to secure the I.V. insertion site, you can apply a transparent semipermeable dressing. Here's how:

• Make sure the insertion site is clean and dry.
• Remove the dressing from the package and, using aseptic technique, remove the protective seal. Avoid touching the sterile surface.
• Place the dressing directly over the insertion site and the hub, as shown. Don't cover the tubing. Also, don't stretch the dressing; doing so *may cause itching.*

• Tuck the dressing around and under the catheter hub *to make the site impervious to microorganisms.*
• To remove the dressing, grasp one corner, then lift and stretch. If removal is difficult, try loosening the edges with alcohol or water.

• You may use a transparent dressing to secure the device. (See *How to apply a transparent semipermeable dressing.*) If you don't use a transparent dressing, apply antiseptic ointment and cover the site with a sterile gauze pad or small adhesive bandage.

• Loop the I.V. tubing on the patient's limb, and secure the tubing with tape. *The loop allows some slack to prevent dislodgment of the catheter from tension on the line.* (See *Methods of taping a venipuncture site,* pages 278 and 279.)

• Label the last piece of tape with the type and gauge of needle or catheter, the date and time of insertion, and your initials. Adjust the flow rate, as ordered.

• If the puncture site is near a movable joint, secure an

(Text continues on page 280.)

Methods of taping a venipuncture site

If you'll be using tape to secure the venipuncture device to the insertion site, use one of the four basic methods described below.

Chevron method

• Cover the venipuncture site with an adhesive strip or a 2″×2″ sterile gauze pad. Then cut a long strip of ½″ (1.3-cm) tape and place it, sticky side up, under the needle and parallel to the short strip of tape (below).

• Cross the ends of the tape over the needle so that the tape sticks to the patient's skin (below).
• Apply a piece of 1″ (2.5-cm) tape across the two wings of the chevron.

• Loop the tubing and secure it with more tape. Write the date and time of insertion, the type and gauge of the needle, and your initials (below).

U method

• Cover the venipuncture site with an adhesive strip or a 2″×2″ sterile gauze pad. Then place a 2″ (5-cm) strip of ½″ tape, sticky side up, under the tubing (below).

• Bring each side of the tape up, folding it over the wings of the needle. Affix it parallel to the tubing (below).
• Now apply tape as you would with the chevron method.

• Write the date and time of insertion, the type and gauge of the needle or catheter, and your initials (below).

Methods of taping a venipuncture site *(continued)*

Two tape method

• Cover the venipuncture site with an adhesive strip or a 2″×2″ gauze pad. Then place a 2″ strip of ½″ tape, sticky side up, under the needle (below).

• Fold the tape ends over and affix them to the patient's skin in a U shape (below).

• Place a second strip of ½″ tape, sticky side down, over the needle hub. On the tape, write the date and time of insertion, the type and gauge of the needle or catheter,

and your initials (below).

With this method, you can remove the upper strip of tape to check the insertion site while the lower strip anchors the needle.

Three tape method

• Cover the venipuncture site with an adhesive strip or a 2″×2″ gauze pad (below). Then cut three strips of 1″ tape.

• Place one strip of tape over each wing, keeping the tape parallel to the needle (below).

• Now place the other strip of tape perpendicular to the first two. Put it either directly on top of the wings or just below the wings, directly on top of the tubing.

• On the last piece of tape, write the date and time of insertion, the type and gauge of the needle or catheter, and your initials (below).

armboard with roller gauze or tape *to provide stability, because excessive movement can dislodge the needle or catheter and increase the risk of thrombophlebitis and infection.*

Removing a peripheral I.V. line

• Performed upon completion of therapy, for needle or catheter changes, and for suspected infection or infiltration, removal of a peripheral I.V. line usually requires an alcohol sponge, a sterile gauze pad, and an adhesive bandage.

• To remove the I.V. line, first clamp the I.V. tubing *to stop the flow of solution.* Then, gently remove all tape from the skin.

• Using aseptic technique, open the gauze pad and adhesive bandage, and place them within reach. Put on gloves. Hold the sterile gauze pad over the puncture site, and use your other hand to withdraw the needle or catheter slowly and smoothly, keeping it parallel to the skin. (Inspect the catheter tip; if it's not smooth, assess the patient immediately, and notify the doctor.)

• Using the gauze pad, apply firm pressure over the puncture site for 1 to 2 minutes after the device has been removed or until bleeding has stopped.

• Clean the site and apply the adhesive bandage. Or if blood oozes from the site, apply a pressure bandage.

• If drainage appears at the puncture site, send the tip of the device and a sample of the drainage to the laboratory to be cultured according to hospital policy. (A draining site may or may not be infected.) Then clean the area and apply antiseptic ointment and a sterile dressing.

• Instruct the patient to restrict activity for about 10 minutes and to leave the dressing in place for at least 8 hours. If the patient feels lingering tenderness at the site, apply warm packs.

Special considerations

If the patient is elderly, apply the tourniquet carefully *to avoid pinching the skin.* If necessary, apply it over the patient's gown. Make sure skin preparation materials are at room temperature *to avoid vasoconstriction resulting from lower temperatures.* If the patient is allergic to iodine-containing compounds, clean the skin with alcohol.

If you fail to see blood flashback after entering the vein, pull back slightly and rotate the device. If you still fail to see flashback, remove the cannula and try again. If you suspect that the device is in the vein, try these measures to facilitate blood flashback: position the I.V. container below needle level, or insert the needle and syringe into the injection port closest to the puncture site. Then close the clamp on the I.V. tubing and attempt to aspirate. (Keep in mind that, if the device is tightly in place or the patient is extremely dehydrated or hypovolemic, you may not see blood flashback.)

Change a gauze or transparent dressing when you change the administration set (every 48 hours or according to hospital policy).

Be sure to rotate the I.V. site, usually every 48 to 72 hours or according to hospital policy.

When a vein cannot be entered percutaneously, venesection may need to be performed.

Home care

Most patients receiving I.V. therapy at home will have a central venous line. But if you care for a patient going home with a peripheral line, you should teach care of the I.V. site and identify certain complications. If the patient must observe movement restrictions, make sure he understands them.

Teach the patient how to examine the site, and instruct him to notify the doctor if redness, swelling, or discomfort develops; if the dressing becomes moist; or if blood is in the tubing.

Also tell the patient to report any problems with the I.V. line; for instance, if the solution stops infusing or if an alarm goes off on an infusion pump or controller. Explain that the I.V. site will be changed at established intervals by a home care nurse.

If the patient is using an intermittent infusion device, such as a heparin lock, teach him how and when to flush it. Finally, teach the patient to document daily whether the I.V. site is free from pain, swelling, and redness.

Complications

Peripheral line complications can result from the needle or catheter (infection, phlebitis, and embolism) or from the solution (circulatory overload, infiltration, sepsis, and allergic reaction). (See *Risks of peripheral I.V. therapy.*)

Documentation

In your notes or on the appropriate I.V. sheets, record the date and time of venipuncture, the type and gauge of needle or catheter, the location of the insertion site, and the reason the site was changed.

Also document the number of attempts at venipuncture (if you made more than one), the type and flow rate of the I.V. solution, the name and amount of medication in the solution (if any), any adverse reactions and actions taken to correct them, patient teaching and evidence of patient understanding, and your initials.

Risks of peripheral I.V. therapy

COMPLICATION	SIGNS AND SYMPTOMS	POSSIBLE CAUSES	NURSING INTERVENTIONS
Local complications			
Phlebitis	• Tenderness at tip of and proximal to venipuncture device • Redness at tip of catheter and along vein • Puffy area over vein • Vein hard on palpation • Elevated temperature	• Poor blood flow around venipuncture device • Friction from catheter movement in vein • Venipuncture device left in vein too long • Clotting at catheter tip (thrombophlebitis) • Drug or solution with high or low pH or high osmolarity	• Remove venipuncture device. • Apply warm soaks. • Notify doctor if patient has fever. • Document patient's condition and your interventions. ***Prevention*** • Restart infusion using larger vein for irritating solution, or restart with smaller-gauge device *to ensure adequate blood flow.* • Use filter *to reduce risk of phlebitis.* • Tape device securely *to prevent motion.*
Extravasation	• Swelling at and above I.V. site (may extend along entire limb) • Discomfort, burning, or pain at site (but may be painless) • Tight feeling at site • Decreased skin temperature around site • Blanching at site • Continuing fluid infusion even when vein is occluded (although rate may decrease) • Absent backflow of blood	• Venipuncture device dislodged from vein, or perforated vein	• Stop the infusion. Infiltrate the site with an antidote, if appropriate. • Apply ice (early) or warm soaks (later) *to aid absorption.* Elevate limb. • Check for pulse and capillary refill periodically *to assess circulation.* • Restart infusion above infiltration site or in another limb. • Document patient's condition and your interventions. ***Prevention*** • Check I.V. site frequently. • Don't obscure area above site with tape. • Teach patient to observe I.V. site and report pain or swelling.
Catheter dislodgment	• Loose tape • Catheter partly backed out of vein • Solution infiltrating	• Loosened tape, or tubing snagged in bed linens, resulting in partial retraction of catheter; pulled out by confused patient	• If no infiltration occurs, retape without pushing catheter back into vein. If pulled out, apply pressure to I.V. site with sterile dressing. ***Prevention*** • Tape venipuncture securely on insertion.
Occlusion	• No increase in flow rate when I.V. container is raised • Blood backflow in line • Discomfort at insertion site	• I.V. flow interrupted • Heparin lock not flushed • Blood backflow in line when patient walks • Line clamped too long	• Use mild flush injection. Don't force it. If unsuccessful, reinsert I.V. line. ***Prevention*** • Maintain I.V. flow rate. • Flush promptly after intermittent piggyback administration. • Have patient walk with his arm bent at the elbow *to reduce risk of blood backflow.*

(continued)

Risks of peripheral I.V. therapy *(continued)*

COMPLICATION	SIGNS AND SYMPTOMS	POSSIBLE CAUSES	NURSING INTERVENTIONS
Local complications *(continued)*			
Vein irritation or pain at I.V. site	• Pain during infusion • Possible blanching if vasospasm occurs • Red skin over vein during infusion • Rapidly developing signs of phlebitis	• Solution with high or low pH or high osmolarity, such as 40 mEq/liter of potassium chloride, phenytoin, and some antibiotics (vancomycin, erythromycin, and nafcillin)	• Decrease the flow rate. • Try using an electronic flow device *to achieve a steady flow.* **Prevention** • Dilute solutions before administration. For example, give antibiotics in 250-ml solution rather than 100 ml. If drug has low pH, ask pharmacist if drug can be buffered with sodium bicarbonate. (Refer to hospital policy.) • If long-term therapy of irritating drug is planned, ask doctor to use central I.V. line.
Severed catheter	• Leakage from catheter shaft	• Catheter inadvertently cut by scissors • Reinsertion of needle into catheter	• If broken part is visible, attempt to retrieve it. If unsuccessful, notify the doctor. • If portion of catheter enters bloodstream, place tourniquet above I.V. site *to prevent progression of broken part.* • Notify doctor and radiology department. • Document patient's condition and your interventions. **Prevention** • Don't use scissors around I.V. site. • Never reinsert needle into catheter. • Remove unsuccessfully inserted catheter and needle together.
Hematoma	• Tenderness at venipuncture site • Bruised area around site • Inability to advance or flush I.V. line	• Vein punctured through opposite wall at time of insertion • Leakage of blood from needle displacement • Inadequate pressure applied when catheter discontinued	• Remove venipuncture device. • Apply pressure and warm soaks to affected area. • Recheck for bleeding. • Document patient's condition and your interventions. **Prevention** • Choose a vein that can accommodate size of venipuncture device. • Release tourniquet as soon as successful insertion achieved.

Risks of peripheral I.V. therapy *(continued)*

COMPLICATION	SIGNS AND SYMPTOMS	POSSIBLE CAUSES	NURSING INTERVENTIONS
Local complications *(continued)*			
Venous spasm	• Pain along vein • Flow rate sluggish when clamp completely open • Blanched skin over vein	• Severe vein irritation from irritating drugs or fluids • Administration of cold fluids or blood • Very rapid flow rate (with fluids at room temperature)	• Apply warm soaks over vein and surrounding area. • Decrease flow rate. ***Prevention*** • Use a blood warmer for blood or packed red blood cells.
Vasovagal reaction	• Sudden collapse of vein during venipuncture • Sudden pallor, sweating, faintness, dizziness, and nausea • Decreased blood pressure	• Vasospasm from anxiety or pain	• Lower head of bed. • Have patient take deep breaths. • Check vital signs. ***Prevention*** • Prepare patient for therapy *to relieve his anxiety.* • Use local anesthetic *to prevent pain.*
Thrombosis	• Painful, reddened and swollen vein • Sluggish or stopped I.V. flow	• Injury to endothelial cells of vein wall, allowing platelets to adhere and thrombi to form	• Remove venipuncture device; restart infusion in opposite limb if possible. • Apply warm soaks. • Watch for I.V. therapy-related infection; thrombi provide an excellent environment for bacterial growth. ***Prevention*** • Use proper venipuncture techniques *to reduce injury to vein.*
Thrombophlebitis	• Severe discomfort • Reddened, swollen, and hardened vein	• Thrombosis and inflammation	• Same as for thrombosis. ***Prevention*** • Check site frequently. Remove venipuncture device at first sign of redness and tenderness.
Nerve, tendon, or ligament damage	• Extreme pain (similar to electrical shock when nerve is punctured) • Numbness and muscle contraction • Delayed effects, including paralysis, numbness, and deformity.	• Improper venipuncture technique, resulting in injury to surrounding nerves, tendons, or ligaments • Tight taping or improper splinting with armboard	• Stop procedure. ***Prevention*** • Don't repeatedly penetrate tissues with venipuncture device. • Don't apply excessive pressure when taping; don't encircle limb with tape. • Pad armboards and tape securing armboards if possible.

(continued)

Risks of peripheral I.V. therapy *(continued)*

COMPLICATION	SIGNS AND SYMPTOMS	POSSIBLE CAUSES	NURSING INTERVENTIONS
Systemic complications			
Circulatory overload	• Discomfort • Neck vein engorgement • Respiratory distress • Increased blood pressure • Crackles • Increased difference between fluid intake and output	• Roller clamp loosened to allow run-on infusion • Flow rate too rapid • Miscalculation of fluid requirements	• Raise the head of the bed. • Administer oxygen as needed. • Notify the doctor. • Administer medications (probably furosemide) as ordered. ***Prevention*** • Use pump, controller, or rate minder for elderly or compromised patients. • Recheck calculations of fluid requirements. • Monitor infusion frequently.
Systemic infection (septicemia or bacteremia)	• Fever, chills, and malaise for no apparent reason • Contaminated I.V. site, usually with no visible signs of infection at site	• Failure to maintain aseptic technique during insertion or site care • Severe phlebitis, which can set up ideal conditions for organism growth • Poor taping that permits venipuncture device to move, which can introduce organisms into bloodstream • Prolonged indwelling time of device • Weak immune system	• Notify the doctor. • Administer medications as prescribed. • Culture the site and device. • Monitor vital signs. ***Prevention*** • Use scrupulous aseptic technique when handling solutions and tubing, inserting venipuncture device, and discontinuing infusion. • Secure all connections. • Change I.V. solutions, tubing, and venipuncture device at recommended times. • Use I.V. filters.
Air embolism	• Respiratory distress • Unequal breath sounds • Weak pulse • Increased central venous pressure • Decreased blood pressure • Loss of consciousness	• Solution container empty • Solution container empties, and added container pushes air down the line (if line not purged first)	• Discontinue infusion. • Place patient in Trendelenburg's position *to allow air to enter right atrium and disperse via pulmonary artery.* • Administer oxygen. • Notify doctor. • Document patient's condition and your interventions. ***Prevention*** • Purge tubing of air completely before starting infusion. • Use air-detection device on pump or air-eliminating filter proximal to I.V. site. • Secure connections.

Risks of peripheral I.V. therapy *(continued)*

COMPLICATION	SIGNS AND SYMPTOMS	POSSIBLE CAUSES	NURSING INTERVENTIONS
Systemic complications *(continued)*			
Allergic reaction	• Itching • Watery eyes and nose • Bronchospasm • Wheezing • Urticarial rash • Edema at I.V. site • Anaphylactic reaction, which may occur within minutes or up to 1 hour after exposure (flushing, chills, anxiety, agitation, itching, palpitations, paresthesia, throbbing in ears, wheezing, coughing, convulsions, cardiac arrest)	• Allergens, such as medications	• If reaction occurs, stop infusion immediately. • Maintain patent airway. • Notify doctor. • Administer antihistaminic steroid, anti-inflammatory, and antipyretic drugs, as ordered. • Give 0.2 to 0.5 ml of 1:1,000 aqueous epinephrine subcutaneously, as ordered. Repeat at 3-minute intervals and as needed. • Administer cortisone if ordered. ***Prevention*** • Obtain patient's allergy history. Be aware of cross-allergies. • Assist with test dosing. • Monitor patient carefully during first 15 minutes of administration of a new drug.

Insertion of a heparin lock

Also called an intermittent infusion device, a heparin lock consists of either a steel winged-tip needle with tubing that ends in a resealable rubber injection port or a catheter with injection cap attached. Filled with dilute heparin to prevent blood clot formation, the device maintains venous access in patients receiving I.V. medication regularly or intermittently, but not requiring continuous infusion of fluids. A heparin lock proves superior to a keep-vein-open line because it minimizes the risk of fluid overload and electrolyte imbalance. It also cuts costs, reduces the risk of contamination by eliminating I.V. solution containers and administration sets, increases patient comfort and mobility, reduces patient anxiety and, if inserted in a large vein, allows collection of multiple blood samples without repeated venipuncture.

Equipment

Heparin lock ■ 25G needle ■ dilute heparin solution in a 1-ml syringe ■ povidone-iodine sponges ■ tourniquet ■ alcohol sponges ■ venipuncture equipment, sterile dressing, and tape ■ optional: transparent semipermeable dressing, stretch net protective sleeve.

Some hospitals use a 100 units/ml heparin flush; others, a 10 units/ml flush; and still others, a normal saline solution instead of heparin. Prefilled heparin or saline cartridges are available in both dosages for use in a syringe cartridge holder.

Implementation

• Wash your hands thoroughly *to prevent contamination of the venipuncture site.*
• Explain the procedure to the patient, and describe the purpose of the heparin lock.
• Remove the set from its packaging, wipe the port with an alcohol sponge, and inject a dilute heparin solution or normal saline solution to fill the tubing and 25G needle. *This removes air from the system, preventing formation of an air embolus.*
• Select a venipuncture site, and clean it first with povidone-iodine sponges, wiping outward from the site in a circular motion. Do not wipe off the povidone-iodine with alcohol *because doing so negates its effect.*
• Perform the venipuncture and ensure correct needle placement in the vein. Then release the tourniquet. (See "Venipuncture" in Chapter 3 for complete instructions.)
• Tape the set in place, using the chevron method or an accepted alternative. Loop the tubing, if applicable, so the injection port is free and easily accessible.

Stabilizing a heparin lock

Before inserting or removing a needle from a heparin lock, you must stabilize the device. To do this, grasp the lock just below the injection cap with the thumb and index finger of your nondominant hand, as shown, and hold the device steady during needle insertion and withdrawal.

• Apply a sterile dressing. On the last piece of tape used to secure the dressing, write the time, date, and your initials.
• Inject dilute heparin solution or normal saline solution every 6 to 12 hours or according to hospital policy *to maintain the patency of the heparin lock.* Inject the heparin slowly *to prevent stinging.*

Special considerations

Whenever inserting or removing a needle from a heparin lock, be sure to stabilize the device to prevent dislodging it from the vein. (See *Stabilizing a heparin lock.*)

If ordered, obtain a blood sample for activated partial thromboplastin time *before* inserting the intermittent infusion set *because small amounts of heparin can alter the results of this test.*

If the patient has a clotting disorder, use 1 to 2 ml of normal saline solution according to hospital policy, instead of a heparin flush.

If the patient feels a burning sensation during injection of heparin, stop the injection and check needle placement. If the needle is in the vein, inject the heparin at a slower rate *to minimize irritation.* If the needle is not in the vein, remove and discard it. Then select a new venipuncture site and, using fresh equipment, restart the procedure.

Change the sterile dressing every 24 to 48 hours and the heparin lock every 72 hours according to hospital policy, using a new venipuncture site. Some hospitals use a transparent semipermeable dressing or a stretch net protective sleeve to cover the entire device. *This allows more patient freedom and better observation of the injection site.*

If the doctor orders an I.V. infusion discontinued and a heparin lock inserted in its place, convert the existing line into a heparin lock by disconnecting the I.V. tubing and inserting a male adapter plug into the device. (See *Converting an I.V. line to a heparin lock.*)

Home care

Most patients receiving I.V. therapy at home will have a central venous line. But if you care for a patient who will be going home with a peripheral line, you should teach the patient how to care for the I.V. site and how to identify complications. If the patient must observe movement restrictions, make sure he understands which movements to avoid.

Because the patient may have special drug delivery equipment that differs from the hospital's, be sure to demonstrate the equipment and have the patient give a return demonstration.

Teach the patient to examine the site and to notify the doctor if the dressing becomes moist, if blood appears in the tubing, or if redness, swelling, or discomfort develops.

Also tell the patient to report any problems with the I.V. line — for instance, if the solution stops infusing or if an alarm goes off on the infusion pump controller. Explain that the I.V. site will be changed at established intervals by a home care nurse.

Teach the patient or caregiver how and when to flush the heparin lock. Finally, teach the patient to document daily whether the I.V. site is free from pain, swelling, and redness.

Complications

Use of a heparin lock set has the same potential complications as the use of a peripheral I.V. line. (See "Insertion of a peripheral I.V. line," page 272.)

Documentation

Record the date and time of insertion, the type and gauge of needle, and the date and time of each heparin flush.

Maintenance of peripheral I.V. sites and systems

Routine maintenance of I.V. sites and systems includes regular assessment and rotation of the site and periodic changes of the dressing, tubing, and solution. These measures help prevent complications, such as thrombophlebitis and infection. They should be performed according to hospital policy. Typically, I.V. dressings are changed every 48 hours or whenever the dressing becomes wet, soiled, or nonocclusive. I.V. tubing is changed every 48 to 72 hours or according to hospital policy, and I.V. solution is changed every 24 hours or as needed. The site should be assessed every 2 hours if a transparent semipermeable dressing is used, with every dressing change otherwise, and should be rotated every 48 to 72 hours. Sometimes limited venous access will prevent frequent site changes; if so, be sure to assess the site frequently.

Equipment
For dressing changes: sterile gloves ▪ povidone-iodine or alcohol sponges ▪ povidone-iodine or other antimicrobial ointment, according to hospital policy ▪ adhesive bandage, sterile 2″ × 2″ gauze pad, or transparent semipermeable dressing ▪ 1″ adhesive tape.

   For solution changes: solution container ▪ alcohol sponge.

   For tubing changes: I.V. administration set ▪ sterile 2″ × 2″ gauze pad ▪ adhesive tape for labeling ▪ sterile gloves ▪ optional: hemostats.

   For I.V. site change: See "Insertion of a peripheral I.V. line," page 272.

   Commercial kits containing the equipment for dressing changes are available.

Preparation of equipment
If your hospital keeps I.V. equipment and dressings in a tray or cart, have it nearby, if possible, *because you may have to select a new venipuncture site, depending on the current site's condition.* If you're changing both the solution and the tubing, attach and prime the I.V. administration set before entering the patient's room.

Implementation
• Wash your hands thoroughly *to prevent the spread of microorganisms.* Remember to wear sterile gloves whenever working near the venipuncture site.
• Explain the procedure to the patient *to allay his fears and ensure cooperation.*

Converting an I.V. line to a heparin lock

Two types of adapter plugs (shown below) allow you to convert an existing I.V. line into a heparin lock. To make the conversion, follow these steps:
• Prime the adapter plug with dilute heparin or normal saline solution, as appropriate.
• Clamp the I.V. tubing and remove the administration set from the catheter or needle hub.
• Insert the male adapter plug.

   Inject the remaining dilute heparin or normal saline solution to fill the line and to prevent clot formation.

Long male adapter
This long adapter plug slides into place.

Short male adapter
This short luer-lock adapter plug twists into place.

To change the dressing
• Remove the old dressing, open all supply packages, and put on sterile gloves.
• Hold the needle or catheter in place with your nondominant hand *to prevent accidental movement or dislodgment, which could puncture the vein and cause infiltration.*
• Assess the venipuncture site for signs of infection (redness and pain at the puncture site), infiltration (coolness, blanching, and edema at the site), and thrombophlebitis (redness, firmness, pain along the path of the vein, and edema). If any such signs are present, apply pressure to the area with a sterile 2″ × 2″ gauze pad and remove the catheter or needle. Maintain pressure on the area until the bleeding stops, and apply an adhesive bandage. Then,

using fresh equipment and solution, start the I.V. in another appropriate site, preferably on the opposite extremity.

• If the venipuncture site is intact, hold the needle or catheter and carefully clean around the puncture site with a povidone-iodine or alcohol sponge. Work in a circular motion outward from the site *to avoid introducing bacteria into the clean area.* Allow the area to dry completely.

• Apply povidone-iodine or other antimicrobial ointment if hospital policy dictates, and cover with an adhesive bandage or sterile 2″ × 2″ gauze pad. Retape the site, or apply a transparent semipermeable dressing.

• When using a transparent semipermeable dressing, you may omit the povidone-iodine ointment. The transparent dressing allows visualization of the insertion site. It maintains sterility and is placed over the insertion site to halfway up the catheter or needle hub.

To change the solution

• Wash your hands.

• Inspect the new solution container for cracks, leaks, and other damage. Check the solution for discoloration, turbidity, and particulates. Note the date and time the solution was mixed and its expiration date.

• Clamp the tubing when inverting it *to prevent air from entering the tubing.* Keep the drip chamber half full.

• If you're replacing a bag, remove the seal or tab from the new bag and remove the old bag from the pole. Remove the spike, insert it into the new bag, and adjust the flow rate.

• If you're replacing a bottle, remove the cap and seal from the new bottle and wipe the rubber port with an alcohol sponge. Clamp the line, remove the spike from the old bottle, and insert the spike into the new bottle. Then hang the new bottle and adjust the flow rate.

To change tubing

• Reduce the I.V. flow rate, remove the old spike from the container, and hang it on the I.V. pole. Place the cover of the new spike loosely over the old one.

• Keeping the old spike in an upright position above the patient's heart level, insert the new spike into the I.V. container, as shown at the top of the next column.

• Prime the system. Hang the new I.V. container and primed set on the pole, and grasp the new adapter in one hand. Then stop the flow rate in the old tubing.

• Put on sterile gloves.

• Place a sterile gauze pad under the needle or catheter hub *to create a sterile field.* Press one of your fingers over the catheter to prevent bleeding.

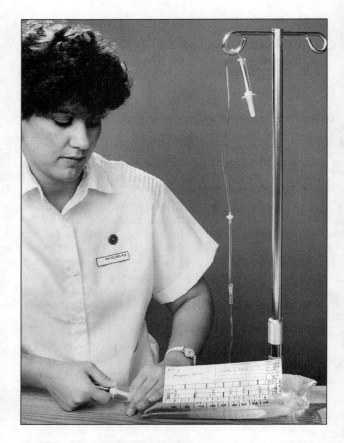

• Gently disconnect the old tubing, being careful not to dislodge or move the I.V. device. (If you have trouble disconnecting the old tubing, use a hemostat to hold the hub securely while twisting the tubing *to remove it.* Or use one hemostat on the venipuncture device and another on the hard plastic end of the tubing. Then pull the hemostats in opposite directions. Don't clamp the hemostats shut; *this may crack the tubing adapter or the venipuncture device.)*

• Remove the protective cap from the new tubing, and connect the new adapter to the needle or catheter. Hold the hub securely *to prevent dislodging the needle or catheter tip.*

• Observe for blood backflow into the new tubing *to verify that the needle or catheter is still in place.* (You may not be able to do this with small-gauge catheters.)

• Adjust the clamp to maintain the appropriate flow rate.

• Retape the needle or catheter hub and I.V. tubing, and recheck the I.V. flow rate *because taping may alter it.*

• Label the new tubing and container with the date and time. Label the solution container with a time strip.

Special considerations

Check the prescribed I.V. flow rate before each solution change *to prevent errors.* If you crack the adapter or hub (or if you accidentally dislodge the needle or catheter from the vein), remove the needle or catheter. Apply pressure and an adhesive bandage to stop any bleeding. Perform a venipuncture at another site and restart the I.V.

Keep in mind that flow rates may change 20% to 40% during an infusion. If you're not using an infusion pump, check the flow rate every hour.

Documentation

Record the time, date, and rate and type of solution (and any additives) on the I.V. flowchart. Also record this information, dressing or tubing changes, and appearance of the site in your notes.

FLOW RATE MANAGEMENT
Flow rate calculation and manual control

Calculated from a doctor's orders, flow rate is usually expressed as the total volume of I.V. solution infused over a prescribed interval or as the total volume given in milliliters per hour (ml/hr). Many devices can regulate the flow of I.V. solution, including clamps, controllers, the flow regulator (or rate minder), and the volumetric pump. (See *Using I.V. clamps,* page 290.)

When regulated by a clamp or controller, flow rate is usually measured in drops per minute; by a volumetric pump, in ml/hr. The flow regulator can be set to deliver the desired amount of solution, also in ml/hr. Less accurate than infusion pumps or controllers, flow regulators are most reliable when used with inactive adult patients. With any device, flow rate can be easily monitored by using a time tape, which indicates the prescribed solution level at hourly intervals.

Equipment

I.V. administration set with clamp ▪ 1″ paper or adhesive tape (or premarked time tape) ▪ infusion pump and controller (if infusing drugs) ▪ watch with second hand ▪ drip rate chart, as necessary ▪ pen.

Standard macrodrip sets deliver 10 to 20 drops/ml, depending on the manufacturer; microdrip sets, 60 drops/ml; and blood transfusion sets, 10 drops/ml. A commer-

Using I.V. clamps

With a roller clamp or screw clamp, you can increase or decrease flow through the I.V. line by turning a wheel or screw.

With a slide clamp, you can open or close the line by moving the clamp horizontally. However, you can't make fine adjustments to flow rate.

cially available adapter can convert a macrodrip set to a microdrip system.

Implementation
● Flow rate requires close monitoring and correction because such factors as venous spasm, venous pressure changes, patient movement or manipulation of the clamp, and bent or kinked tubing can cause the rate to vary markedly.

To calculate and set the drip rate
● Follow the steps in *Calculating flow rates* to determine the proper drip rate, or use your unit's drip rate chart.
● After calculating the desired drip rate, remove your watch and hold it next to the drip chamber of the I.V. administration set *to allow simultaneous observation of the watch and the drops.*
● Release the clamp to the approximate drip rate. Then count drops for 1 minute *to account for flow irregularities.*
● Adjust the clamp, as necessary, and count drops for 1 minute. Continue to adjust the clamp and count drops until the correct rate is achieved.

To make a time tape
● Calculate the number of milliliters to be infused per hour. Place a piece of tape vertically on the container alongside the volume-increment markers.
● Starting at the current solution level, move down the number of milliliters to be infused in 1 hour, and mark the appropriate time and a horizontal line on the tape at this level. Then continue to mark 1-hour intervals until you reach the bottom of the container.
● Check the flow rate every 15 minutes until it is stable. Then recheck it every hour or according to hospital policy, and adjust as necessary.
● With each check, inspect the I.V. site for complications and assess the patient's response to therapy.

Special considerations
If the infusion rate slows significantly, a slight rate increase may be necessary. If the rate must be increased by more than 30%, consult the doctor. When infusing drugs, use an I.V. pump or controller, if possible, *to avoid flow rate inaccuracies.* Always use a pump or controller when infusing solutions via a central line.

Large-volume solution containers have approximately 10% more fluid than the amount indicated on the bag, to allow for tubing purges. Thus, a 1,000-ml bag or bottle will contain an additional 100 ml; similarly, a 500-ml container will hold an extra 50 ml; and a 250-ml container, 25 ml.

Complications
An excessively slow flow rate may cause insufficient intake of fluids, drugs, and nutrients; an excessively rapid rate of fluid or drug infusion may cause circulatory overload—possibly leading to congestive heart failure and pulmonary edema, as well as drug side effects. (See *Managing I.V. flow rate deviations,* page 292.)

Calculating flow rates

When calculating the flow rate of I.V. solutions, remember that the number of drops required to deliver 1 ml varies with the type and manufacturer of the administration set used. The illustration on the left shows a standard (macrodrip) set, which delivers from 10 to 20 drops/ml. The illustration in the center shows a pediatric (microdrip) set, which delivers about 60 drops/ml. The illustration on the right shows a blood transfusion set, which delivers about 10 drops/ml.

To calculate the flow rate, you must know the calibration of the drip rate for each manufacturer's product. As a quick guide, refer to the chart below. Use this formula to calculate specific drip rates:

$$\frac{\text{Volume of infusion (in ml)}}{\text{time of infusion (in minutes)}} \times \text{drip factor (in drops/ml)} = \text{drops/minute}$$

ADMINISTRATION SET	DRIP FACTOR	ORDERED VOLUME 500 ml/ 24 hr or 21 ml/hr	1,000 ml/ 24 hr or 42 ml/hr	1,000 ml/ 20 hr or 50 ml/hr	1,000 ml/ 10 hr or 100 ml/hr	1,000 ml/ 8 hr or 125 ml/hr	1,000 ml/ 6 hr or 166 ml/hr
		DROPS/MINUTE TO INFUSE					
Macrodrip							
Abbott	15	5	10	12	25	31	42
Baxter Healthcare	10	3	7	8	17	21	28
Cutter	20	7	14	17	34	42	56
IVAC	20	7	14	17	34	42	56
McGaw	15	5	10	12	25	31	42
Microdrip							
Various manufacturers	60	21	42	50	100	125	166

Managing I.V. flow rate deviations

PROBLEM	CAUSE	INTERVENTION
Flow rate too fast	• Patient or visitor manipulates the clamp	• Instruct the patient not to touch the clamp, and place tape over it. Restrain the patient or administer the I.V. with an infusion pump or a controller, if necessary.
	• Tubing disconnected from the catheter	• Wipe the distal end of the tubing with alcohol, reinsert firmly into the catheter hub, and tape at the connection site. Consider using tubing with luer connections.
	• Change in patient position	• Administer the I.V. with an infusion pump or a controller to ensure the correct flow rate.
	• Bevel against vein wall (positional cannulation)	• Manipulate the cannula, and place a 2″ × 2″ gauze pad under or over the catheter hub to change the angle. Reset the flow clamp at the desired rate. If necessary, remove the cannula and reinsert.
	• Flow clamp drifting as a result of patient movement	• Place tape below the clamp.
Flow rate too slow	• Venous spasm after insertion	• Apply warm soaks over site.
	• Venous obstruction from bending arm	• Secure with an armboard if necessary.
	• Pressure change (decreasing fluid in bottle causes solution to run slower due to decreasing pressure)	• Readjust the flow rate.
	• Elevated blood pressure	• Readjust the flow rate. Use an infusion pump or a controller to ensure correct flow rate.
	• Cold solution	• Allow the solution to warm to room temperature before hanging.
	• Change in solution viscosity from medication added	• Readjust the flow rate.
	• I.V. container too low or patient's arm or leg too high	• Hang the container higher or remind the patient to keep his arm below heart level.
	• Bevel against vein wall (positional cannulation)	• Withdraw the needle slightly, or place a folded 2″ × 2″ gauze pad over or under the catheter hub to change the angle.
	• Excess tubing dangling below insertion site	• Replace the tubing with a shorter piece, or tape the excess tubing to the I.V. pole, below the flow clamp (make sure the tubing is not kinked).
	• Cannula too small	• Remove the cannula in use and insert a larger-bore cannula, or use an infusion pump.
	• Infiltration or clotted cannula	• Remove the cannula in use and reinsert a new cannula.
	• Kinked tubing	• Check the tubing over its entire length and unkink it.
	• Clogged filter	• Remove the filter and replace with a new one.
	• Tubing memory (tubing compressed at area clamped)	• Massage or milk the tubing by pinching and wrapping it around a pencil four or five times. Quickly pull the pencil out of the coiled tubing.

Documentation

Record the original flow rate when setting up a peripheral line. If you adjust the rate, record the change, the date and time, and your initials.

Use of I.V. controllers and pumps

Various types of controllers and pumps electronically regulate the flow of I.V. solutions or drugs with extreme accuracy. (See *Regulating flow rate electronically.*) Controllers regulate gravity flow by counting drops and achieve the desired infusion rate by compressing the I.V. tubing. However, because controllers simply count drops, which aren't always of equal size, these devices fail to achieve the accuracy of volumetric pumps, which measure flow rate in milliliters per hour.

Volumetric pumps, used for high-pressure infusion of drugs or for highly accurate delivery of fluids or drugs, have mechanisms to propel the solution at the desired rate under pressure. (Pressure is brought to bear only when gravity flow rates are insufficient to maintain preset infusion rates.) The peristaltic pump applies pressure to the I.V. tubing to force the solution through it. (Not every peristaltic pump is volumetric; some count drops.) The piston-cylinder pump pushes the solution through special disposable cassettes; most of these pumps operate at high pressures (up to 45 psi) and can deliver 1 to 999 ml/hour with a 97% to 98% accuracy. (Some newer pumps operate at 10 to 25 psi.) The portable syringe pump, another type of volumetric pump, delivers very small amounts of fluid over a long duration. It's used for administering fluids to infants and for delivering intra-arterial drugs. Other special devices include the controlled release infusion system, secondary syringe converter, and patient-controlled analgesia device. (See *Devices for intermittent infusion*, page 294, and *Understanding patient-controlled analgesia*, page 295.)

Controllers and pumps have various detectors and alarms that automatically signal or respond to the completion of an infusion, air in the line, low battery power, and occlusion or inability to deliver at the set rate. Depending on the problem, these devices may sound or flash an alarm, shut off, or switch to a keep-vein-open rate.

Equipment

Controller or peristaltic pump ■ I.V. pole ■ I.V. solution ■ sterile administration set ■ sterile peristaltic tubing or cassette, if needed ■ alcohol sponges ■ adhesive tape.

Tubing and cassette vary with each manufacturer.

Preparation of equipment

To set up a controller: First, attach the controller to the

(Text continues on page 296.)

EQUIPMENT

Regulating flow rate electronically

Controllers and infusion pumps, such as the two shown below, electronically regulate the flow of I.V. solutions and drugs. You'll use them when a precise flow rate is required—for instance, when administering total parenteral nutrition solutions and chemotherapeutic or cardiovascular agents.

Controller

- Rate clip regulator
- Drop rate display
- Power button
- Start button
- Drop rate select button

Infusion pump

- Pump door panel
- Flow rate display (ml/hr)
- Flow rate control
- Power button

Devices for intermittent infusion

The devices shown below allow you to deliver precise drug amounts over a prescribed time period from a vial or a syringe.

Controlled release infusion system
Place this device between the I.V. container and the tubing, then attach the drug vial to its side, as shown. The I.V. fluid passes into the device where it mixes with the drug from the vial to deliver a controlled amount of medication to the patient.

Secondary syringe converter
This special administration set converts any syringe into a piggyback container. The tubing connects to the syringe instead of to a bag or bottle. Follow the same procedure as you would with a minibag, substituting the syringe for the minibag.

Syringe pump
Battery-operated mini-infusion syringe pumps can be used to infuse small volumes intermittently or continuously. You'll find them especially useful for pediatric patients. The syringe and microbore tubing replace the minibag and piggyback tubing to deliver a precise volume over the prescribed time.

The major disadvantage of the syringe pump is that you need tubing to connect it to the venipuncture device. So when you give a small-volume dose, a portion of the drug remains in the tubing. You can help to limit the amount of drug remaining by using small-volume tubing. (Standard I.V. tubing holds 1.9 ml/foot; small-volume tubing has a smaller lumen and holds only 0.06 ml/foot.)

Also, remember that syringe pumps don't have air detectors. So be sure to eliminate all air from the syringe, tubing, and needle. Use luer-locks and tape all connections. This helps prevent partial disconnections that could cause an air infusion and drug leaks.

Understanding patient-controlled analgesia

In patient-controlled analgesia (PCA), the patient controls I.V. delivery of an analgesic (usually morphine) by pressing the button on a delivery device. The patient therefore receives analgesia at the level he needs and at the time he needs it. The device prevents the patient from accidentally overdosing by imposing a lock-out time between doses—usually 6 to 10 minutes. During this interval, the patient will not receive any analgesic, even if he pushes the button. The accompanying illustrations show two of the more commonly used PCA devices.

The first device, shown below, is a reusable, battery-operated pump that delivers a drug dose when the patient presses a call button at the end of a cord.

The other device, shown below, is disposable and mechanically operated. It contains an infusor and a unit that's worn like a wristwatch. The patient pushes a button on the device to receive the analgesic from a collapsible chamber. No more than 0.5 ml of solution can be delivered in 6 minutes.

Indications and advantages
Indicated for patients who need parenteral analgesia, PCA therapy is typically given to trauma patients post-operatively and to terminal cancer patients and others with chronic diseases. To receive PCA therapy, a patient must be mentally alert, able to understand and comply with instructions and procedures, and have no history of allergy to the analgesic. Patients ineligible for therapy include those with limited respiratory reserve, a history of drug abuse or chronic sedative or tranquilizer use, or a psychiatric disorder. PCA therapy's advantages include:
• no need for I.M. analgesics
• pain relief tailored to patient's size and pain tolerance
• a sense of control over pain
• ability to sleep at night with minimal daytime drowsiness
• lower narcotic use compared with patients not on PCA
• improved postoperative deep-breathing, coughing, and ambulation.

PCA setup
To set up a PCA system, the doctor's order should include:
• a loading dose, given by I.V. push at the start of PCA therapy (typically 25 mg meperidine [Demerol] or 2 mg morphine)
• the appropriate lock-out interval
• the maintenance dose (also called the basal dose)
• the amount the patient will receive when he activates the device (typically 10 mg meperidine or 1 mg morphine)
• the maximum amount the patient can receive within a specified time (if an adjustable device is used).

Nursing considerations
Because the primary adverse effect of analgesics is respiratory depression, you must monitor your patient's respiratory rate routinely. Also, check for infiltration into the subcutaneous tissues and for catheter occlusion, which may cause the drug to back up in the primary I.V. tubing. If the analgesic nauseates your patient, you may need to administer an antiemetic drug.

Before your patient starts using the PCA device, teach him how it works. Then have the patient practice with a sample device. Explain that he should take enough analgesic to relieve acute pain but not enough to induce drowsiness.

During therapy, monitor and record the amount of analgesic infused, the patient's respiratory rate, and the patient's assessment of pain relief. If the patient reports insufficient pain relief, notify the doctor.

I.V. pole. Then clean the port on the I.V. solution container with an alcohol sponge, insert the administration set spike, and fill the drip chamber no more than halfway *to avoid miscounting the drops.* Rotate the chamber so the fluid touches all sides *to remove any vapor that could interfere with correct drop counting.* Now, prime the tubing and close the clamp. Position the drop sensor above the fluid level in the drip chamber and below the drop port *to ensure correct drop counting.* Insert the peristaltic tubing into the controller, close the door, and open the flow clamp completely.

To set up a volumetric pump: First, attach the pump to the I.V. pole. Then, swab the port on the I.V. container with alcohol, insert the administration set spike, and completely fill the drip chamber *to prevent air bubbles from entering the tubing.* Next, prime the tubing and close the clamp. Now, follow the manufacturer's instructions for placement of tubing.

Implementation
• Position the controller or pump on the same side of the bed as the I.V. or anticipated venipuncture site *to avoid crisscrossing I.V. lines over the patient.* If necessary, perform the venipuncture.
• Plug in the machine and attach its tubing to the needle or catheter hub. If you're using a controller, position the drip chamber 30″ (76.2 cm) above the infusion site *to ensure accurate gravity flow.*
• Depending on the machine, turn it on and press the start button. Set the appropriate dials on the front panel to the desired infusion rate and volume. Always set the volume dial at 50 ml less than the prescribed volume or 50 ml less than the volume in the container *so that you can hang a new container before the old one empties completely.*
• Check the patency of the I.V. line and watch for infiltration. If you're using a controller, monitor the accuracy of the infusion rate.
• Tape all connections and recheck the controller's drip rate *because taping may alter it.*
• Turn on the alarm switches. Then explain the alarm system to the patient *to prevent anxiety when a change in the infusion activates the alarm.*

Special considerations
Monitor the pump or controller and the patient frequently *to ensure the device's correct operation and flow rate, and to detect infiltration and such complications as infection and air embolism.*

If electrical power fails, the pumps will automatically switch to battery power.

Check the manufacturer's recommendations before administering opaque fluids, such as blood, because some pumps fail to detect opaque fluids and others may cause hemolysis of infused blood.

Move the tubing in controllers every few hours *to prevent permanent compression or tubing damage.* Change the tubing and cassette every 48 hours or according to hospital policy.

Remove I.V. solutions from the refrigerator 1 hour before infusing them to help release small gas bubbles from the solutions. *Small bubbles in the solution can join to form larger bubbles, which can activate the pump's air-in-line alarm.*

Home care
Be sure the patient and his family understand the purpose of using the pump or controller. If necessary, demonstrate how the device works. Also demonstrate how to maintain the system (tubing, solution, and site assessment and care) until you're confident that the patient and family can proceed safely. As time permits, have the patient repeat the demonstration. Discuss which complications to watch for, such as infiltration, and review what measures to take if complications occur. Schedule a teaching session with the patient or family so you can answer questions they may have about the procedure before the patient's discharge.

Complications
Complications associated with I.V. controllers and pumps are the same as those associated with peripheral lines. (See "Insertion of a peripheral I.V. line," page 272.) Keep in mind that infiltration can develop rapidly with infusion by a volumetric pump because the increased subcutaneous pressure won't slow the infusion rate until significant edema occurs.

Documentation
In addition to routine documentation of the I.V. infusion, record the use of a controller or pump on the I.V. record and in your notes.

PARENTERAL NUTRITION
Equipment preparation and site care for total parenteral nutrition

Total parenteral nutrition (TPN) is the parenteral administration of a solution of dextrose, proteins, electrolytes, vitamins, and trace elements in amounts that exceed the patient's energy expenditure and thereby achieve anabolism. Because this solution has about six times the solute concentration of blood, it requires dilution by delivery into a high-flow central vein to avoid injury to the peripheral vasculature. Typically, the solution is delivered to the superior vena cava through an indwelling subclavian vein catheter inserted by the infraclavicular approach or, less commonly, by the supraclavicular, internal jugular, or antecubital fossa approach.

A patient may receive TPN for any of the following reasons:
• debilitating illness lasting longer than 2 weeks
• limited or no oral intake for longer than 7 days, such as in cases of multiple traumatic injuries, severe burns, or anorexia nervosa
• loss of 10% or more of pre-illness weight
• serum albumin level below 3.5 g/dl
• poor tolerance of long-term enteral feedings
• chronic vomiting or diarrhea
• continued weight loss despite adequate oral intake
• GI disorders that prevent or severely reduce absorption, such as bowel obstruction, Crohn's disease, ulcerative colitis, short bowel sydrome, cancer malabsorption syndrome, and bowel fistulas
• inflammatory GI disorders, such as pancreatitis and peritonitis
• excessive nitrogen loss resulting from wound infection, fistulas, or abscesses
• renal or hepatic failure.

TPN also promotes normal growth and development in infants with congenital anomalies, such as tracheo-esophageal fistula, gastroschisis, duodenal atresia, cystic fibrosis, meconium ileus, diaphragmatic hernia, volvulus, malrotation of the gut, and annular pancreas.

Because TPN solution supports bacterial growth and the central venous (CV) line gives systemic access, contamination and sepsis are always a risk. Strict surgical asepsis is required during solution, dressing, tubing, and filter changes. Site care and dressing changes should be performed according to hospital policy, usually at least three times weekly (once weekly for transparent dressings), and whenever the dressing becomes wet, soiled, or nonocclusive. Tubing and filter changes are performed every 24 to 48 hours according to hospital policy.

Equipment
Infusion pump and sterile tubing ▪ extension tubing ▪ two pairs of sterile gloves ▪ organic solvent (such as 70% alcohol) ▪ alcohol sponges ▪ antimicrobial solution (such as povidone-iodine) ▪ povidone-iodine ointment (or substitute) ▪ bags or bottles of TPN solution ▪ sterile 4″ × 4″ gauze pads ▪ cotton-tipped applicators ▪ transparent semipermeable dressing ▪ antiseptic adhesive balsam ▪ nonallergenic tape ▪ time tape ▪ optional: two face masks, sterile scissors, sterile drape, precut drain dressing, dex-

trose 10% in water, 0.22-micron cellulose membrane filter (1.2 microns if solution contains lipid emulsions or albumin), and luer-lock connections.

Some administration sets include single tubing with an in-line filter incorporated into the tubing. Prepackaged dressing kits are available commercially.

Preparation of equipment
Remove the 1-liter, 2-liter, or 3-liter bags or bottles of TPN solution from the refrigerator at least 1 hour before use *because delivery of a chilled solution can cause pain, hypothermia, venous spasm, and venous constriction.*

Double-check the contents of the solution and the doctor's orders. Then observe the solution for cloudiness, turbidity, and particles and the container for cracks; if any of these are present, return the solution to the pharmacy. (See *Types of parenteral nutrition*, pages 298 and 299, to compare solutions.)

Always maintain strict aseptic technique when preparing and handling equipment. Connect, in sequence, the pump tubing, cellulose membrane filter (if applicable), and extension tubing. Tape the tubing connections or use the luer-lock connections, if available, *to prevent accidental separation, which can lead to air embolism, exsanguination, and sepsis.* Squeeze the drip chamber of the tubing before spiking the bag or bottle, turn it upright and, using strict aseptic technique, insert the tubing spike into the port of the TPN container and release the drip chamber. *This prevents accidental dripping of TPN solution from a bottle (bags won't drip).* Start the flow of solution *to prime the tubing and remove air.* Gently tap the tubing *to dislodge air bubbles trapped in the Y ports.* If necessary, attach a time tape to the TPN container *to allow approximate measurement of fluid intake.* Attach the set-up to the infusion pump and prepare it according to the manufacturer's instructions.

Implementation
• Explain the procedure, make sure the bedside area is clean, and open the equipment.
• If required, put on a mask (especially if the patient is immunodeficient), and position the patient supine, with his head turned away from the catheter insertion site. If hospital policy dictates and the patient can tolerate it, place a mask over his nose and mouth. Place a sterile drape over the patient if he's being mechanically ventilated.
• Put on gloves.
• Remove the dressing carefully, pulling the tape gently from the skin *to minimize traumatic injury.* Then inspect the skin for signs of infection and the catheter for leaks or other mechanical problems. Remove your gloves.

(Text continues on page 300.)

Types of parenteral nutrition

TYPE	SOLUTION COMPONENTS/LITER	USES	SPECIAL CONSIDERATIONS
Standard I.V. therapy	• Dextrose, water, electrolytes in varying amounts. For example: $D_5W = 170$ calories/liter, $D_{10}W = 340$ calories/liter, 0.9% sodium chloride = 0 calories • Vitamins as ordered	• Less than 1 week as nutrition source • Maintains hydration (main function) • Facilitates and maintains normal metabolic function	• Nutritionally incomplete; does not provide sufficient calories to maintain adequate nutritional status
Total parenteral nutrition (TPN) via central venous (CV) line	• Dextrose 20% to 25% in water (1 liter dextrose 25% = 850 nonprotein calories) • Crystalline amino acids 2.5% to 8.5% • Electrolytes, vitamins, trace elements, insulin, and heparin, as ordered • Lipid emulsion 10% to 20% (usually infused as a separate solution, but an infusion system is available in which dextrose, protein, and lipids are mixed in the same container)	• 3 weeks or more • For patients with large caloric and nutrient needs • Provides calories, restores nitrogen balance, and replaces essential vitamins, electrolytes, minerals, and trace elements • Promotes tissue synthesis, wound healing, and normal metabolic function • Allows bowel rest and healing; reduces activity in the gallbladder, pancreas, and small intestine • Improves tolerance of surgery	***Basic solution*** • Nutritionally complete • Requires minor surgical procedure for CV line insertion (can be done at bedside by the doctor) • Highly hypertonic solution • May cause metabolic complications (glucose intolerance, electrolyte imbalance, essential fatty acid deficiency) ***I.V. lipid emulsion*** • May not be used effectively in severely stressed patients (especially burn patients) • May interfere with immune mechanisms • Given via CV line; irritates peripheral vein in long-term use
Total nutrient admixture	• One day's nutrients are contained in a single, 3-liter bag (also called 3:1 solution) • Combines lipids with other parenteral solution components	• 3 weeks or more • For relatively stable patients because solution components can be adjusted just once daily • For other uses, see TPN (above)	• See TPN (above) • Reduces need to handle bag, cutting risk of contamination • Decreases nursing time and reduces need for infusion sets and electronic devices, lowering hospital costs, increasing patient mobility, and allowing easier adjustment to home care • Precludes use of certain infusion pumps because they can't accurately deliver large volumes of solution; precludes use of standard I.V. tubing filters because a 0.22-micron filter blocks lipid and albumin molecules

Types of parenteral nutrition *(continued)*

TYPE	SOLUTION COMPONENTS/LITER	USES	SPECIAL CONSIDERATIONS
Peripheral parenteral nutrition (PPN)	• Dextrose 5% to 12.5% • Crystalline amino acids 2.75% to 4.25% • Electrolytes, trace elements, and vitamins as ordered • Lipid emulsion 10% or 20% (1 liter dextrose 10% and amino acids 3.5% infused at the same time as 1 liter lipid emulsion = 1,440 nonprotein calories [340 from dextrose and 1,100 from lipid emulsion]) • Heparin or hydrocortisone, as ordered	• 3 weeks or less • Maintains nutritional state in patients who can tolerate relatively high fluid volume, in those who usually resume bowel function and oral feedings after a few days, and in those who are susceptible to infections of the CV catheter	***Basic solution*** • Nutritionally complete for a short time • Cannot be used in nutritionally depleted patients • Can't be used in volume-restricted patients because PPN exceeds CV line volume • Doesn't cause weight gain • Avoids insertion and care of CV line, but requires adequate venous access; site must be changed every 48 hours • Delivers less hypertonic solutions than CV line TPN • May cause phlebitis • Less chance of metabolic complications than with central line TPN ***I.V. lipid emulsion*** • As effective as dextrose for caloric source • Diminishes phlebitis if infused at the same time as basic nutrient solution • Irritates vein in long-term use • Reduces carbon dioxide buildup when pulmonary compromise is present
Protein-sparing therapy	• Crystalline amino acids in same amounts as TPN • Electrolytes, vitamins, and minerals as ordered	• 2 weeks or less • May preserve body protein in a stable patient • Augments oral or tube feedings	• Nutritionally complete • Requires little mixing • May be started or stopped any time during the hospital stay • Other I.V. fluids, medications, and blood by-products may be administered through the same I.V. line • Not as likely to cause phlebitis as PPN • Adds a major expense; has limited benefits

• Wash your hands, put on sterile gloves, and clean the catheter insertion site three times with alcohol sponges or cotton-tipped applicators soaked in an organic solvent, such as 70% alcohol. Work in a circular motion, moving from the insertion site outward to the edge of the adhesive border *to avoid introducing contaminants from the unclean area.*

• Working in a circular motion, as before, clean the insertion site and the catheter three times with the povidone-iodine solution.

• Instruct the patient to perform Valsalva's maneuver or to hold his breath on deep inspiration as you change the I.V. tubing. If the patient is being mechanically ventilated, change the I.V. tubing immediately after the machine delivers a breath at peak inspiration. *These measures increase intrathoracic pressure and prevent air embolism.*

• Set the infusion pump at the ordered flow rate and start the infusion.

• Ensure that the junction of the catheter tubing is secure (you may use luer-lock connections), remove the contaminated gloves, and put on a sterile pair.

• Following your hospital's policy, use a sterile cotton-tipped applicator or pad to apply povidone-iodine ointment to the skin at the insertion site and to the hub of the catheter at the catheter-tubing junction, being careful not to loosen the connections.

• Do not remove the povidone-iodine solution from the skin *because its antimicrobial effects are long-lasting and continue after drying.*

• Arrange the sterile dressing pads *to shield the catheter and skin from airborne contaminants.* A precut drain dressing may be used around the catheter.

• Apply adhesive balsam to the skin at the perimeter of the drain dressings.

• Tape the dressing securely to the skin.

• You may use a transparent semipermeable dressing instead of the gauze drain dressings and tape. *These allow visualization of the insertion site.* When using these dressings, do not use povidone-iodine ointment at the insertion site.

• Write the catheter insertion date, the date of the dressing change, and your initials on a strip of tape and apply this to the dressing.

• Loop and tape the administration tubing (but not the filter) over the intact dressing *to prevent tension on the catheter and its inadvertent removal if the tubing is pulled.*

Special considerations

If the patient is sensitive or allergic to iodine, use 70% alcohol as the antimicrobial agent. Scrub for 30 seconds or until the applicator comes away visibly clean.

When using a CV line for TPN, the following are contraindicated: infusion of blood or blood products, bolus injection of drugs, simultaneous administration of I.V. solutions, measurement of CV pressure, aspiration of blood for routine laboratory tests, addition of medication to a TPN solution container, and use of three-way stopcocks.

If the patient develops a fever, discontinue the TPN solution and replace it with dextrose 10% in water, infusing it at the same rate as the TPN solution. Change the I.V. tubing and dressing and notify the doctor, who may order bacterial and fungal cultures of the TPN solution, tubing, and blood. Reduction of fever within 4 to 6 hours after withdrawal implicates the solution or the delivery apparatus. If the fever persists, suspect catheter-related sepsis and again notify the doctor, who may then order blood and urine cultures to help determine the cause of infection. If necessary, the doctor will remove the catheter and order fungal and bacterial cultures. Fever usually subsides within 12 to 24 hours after catheter removal.

Observe the patient for signs of thrombosis or thrombophlebitis, such as erythema and edema at the catheter insertion site; ipsilateral swelling of the arm, neck, or face; pain along the course of the vein; and other systemic manifestations. If such signs occur, notify the doctor immediately; he may remove the catheter and start heparin infusion at a peripheral site.

Be alert for swelling at the catheter insertion site *because it indicates extravasation of the TPN solution, which can cause necrosis.* Check the catheter tubing for leaks from mechanical or chemical disruption.

Watch for signs and symptoms of air embolism: dyspnea, apprehension, chest pain, tachycardia, hypotension, cyanosis, seizures, loss of consciousness, and cardiopulmonary arrest. If you suspect air embolism, position the patient in left Trendelenburg's position *to allow air to pass from the pulmonary artery,* and administer supplemental oxygen. It may take several minutes for the air to dissipate.

Observe for catheter retraction from the vein, which may result from loosening of the sutures at the insertion site. Measure catheter length from the insertion site to the hub during dressing changes for verification.

Complications

Catheter-related sepsis is the most serious complication of TPN. Although uncommon, subclavian or jugular vein thrombosis can result from a malpositioned catheter and can precede septicemia. Air embolism, a potentially fatal complication, can occur during tubing replacement, from inadvertent disconnection of tubing and from undetected hairline cracks in the tubing. Extravasation of TPN solution can cause necrosis, with sequential sloughing of the epidermis and dermis.

Documentation
Record the times of dressing, filter, and solution changes; the condition of the catheter insertion site; your observations on the patient's condition; and any complications and resulting treatments.

Patient monitoring during total parenteral nutrition

Total parenteral nutrition (TPN) requires careful monitoring to assess the patient's response to the nutrient solution and to detect early signs of complications. Because the typical patient is in a protein-wasting state, TPN therapy causes marked changes in fluid and electrolyte status and in glucose, amino acid, mineral, and vitamin levels. If the patient displays an adverse reaction or signs of complications, the TPN regimen can be changed as needed.

Assessment of the patient's nutritional status includes physical examination, anthropometric measurements, biochemical determinations, and tests of cell-mediated immunity. Assessment of the patient's condition to detect complications requires recognition of the signs and symptoms of possible complications, understanding of laboratory test results, and careful record keeping.

Because the TPN solution is high in glucose, the infusion must start slowly to allow the patient's pancreatic beta cells to adapt to it by increasing insulin output. Usually, if the adult patient tolerates the TPN solution the first day, the doctor increases the intake to 1 liter every 12 hours for at least 2 days. Within the first 3 to 5 days of TPN, the typical adult patient can tolerate 3 liters of solution daily without adverse reactions. Lipid emulsions also require monitoring. (See *Precautions for giving lipid emulsions*, page 302.)

Equipment
Test kits for blood and urine glucose and urine ketones ▪ stethoscope ▪ sphygmomanometer ▪ watch with second hand ▪ scale ▪ input and output chart ▪ time tape ▪ additional equipment for nutritional assessment, as ordered ▪ optional: 10% dextrose in water.

If the patient is receiving cephalosporins, methyldopa, aspirin, or large doses of ascorbic acid, Tes-Tape should be used in place of Clinitest reagent tablets *to avoid false positive results in urine glucose and ketone determinations.*

Preparation of equipment
For preparation of the infusion pump and TPN solution, see appropriate sections of this chapter. Attach a time tape to the TPN container to allow approximate measurement of fluid intake. Make sure each bag or bottle has a label listing the expiration date, glucose concentration, and total volume of solution. (If the bag or bottle is damaged and you don't have an immediate replacement, hang a bag of dextrose 10% in water until the new container is ready.)

Implementation
● Explain the procedure to the patient *to diminish his anxiety and encourage cooperation.* Instruct the patient to inform you if he experiences any unusual sensations during the infusion. Begin the infusion at a slow rate (usually 40 ml/hour), as ordered, *to reduce the risk of hyperglycemia.* Then, as ordered, increase the adult patient's infusion rate (usually in 25 ml/hour increments) *to allow the pancreatic beta cells to increase endogenous insulin production, and to establish carbohydrate and water tolerances.*
● Record vital signs every 4 hours, or more often if necessary, *because increased temperature is one of the earliest signs of catheter-related sepsis.*
● Watch for swelling at the catheter site, *which may indicate extravasation of the TPN solution, possibly leading to tissue necrosis.*
● Check blood or urine for glucose and notify the doctor as appropriate.
● Perform I.V. site care and dressing changes at least three times a week (once a week for transparent semipermeable dressings), or whenever the dressing becomes wet, soiled, or nonocclusive. Use strict aseptic technique.
● Expect to change the tubing and filter every 24 to 48 hours, using strict aseptic technique. Make sure all tubing junctions are secure.
● Maintain flow rates, as prescribed, even if the flow falls behind schedule.
● Record daily fluid intake and output accurately. Specify the volume and type of each fluid, and calculate the daily caloric intake. *This record is a diagnostic tool for prompt, precise replacement of fluid and electrolyte deficits.*
● Physically assess the patient daily. If ordered, measure arm circumference and skinfold thickness over the triceps. Weigh the patient at the same time each morning (after voiding), in similar clothing, and on the same scale. Suspect fluid imbalance if the patient gains more than 1.1 lb (0.5 kg) daily.
● Monitor the results of routine laboratory tests and report abnormal findings to the doctor *to allow appropriate changes in the TPN solution.* Laboratory tests usually include serum electrolytes, blood urea nitrogen, and blood glucose at least three times weekly; and liver function

Precautions for giving lipid emulsions

You may administer lipid emulsions as part of a total parenteral nutrition (TPN) solution along with a peripheral parenteral nutrition (PPN) solution, or separately through either a central venous line or a peripheral I.V. line. No matter which of these methods you use, be sure to observe these precautions.

Before the infusion
• Use a particulate filter according to the manufacturer's recommendations (usually a 1.2-micron filter). Standard 0.22-micron filters are insufficient because lipid particles clog the filter and disturb the emulsion.
• Aways check the lipid emulsion for separation or an oily appearance. If either condition exists, the emulsion may have been disturbed and should not be used. Never shake the lipid container excessively or use the emulsion if you see any inconsistency in texture or color.
• Never add anything to the lipid emulsion; doing so could cause instability. Also, protect the emulsion from freezing.

During the infusion
• Monitor the patient's vital signs. The flow rate should not exceed 1 ml/minute for the first 30 minutes.

• Check for signs and symptoms of an adverse reaction. Indications of an immediate adverse reaction, which can occur within 2½ hours, include increased temperature, flushing, sweating, pressure sensations over the eyes, nausea, vomiting, headache, chest and back pain, dyspnea, and cyanosis. Indications of a delayed reaction, which occurs up to 10 days after the infusion, include hepatomegaly, splenomegaly, thrombocytopenia, focal seizures, hyperlipidemia, hepatic damage, jaundice, hemorrhagic diathesis, and gastroduodenal ulcer.

After the infusion
• Be aware of the biochemical and clinical signs and symptoms of essential fatty acid disease that may be associated with impaired wound healing, adverse effects on red blood cells, and ineffective prostaglandin synthesis. Check for dry or scaly skin, thinning hair, liver function abnormalities, and thrombocytopenia.
• Discard any unused emulsion; if contaminated, it can support microbial growth. The Centers for Disease Control guidelines recommend allowing lipid emulsions to hang no longer than 12 hours. Follow the manufacturer's recommendations.

studies, complete blood count and differential, and serum albumin, phosphorus, calcium, magnesium, and creatinine once weekly. Studies ordered less frequently include serum transferrin, prothrombin time, creatinine-height index, nitrogen balance, total lymphocyte count, and skin tests.
• Monitor the patient for signs and symptoms of glucose metabolism disturbance, fluid and electrolyte imbalances, and nutritional aberrations. Remember that some patients may require supplementary insulin for the duration of TPN; the pharmacy usually adds insulin directly to the TPN solution.
• Provide emotional support. Keep in mind that patients often associate eating with positive feelings and become disturbed when eating is prohibited.
• Provide frequent mouth care.
• Keep the patient active *to enable him to utilize nutrients more fully.*
• When discontinuing TPN, decrease the infusion rate slowly, depending on the patient's current glucose intake, *to minimize the risk of hyperinsulinemia and resulting hypoglycemia.* Weaning usually takes place over 24 to 48 hours but can be completed in 4 to 6 hours if the patient

receives sufficient oral or I.V. carbohydrates. You may use a cyclic administration schedule, as ordered, to wean the patient from TPN to enteral feedings.

Special considerations
Always maintain strict aseptic technique when handling the equipment used to administer therapy. *Because the TPN solution serves as a medium for bacterial growth and the central venous (CV) line provides systemic access, the patient risks infection and sepsis.*

When using a filter, position it as close to the access site as possible. Check the filter's porosity and psi capacity to make sure it exceeds the psi exerted by the infusion pump.

Don't allow TPN solutions to hang for more than 24 hours.

Be careful when using the TPN line for other functions. If using a single-lumen CV catheter, do not use the line to infuse blood or blood products, to give a bolus injection, to administer simultaneous I.V. solutions, to measure CV pressure, or to draw blood for laboratory tests. Never add medication to a TPN solution container.

Also, do not use a three-way stopcock, if possible, *because add-on devices increase the risk of infection.*

Complications
Catheter-related, metabolic, and mechanical complications can occur during TPN administration. (See *Dealing with TPN hazards,* pages 304 and 305.)

Documentation
Record serial monitoring indices on the appropriate flowchart to determine the patient's progress and response. Note any abnormal, adverse, or altered responses.

 # Peripheral parenteral nutrition

Using a solution that combines amino acids, dextrose (5% to 12.5%) in water, and a lipid emulsion, peripheral parenteral nutrition (PPN) can supply full caloric needs without the risks associated with a central venous (CV) line. Because this combined solution has a lower tonicity than a total parenteral nutrition solution, the success of PPN depends on the patient's tolerance for the large volumes of fluid necessary to supply full nutritional needs. PPN that includes a lipid emulsion is associated with a lower incidence of phlebitis than a solution that contains only amino acids and dextrose.

Patients who don't need to gain weight yet need nutritional support may receive PPN for as long as 2 to 3 weeks. It's used to maintain or restore fluid and electrolyte balance, to maintain homeostasis before and after surgery, and to help a patient meet minimum calorie and protein requirements.

This therapy may also be used as an adjunct to oral or enteral feedings for a patient who needs to supplement his low-calorie intake. Or PPN may be given to a patient who's unable to absorb enteral therapy.

PPN should be used cautiously in patients with severe hepatic damage, coagulation disorders, anemia, and pulmonary disease, and in those at increased risk for fat embolism. It should not be used for patients with malnutrition or metabolic disorders, such as pathologic hyperlipidemia, lipid nephrosis, and acute pancreatitis accompanied by hyperlipidemia.

Equipment
Amino acid-dextrose solution at room temperature (dextrose should not exceed 12.5%) ▪ lipid emulsion ▪ two controllers or pumps ▪ Y-type nonphthalate administration set ▪ alcohol sponges ▪ adhesive tape ▪ I.V. pole and venipuncture equipment, if necessary ▪ sterile gloves.

The only additive allowed to the lipid emulsion is sodium heparin (in a small dose), which activates lipase, the enzyme needed to oxidize fatty acids and enhance clearance of fat from the blood. An excessive amount of sodium heparin can deplete the body's stores of lipase.

A nonphthalate administration set, designed especially for simultaneous infusion of lipid emulsion and amino acid-dextrose solution, consists of two lines in a Y configuration. (See *Giving lipids and amino acids together,* page 306.) The vented line is used for the lipid emulsion; the nonvented line, containing a filter, for the amino acid-dextrose solution. This special nonphthalate tubing is necessary because lipids can extract small amounts of phthalates from phthalate-plasticized polyvinylchloride tubing.

Controllers that can accommodate the special tubing are needed to ensure the correct infusion rate *because the risk of phlebitis is smaller when two components are administered at approximately the same rate.*

Preparation of equipment
Inspect the lipid emulsion for opacity and consistency of color and texture. If the emulsion looks frothy, oily, or contains particles, or if its stability or sterility is questionable, return the bottle to the pharmacy. Avoid shaking the bottle excessively *to prevent aggregation of fat globules.*

Similarly, inspect the amino acid-dextrose solution for cloudiness, turbidity, and particles and the bottle for cracks; if any of these are present, return the bottle to the pharmacy.

Wash your hands and, using aseptic technique, take the nonphthalate tubing from its package. Close the flow clamp *to equalize pressure in the tubing.* Remove the protective cap from the lipid emulsion bottle, and wipe the rubber stopper with an alcohol sponge. Hold the bottle upright, and insert the vented spike through the inner circle of the rubber stopper. Invert the bottle, and squeeze the drip chamber until it fills to the level indicated in the tubing package instructions. Open the flow clamp, allow fat emulsion to flow through to the Y connector, and then close the clamp.

Remove the protective cap from the container of amino acid-dextrose solution, and wipe the rubber stopper with an alcohol sponge. Hold the bottle upright and insert the nonvented spike. Squeeze the drip chamber to eliminate dripping of solution, invert the bottle, and squeeze the drip chamber until the fluid reaches the desired level. Hold the filter with the Y connector facing upward and the air vent downward, and open the clamp. Start the solution flow *to remove air from the filter and line.* Then close the clamp.

Dealing with TPN hazards

COMPLICATIONS	SIGNS AND SYMPTOMS	INTERVENTIONS
Metabolic hazards		
Hyperglycemia	Fatigue, restlessness, confusion, anxiety, weakness, and (in severe cases) delirium or coma; polyuria; dehydration; elevated glucose levels	• Start insulin therapy or adjust total parenteral nutrition (TPN) flow rate.
Hypoglycemia	Sweating, shaking, irritability when infusion is stopped	• Infuse dextrose 10% in water.
Hyperosmolar nonketotic syndrome	Confusion, lethargy, seizures, coma, hyperglycemia, dehydration, glycosuria	• Stop the dextrose infusion. • Give insulin and 0.45% sodium chloride to rehydrate.
Hypokalemia	Muscle weakness, paralysis, paresthesia, arrhythmias	• Increase potassium supplementation.
Hypomagnesemia	Tingling around mouth, paresthesia in fingers, mental changes, hyperreflexia	• Increase magnesium supplementation.
Hypophosphatemia	Irritability, weakness, paresthesia, coma, respiratory arrest	• Increase phosphate supplementation.
Hypocalcemia	Polyuria, dehydration, elevated blood and urine glucose levels	• Increase calcium supplementation.
Metabolic acidosis	Increased serum chloride level, decreased serum bicarbonate level	• Use acetate or lactate salts of sodium or hydrogen.
Hepatic dysfunction	Increased serum transaminase, lactate dehydrogenase, and bilirubin levels	• Use special hepatic formulations. • Decrease carbohydrates and add I.V. lipids.
Mechanical hazards		
Clotted catheter	Interrupted flow rate, hypoglycemia	• Reposition the catheter. Attempt to aspirate clot. • If unsuccessful, instill urokinase to clear catheter lumen, as ordered.
Dislodged catheter	Catheter out of the vein	• Place a sterile gauze pad on the site and apply pressure.
Air embolism	Apprehension, chest pain, tachycardia, hypotension, cyanosis, seizures, loss of consciousness, cardiac arrest	• Clamp the catheter. • Place patient in Trendelenburg's position on left side. Give oxygen as ordered. • If cardiac arrest occurs, begin cardiopulmonary resuscitation.

Dealing with TPN hazards *(continued)*

COMPLICATIONS	SIGNS AND SYMPTOMS	INTERVENTIONS
Mechanical hazards *(continued)*		
Thrombosis	Erythema and edema at insertion site; ipsilateral swelling of arm, neck, and face; pain at the insertion site and along vein; malaise; fever; tachycardia	• Remove the catheter promptly. • Administer heparin if ordered. • Venous flow studies may be done.
Too-rapid infusion	Nausea, headache, lethargy	• Check the infusion rate. • Check the infusion pump if you're using one.
Extravasation	Swelling of tissue around the insertion site; pain	• Stop the I.V. infusion. • Assess the patient for cardiopulmonary abnormalities. • Chest X-ray may be performed.
Phlebitis	Pain, tenderness, redness, and warmth	• Apply gentle heat to the insertion site. • Elevate the insertion site if possible.
Cracked or broken tubing	Fluid leaking from the tubing	• Apply a padded hemostat above the break to prevent air from entering the line.
Pneumothorax and hydrothorax	Dyspnea, chest pain, cyanosis, decreased breath sounds	• Apply suction. • Chest tube will be inserted.
Sepsis	Fever, chills, leukocytosis, erythema or pus at the insertion site	• Remove the catheter and culture the tip. • Give appropriate antibiotics.

If your administration set contains a second Y injection site, insert it and tap gently *to remove all air from the tubing* before closing the clamp.

If you're initiating the infusion, hang the containers on the I.V. pole after inserting the spikes. Always hang the lipid emulsion container higher than the amino acid-dextrose container *so that the lipid emulsion doesn't backflow into the amino acid set.* Then attach the controllers to the I.V. pole, and prepare them according to manufacturer's instructions.

Implementation

• Explain the procedure to the patient *to ease his anxiety and promote his cooperation.*
• Obtain baseline vital signs, as ordered. If necessary, perform a venipuncture. Select the patient's largest available vein as the insertion site *to ensure hemodilution of the irritating PPN solution.* When using a short-term catheter that requires 48- to 72-hour site rotation, try applying heat to the site to facilitate insertion.

To start the infusion
• Connect the administration set to the I.V. needle or catheter hub. Then turn on the controllers and set them to the desired flow rate (start the infusion slowly and increase gradually to ensure tolerance to the hypertonic solution). Next, completely open the flow clamps *to allow the controllers to regulate the flow rate.*
• Monitor vital signs every 10 minutes for the first 30 minutes and every hour thereafter.

To change the solutions
• Remove the protective caps, and wipe the stoppers of the solution containers with alcohol sponges.

Giving lipids and amino acids together

The illustration below shows the setup you'll use to administer lipid emulsions with amino acids. Note that the lipid emulsion container is higher than the amino acid container.

Lipid emulsion container

Amino acid container

Vent

Vented line (60 gtt/ml)

Filtered line (10 gtt/ml)

Roller clamps

0.22 micron filter

Y connector

• Turn off the controllers, and close the flow clamps. Using strict aseptic technique, remove each spike and insert it in the new container.
• Hang the containers, turn on the controllers, and set the flow rate. Open the flow clamps completely.

To change the solutions and tubing
• Hang the new solution container and tubing alongside the old ones.
• Put on sterile gloves. Examine the skin above the insertion site for signs of phlebitis, such as redness, warmth, and pain. If such signs are present, remove the existing I.V. line and start a line in a different vein, using venipuncture equipment.
• Turn off the controllers, and close the flow clamps on the old tubing. Disconnect the tubing from the needle or catheter hub, and connect the new tubing.
• Open the flow clamps on the new containers to equal, slow flow rates *to prevent clot formation in the needle or catheter while you're inserting the tubing into the controllers.*
• Remove the old tubing from the controllers, and insert the new tubing according to the manufacturer's instructions.
• Turn on the controllers, set them to the desired flow rate, and open the flow clamps completely.
• Remove the old equipment and dispose of it properly.

To change a dressing and needle or catheter
• Change the dressing at intervals specified by hospital policy (usually every 24 to 48 hours), and inspect the insertion site for signs of phlebitis.
• Change the needle or catheter according to hospital policy or at the onset of signs of phlebitis.
• Loop and tape the tubing *to prevent its dislodging from the needle or catheter hub.*

Special considerations
Always use strict aseptic technique when handling equipment, and never reuse a partially empty bottle of lipid emulsion *because it is an excellent medium for bacterial growth.* All bottles, bags, tubing, and filters should be changed every 24 hours. Be alert for signs of sepsis, such as elevated temperature, chills, malaise, leukocytosis, and altered level of consciousness.

Observe the patient's reaction to the lipid emulsion; usually, the patient experiences a feeling of satiety but occasionally reports an unpleasant metallic taste in his mouth. Monitor the patient's lipid tolerance rate closely. Cloudy plasma in a centrifuged sample of citrated blood indicates that the fat hasn't been cleared from the bloodstream. Lipid emulsion may clear from the blood at an accelerated rate in a patient with full-thickness burns, multiple traumatic injuries, and metabolic imbalance *because catecholamines, adrenocortical hormones, thyroxine, and growth hormone enhance lipolysis and mobilization of fatty acids.*

Check serum triglyceride levels; these should return to normal within 18 hours after infusion of a bottle of lipid emulsion. As ordered, obtain blood samples for laboratory analysis; typically, aspartate aminotransferase (formerly SGOT), alanine aminotransferase (formerly SGPT), alkaline phosphatase, cholesterol, triglyceride, plasma free fatty acid, and coagulation tests are performed weekly *to monitor the patient's response.*

Because lipase synthesis increases insulin requirements, increase the insulin dosage of the patient with diabetes, as ordered. For the patient with hypothyroidism, administer thyroid-stimulating hormone — which affects lipase activity — as ordered, *to prevent intravascular accumulations of triglycerides.*

Monitor for signs and symptoms of adverse reactions to lipid emulsion therapy.

Complications

Immediate or early adverse reactions to lipid emulsion therapy, which reportedly occur in fewer than 1% of patients, include fever, dyspnea, cyanosis, nausea, vomiting, headache, flushing, diaphoresis, lethargy, syncope, chest and back pain, slight pressure over the eyes, irritation at the infusion site, hyperlipemia, hypercoagulability, and thrombocytopenia. Thrombocytopenia has been reported in infants receiving 20% I.V. lipid emulsion.

Delayed but uncommon complications associated with prolonged administration of lipid emulsion include hepatomegaly, splenomegaly, jaundice secondary to central lobular cholestasis, and blood dyscrasias (thrombocytopenia, leukopenia, and transient increases in liver function studies). For unknown reasons, a few patients receiving 20% I.V. lipid emulsion have developed brown pigmentation (I.V. fat pigment) in the reticuloendothelial system.

In a premature or low-birth-weight infant, PPN with lipid emulsion may cause lipid accumulation in the lungs.

Documentation

Record the dates and times of all dressing and cannula changes, the duration and amount of each infusion, and the patient's condition and response to therapy.

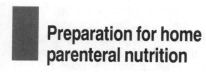

Preparation for home parenteral nutrition

Home parenteral nutrition (HPN) makes possible prolonged or indefinite I.V. total parenteral nutrition (TPN). This technique has dramatically improved the health of patients with such chronic conditions as Crohn's disease and malabsorption syndrome, and with such acute conditions as incomplete bowel obstruction and antineo-

plastic therapy. It has also decreased the duration of hospitalization. Although peripheral parenteral nutrition may be administered at home, long-term TPN is the primary home care therapy.

To prepare for HPN, a barium-impregnated silicone rubber catheter with a Dacron cuff is implanted, usually in the superior vena cava. Its entrance site is on the anterior abdomen to allow the patient to care for the catheter. About 2 to 3 weeks after implantation, firm tissue covers the catheter cuff to provide a physical barrier to microbial contamination.

Preparation for HPN usually necessitates extensive patient teaching and, when possible, instructions for the patient's family.

Typically, patients receiving HPN can ingest part of their caloric requirements during the day and require about 10 to 14 hours of infusion nightly to supply the remaining nutrients. If all the patient's nutrition must be received I.V., a continuous infusion may be necessary. For intermittent and continuous infusion, patient teaching must include techniques for proper care. (See *Teaching topics for home parenteral nutrition,* page 308.)

Equipment

Teaching aids (including audiovisual teaching aids and mannequins) as available ■ I.V. infusion apparatus ■ dressings ■ TPN solution ■ volumetric infusion pump ■ portable I.V. pole or ambulatory TPN vest ■ HPN supplies (including tubing, dressings, TPN solution).

Implementation

• Assess the patient's ability to perform the care routines necessary for HPN, and determine if family members or friends can assist with or perform them. Consider the patient's motivation, mental aptitude, job or other daily activities, home environment, and the accessibility of hospitals, home nursing services, and other health care support systems.

• Formulate a teaching plan based on this assessment and on the patient's expectations. Be sure the plan incorporates goals, specifies criteria for meeting them, and proceeds from simple to complex tasks *to allow the patient to develop confidence.* Avoid placing time limits on goals *because learning ability and mastery of tasks requiring manual dexterity vary from patient to patient.*

• If desired, develop a written contract between you and the patient that specifies the goals of HPN and the means to achieve them. Revise the contract as necessary *to reflect changes in the patient's needs and performance. Use of the contractual relationship enhances the patient's independence, minimizes conflict and frustration between patient and nurse, encourages open communication, and promotes a cooperative patient-nurse relationship.*

Teaching topics for home parenteral nutrition

Techniques
☐ Catheter heparinization
☐ How to destroy contaminated needles and syringes
☐ Dressing changes
☐ Drug administration
☐ Hand washing
☐ Lipid emulsion administration
☐ Tubing changes
☐ Pump operation
☐ Self-monitoring of intake and output, weight, temperature, diet
☐ Solution preparation
☐ Use of sterile equipment

Related topics
☐ How to detect complications, such as air embolism, thrombosis, clotted or fractured catheter, pump malfunction, metabolic disturbance, solution contamination
☐ Financial support, home referral, medical alert, and networking services
☐ Follow-up appointments
☐ How to maintain procedures when traveling
☐ How to find, buy, and store supplies
☐ How to schedule infusions
☐ Weaning

• Conduct teaching sessions in a quiet area and, if possible, arrange to have a family member present. *When the family member understands the patient's pathophysiology, medical management, and progress, he tends to be less anxious, more satisfied with the quality of health care, and more able to acknowledge the limitations and constraints of HPN.*
• Use a variety of teaching aids *to accommodate differences in the patient's ability.* When teaching the mature patient, use an extensively illustrated manual (if available) that includes goals, equipment, procedures with rationales, suggested learning activities, and evaluations of HPN equipment. Give demonstrations with mannequins (if available) and real equipment *to involve the patient actively and reduce anxiety about performing the HPN tasks.* Stimulate the patient's interest with audiovisual teaching aids.
• Offer positive feedback during all teaching phases.

• Before discharge, critically evaluate the patient's ability to perform HPN tasks and ensure that all essential learning goals have been met.
• Remind the patient to change the catheter site dressing as ordered (usually every 2 to 3 days) or whenever it becomes soiled or nonocclusive and to change administration tubing as scheduled. Tell the patient to wash gently around the site and to take only sponge baths. Tell him he may be allowed to remove his dressing and bathe or shower after the implanted catheter has been in place for 1 month or longer.
• Also remind the patient to prevent contact between the catheter and granular or lint-producing surfaces *to avoid local tissue reaction from airborne particles and surface contaminants.*
• Discuss a suitable TPN schedule with the patient, considering his nutritional needs as well as his life-style. Emphasize his adherence to the prescribed schedule and volume *to prevent glucose imbalance.*
• Arrange for a home care agency to help the patient adjust to HPN and resolve any difficulties (including how to obtain supplies), or notify the hospital's discharge planner *so the appropriate referrals can be made.*

Special considerations
Suggest that the patient wear a medical identification bracelet or subscribe to a medical alert service. Tell the patient that a nurse from the home health care team will always be available in case of emergency.

To preserve as much patient mobility as possible, equipment such as the ambulatory TPN vest is available. This vest is made from lightweight materials and is adjustable to individual specifications. Breast pockets accommodate bags of nutrient solution, which are attached to the front of each shoulder. The pockets vary with the size of the nutrient bags. Y tubing connects these bags to a portable volumetric pump, located in a zippered pocket. To provide balance and enhance patient comfort, the pump empties both bags at the same rate. When the patient is wearing the vest, the administration tubing is coiled in one of the pockets. When the patient is not wearing the vest, the nutrient bags can hang from a clothes hanger.

Because the financial burden of long-term or permanent HPN can be devastating—even for the patient with health insurance—make a social service referral. Inform the elderly patient that Medicare may assume the cost of supplies and pharmaceuticals if he meets eligibility requirements.

Documentation
Record your patient teaching measures and the patient's learning progress in your notes.

BLOOD AND BLOOD COMPONENTS

Transfusion of whole blood and packed cells

Whole-blood transfusion replenishes both the volume and the oxygen-carrying capacity of the circulatory system. Transfusion of packed red blood cells (RBCs), from which 80% of the plasma has been removed, restores only the oxygen-carrying capacity. Both types of transfusion treat decreased hemoglobin and hematocrit levels. Whole blood is usually transfused only when decreased levels result from hemorrhage; packed RBCs are transfused when such depressed levels accompany normal blood volume, avoiding possible fluid and circulatory overload. Both whole blood and packed RBCs contain cellular debris, necessitating in-line filtration during administration. (Washed packed RBCs—commonly used for patients previously sensitized by transfusions—are rinsed with a special solution that removes white blood cells and platelets, thus decreasing the chance of transfusion reaction.)

Depending on hospital policy, two nurses may have to identify the patient and blood product before administering a transfusion to prevent errors and a potentially fatal reaction. The procedure also usually requires a signed patient consent form. If the patient is a Jehovah's Witness, transfusion requires special written permission.

Equipment

Blood recipient set (filter and tubing with drip chamber for blood, or combined set) ▪ I.V. pole ▪ gloves ▪ multiple-lead tubing ▪ whole blood or packed RBCs ▪ 250 ml of normal saline solution ▪ venipuncture equipment, if necessary (should include 18G catheter or 19G needle) ▪ optional: ice bag, warm compresses.

Straight-line and Y-type blood administration sets are commonly used. Although filters come in mesh and microaggregate types, the latter type is preferred, especially when transfusing multiple units of blood. New, highly effective leukocyte removal filters are available for use when transfusing blood and packed RBCs. Use of these filters delays a patient from becoming sensitive to transfusion therapy.

For some patients, you may need to use a blood warmer. (See *Using a dry-heat blood warmer,* page 310.)

Administer packed RBCs with a Y-type set. Using a straight-line set forces you to piggyback the tubing *so you can stop the transfusion if necessary but still keep the vein open.* Piggybacking increases the chance of harmful microorganisms entering the tubing as you're connecting the blood line to the established line.

Multiple-lead tubing minimizes the risk of contamination, especially when transfusing multiple units of blood (a straight-line set would require multiple piggybacking). A Y-type set gives you the option of adding normal saline solution to packed cells—decreasing their viscosity—if the patient can tolerate the added fluid volume.

Preparation of equipment

Avoid obtaining either whole blood or packed RBCs until you're ready to begin the transfusion *because RBCs deteriorate after 2 hours when stored at room temperature.* Prepare equipment when you're ready to start the infusion.

Implementation

• Explain the procedure to the patient. Ascertain that he has signed an informed consent form before transfusion therapy.

• Record the patient's vital signs *to serve as baseline values.*

• Obtain whole blood or packed RBCs from the blood bank within 30 minutes of the transfusion start time. Check the expiration date on the blood bag, and observe for abnormal color, RBC clumping, gas bubbles, and extraneous material. Return outdated or abnormal blood to the blood bank.

• Compare the name and number on the patient's wristband with those on the blood bag label. Check the blood bag identification number and ABO blood group and Rh compatibility. Also, compare the patient's blood bank identification number, if present, with the number on the blood bag. Identification of blood and blood products is performed at the patient's bedside by two licensed professionals according to hospital policy.

• Put on gloves. Using a Y-type set, close all the clamps on the set. Then insert the spike of the line you're using for the normal saline solution into the bag of saline solution. Next, open the port on the blood bag and insert the spike of the line you're using to administer the blood or cellular component into the port. Hang the normal saline solution and blood or cellular component on the I.V. pole, open the clamp on the line of saline solution, and squeeze the drip chamber until it's half full of saline solution. Then remove the adapter cover at the tip of the blood administration set, open the main flow clamp, and prime the tubing with saline solution.

• If you're administering packed RBCs with a Y-type set, you can add saline solution to the bag *to dilute the cells* by closing the clamp between the patient and the drip chamber and opening the clamp from the blood. Then lower the blood bag below the saline container and let

Using a dry-heat blood warmer

Rapid transfusion of cold blood can lead to hypothermia and may cause arrhythmias. Depending on hospital policy, you may use a dry-heat blood warmer for massive, rapid transfusions and for exchange transfusions in neonates. You can also use this device for transfusions in patients with increased cold agglutinin titers. The warmer maintains a constant temperature of 98.6° F (37° C). To use the blood warmer, follow these steps:
• Attach the blood warmer to an I.V. pole at mattress height. Plug in the device. Prepare and hang a Y-set with a blood bag and normal saline solution.
• Insert the warming bag into the blood warmer. The lead at the bottom of the warming bag is attached to the Y-set. The lead at the top of the warming bag is connected to the patient. Match these leads to the corresponding openings and mount the warming bag on the support pins, keeping the bag flat against the back panel. Then secure the pins.
• Close the blood warmer door and secure the latch. Turn the machine on, and allow it to operate for at least 2 minutes to warm up. (Avoid opening the door at any time during the transfusion. Otherwise, you'll break the vacuum and will have to replace the warming bag.)
• While the blood warmer is heating up, connect the blood-line adapter to the female adapter on the bottom lead. When the desired temperature is indicated on the machine, open the saline line to fill the bag with normal saline solution. Squeeze the outlet chamber until it's flat; continue to hold the chamber. When saline solution appears in the chamber, close the main flow clamp and release the chamber. The chamber then automatically fills halfway with saline solution.
• Remove the adapter cover on the top lead and open the clamp. Expel residual air from the line. Proceed as you would when administering blood with a Y-type set.

Blood

Normal saline solution

Microaggregate filter

Top lead connector

Temperature gauge

On/off switch

Outlet chamber

Main flow clamp

30 to 50 ml of saline flow into the packed cells. Finally, close the clamp to the blood bag, rehang the bag, rotate it gently *to mix the cells and saline solution,* and close the clamp to the saline container.
• If the patient doesn't have an I.V. line in place, perform venipuncture, preferably using an 18G catheter or 19G needle. Avoid using an existing line if the needle or catheter lumen is smaller than 20G. Central venous access devices also may be used for transfusion therapy.
• If you're administering whole blood, gently invert the bag several times *to mix the cells.*
• Attach the prepared blood administration set to the venipuncture device and flush it with normal saline solution.

Transfusing blood under pressure

Transfuse blood under pressure only when rapid replacement is necessary. Begin this procedure by selecting the proper equipment—a pressure cuff or a positive-pressure set. The *pressure cuff,* which resembles a sleeve, is placed over the blood bag and inflated; a pressure gauge, attached to the cuff, is calibrated in millimeters of mercury (mm Hg). The *positive-pressure set* is a gravity administration set containing a built-in pressure chamber that increases the flow rate when manual pressure is applied externally to the chamber.

Prepare the patient and set up the equipment just as you would a standard administration set. Connect the tubing to the needle or catheter hub. Throughout the transfusion, watch the patient closely for complications, such as infiltration or extravasation, which can occur quite rapidly.

To use a pressure cuff
• Insert your hand into the pressure-cuff sleeve and pull the blood bag upward through the center opening. Then grasp one loop of the sleeve, slip it through the blood bag loop, and pull the other sleeve loop through it.
• Hang the blood bag on the I.V. pole. Open the flow clamp on the tubing.
• To set the flow rate, turn the screw clamp on the pressure cuff counterclockwise, as shown at upper right.
• Compress the pressure bulb of the cuff to inflate the bag until you achieve the desired flow rate. Then turn the screw clamp clockwise *to maintain this constant flow rate. Note:* As the blood bag empties, the pressure decreases, so check the flow rate regularly and adjust the pressure in the pressure cuff as necessary *to maintain a constant flow rate.* Don't allow the cuff needle to exceed 300 mm Hg *because excessively high pressure may cause hemolysis of red blood cells or even rupture the blood bag.*

To use a positive-pressure set
• Open the upper and lower flow clamps on the administration set. Manually compress and release the pump chamber *to force the blood down the tubing and into the patient,* as shown at right. Allow the pump chamber to refill completely before compressing it again.
• Continue to compress and release the chamber until the blood bag empties or until rapid administration is no longer necessary. *To discontinue transfusion under pressure,* stop compressing the chamber and adjust the flow rate as for standard administration.

Pressure cuff

Positive-pressure set

Administering transfusions in the home

To administer transfusions to patients at home, follow this procedure:
• Transport blood products in a container with the appropriate coolant for the product. The proper temperature for transporting blood is between 33.8° and 50° F (1° and 10° C); for platelets, between 68° and 75° F (20° and 24° C).
• Encourage the patient to void before beginning the procedure *because the transfusion may take up to 2 hours.*
• Set up and transfuse the product according to your agency's or institution's policy.
• After stopping the infusion, keep the I.V. line open and remain with the patient for at least 30 minutes *to watch for delayed reaction to the procedure.* Take a final set of vital signs, and complete all charting.
• If no reactions occur after 30 minutes, remove the I.V. and give the patient or a caretaker posttransfusion instructions. Place all equipment, including the containers and infusion devices, in a biohazard bag and then into the transport container. Return the container to the blood bank for proper disposal.
• If a transfusion reaction occurs, notify the transfusion service and the patient's doctor immediately.

• Then close the clamp to the saline solution and open the clamp between the blood bag and the patient. Adjust the flow clamp closest to the patient to deliver the blood at the calculated drip rate.
• Be sure to remain with the patient, and watch for signs of transfusion reaction. If such signs develop, record vital signs, stop the transfusion, infuse the saline solution at a keep-vein-open rate, and notify the doctor immediately. If no signs of a reaction appear within 15 minutes, you'll need to adjust the flow clamp to the ordered infusion rate. Raising and lowering the blood bag *to adjust the rate reduces the risk of hemolysis from pressure on the tubing.* A unit of RBCs may be given over a period of 1 to 4 hours, as ordered.
• After completing the transfusion, you'll need to put on gloves and flush the filter and tubing with normal saline solution, if this is recommended by the manufacturer. Then remember to reconnect the original I.V. fluid or discontinue the I.V.

• Return the empty blood bag to the blood bank, and discard the tubing and filter.
• Record the patient's vital signs.

Special considerations
Although some microaggregate filters can be used for up to 10 units of blood, always replace the filter and tubing if more than 1 hour elapses between transfusions. When administering multiple units of blood under pressure, use a blood warmer *to avoid hypothermia.*

For rapid blood replacement, you may need to use a pressure bag. Be aware, however, that excessive pressure may develop, leading to broken blood vessels and extravasation, with hematoma and hemolysis of the infusing RBCs. (See *Transfusing blood under pressure,* page 311.)

If the transfusion stops, take the following steps as needed:
• Check that the I.V. container is at least 3' (1 m) above the level of the I.V. site.
• Make sure that the flow clamp is open and that the blood completely covers the filter. If it doesn't, squeeze the drip chamber until it does.
• Gently rock the bag back and forth, agitating any blood cells that may have settled on the bottom.
• Untape the dressing over the I.V. site to check needle placement. Reposition the needle if necessary.
• Flush the line with saline solution and restart the transfusion. Using a Y-type set, close the flow clamp to the patient and lower the blood bag. Next, open the saline clamp and allow some saline solution to flow into the blood bag. Rehang the blood bag, open the flow clamp to the patient, and reset the flow rate.

If a hematoma develops at the I.V. site, immediately stop the infusion. Remove the needle or catheter. Notify the doctor and expect to place ice intermittently on the site for 8 hours; then apply warm compresses. Promote reabsorption of the hematoma by having the patient gently exercise the affected limb. Document your observations and actions.

If the blood bag empties before the next one arrives, administer normal saline solution slowly. If you're using a Y-type set, close the blood-line clamp, open the saline-line clamp, and let the saline solution run slowly until the new blood arrives. Decrease the flow rate or clamp the line before attaching the new unit of blood.

Home care
Standards established by the American Association of Blood Banks, in accordance with federal, state, and local regulations, allow a doctor to order transfusions of blood products (not whole blood) for home care patients. To qualify, a patient must be unable to leave his home without assistance and must have received previous trans-

Understanding autotransfusion

Autotransfusion is the collection, filtration, and reinfusion of the patient's own blood. The procedure has several advantages over transfusion of bank blood. Autotransfusion uses blood that is warm, safe, and readily available. Most important, because autotransfused blood is autologous, it eliminates disease transmission, transfusion reactions, isoimmunization and, postoperatively, the addition of anticoagulants. Autotransfusion can overcome the objections of certain religious groups who oppose transfusions of donor blood. Unlike bank blood, autologous blood contains normal levels of 2,3-diphosphoglycerate advantageous for tissue oxygenation, potassium, ammonia, and clotting factors (except for fibrinogen); has a normal pH; and appears to have viable platelets. Occasionally, autologous blood causes transient hemoglobinuria because of traumatic injury to red blood cells (RBCs) during collection.

Indications and use

Autotransfusion techniques are used after traumatic injury and before, during, and after surgery. The trauma technique, most commonly used for hemothorax, can also be used in primary injuries of the lungs, liver, chest wall, heart, pulmonary vessels, spleen, kidneys, inferior vena cava, and iliac, portal, and subclavian veins. In this technique, the collection system uses citrated phosphate dextrose to prevent clotting of the collected blood.

The preoperative technique, also called autologous blood donation, is performed primarily for the patient with a rare blood type before major surgery or the patient for whom isoimmunization may complicate future transfusion needs. This technique follows standard blood-bank donation and transfusion procedures.

The intraoperative technique, used most often for thoracic and cardiovascular surgery, can also be used in hip and knee resection, spinal fusion, liver resection, and ruptured ectopic pregnancy. In this technique, a commercial cell washer-processor reduces anticoagulated collected whole blood to washed, packed RBCs for later reinfusion. The postoperative technique is used solely to collect shed mediastinal blood after cardiac surgery.

Autotransfusion is contraindicated in patients with malignant neoplasms, intrathoracic or systemic infections and infestations, coagulopathies, enteric contamination, excessive hemolysis, and when using an antibiotic at a site unsuitable for I.V. administration.

Nursing interventions

• Monitor vital signs, particularly the cardiovascular and respiratory signs.
• Maintain equipment sterility. Monitor and correct problems in the system.
• Monitor controlled suction.
• If an anticoagulant is ordered, ensure the proper ratio of anticoagulant to shed blood. (Consult the manufacturer's guidelines or doctor's order.)
• Monitor laboratory data during and after autotransfusion, particularly the coagulation profile, hemoglobin and hematocrit, arterial blood gas, and calcium levels.
• Document the amount of blood retrieved and reinfused in intake and output records.
• Infuse collected blood within 4 hours of collection.
• Follow the manufacturer's recommendations for proper use of the autotransfusion device.

---

fusions without difficulties. (See *Administering transfusions in the home*.)

Complications

Despite increasingly accurate crossmatching precautions, transfusion reactions can occur. (See *Understanding autotransfusion*.)

Unlike a transfusion reaction, an infectious disease transmitted during a transfusion may go undetected until days, weeks, or even months later, when it produces signs and symptoms. Measures to prevent disease transmission include laboratory testing of blood products and careful screening of potential donors, neither of which is guaranteed.

Hepatitis C (non-A, non-B) accounts for the majority of posttransfusion hepatitis cases. The tests that detect hepatitis B and hepatitis C can produce false-negative results and may allow some hepatitis cases to go undetected.

When testing for antibodies to human immunodeficiency virus (HIV), keep in mind that antibodies do not appear until about 6 to 12 weeks after exposure. Consequently, blood from a donor exposed to HIV but who has not yet developed antibodies could infect the recipient. The estimated risk of acquiring HIV from blood products varies from 1 in 40,000 to 1 in 153,000, depending on the source.

(Text continues on page 316.)

Reviewing transfusion products

PRODUCT	DESCRIPTION	NURSING CONSIDERATIONS
Whole blood	500-ml unit contains about 200 ml of red blood cells (RBCs) and about 300 ml of plasma.	• Indicated for massive blood loss and exchange transfusion in neonates. • Multiple-lead tubing (preferably a Y-type set) is recommended over piggybacking on a straight-line set. • Monitor vital signs frequently throughout transfusion. • Administer ABO group- and Rh type-specific product.
RBCs (packed)	350- to 400-ml unit contains about 200 to 250 ml of RBCs (with same amount of hemoglobin as whole blood) and 150 ml of plasma and additive solution (normal saline, adenine, glucose, and mannitol).	• Indicated for inadequate oxygen-carrying capacity. • A filter with larger surface area may be used to increase transfusion rate. • Administer ABO group- and Rh type-specific product, if possible. If not, group- and type-compatible product can be transfused safely.
RBCs (deglycerolized or leukocyte-poor)	200-ml unit contains RBCs suspended in 50 ml of normal saline, with virtually all leukocytes and plasma proteins removed. Deglycerolized RBCs, taken from donors with rare blood types, are first frozen (with glycerol added to preserve RBCs), then thawed and deglycerolized before transfusion. Leukocyte-poor RBCs aren't frozen.	• Same indications as for packed RBCs. Also used to prevent febrile reactions from leukocyte antibodies and to treat immunosuppressed patients. • All tubing should be rubber-free to prevent platelets from sticking. • Transfuse more rapidly than whole blood to prevent platelets from clumping and sticking to side of bag. • Administer ABO group- and Rh type-compatible product if possible. • Inspect unit for color. It should have a yellow tinge. • Agitate bag more often than other blood products because platelets tend to clump. • Adverse reactions are usually slight. • American Red Cross recommends that units of platelet concentrates be pooled in blood bank into transfer packs, rather than administered as single-donor units. Expiration date is usually 2 to 5 days from date of collection, depending on method of storage.
Platelets	30- to 60-ml unit contains about half the number of platelets originally found in 1 unit of whole blood.	• Indicated to treat thrombocytopenia, acute leukemia and marrow aplasia, and to restore platelet count preoperatively in a patient with a count of 100,000/mm³ or less. • ABO compatibility not necessary but recommended for repeated platelet transfusions. • Use a component drip administration set; infuse 100 ml over 15 minutes. • Patients with a history of platelet reaction require premedication with antipyretics and antihistamines. • Avoid administering when the patient has a fever.
Fresh frozen plasma	200- to 250-ml unit contains all coagulation factors and 250 mg of fibrinogen.	• Indicated to expand plasma volume, treat postoperative hemorrhage or shock, and correct coagulation factor deficiencies. • ABO compatibility not necessary. • Use a straight-line set and administer rapidly. • Large volume transfusions may require correction for hypocalcemia.

Reviewing transfusion products *(continued)*

PRODUCT	DESCRIPTION	NURSING CONSIDERATIONS
Cryoprecipitated antihemophilic factor	Frozen 20-ml unit contains mostly coagulation Factor VIII, plus 250 mg of fibrinogen.	• Indicated for hemophilia A, von Willebrand's disease, hypofibrinogenemia, and "fibrin glue." • Smaller needle or catheter size (22G or 23G for adults) may be used because product is not viscous. • Use component Y-type set if available. Tubing doesn't have to be rubber-free because product won't stick. • Transfuse more rapidly than whole blood because coagulation factors become unstable after thawing. • Administer ABO group-compatible product. • Patient usually receives multiple units. American Red Cross recommends that they be pooled into transfer packs. Administer all units within 6 hours. • Because product has short half-life, transfusions may need to be repeated frequently, depending on the patient's clinical status.
Granulocytes	Unit volume varies (200-500 ml), but units contain mostly granulocytes (exact number depends on method of salvage) and RBCs, plasma, and platelets.	• Indicated in severe gram-negative infection or severe neutropenia unresponsive to routine forms of therapy in immunosuppressed patient. Also indicated in severe granulocyte dysfunction. • Microaggregate filter is contraindicated because it traps granulocytes. • Administer ABO group-compatible and, when possible, Rh type-compatible and human leukocyte antigen-compatible products. • For best results, administer as soon as possible after salvage. • Procedure must be repeated daily for 4 days or longer to be effective. • Because product consists of white blood cells, watch for chills and fever. Other adverse reactions include coughing and shortness of breath. Continue transfusion if possible but, if severe dyspnea develops, stop transfusion, keep vein open, and notify the doctor.
Serum albumin (5% and 25%) and plasma protein fraction (PPF)	25% albumin comes in 50-ml and 100-ml units. 5% albumin and PPF (essentially the same product) come in 250-ml units.	• Indicated in hypovolemia and hypoproteinemia (in burns, for example). • Because product comes in glass bottle, use administration set supplied with it. The set will have a filtered air inlet. Normal saline solution is not needed as a starter. Product needs no blood filter. • 25% albumin is not usually given at more than 1 ml/minute because of the danger of fluid overload. PPF given at over 10 ml/minute may produce hypotension. • Compatibility testing isn't required because product contains no RBCs or plasma antibodies. • Product is free from HIV and hepatitis viruses. • 25% albumin is used for patient with depleted vascular volume but extravascular fluid accumulation. • Because 25% albumin rapidly mobilizes large volumes of fluid into circulation, watch for pulmonary edema and other signs and symptoms of fluid overload. • Product is stored at room temperature and has an extremely long shelf life. Always check expiration date before administering.

Many blood banks screen blood for cytomegalovirus (CMV). Blood with CMV is especially dangerous for an immunosuppressed, seronegative patient. Blood banks also test blood for syphilis, although the routine practice of refrigerating blood kills the syphilis organism and virtually eliminates the risk of transfusion-related syphilis.

Circulatory overload and hemolytic, allergic, febrile, and pyogenic reactions can result from any transfusion. Coagulation disturbances, citrate intoxication, hyperkalemia, acid-base imbalance, loss of 2,3-diphosphoglycerate, ammonia intoxication, and hypothermia can result from massive transfusion.

Documentation

Record the date and time of transfusion, the type and amount of transfusion product, the patient's vital signs, and your check of all identification data, and the patient's response. (See *Reviewing transfusion products,* pages 314 and 315.) Document any transfusion reaction and treatment.

Management of transfusion reactions

A transfusion reaction typically stems from a major antigen-antibody reaction and can result from a single or massive transfusion of blood or blood products. Although many reactions occur during transfusion or within 96 hours afterward, infectious diseases transmitted during a transfusion may go undetected until days, weeks, or months later, when signs and symptoms appear.

Transfusion reaction requires immediate recognition and prompt nursing action to prevent further complications and possible death—particularly if the patient is unconscious or so heavily sedated that he can't report the common symptoms.

Equipment

Normal saline solution ■ I.V. administration set ■ sterile urine specimen container ■ needle, syringe, and tubes for blood samples ■ transfusion reaction report form ■ optional: oxygen, epinephrine, hypothermia blanket, leukocyte removal filter.

Implementation

● As soon as you suspect an adverse reaction, stop the transfusion and start the saline infusion at a keep-vein-open rate *to maintain venous access.* Don't discard the blood bag or administration set.
● Notify the doctor.
● Monitor vital signs every 15 minutes or as indicated by the severity and type of reaction.
● Compare the labels on all blood containers to corresponding patient identification forms *to verify that the transfusion was the correct blood or blood product.*
● Notify the blood bank of a possible transfusion reaction and collect blood samples, as ordered. Immediately send these samples, all transfusion containers (even if empty), and the administration set to the blood bank. The blood bank will test these materials to further evaluate the reaction.
● Collect the first posttransfusion urine specimen, mark the collection slip "Possible transfusion reaction," and send it to the laboratory immediately. *The laboratory tests this urine specimen for the presence of hemoglobin, which indicates a hemolytic reaction.*
● Closely monitor intake and output. Note evidence of oliguria or anuria *because hemoglobin deposition in the renal tubules can cause renal damage.*
● If ordered, administer oxygen, epinephrine, or other drugs. If ordered, apply a hypothermia blanket *to reduce fever.*
● Make the patient as comfortable as possible and provide reassurance as necessary. (For specific steps, see *Managing transfusion reactions.*)

Special considerations

Treat all transfusion reactions as serious until proven otherwise. If the doctor anticipates a transfusion reaction, such as one that may occur in a leukemia patient, he may order prophylactic treatment with antihistamines or antipyretics to precede blood administration.

To avoid a possible febrile reaction, the doctor may order the blood washed *to remove as many leukocytes as possible,* or a leukocyte removal filter may be used during the transfusion.

Documentation

Record the time and date of the transfusion reaction, the type and amount of infused blood or blood products, the clinical signs of the transfusion reaction in order of occurrence, the patient's vital signs, any specimens sent to the laboratory for analysis, any treatment given, and the patient's response to treatment. If required by hospital policy, complete the transfusion reaction form.

Managing transfusion reactions

REACTION AND CAUSE	SIGNS AND SYMPTOMS	NURSING INTERVENTIONS
Reactions from single transfusion		
Hemolytic ABO or Rh incompatibility, intradonor incompatibility, or improper blood storage	• Shaking, chills, fever, nausea, vomiting, chest pain, dyspnea, hypotension, oliguria, hemoglobinuria, flank pain, abnormal bleeding • May progress to shock and renal failure	• Monitor blood pressure. • Treat shock as indicated by the patient's condition, using I.V. fluids, oxygen, epinephrine, a diuretic, and a vasopressor. • Obtain posttransfusion reaction blood sample and urine specimen for evaluation. • Observe for signs of hemorrhage resulting from disseminated intravascular coagulation. ***Prevention*** • Before transfusion, check donor and recipient blood types to ensure blood compatibility; identify patient with another nurse or doctor present. • Transfuse blood slowly for first 15 to 20 minutes while observing the patient closely.
Febrile Bacterial lipopolysaccharides	• Fever, chills, headache, flank pain	• Relieve symptoms with an antipyretic, antihistamine, or analgesic, as ordered. ***Prevention*** • Premedicate with an antipyretic, antihistamine and, possibly a steroid. • Use leukocyte-poor or washed red blood cells (RBCs).
Allergic Allergen in donor's blood	• Pruritus, urticaria, fever, chills, nausea, vomiting, facial swelling, wheezing, laryngeal edema • May progress to anaphylaxis	• Administer antihistamines. • Monitor for anaphylactic reaction and administer epinephrine and steroids, if indicated. ***Prevention*** • Premedicate with antihistamine if patient has a history of allergic reactions. • Observe the patient closely for the first 20 minutes of the transfusion.
Bacterial contamination Cold-growing, gram-negative organisms, such as species of *Pseudomonas*	• Chills, fever, vomiting, abdominal cramping, diarrhea, shock, signs of renal failure	• Treat with broad-spectrum antibiotic and steroid. ***Prevention*** • Observe blood before transfusion for gas, clots, and dark purple color. • Use air-free, touch-free method to draw and deliver blood. • Maintain strict storage control. • Change blood tubing and filter every 4 hours. • Infuse each unit of blood over 2 to 4 hours; terminate the infusion if time exceeds 4 hours. • Maintain aseptic technique during administration.

(continued)

Managing transfusion reactions *(continued)*

REACTION AND CAUSE	SIGNS AND SYMPTOMS	NURSING INTERVENTIONS
Reactions from single transfusion *(continued)*		
Plasma protein incompatibility Immunoglobulin A (IgA) incompatibility	• Flushing, abdominal pain, diarrhea, chills, fever, dyspnea, hypotension	• Treat for shock by administering oxygen, fluids, epinephrine and, possibly, a steroid, as ordered. ***Prevention*** • Transfuse only IgA-deficient blood or well-washed RBCs.
Reactions from multiple transfusions		
Hemosiderosis Increased hemosiderin (iron-containing pigment) from RBC destruction, especially after receiving chronic transfusions	• Plasma iron level greater than 200 mg/dl	• Perform a phlebotomy to remove excess iron. ***Prevention*** • Administer blood only when absolutely necessary.
Bleeding tendencies Low platelet count in stored blood, causing dilutional thrombocytopenia	• Abnormal bleeding and oozing from cut or break in skin surface	• Administer platelets. • Monitor platelet count. ***Prevention*** • Use only fresh blood (less than 7 days old) when possible.
Elevated blood ammonia level Increased level of ammonia in stored blood	• Forgetfulness, confusion	• Monitor ammonia level. • Decrease the amount of protein in diet. • If indicated, give neomycin sulfate. ***Prevention*** • Use only RBCs, fresh frozen plasma, or fresh blood, especially if patient has hepatic disease.
Increased oxygen affinity for hemoglobin Decreased level of 2,3-diphosphoglycerate in stored blood. When oxygen's affinity for hemoglobin rises, oxygen stays in the bloodstream and isn't released into tissues.	• Depressed respiratory rate, especially in patients with chronic lung disease	• Monitor arterial blood gas levels and give respiratory support as needed. ***Prevention*** • Use only RBCs or fresh blood if possible.
Hypothermia Rapid infusion of large amounts of cold blood, which decreases myocardial temperature	• Shaking, chills, hypotension, ventricular fibrillation • Cardiac arrest if core temperature falls below 86° F (30° C)	• Stop transfusion. • Warm the patient with blankets. • Obtain an ECG. ***Prevention*** • Warm blood to 95° to 98.6° F (35° to 37° C), especially before massive transfusions.

Managing transfusion reactions *(continued)*

REACTION AND CAUSE	SIGNS AND SYMPTOMS	NURSING INTERVENTIONS
Reactions from multiple transfusions *(continued)*		
Hypocalcemia Citrate toxicity occurs when citrate-treated blood is infused rapidly. Citrate binds with calcium, causing a calcium deficiency, or normal citrate metabolism becomes hindered by hepatic disease.	• Tingling in fingers, muscle cramps, nausea, vomiting, hypotension, cardiac arrhythmias, convulsions	• Slow or stop transfusion, depending on reaction. Expect a worse reaction in hypothermic patients or in patients with elevated potassium levels. • Slowly administer calcium gluconate I.V. ***Prevention*** • Infuse blood slowly. • Monitor potassium and calcium levels. • Use blood less than 2 days old if administering multiple units.
Hyperkalemia An abnormally high level of potassium in stored plasma caused by RBC lysis	• Intestinal colic, diarrhea, muscle twitching, oliguria, renal failure, ECG changes with tall peaked T waves, bradycardia proceeding to cardiac standstill.	• Obtain an ECG. • Administer sodium polystyrene sulfonate (Kayexalate) orally or by enema. ***Prevention*** • Use fresh blood when administering massive transfusions.

Selected references

American Association of Blood Banks. "Blood Transfusion Outside the Hospital," *AJN* 89(4):486-89, April 1989.

Bartlett, K., and Burgoon, D. "Venous Access Devices: Appropriate for Home Use," *Home Healthcare Nurse* 8(2):38-41, March-April 1990.

Brown, J.M. "Evaluation of Surecath Access Devices," *Journal of Intravenous Nursing* 12(5):298-301, September-October 1989.

Freedman, S., et al. "Nursing Considerations in the Administration of Blood Component Therapy," *Seminars in Oncology Nursing* 6(2):155-62, May 1990.

Hadaway, L.C. "Evaluation and Use of Advance I.V. Technology: Central Venous Access Devices," Part I. *Journal of Intravenous Nursing* 12(2):73-82, March-April 1989.

Handy, C.M. "Vascular Access Devices: Hospital to Home Care," *Journal of Intravenous Nursing* 12(Supp.):S10-S18, January-February 1989.

Intravenous Nurses Society. "Intravenous Nursing Standards of Practice," *Journal of Intravenous Nursing* 13(Supp.):S1-S98, April 1990.

Lichtor, J.L. "Transfusion Reactions," Part 2. *Current Reviews for Nurse Anesthetists* 12(4):27-32, July 27, 1989.

Newman, L.N. "A Side-by-Side Look at Two Venous Access Devices," *AJN* 89(6):826-35, June 1989.

Nursing94 Drug Handbook. Springhouse, Pa.: Springhouse Corp., 1994.

CHAPTER 7

CARDIOVASCULAR CARE

CHERYL MILFORD, RN, MS, CCRN

Introduction

Cardiovascular disorders, the leading cause of death in the United States, affects millions of Americans each year. The responsibility of caring for patients with these disorders pervades nearly every area of nursing practice. As a result, cardiovascular care ranks as one of the most rapidly growing areas of nursing. What's more, it's one of the most rapidly changing fields, with the continuing proliferation of new diagnostic tests, new drug and other treatments, and sophisticated monitoring equipment. Consequently, nurses face a constant challenge to keep up with the latest developments.

Patient teaching

Today, nurses assume much of the responsibility for preparing patients physically and psychologically for their hospitalization and ongoing care. Specifically, they play a pivotal role in teaching patients and their families about test and procedure preparation and follow-up care, drug and other treatments, disease prevention, and life-style modification. Through patient teaching, nurses can help patients reduce stress and comply with prescribed therapy.

Monitoring

Cardiac monitoring involves either hardwire or telemetric systems that continuously record the patient's cardiac activity. This makes monitoring useful not only for assessing cardiac rhythm, but also for gauging a patient's response to drug therapy and for preventing complications associated with diagnostic and therapeutic procedures. Once used only in critical care areas, cardiac monitoring is now performed in high-risk obstetric, general medical, pediatric, and transplantation departments.

Treatment

In cardiovascular emergencies, nurses may perform or assist with cardiopulmonary resuscitation. Carrying out this life-saving procedures calls for in-depth knowledge of cardiovascular anatomy and physiology as well as sound assessment and intervention techniques.

Monitoring
Electrocardiography

One of the most valuable and frequently used diagnostic tools, electrocardiography (ECG) measures the heart's electrical activity. Impulses moving through the heart's conduction system create electric currents that can be monitored on the body's surface. Electrodes attached to the skin can detect these electric currents and transmit them to an instrument that produces a record (the electrocardiogram) of cardiac activity.

ECG helps identify myocardial ischemia and infarction, rhythm and conduction disturbances, chamber enlargement, electrolyte imbalances, and drug toxicity.

The standard 12-lead ECG uses a series of electrodes placed on the extremities and the chest wall to assess the heart from 12 different views (leads). The 12 leads consist of 3 standard bipolar limb leads (designated I, II, III), 3 unipolar augmented leads (aV_R, aV_L, aV_F), and 6 unipolar precordial leads (V_1 to V_6). The limb leads and augmented leads show the heart from the frontal plane. The precordial leads show the heart from the horizontal plane.

The ECG device measures and averages the differences between the electrical potential of the electrode sites for each lead and graphs them over time. This creates the standard ECG complex, called P-QRS-T. The P wave represents atrial depolarization; the QRS complex, ventricular depolarization; and the T wave, ventricular repolarization. (See *Reviewing ECG waveform components*, page 322.)

Variations of standard ECG include exercise ECG (stress ECG) and ambulatory ECG (Holter monitoring). Exercise electrocardiography monitors heart rate, blood pressure, and ECG waveforms as the patient walks on a treadmill or pedals a stationary bicycle. For ambulatory ECG, the patient wears a portable Holter monitor to record heart activity continuously over 24 hours.

ECG may be accomplished using a multichannel or a single-channel method. For the multichannel method, all electrodes are attached to the patient at once and the machine prints a simultaneous view of all leads. The single-channel method requires systematic attachment and removal of selected electrodes and stopping and starting the tracing each time.

Equipment

ECG machine ■ recording paper ■ pre-gelled disposable electrodes or reusable electrodes with suction bulbs, electrode gel, and rubber straps ■ 4″ × 4″ gauze pads ■ moist

Reviewing ECG waveform components

An electrocardiogram (ECG) waveform has three basic components: P wave, QRS complex, and T wave. These elements can be further divided into a PR interval, J point, ST segment, U wave, and QT interval.

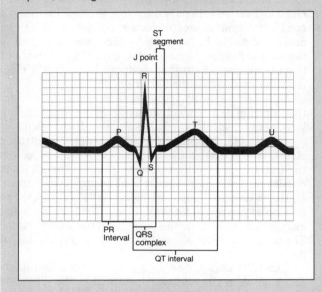

P wave and PR interval

The P wave represents atrial depolarization. The PR interval represents the time it takes an impulse to travel from the atria through the AV node and bundle of His. The PR interval measures from the beginning of the P wave to the beginning of the QRS complex.

QRS complex

The QRS complex represents ventricular depolarization (the time it takes for the impulse to travel through the bundle branches to the Purkinje fibers).

The Q wave appears as the first negative deflection in the QRS complex; the R wave, as the first positive deflection. The S wave appears as the second negative deflection or the first negative deflection after the R wave.

J point and ST segment

Marking the end of the QRS complex, the J point also indicates the beginning of the ST segment. The ST segment represents part of ventricular repolarization.

T wave and U wave

Usually following the same deflection pattern as the P wave, the T wave represents ventricular repolarization. The U wave follows the T wave, but is not always seen.

QT interval

The QT interval represents ventricular depolarization and repolarization. It extends from the beginning of the QRS complex to the end of the T wave.

---

cloth towel ■ sterile drape ■ optional: shaving supplies, marking pen.

Preparation of equipment

Before using the ECG machine, check the date of its last inspection by the hospital's engineering department. If the period for authorized use has elapsed, avoid using the machine *because even a miniscule leakage of electric current (10 microamperes) may put the patient at risk for life-threatening arrhythmias.*

Implementation

• Explain the procedure to the patient *to allay his fears and promote cooperation.* Inform him that no special preparation is required and that the procedure takes no longer than 15 minutes. Instruct him to relax, lie still, and breathe normally. Advise him not to talk during the procedure *because the movement of his muscles may distort the ECG tracing.*

• Check the patient's history for cardiac medications, and note any current therapy on the test request form.
• Place the patient in the supine position. If he can't tolerate lying flat, help him to assume a semi-Fowler's position.
• Instruct the patient to expose his chest, both ankles, and both wrists for electrode placement. Drape the female patient's chest until chest leads are applied.
• Turn on the machine *to warm up the stylus mechanism.* Check the paper supply.

Multichannel ECG

• Place electrodes on the inner aspect of the wrists, the medial aspect of the lower legs, and the chest. (See *Positioning chest electrodes.*) If using disposable electrodes, remove the paper backing before positioning. Then connect the lead wires after all electrodes are in place. For reusable electrodes, apply electrode gel and affix the electrodes with suction bulbs. Secure the limb electrodes with rubber straps, but avoid tightening them *to prevent circulatory impairment and distortion on the recording.*

• If frequent ECGs will be necessary, use a marking pen to indicate lead positions on the patient's chest *to ensure consistent placement.*

• Set the paper speed to 25 mm/second or as ordered. Calibrate the machine by adjusting the sensitivity to normal and checking the quality and baseline position of the tracing.

• Press the start button and the machine will produce a printout showing all 12 leads simultaneously on thermal or pressure-sensitive recording paper.

• As the machine records the ECG, check to be sure that all leads are represented in the tracing. If not, determine which one has come loose, reattach it, and restart the tracing. Check for artifact in the tracing.

• Also observe to be sure that the wave doesn't peak beyond the top edge of the recording grid. If it does, adjust the machine to bring the wave inside the boundaries.

• When the machine finishes the tracing, remove the electrodes and reposition the patient's gown and bed covers.

Single-channel ECG

• Apply either disposable or standard electrodes to the inner aspects of the wrists and medial aspects of the lower legs.

• Connect each lead wire to the corresponding electrode by inserting the wire prong into the terminal post and tightening the screw.

• Set the paper speed to 25 mm/second or as ordered. Calibrate the machine by adjusting the sensitivity to normal and checking the quality and baseline position of the tracing. Recalibrate the machine after running each lead *to provide a consistent test standard.*

• Turn the lead selector to I. Then mark the lead by writing "I" on the paper strip or by depressing the marking button on the machine (some machines do this automatically). Record for 3 to 6 seconds and then return the machine to the standby mode. Repeat this procedure for leads II, III, aV_R, aV_L, and aV_F.

• Determine proper placement for the chest electrodes. If frequent ECGs are necessary, use a marking pen to indicate lead positions on the patient's chest *to ensure consistent placement.*

• Connect the chest lead wire to the suction bulb in the same manner as you connected the limb electrodes. Apply gel to each of the six chest positions, then firmly press the suction bulb to attach the chest lead to the V_1 position. Mark the strips as before. Then turn the lead selector to V and record V_1 for 3 to 6 seconds. Return the lead

---

Positioning chest electrodes

To ensure accurate test results, position chest electrodes as follows:

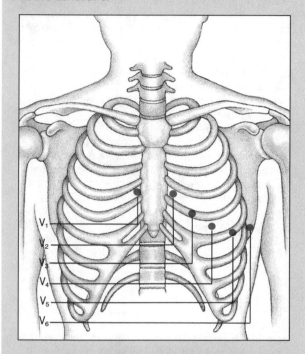

V_1: Fourth intercostal space at right border of sternum
V_2: Fourth intercostal space at left border of sternum
V_3: Halfway between V_2 and V_4
V_4: Fifth intercostal space at midclavicular line
V_5: Fifth intercostal space at anterior axillary line (halfway between V_4 and V_6)
V_6: Fifth intercostal space at midaxillary line, level with V_4

---

selector to standby. Reposition the electrode and repeat the procedure for V_2 to V_6.

• After completing V_6, run a rhythm strip on lead II for at least 6 seconds.

• Assess the quality of the tracings and repeat any that are unclear.

• Disconnect the equipment, remove the electrodes, and wipe the gel from the patient with a moist cloth towel. Wash the gel from the electrodes and dry them thoroughly.

EQUIPMENT

Setting up for telemetry

Telemetry detects arrhythmias that occur during sleep, or when the patient is resting, performing mild exercise, or undergoing stress. It's especially useful for the ambulatory patient because it permits greater freedom than hardwire monitoring and avoids electrical hazards by isolating the monitor system from leakage and accidental shock. To set up a telemetry monitor:

• Insert a battery in the telemetry transmitter, matching the polarity markings on the transmitter case with those on the battery.

• Test the battery's charge by observing the oscilloscope screen, which registers no cardiac activity if the battery is low. In some models, check the battery by pushing the test-light button on the back of the transmitter. If the test light fails to go on, replace the battery. Make sure the lead wire cable is securely attached to the transmitter.

• Show the transmitter to the patient and explain how it works. Before proceeding, answer any questions he may have.

• Apply electrodes to the patient's chest and attach the lead wires to them.

• Place the transmitter in the pouch provided by the manufacturer or hospital. Tie the pouch strings around the patient's neck and waist. Make sure the pouch fits snugly without making the patient uncomfortable. If no pouch is available, place the transmitter in the patient's bathrobe pocket.

• After locating the patient's telemetry monitor in the central console, calibrate it and adjust the heart-rate alarms as you would a hardwire monitor.

• Some units have a button that can be pushed if the patient has symptoms. This causes the central console to print a rhythm strip. Tell the patient how and when to use this button.

• Tell the patient to remove the transmitter if he takes a shower or bath.

Special considerations

In place of the electrodes and straps on the extremities, suction bulbs may be used *to enhance baseline stability.*

Small areas of hair on the patient's chest or extremities may be shaved, but this usually isn't necessary.

If the patient's skin is exceptionally oily, scaly, or diaphoretic, rub the electrode site with a dry 4″ × 4″ gauze pad before applying the electrode *to help reduce interference in the tracing.* During the procedure, ask the patient to breathe normally. If his respirations distort the recording, ask him to hold his breath briefly *to reduce baseline wander in the tracing.*

If the patient has a pacemaker, you can perform ECG with or without a magnet. Be sure to note the presence of a pacemaker and the use of the magnet (to turn off the pacemaker) on the strip.

Documentation

Label the ECG recording with the patient's name, room number, and hospital identification number. If you're sending the ECG to another department for interpretation and mounting, complete all information on the request form. Document in your notes the test's date and time and significant responses by the patient as well.

Cardiac monitoring

Because it allows continuous observation of the heart's electrical activity, cardiac monitoring is used in patients with conduction disturbances or in those at risk for life-threatening arrhythmias. It's also used to evaluate the effects of therapy.

Like other forms of electrocardiography (ECG), cardiac monitoring uses electrodes placed on the patient's chest to transmit electrical signals that are converted into a tracing of cardiac rhythm on an oscilloscope.

Two types of monitoring may be performed: hardwire or telemetry. In *hardwire* monitoring, the patient is connected to a monitor at bedside. The rhythm display appears at bedside, but it may also be transmitted to a console at a remote location. *Telemetry* uses a small transmitter connected to the ambulatory patient to send electrical signals to another location where they are displayed on a monitor screen. (See *Setting up for telemetry*.)

Regardless of the type, cardiac monitors can display the patient's rhythm and heart rate; produce a printed record of cardiac rhythm; and sound an alarm if the patient's heart rate rises above or falls below specified limits. Some monitors can also recognize and count abnormal heartbeats and trigger an alarm if the heartbeats exceed a set limit.

Equipment

Cardiac monitor ▪ lead wires ▪ patient cable ▪ disposable pre-gelled electrodes (the number of electrodes varies from three to five, depending on the manufacturer) ▪ alcohol sponges ▪ 4″ × 4″ gauze pads ▪ optional: shaving supplies, washcloth.

Identifying cardiac monitor problems

PROBLEM	POSSIBLE CAUSES	SOLUTIONS
False-high-rate alarm	• Monitor interpreting large T waves as QRS complexes, which doubles the rate • Skeletal muscle activity	• Reposition electrodes to lead where QRS complexes are taller than T waves. • Place electrodes away from major muscle masses.
False-low-rate alarm	• Shift in electrical axis from patient movement, making QRS complexes too small to register • Low amplitude of QRS • Poor contact between electrode and skin	• Reapply electrodes. Set gain so height of complex is greater than 1 millivolt. • Increase gain. • Reapply electrodes.
Low amplitude	• Gain dial set too low • Poor contact between skin and electrodes; dried gel; broken or loose lead wires; poor connection between patient and monitor; malfunctioning monitor; physiologic loss of QRS amplitude	• Increase gain. • Check connections on all lead wires and monitoring cable. Replace electrode as necessary. Reapply electrodes, if required.
Wandering baseline	• Poor position or contact between electrodes and skin • Thoracic movement with respirations	• Reposition or replace electrodes. • Reposition electrodes.
Artifact (waveform interference)	• Patient having seizures, chills, or anxiety • Patient movement • Electrodes applied improperly • Static electricity • Electrical short circuit in lead wires or cable • Interference from decreased room humidity	• Notify doctor and treat patient as ordered. Keep patient warm and reassure him. • Help patient relax. • Check electrodes and reapply, if necessary. • Make sure cables don't have exposed connectors. Change static-causing bedclothes. • Replace broken equipment. Use stress loops when applying lead wires. • Regulate humidity to 40%.
Broken lead wires or cable	• Stress loops not used on lead wires • Cables and lead wires cleaned with alcohol or acetone, causing brittleness	• Replace lead wires and retape them, using stress loops. • Clean cable and lead wires with soapy water. *Do not allow cable ends to become wet.* Replace cable as necessary.
60-cycle interference (fuzzy baseline)	• Electrical interference from other equipment in room • Patient's bed improperly grounded	• Attach all electrical equipment to common ground. Check plugs to make sure prongs aren't loose. • Attach bed ground to the room's common ground.
Skin excoriation under electrode	• Patient allergic to electrode adhesive • Electrode on skin too long	• Remove electrodes and apply nonallergenic electrodes and nonallergenic tape. • Remove electrode, clean site, and reapply electrode at new site.

Understanding lead placement

You'll have several leads and electrodes to place depending on the cardiac monitoring system you're using. The most typical system is the three-electrode system, which uses standard limb leads and a modified version of standard chest leads. To increase monitoring capability, you may need to use the four- or five-electrode system. Review the manufacturer's instructions for your particular system and use the following guidelines to place the leads precisely.

Three-electrode system

In this system, the most commonly used limb lead is lead II, and typically used modified chest leads are MCL_1 and MCL_6 (modified versions of V_1 and V_6). In general, a three-electrode monitoring system has one positive lead and one negative lead. A third lead serves as a ground.

Lead II

For lead II, you'll place the negative electrode at the first intercostal space on the right sternal border, the positive electrode at the fourth intercostal space on the left midclavicular line, and the ground electrode at the fourth intercostal space at the right sternal border.

Lead II measures the electrical flow from the RA ($-$) to the LL ($+$), producing good QRS complexes, which reflect ventricular activity, and positive P waves, which show atrial activity.

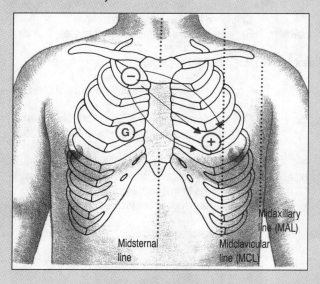

Lead MCL₁

Using MCL_1, the negative electrode would be positioned on the left side of the patient's chest just below the clavicle. The positive electrode would be positioned on the right sternal border at the fourth intercostal space, and the ground electrode would be positioned on the right side of the chest just below the clavicle.

Lead MCL_1 records the sequence of ventricular depolarization better, so it's used to differentiate between right or left bundle-branch block and ectopy. Note that in MCL_1, the positive electrode should be positioned directly over the right ventricle.

Lead MCL₆

With lead MCL_6, the negative electrode would be positioned just below the left clavicle on the midclavicular line. The positive electrode would be positioned at the left fifth intercostal space on the midaxillary line, and the ground electrode would be positioned just below the right clavicle on the midclavicular line.

Lead MCL_6 allows you to easily see tall QRS complexes so that you can identify right bundle-branch block and ST segment and T wave changes. In MCL_6, the positive electrode lies over the apex of the left ventricle.

Four- and five-electrode systems

In a four-electrode system, a right leg (RL) electrode is added to provide a permanent ground for all leads used in the three-electrode system. Place this electrode on the 4th or 5th intercostal space, right midclavicular line.

A five-electrode system uses an additional exploratory chest electrode. This lets the examiner obtain any of the six modified chest leads and the standard limb leads as well. Place this lead (marked C or V) on the 3rd or 4th intercostal space, left sternal border.

Preparation of equipment

Plug the monitor into an electrical outlet and turn it on *to warm up the unit while you prepare the equipment and the patient.* Insert the cable into the appropriate socket in the monitor.

Connect the lead wires to the cable. In some systems, the lead wires are permanently secured to the cable. (Each lead wire should indicate the location for attachment to the patient: right arm [RA], left arm [LA], right leg [RL], left leg [LL], and ground [C or V]). This should appear on the lead wire — if it's permanently connected — or at the connection of the lead wires and cable to the patient. Then connect an electrode to each of the lead wires, carefully checking that each lead wire is in its correct outlet.

Implementation

• Explain the procedure to the patient, provide privacy, and ask the patient to expose his chest. Wash your hands.
• Determine electrode positions on the patient's chest, based on the system and lead you're using. (See *Understanding lead placement.*)
• If the lead wires and patient cable aren't permanently attached, verify that the electrode placement corresponds to the label on the patient cable.
• If necessary, shave an area about 4″ (10 cm) in diameter around each electrode site. Clean the area with an alcohol sponge and dry it completely *to remove skin secretions that may interfere with electrode function.* Gently abrade the dried area by rubbing it briskly until it reddens *to remove dead skin cells and to promote better electrical contact with living cells.* (Some electrodes have a small, rough patch for abrading the skin; otherwise, use a dry washcloth or a dry gauze pad.)
• Remove the backing from the pre-gelled electrode. Check the gel for moistness. If the gel is dry, discard it and replace it with a fresh electrode.
• Apply the electrode to the site and press firmly *to ensure a tight seal.* Repeat with the remaining electrodes.
• When all the electrodes are in place, check for a tracing on the cardiac monitor. Assess the quality of the ECG. (See *Identifying cardiac monitor problems,* page 325.) To verify that each beat is being detected by the monitor, compare the digital heart rate display with your count of the patient's heart rate.
• If necessary, use the gain control to adjust the size of the rhythm tracing, and the position control to adjust the waveform position on the recording paper.
• Set the upper and lower limits of the heart rate alarm, based on unit policy. Turn the alarm on.

Special considerations

Make sure that all electrical equipment and outlets are grounded *to avoid electric shock and interference (artifacts)*. Also ensure that the patient is clean and dry *to prevent electric shock.*

Avoid opening the electrode packages until just before using *to prevent the gel from drying out.*

Avoid placing the electrodes on bony prominences, hairy areas, areas where defibrillator pads will be placed, or areas for chest compression.

If the patient's skin is exceptionally oily, scaly, or diaphoretic, rub the electrode site with a dry 4″ × 4″ gauze pad before applying the electrode *to help reduce interference in the tracing.* During the procedure, ask the patient to breathe normally. If his respirations distort the recording, ask him to hold his breath briefly *to reduce baseline wander in the tracing.*

Assess skin integrity, and reposition the electrodes every 24 hours or as necessary.

Documentation

Record the date and time that monitoring begins and the monitoring lead in your notes. Document a rhythm strip at least every 8 hours with any changes in the patient's condition (or as stated by hospital policy). Label the rhythm strip with the patient's name, room number, the date, and time.

If cardiac monitoring will continue after the patient's discharge, ensure that all caregivers have some knowledge of rhythm interpretation and cardiopulmonary resuscitation. Also discuss troubleshooting techniques to use if the monitor malfunctions. As needed, contact the monitor supplier to help in discharge planning.

◼ *TREATMENT*
⊾⊿ Cardiopulmonary resuscitation

Cardiopulmonary resuscitation (CPR) seeks to restore and maintain the patient's respiration and circulation after his heartbeat and breathing have stopped. CPR is a basic life support (BLS) procedure performed on victims of cardiac arrest. Other BLS procedures include clearing an obstructed airway (see "Obstructed airway management" in Chapter 8).

Most adults in sudden cardiac arrest develop ventricular fibrillation and require defibrillation; CPR alone does not improve their chances of survival. Therefore, you must assess the victim and then contact emergency medical services (EMS) or call a code *before* starting

CPR. Timing is critical. Early access to EMS, early CPR, and early defibrillation greatly improve chances of survival.

In most instances, you perform CPR to keep the patient alive until advanced life support (ACLS) can begin. Basic CPR procedure consists of assessing the victim, calling for help, and then following the ABC scheme: opening the **a**irway, restoring **b**reathing, then restoring **c**irculation. After the airway has been opened and breathing and circulation have been restored, drug therapy, diagnosis by electrocardiogram (ECG), or defibrillation may follow. CPR is contraindicated in "no code" patients.

Equipment

CPR requires no special equipment except a hard surface on which to place the patient.

Implementation

● The following illustrated instructions provide a step-by-step guide for CPR as currently recommended by the American Heart Association.

One-person rescue

● If you're the sole rescuer, expect to open the patient's airway, check for breathing, assess for circulation, and call for help before beginning compressions.

Open the airway

● As shown below, assess the victim to determine if he's unconscious. Gently shake his shoulders and shout, "Are you okay?" This helps ensure that you don't start CPR on a person who's conscious. Check whether he has an injury, particularly to the head or neck. If you suspect a head or neck injury, move him as little as possible to reduce the risk of paralysis.

• Call out for help. Send someone to contact the EMS or call a code, if appropriate. Place the victim in a supine position on a hard, flat surface. When moving him, roll his head and torso as a unit. Avoid twisting or pulling his neck, shoulders, or hips.

• Kneel near his shoulders. This position will give you easy access to his head and chest.

• In many cases, the muscles controlling the victim's tongue will be relaxed, causing the tongue to obstruct the airway. If the victim doesn't appear to have a neck injury, use the *head-tilt/chin-lift maneuver* to open his airway. To accomplish this, first place your hand that's closer to the victim's head on his forehead. Then apply firm pressure. The pressure should be firm enough to tilt the victim's head back. Next place the fingertips of your other hand under the bony part of his lower jaw near the chin. Now lift the victim's chin. At the same time, keep his mouth partially open (as shown below).

• Avoid placing your fingertips on the soft tissue under the victim's chin *because this maneuver may inadvertently obstruct the airway you're trying to open.*

• If you suspect a neck injury, use the *jaw-thrust maneuver* instead of the *head-tilt/chin-lift maneuver.* Kneel at the victim's head with your elbows on the ground. Rest your thumbs on his lower jaw near the corners of the mouth, pointing your thumbs toward his feet. Then place your fingertips around the lower jaw. To open the airway, lift the lower jaw with your fingertips. (See illustration on page 330 at the top of the left column.)

Check for breathing

• While maintaining the open airway, place your ear over the victim's mouth and nose. Now, listen for the sound of air moving, and note whether his chest rises and falls. You may also feel airflow on your cheek. If he starts to breathe, keep the airway open and continue checking his breathing until help arrives.

• If the victim doesn't start breathing after you open his airway, begin rescue breathing. Pinch his nostrils shut with the thumb and index finger of the hand you've had on his forehead. (See illustration at the top of the right column.)

• Take a deep breath and place your mouth over the victim's mouth, creating a tight seal. Give two full ventilations, taking a deep breath after each to allow enough time for his chest to expand and relax and to prevent gastric distention. Each ventilation should last 1½ to 2 seconds.

• If the first ventilation isn't successful, reposition the victim's head and try again. If you're still not successful, he may have a foreign-body airway obstruction. Check for loose dentures. If dentures or any other objects are blocking the airway, follow the procedure for clearing an airway obstruction. (See "Obstructed airway management," Chapter 8.)

Assess circulation

• Keep one hand on the victim's forehead so his airway remains open. With your other hand, palpate the carotid artery that's closer to you. To do this, place your index and middle fingers in the groove between the trachea and the sternocleidomastoid muscle. Palpate for 5 to 10 seconds.

• If you detect a pulse, don't begin chest compressions. Instead, perform rescue breathing by giving the victim 12 ventilations per minute (or one every 5 seconds). After every 12 ventilations, recheck his pulse.
• If there's no pulse, start giving chest compressions. Make sure your knees are apart for a wide base of support. Using the hand closer to his feet, locate the lower margin of the rib cage. Then move your fingertips along the margin to the notch where the ribs meet the sternum.

• Place your middle finger on the notch and your index finger next to your middle finger. Your index finger will now be on the bottom of the sternum.

• Put the heel of your other hand on the sternum, next to the index finger. The long axis of the heel of your hand will be aligned with the long axis of the sternum.

• Take the first hand off the notch and put it on top of the hand on the sternum. Make sure you have one hand directly on top of the other and your fingers aren't on his chest. This position will keep the force of the compression on the sternum and reduce the risk of a rib fracture, lung puncture, or liver laceration.

• With your elbows locked, arms straight, and your shoulders directly over your hands, you're ready to give chest compressions. Using the weight of your upper body, compress the victim's sternum 1½" to 2" (3.8 to 5 cm), delivering the pressure through the heels of your hands. After each compression, release the pressure and allow the chest to return to its normal position so that the heart can fill with blood. Don't change your hand position during compressions — you might injure the victim.

• Give 15 chest compressions at a rate of 80 to 100 per minute. Count, "One and two and three and..." up to 15. Open the airway and give 2 ventilations. Then find the proper hand position again and deliver 15 more compressions. Do four complete cycles of 15 compressions and 2 ventilations.

• Palpate the carotid pulse again. If there's still no pulse, continue performing CPR in cycles of 15 compressions and 2 ventilations. Every few minutes, check for breathing and a pulse at the end of a complete cycle of compressions and ventilations. If you detect a pulse but he isn't breathing, give 12 ventilations per minute and monitor his pulse. If he has a pulse and is breathing, monitor his respirations and pulse closely. You should stop performing CPR only when his respirations and pulse return, he's turned over to the EMS, or you're exhausted.

Two-person rescue

If another rescuer arrives while you're giving CPR, follow these steps:

• If the EMS team hasn't arrived, tell the second rescuer to repeat the call for help. If he's not a health care professional, ask him to stand by. Then, if you become fatigued, he can take over one-person CPR.

• Have him begin by checking the victim's pulse for 5 seconds after you've given two ventilations. If he doesn't feel a pulse, he should give two ventilations and begin chest compressions.

• If the rescuer is another health care professional, the two of you can perform two-person CPR. He should start assisting after you've finished a cycle of 15 compressions, two ventilations, and a pulse check.

• The second rescuer should get into place opposite you. While you're checking for a pulse, he should be finding the proper hand placement for delivering chest compressions.

• If you don't detect a pulse, say, "No pulse, continue CPR," and give one ventilation (as shown above at right). Then the second rescuer should begin delivering compressions at a rate of 80 to 100 per minute. Compressions and ventilations should be administered at a ratio of 5 compressions to 1 ventilation. The compressor (at this point, the second rescuer) should count out loud so the ventilator can anticipate when to give ventilations. To ensure that the ventilations are effective, the rescuer performing the chest compressions should stop briefly or at least long enough to observe the victim's chest rise with the air supplied by the rescuer giving ventilations.

• As the ventilator, you must check for breathing and a pulse. Signal the compressor to stop giving compressions for 5 seconds so you can make these assessments.

• After a minimum of 10 cycles, the compressor (second rescuer) may call for a switch. This should be done clearly to allow for a smooth transition. The compressor can substitute the word "switch" for the word "one" as he counts compressions. In other words, he'd say, "Switch and two and three and four and five." You'd then give a ventilation and become the compressor by moving down to the victim's chest and placing your hands in the proper position.

• The second rescuer would become the ventilator and move to the victim's head. He'd check the pulse for 5 seconds. If he found no pulse, he'd say, "No pulse," and give a ventilation. You'd then give compressions at a rate of 80 to 100 per minute — or five compressions for each ventilation. As shown at right above, both of you should continue giving CPR in this manner until the victim's respirations and pulse return, he's turned over to the EMS, or both of you are exhausted.

Special considerations

Although acquired immunodeficiency syndrome (AIDS) isn't known to be transmitted in saliva, some health care professionals may hesitate to give rescue breaths — especially if the victim has AIDS. For this reason, the American Heart Association recommends that all health care professionals learn how to use disposable airway equipment.

A second rescuer may instinctively take the victim's pulse without waiting for the end of a cycle. This is *not*

part of the American Heart Association recommendations and may confuse some rescuers. The recommendations aim to have all rescuers act in the same way so that time isn't wasted and all efforts help restore the victim's respirations and heartbeat.

Complications

CPR can cause certain complications — especially if the compressor doesn't place her hands properly on the sternum. These complications include fractured ribs, a lacerated liver, and punctured lungs. Gastric distention, a common complication, results from giving too much air during ventilation. (For more information, see *Managing hazards of CPR*.)

Documentation

Whenever you perform CPR, document why you initiated it, whether the victim suffered from cardiac or respiratory arrest, when you found the victim and started CPR, and how long the victim received CPR. Note his response and any complications. Also include any interventions taken to correct complications.

If the victim also received advanced cardiac life support, document which interventions were performed, who performed them, when they were performed, and what equipment was used.

Managing hazards of CPR

To prevent complications, make sure to position your hands properly for chest compressions, and check that you're not delivering excessive ventilation. If you suspect the following complications, tell the doctor, but don't stop cardiopulmonary resuscitation (CPR).

Fractured ribs

Once the victim's condition has stabilized, you can detect fractured ribs by palpating for bone displacement and crepitus (a crunching sound). The victim will need rest and pain medication for a fractured rib. If he has a serious fracture, he may need his rib cage splinted.

Liver laceration

Although rare, liver laceration poses a much more serious threat. It usually causes hemorrhage, resulting in shock, decreased blood pressure, increased heart rate, and abdominal distention. You may have trouble distinguishing it from shock caused by respiratory or cardiac arrest. If you suspect liver laceration, tell the doctor. After the victim is stabilized, diagnostic studies, such as peritoneal fluid analysis, may be ordered. Treatment includes fluid resuscitation and surgical repair.

Punctured lung

If the victim has a punctured lung from a broken rib, he may develop a tension pneumothorax. With this compli-cation, air enters—but can't escape—the pleural space, building up positive pressure in the thoracic cavity and collapsing the lung. You may have trouble ventilating a victim with a punctured lung.

Other signs of a tension pneumothorax include asymmetrical chest movement, absent breath sounds on the side where the pneumothorax has developed and, as the condition grows worse, a shift of the trachea away from the affected side. A chest X-ray will be needed to confirm the diagnosis.

The victim will need to have a chest tube or a large-bore needle inserted into the pleural space (at about the second intercostal space) to relieve the pressure caused by trapped air.

Gastric distention

A more common complication of CPR—also signaled by difficulty in giving resuscitative breaths—is gastric distention. Caused by delivering too much air during ventilation, gastric distention can lead to vomiting, which increases the risk of aspiration.

If you notice the victim's stomach becoming distended during CPR, reposition his airway and make sure that his chest, not his stomach, rises and falls during ventilation. If the victim vomits, turn him on his side—preferably away from you. Suction his airway and continue to perform CPR.

Selected references

American Heart Association. "Guidelines for Cardiopulmonary Resuscitation and Emergency Cardiac Care, I: Introduction," *JAMA* 16(268):2172-83, October 1992.

Deciphering Difficult ECGs. Advanced Skills Series. Springhouse, Pa.: Springhouse Corp., 1993.

Illustrated Manual of Nursing Practice, 2nd ed. Springhouse, Pa.: Springhouse Corp., 1994.

Jaffe, A., ed. *Textbook of Advanced Cardiac Support,* 2nd ed. Dallas: American Heart Association, 1990.

Lewis, S., and Collier, I. *Medical-Surgical Nursing: Assessment and Management of Clinical Problems,* 3rd ed. St. Louis: Mosby, Inc., 1992.

Nursing94 Drug Handbook. Springhouse, Pa.: Springhouse Corp., 1994.

CHAPTER 8

RESPIRATORY CARE

VICKI L. BUCHDA, RN, MS

Introduction

No matter where you work, you're sure to encounter patients with respiratory conditions. Such conditions may be acute or chronic, may have developed as primary disorders, or may result from cardiac or other disorders.

Caring for the patient with a respiratory condition will challenge your nursing skills. Not only is the patient's oxygenation compromised, but he may develop other problems as well. For instance, the patient may experience ineffective airway clearance and gas exchange, altered cardiac output, altered fluid volume, impaired thermoregulation, and decreased mobility. He may be anxious, cope ineffectively, and have an impaired ability to communicate. In addition, his nutritional status may be compromised. For such a patient, you'll need to develop an individual plan of care to ensure that he achieves optimum gas exchange and physical function.

To meet your care goals, you need to have a working knowledge of the many therapies available to respiratory patients. Although many hospitals have staff who specialize in respiratory procedures, you still need to keep your knowledge up-to-date. That way, you'll understand the rationales behind the patient's treatment, perform or assist with procedures if necessary, recognize complications, and detect the need for additional therapy. You'll also work with other members of the health care team to teach the patient and his family about equipment and procedures necessary for his care.

AIRWAY MANAGEMENT
Obstructed airway management

Sudden airway obstruction may occur when a foreign body lodges in the throat or bronchus; when the patient aspirates blood, mucus, or vomitus; when the tongue blocks the pharynx; or when the patient experiences traumatic injury, bronchoconstriction, or bronchospasm.

An obstructed airway causes anoxia, which in turn leads to brain damage and death in 4 to 6 minutes. The Heimlich maneuver uses an upper-abdominal thrust to create diaphragmatic pressure in the static lung below the foreign body sufficient to expel the obstruction. The Heimlich maneuver is used in conscious adult patients; if the patient is unconscious, an abdominal thrust should be used. However, the abdominal thrust is contraindicated in pregnant women, markedly obese patients, and patients who have recently undergone abdominal surgery. For such patients, a chest thrust, which forces air out of the lungs to create an artificial cough, should be used. The finger sweep maneuver is then used to manually remove the foreign body from the mouth.

These maneuvers are contraindicated in a patient with incomplete or partial airway obstruction or when the patient can maintain adequate ventilation to dislodge the foreign body by effective coughing. However, the patient's inability to speak, cough, or breathe demands immediate action to dislodge the obstruction. (Also see "Cardiopulmonary resuscitation" in Chapter 7.)

Implementation

• Determine the patient's level of consciousness by tapping his shoulder and asking, "Are you choking?" If he has a complete airway obstruction, he won't be able to answer because airflow to his vocal cords will be blocked. If he makes crowing sounds, his airway is partially obstructed, and you should encourage him to cough. This will either clear the airway or make the obstruction complete. For a complete obstruction, intervene as follows, depending on whether the patient is conscious or unconscious.

Conscious adult

• Tell the patient that you'll try to dislodge the foreign body.
• Standing behind the patient, wrap your arms around her waist. Make a fist with one hand and place the thumb side against her abdomen, slightly above the umbilicus and well below the xiphoid process. Then grasp your fist with the other hand.

● Squeeze the patient's abdomen 6 to 10 times with quick inward and upward thrusts. Each thrust should be a separate and distinct movement; each should be forceful enough to create an artificial cough that will dislodge an obstruction.

● Make sure you have a firm grasp on the patient because she may lose consciousness and need to be lowered to the floor. Look around the floor for objects that may harm her. Then, if she does lose consciousness, lower her carefully to the floor. Support her head and neck to prevent injury, and continue as described below.

Unconscious adult
● If you come upon an unconscious patient, ask any witnesses what happened. Begin cardiopulmonary resuscitation (CPR) and attempt to ventilate the patient. If you're unable to ventilate her, reposition her head and try again.

● If you still can't ventilate the patient, or if a conscious patient loses consciousness during abdominal thrusts, kneel astride her thighs.
● Place the heel of one hand on top of the other. Then place your hands between her umbilicus and the tip of her xiphoid process at the midline. Push inward and upward with 6 to 10 quick abdominal thrusts.

● After delivering the abdominal thrusts, open the patient's airway by grasping the tongue and lower jaw with your thumb and fingers. Lift the jaw *to draw the tongue away from the back of the throat and away from any foreign body.*

• If you can see the object, remove it by inserting your index finger deep into the throat at the base of her tongue. Using a hooking motion, remove the obstruction. Keep in mind that some clinicians object to a blind finger sweep—using your finger when you can't see the obstruction—*because your finger acts as a second obstruction.* They believe that, in most cases, the tongue-jaw lift described above should be enough to dislodge the obstruction.

• After the object is removed, try to ventilate the patient. Then assess for spontaneous respirations, and check for a pulse. Proceed with CPR if necessary.
• If the object is not removed, try to ventilate the patient. If you can't, repeat the abdominal thrust maneuver described above in sequence until you clear the airway.

Obese or pregnant adult
• If the patient is conscious, stand behind her and place your arms under her armpits and around her chest.
• Place the thumb side of your clenched fist against the middle of the sternum, avoiding the margins of the ribs and the xiphoid process. Grasp your fist with your other hand and perform a chest thrust with enough force to expel the foreign body. Continue until the patient expels the obstruction or loses consciousness (top right).

• If the patient loses consciousness, carefully lower her to the floor.
• Kneel close to the patient's side and place the heel of one hand just above the bottom of the patient's sternum. The long axis of the heel of your hand should align with the long axis of the patient's sternum. Place the heel of your other hand on top of that, making sure your fingers don't touch the patient's chest. Deliver each thrust forcefully enough to remove the obstruction.

Child

• If the child is conscious and can stand, perform abdominal thrusts using the same technique as you would with an adult, but with less force.
• If he's unconscious or lying down, kneel at his feet; if he's a large child, kneel astride his thighs. If he's lying on a treatment table, stand by his side. Deliver abdominal thrusts as you would for an adult patient, but use less force. (Never perform a blind finger sweep on a child *because you risk pushing the foreign body further back into the airway.)*

Infant

• Whether the infant is conscious or not, place him face down so that he's straddling your arm with his head lower than his trunk. Rest your forearm on your thigh and deliver four back blows with the heel of your hand between the infant's shoulder blades.

• If you haven't removed the obstruction, place your free hand on the infant's back. Supporting his neck, jaw, and chest with your other hand, turn him over onto your thigh. Keep his head lower than his trunk.

• Position your fingers. To do so, imagine a line between the infant's nipples and place the index finger of your free hand on his sternum, just below this imaginary line. Then place your middle and ring fingers next to your index finger and lift the index finger off his chest. Deliver four chest thrusts as you would for chest compression, but at a slower rate. (As with a child, never perform a blind finger sweep.)

Special considerations

If your patient vomits during abdominal thrusts, quickly wipe out his mouth with your fingers and resume the maneuver as necessary.

Even if your efforts to clear the airway don't seem to be effective, keep trying. As oxygen deprivation increases, smooth and skeletal muscles relax, making your maneuvers more likely to succeed.

Complications

Nausea, regurgitation, and achiness may develop after the patient regains consciousness and can breathe independently. He may also be injured, possibly from incorrect placement of the rescuer's hands or because of osteoporosis or metastatic lesions that increase the risk of fracture. Examine the patient for injuries, such as ruptured or lacerated abdominal or thoracic viscera.

Documentation

Record the date and time of the procedure, the patient's actions before the obstruction, the approximate length of time it took to clear the airway, and the type and size of the object removed. Also note his vital signs after the procedure, any complications that occurred and nursing actions taken, and his tolerance of the procedure.

⬙⬙ Oropharyngeal airway

An oropharyngeal airway, a curved rubber or plastic device, is inserted into the mouth to the posterior pharynx to establish or maintain a patent airway. In an unconscious patient, the tongue usually obstructs the posterior pharynx. The oropharyngeal airway conforms to the curvature of the palate, removing the obstruction and allowing air to pass around and through the tube. It also facilitates oropharyngeal suctioning. The oropharyngeal airway is intended for short-term use, as in the postanesthesia or postictal stage. It may be left in place longer as an airway adjunct to prevent the orally intubated patient from biting the endotracheal tube.

The oropharyngeal airway is not the airway of choice for the patient with loose or avulsed teeth or recent oral surgery. Inserting this airway in the conscious or semiconscious patient may stimulate vomiting and laryngospasm; therefore, you'll usually insert the airway only in unconscious patients.

Equipment

For inserting: oral airway of appropriate size ▪ tongue blade ▪ padded tongue blade ▪ gloves ▪ optional: suction equipment, hand-held resuscitation bag or oxygen-powered breathing device.

For cleaning: hydrogen peroxide ▪ water ▪ basin ▪ optional: pipe cleaner.

For reflex testing: cotton-tipped applicator.

Preparation of equipment

Select an airway of appropriate size for your patient; *an oversized airway can obstruct breathing by depressing the epiglottis into the laryngeal opening.* Usually, you'll select a small size (size 1 or 2) for an infant or child, a medium size (size 4 or 5) for the average adult, and a large size (size 6) for the large adult. Be sure to confirm the correct size of the airway by placing the airway flange beside the patient's cheek, parallel to his front teeth. If the airway is the right size, the airway curve should reach to the angle of the jaw.

Implementation

• Explain the procedure to the patient even though he may not appear to be alert. Provide privacy and put on gloves *to prevent contact with body fluids.* If the patient is wearing dentures, remove them *so they don't cause further airway obstruction.*
• If necessary, suction the patient.
• Place the patient in the supine position with his neck hyperextended, if this is not contraindicated.
• Insert the airway using the cross-finger or the tongue blade technique. (See *Inserting an oral airway.*)
• Auscultate the lungs to ensure adequate ventilation.
• After the airway is inserted, position the patient on his side *to decrease the risk of aspiration of vomitus.*
• Perform mouth care every 2 to 4 hours, as needed. Begin by holding the patient's jaws open with a padded tongue blade and gently removing the airway. Place the airway in a basin and rinse it with hydrogen peroxide followed by water. If secretions remain, use a pipe cleaner to remove them. Complete standard mouth care and reinsert the airway.
• While the airway is removed for mouth care, observe the mouth's mucous membranes *because tissue irritation or ulceration can result from prolonged airway use.*

Inserting an oral airway

Unless this position is contraindicated, hyperextend the patient's head as shown below before using either the cross-finger or tongue blade insertion method.

To insert an oral airway using the cross-finger method, place your thumb on the patient's lower teeth and your index finger on his upper teeth. Gently open his mouth by pushing his teeth apart.

Insert the airway upside down to avoid pushing the tongue towards the pharynx, and slide it over the tongue toward the back of the mouth. Rotate the airway as it approaches the posterior wall of the pharynx so that it points downward, as shown below.

To use the tongue blade technique, open the patient's mouth and depress his tongue with the blade. Guide the airway over the back of the tongue as you did for the cross-finger technique.

• Frequently check the position of the airway *to ensure correct placement.*

• When the patient regains consciousness and is able to swallow, remove the airway by pulling it outward and downward, following the mouth's natural curvature. After the airway is removed, test the patient's cough and gag reflexes *to ensure that removal of the airway wasn't premature, and that the patient can maintain his own airway.*

• To test for gag reflex, use a cotton-tipped applicator to touch both sides of the posterior pharynx. To test for cough reflex, gently touch the posterior oropharynx with the cotton-tipped applicator.

Special considerations

Clear breath sounds on auscultation indicate that the airway is the proper size and that it's in the correct position.

Avoid taping the airway in place *because untaping it could delay airway removal, thus increasing the risk of aspiration.*

Evaluate the patient's behavior *to provide the cue for airway removal.* The patient is likely to gag or cough as he becomes more alert, indicating that he no longer needs the airway.

Complications

Tooth damage or loss, tissue damage, and bleeding may result from insertion.

If the airway is too long, it may press the epiglottis against the entrance of the larynx, producing complete airway obstruction. If the airway is not inserted properly, it may push the tongue posteriorly, aggravating the problem of upper airway obstruction.

To prevent traumatic injury, make sure that the patient's lips and tongue are not between his teeth and the airway.

Immediately after inserting the airway, check for respirations. If respirations are absent or inadequate, initiate artificial positive pressure ventilation by using a mouth-to-mask technique, a hand-held resuscitation bag, or an oxygen-powered breathing device. (See "Manual ventilation" in this chapter.)

Documentation

Record the date and time of the airway's insertion; size of the airway; removal and cleaning of the airway; condition of mucous membranes; any suctioning; any adverse reactions and the nursing action taken; and the patient's tolerance of the procedure.

Nasopharyngeal airway

Insertion of a nasopharyngeal airway — a soft rubber or latex uncuffed catheter — establishes or maintains a patent airway. This airway is the typical choice for patients who've had recent oral surgery or facial trauma, and for patients with loose, cracked, or avulsed teeth. It's also used to protect the nasal mucosa from injury when the patient needs frequent nasotracheal suctioning.

The airway follows the curvature of the nasopharynx, passing through the nose and extending from the nostril to the posterior pharynx. The bevel-shaped pharyngeal end of the airway facilitates insertion, and its funnel-shaped nasal end helps prevent slippage.

Insertion of a nasopharyngeal airway is preferred when an oropharyngeal airway is contraindicated or fails to maintain a patent airway. A nasopharyngeal airway is contraindicated if the patient is receiving anticoagulant therapy or has a hemorrhagic disorder, sepsis, or pathologic nasopharyngeal deformity.

Equipment

For insertion: nasopharyngeal airway of proper size ▪ tongue blade ▪ water-soluble lubricant ▪ gloves ▪ optional: suction equipment.

For cleaning: hydrogen peroxide ▪ water ▪ basin ▪ optional: pipe cleaner.

Preparation of equipment

Measure the diameter of the patient's nostril and the distance from the tip of his nose to his earlobe. Select an airway of slightly smaller diameter than the nostril and of slightly longer length (1" [2.5 cm]) than measured. The sizes for this type of airway are labeled according to their internal diameter.

The recommended size for a large adult is 8 to 9 mm; for a medium adult, 7 to 8 mm; for a small adult, 6 to 7 mm. Lubricate the distal half of the airway's surface with a water-soluble lubricant *to prevent traumatic injury during insertion.*

Implementation

• Put on gloves.

• In nonemergency situations, explain the procedure to the patient.

• Properly insert the airway. (See *Inserting a nasopharyngeal airway.*)

• Once the airway is inserted, check it regularly *to detect dislodgment or obstruction.*

• When the patient's natural airway is patent, remove the airway in one smooth motion. If the airway sticks, apply lubricant around the nasal end of the tube and around the nostril; then gently rotate the airway until it's free.

Special considerations
If the patient coughs or gags, the tube may be too long. If so, remove the airway and insert a shorter one. At least once every 8 hours, remove the airway *to check nasal mucous membranes for irritation or ulceration.* Clean the airway by placing it in a basin and rinsing it with hydrogen peroxide and then with water. If secretions remain, use a pipe cleaner to remove them. Reinsert the clean airway into the other nostril (if it's patent) *to avoid skin breakdown.*

Complications
Sinus infection may result from obstruction of sinus drainage. Insertion of the airway may injure the nasal mucosa and cause bleeding and possible aspiration of blood into the trachea. Suction as necessary to remove secretions or blood. If the tube is too long, it may enter the esophagus and cause gastric distention and hypo-ventilation during artificial ventilation.

Semiconscious patients usually tolerate this type of airway better than conscious patients; however, it may still precipitate laryngospasm and vomiting.

When you insert the airway, remember to use a chin-lift or jaw-thrust technique to anteriorly displace the patient's mandible. Immediately after insertion, assess the patient's respirations. If absent or inadequate, initiate artificial positive-pressure ventilation with a mouth-to-mask technique, a hand-held resuscitation bag, or an oxygen-powered breathing device.

Documentation
Record the date and time of the airway's insertion; size of the airway; removal and cleaning of the airway; shifts from one nostril to the other; condition of the mucous membranes; suctioning; complications and nursing action taken; and the patient's reaction to the procedure.

Oronasopharyngeal suction

Oronasopharyngeal suction removes secretions from the pharynx by means of a suction catheter inserted through the mouth or nostril. Used to maintain a patent airway, this procedure is indicated for the patient who's unable to clear his airway effectively with coughing and ex-pectoration; for example, the unconscious or severely de-

Inserting a nasopharyngeal airway

First, hold the airway beside the patient's face to be sure it's the proper size, as shown here. It should be slightly smaller than the patient's nostril diameter and slightly longer than the distance from the tip of his nose to his earlobe.

To insert the airway, hyperextend the patient's neck (unless contraindicated). Then, push up the tip of his nose and pass the airway into his nostril, as shown below. Avoid pushing against any resistance *to prevent tissue trauma and airway kinking.*

To check for correct airway placement, first close the patient's mouth. Then, place your finger over the tube's opening to detect air exchange. Also de-press the patient's tongue with a tongue blade and look for the airway tip behind the uvula.

bilitated patient, or the intubated patient who has secretions pooled above the cuff of the artificial airway.

The procedure should be done as often as necessary, depending on the patient's condition.

Because the catheter may inadvertently slip into the lower airway or esophagus, oronasopharyngeal suction is an aseptic procedure that requires sterile equipment. However, clean technique may be used for a tonsil tip suction device. In fact, an alert patient can use a tonsil tip suction device himself to remove secretions.

Nasopharyngeal suctioning should be used with caution in patients who have nasopharyngeal bleeding or spinal fluid leakage into the nasopharyngeal area. Also be alert when performing this procedure on patients receiving anticoagulant therapy or who have blood dyscrasias because these conditions increase the risk for bleeding.

Equipment

Wall suction or portable suction apparatus ■ collection bottle ■ connecting tubing ■ water-soluble lubricant ■ normal saline solution or sterile water ■ disposable sterile container ■ sterile suction catheter (a #12 or #14 French for an adult, #8 or #10 French for a child, or pediatric feeding tube for an infant) ■ sterile gloves ■ tonsil tip suction device ■ clean gloves ■ nasopharyngeal or oropharyngeal airway (optional for frequent suctioning) ■ overbed table ■ waterproof trash bag ■ soap, water, and 70% alcohol for cleaning catheters.

A sterile catheter, disposable container, and sterile gloves are available in a commercially prepared kit.

Preparation of equipment

Before beginning, check your hospital's policy to determine whether a doctor's order is required for oronasopharyngeal suctioning. Also review the patient's blood gas or oxygen saturation values, and check vital signs. Evaluate the patient's ability to cough and deep breathe *to determine his ability to move secretions up the tracheobronchial tree.* Check the patient's history for a deviated septum, nasal polyps, nasal obstruction, traumatic injury, epistaxis, or mucosal swelling.

If no contraindications exist, gather and place the suction equipment on the patient's overbed table or bedside stand. Position the table or stand on your preferred side of the bed *to facilitate suctioning.* Attach the collection bottle to the suctioning unit, and attach the connecting tubing to it. Date and then open the bottle of normal saline solution or sterile water. Open the waterproof trash bag.

Implementation

• Explain the procedure to the patient, even if he is unresponsive. Inform the patient that suctioning may stimulate transient coughing or gagging, but tell him that coughing helps to mobilize secretions. If the patient has been suctioned previously, simply summarize the reasons for the procedure. Continue to reassure the patient throughout the procedure *to minimize anxiety and fear. Anxiety and fear can increase oxygen consumption.* Also ask the patient which nostril is more patent.

• Wash your hands.

• Place the patient in semi-Fowler's or high Fowler's position, if tolerated, *to promote lung expansion and effective coughing.*

• Turn on the suction from the wall or portable unit and set the pressure according to hospital policy. Usually, the pressure may be set between 80 and 120 mm Hg; higher pressures cause excessive trauma without enhancing secretion removal. Occlude the end of the connecting tubing *to check suction pressure.*

• Using strict aseptic technique, open the suction catheter kit or the sterile catheter, container, and gloves. Put on the gloves and consider your dominant hand sterile and your nondominant hand nonsterile. Using your nondominant (nonsterile) hand, pour the sterile water or saline into the sterile container.

• With your nondominant hand, place a small amount of water-soluble lubricant on the sterile area. The lubricant is used *to facilitate passage of the catheter during nasopharyngeal suctioning.*

• Pick up the catheter with your dominant (sterile) hand and attach it to the connecting tubing. Use your nondominant hand to control the suction valve while your dominant hand manipulates the catheter.

• Instruct the patient to cough and breathe slowly and deeply several times before beginning suction. *Coughing helps loosen secretions and may decrease the amount of suctioning necessary, while deep breathing helps minimize or prevent hypoxia.* (See *Tips on airway clearance.*)

For nasal insertion

• Raise the tip of the patient's nose with your nondominant hand *to straighten the passageway and facilitate insertion of the catheter.* Without applying suction, gently insert the suction catheter into the patient's nares. Roll the catheter between your fingers *to help it advance through the turbinates.* Continue to advance the catheter approximately 5″ to 6″ (12.7 to 15 cm) until you reach the pool of secretions or the patient begins to cough.

For oral insertion

• Without applying suction, gently insert the catheter into the patient's mouth. Advance the catheter approximately 3″ to 4″ (7.6 to 10 cm) along the side of the patient's mouth until you reach the pool of secretions or the patient begins to cough. Suction both sides of the patient's mouth and pharyngeal area.

• Using intermittent suction, withdraw the catheter from either the mouth or the nose with a continuous rotating motion *to minimize invagination of the mucosa into the catheter's tip and side ports.* Apply suction for only 10 to 15 seconds at a time *to minimize tissue trauma.*

• Between passes, wrap the catheter around your dominant hand *to prevent contamination.*

• If secretions are thick, clear the lumen of the catheter by dipping it in water and applying suction.

• Repeat the procedure until gurgling or bubbling sounds stop and respirations are quiet.

• After completing suctioning, pull your sterile glove off over the coiled catheter and discard it and the nonsterile glove along with the container of water.

• Flush the connecting tubing with normal saline solution or water.

• Replace the used items *so they're ready for the next suctioning,* and wash your hands.

Special considerations

If the patient has no history of nasal problems, alternate suctioning between nostrils *to minimize traumatic injury.* If repeated oronasopharyngeal suctioning is required, the use of a nasopharyngeal or oropharyngeal airway will *help with catheter insertion, reduce traumatic injury, and promote a patent airway. To facilitate catheter insertion for oropharyngeal suctioning,* depress the patient's tongue with a tongue blade, or ask another nurse to do so. *This helps you to visualize the back of the throat and also prevents the patient from biting the catheter.*

If the patient has excessive oral secretions, consider using a tonsil tip catheter *because this allows the patient to remove oral secretions independently, as needed.*

Let the patient rest after suctioning while you continue to observe him. The frequency and duration of suctioning depends on the patient's tolerance for the procedure and on any complications.

Home care

Oronasopharyngeal suctioning may be performed in the home using a portable suction machine. Under these circumstances, suctioning is a clean rather than a sterile procedure. Properly cleaned catheters can be reused, putting less financial strain on patients.

Catheters should be cleaned by first washing them in soapy water and then boiling them for 10 minutes or soaking them in 70% alcohol for 3 to 5 minutes. The catheters should then be rinsed with normal saline solution or tap water.

Tips on airway clearance

Deep breathing and coughing are vital for removing secretions from the lungs. Additional methods to help clear the airway include diaphragmatic breathing and forced expiration. Here's how to teach these methods to your patients.

Diaphragmatic breathing

First, tell the patient to lie supine, with his head elevated 15 to 20 degrees on a pillow. Tell him to place one hand on his abdomen, and then to inhale so that he can feel his abdomen rise. Explain that this is what's known as "breathing with the diaphragm."

Next, instruct the patient to exhale slowly through his nose — or, even better, through pursed lips — while letting his abdomen collapse. Explain that this action decreases his respiratory rate and increases his tidal volume.

Suggest that the patient perform this exercise for 30 minutes several times a day. After he becomes accustomed to the position, and after he's learned to breathe using his diaphragm, he may apply abdominal weights of 4 to 5 kg. The weights enhance the movement of the diaphragm toward the head during expiration.

To enhance the effectiveness of exercise, the patient may also manually compress the lower costal margins, perform straight leg lifts, and coordinate the breathing technique with a physical activity, such as walking.

Forced expiration

Another technique you should teach the patient is forced expiration. First, explain that forced expiration helps clear secretions while causing less traumatic injury than does a cough.

To perform the technique, tell the patient to forcefully expire without closing his glottis, starting with a mid- to low-lung volume. Tell him to follow this expiration with a period of diaphragmatic breathing and relaxation.

Advise the patient that if his secretions are in the central airways, he may have to use a more forceful expiration or a cough to clear them.

Whether the patient requires disposable or reusable suction equipment, you should make sure that the patient and his caregivers have received proper teaching and support.

Complications

Increased dyspnea caused by hypoxia and anxiety may result from this procedure. Hypoxia can result because oxygen from the oronasopharynx is removed with the secretions. The amount of oxygen removed varies, depending upon the duration of the suctioning, suction flow and pressure, the size of the catheter in relation to the size of the patient's airway, and the patient's physical condition.

In addition, bloody aspirate can result from prolonged or traumatic suctioning. Water-soluble lubricant can help to minimize traumatic injury.

Documentation

Record the date, time, reason for suctioning, and technique used; amount, color, consistency, and odor (if any) of the secretions; the patient's respiratory status before and after the procedure; any complications and the nursing action taken; and the patient's tolerance for the procedure.

 Tracheal suction

This procedure involves the removal of secretions from the trachea or bronchi by means of a catheter inserted through the mouth, nose, tracheal stoma, tracheostomy tube, or endotracheal tube. Besides removing secretions, tracheal suctioning also stimulates the cough reflex. This procedure helps maintain a patent airway to promote optimal exchange of oxygen and carbon dioxide and to prevent pneumonia that results from pooling of secretions. Performed as frequently as the patient's condition warrants, tracheal suction calls for strict aseptic technique.

Equipment

Oxygen source (wall or portable unit, and hand-held resuscitation bag with a mask, 15-mm adapter, or a positive end-expiratory pressure [PEEP] valve, if indicated) ■ wall or portable suction apparatus ■ collection container ■ connecting tube ■ suction catheter kit, or a sterile suction catheter, one sterile glove, one clean glove, and a disposable sterile solution container ■ 1-liter bottle of sterile water or normal saline solution ■ sterile water-soluble lubricant (for nasal insertion) ■ syringe for deflating cuff of endotracheal or tracheostomy tube ■ waterproof trash bag ■ optional: sterile towel.

Preparation of equipment

Choose a suction catheter of appropriate size. The diameter should be no larger than half the inside diameter of the tracheostomy or endotracheal tube *to minimize hypoxia during suctioning.* (A #12 or #14 French catheter may be used for an 8-mm or larger tube.) Place the suction apparatus on the patient's overbed table or bedside stand. Position the table or stand on your preferred side of the bed *to facilitate suctioning.*

Attach the collection container to the suction unit and the connecting tube to the collection container. Label and date the normal saline solution or sterile water. Open the waterproof trash bag.

Implementation

● Before suctioning, determine whether your hospital requires a doctor's order and obtain one, if necessary.
● Assess the patient's vital signs, breath sounds, and general appearance *to establish a baseline for comparison after suctioning.* Review the patient's arterial blood gas values and oxygen saturation levels if they're available. Evaluate the patient's ability to cough and deep breathe *because this will help move secretions up the tracheobronchial tree.* If you'll be performing nasotracheal suctioning, check the patient's history for a deviated septum, nasal polyps, nasal obstruction, nasal trauma, epistaxis, or mucosal swelling.
● Wash your hands. Explain the procedure to the patient, even if he is unresponsive. Tell him that suctioning usually causes transient coughing or gagging, but that coughing is helpful for removal of secretions. If the patient has been suctioned previously, summarize the reasons for suctioning. Continue to reassure the patient throughout the procedure *to minimize anxiety, promote relaxation, and decrease oxygen demand.*
● Unless contraindicated, place the patient in the semi-Fowler's or high Fowler's position *to promote lung expansion and productive coughing.*
● Remove the top from the normal saline solution or water bottle. Then open the package containing the sterile solution container.
● Using strictly aseptic technique, open the suction catheter kit and put on the gloves. If using individual supplies, open the suction catheter and the gloves, placing the nonsterile glove on your nondominant hand and then the sterile glove on your dominant hand.
● Using your nondominant (nonsterile) hand, pour the normal saline solution or sterile water into the container.
● Place a small amount of water-soluble lubricant on the sterile area. *Lubricant may be used to facilitate passage of the catheter during nasotracheal suctioning.*
● Place a sterile towel over the patient's chest, if desired, *to provide an additional sterile area.*

• Using your dominant (sterile) hand, remove the catheter from its wrapper. Keep it coiled *so it can't touch a nonsterile object*. Using your other hand to manipulate the connecting tubing, attach the catheter to the tubing.

• Using your nondominant hand, set the suction pressure according to hospital policy. Typically, pressure may be set between 80 and 120 mm Hg. *Higher pressures don't enhance secretion removal and may cause traumatic injury.* Occlude the suction port *to assess suction pressure* (see below).

• Dip the catheter tip in the saline solution *to lubricate the outside of the catheter and reduce tissue trauma during insertion.*

• With the catheter tip in the sterile solution, occlude the control valve with the thumb of your nondominant hand. Suction a small amount of solution through the catheter, as shown below, *to lubricate the inside of the catheter to facilitate passage of secretions through it.*

• For nasal insertion of the catheter, lubricate the tip of the catheter with the sterile, water-soluble lubricant *to reduce tissue trauma during insertion.*

• If the patient is not intubated, or is intubated but is not receiving supplemental oxygen or aerosol, instruct him to take three to six deep breaths *to help minimize or prevent hypoxia during suctioning.*

• If the patient is not intubated but is receiving oxygen, evaluate his need for preoxygenation. If indicated, instruct the patient to take three to six deep breaths while using his supplemental oxygen. (If needed, the patient may continue to receive supplemental oxygen during suctioning by leaving his nasal cannula in one nostril or by keeping the oxygen mask over his mouth.)

• If the patient is being mechanically ventilated, preoxygenate him by using either a hand-held resuscitation bag or the sigh mode on the ventilator. To use the resuscitation bag, set the oxygen flow meter at 15 liters/minute, disconnect the patient from the ventilator, and deliver three to six breaths with the resuscitation bag, as shown on page 348.

• If the patient is being maintained on PEEP, evaluate the need to use a resuscitation bag with a PEEP valve.
• To preoxygenate using the ventilator, first adjust the fraction of inspired oxygen (FIO_2) and tidal volume according to hospital policy and patient need. Then, either use the sigh mode or manually deliver three to six breaths. If you have an assistant for the procedure, the assistant can manage the patient's oxygen needs while you perform the suctioning.

Nasotracheal insertion in a nonintubated patient
• Disconnect the oxygen from the patient, if applicable.
• Using your nondominant hand, raise the tip of the patient's nose *to straighten the passageway and facilitate insertion of the catheter.*
• Insert the catheter into the patient's nostril while gently rolling it between your fingers *to help it advance through the turbinates.*
• As the patient inhales, quickly advance the catheter as far as possible. Do not apply suction during insertion *to avoid oxygen loss and tissue trauma.*
• If the patient coughs as the catheter passes through the larynx, briefly hold the catheter still and then resume advancement when the patient inhales.

Insertion in an intubated patient
• If you are using a closed system, see *Closed tracheal suctioning.*
• Using your nonsterile hand, disconnect the patient from the ventilator.
• Using your sterile hand, gently insert the suction catheter into the artificial airway, as shown at upper right. Advance the catheter, without applying suction, until you

meet resistance. If the patient coughs, pause briefly and then resume advancement.

Suctioning the patient
• After inserting the catheter, apply suction intermittently by removing and replacing the thumb of your nondominant hand over the control valve. Simultaneously use your dominant hand to withdraw the catheter as you roll it between your thumb and forefinger. *This rotating motion prevents the catheter from pulling tissue into the tube as it exits, thus avoiding tissue trauma.* Never suction more than 5 to 10 seconds at a time *to prevent hypoxia.*
• If the patient is intubated, use your nondominant hand to stabilize the tip of the endotracheal tube as you withdraw the catheter *to prevent mucous membrane irritation or accidental extubation.*
• If applicable, resume oxygen delivery by reconnecting the source of oxygen or ventilation, and hyperoxygenating the patient's lungs before continuing *to prevent or relieve hypoxia.*
• Observe the patient and allow him to rest for a few minutes before the next suctioning. The timing of each suctioning and the length of each rest period depend on his tolerance for the procedure and the absence of complications. *To enhance secretion removal,* encourage the patient to cough between suctioning attempts.
• Observe the secretions. If they're thick, clear the catheter periodically by dipping the tip in the saline solution and applying suction. Normally, sputum is watery and tends to be sticky. Tenacious or thick sputum usually indicates dehydration. Watch for color variations. White or translucent color is normal; yellow indicates pus; green indicates retained secretions or *Pseudomonas* infection; brown usually indicates old blood; red indicates fresh

Closed tracheal suctioning

The closed tracheal suction system eliminates the need to disconnect the patient from the mechanical ventilator for suctioning.

T-piece

Suction catheter

Catheter sleeve

As a result, the patient can maintain the tidal volume, oxygen concentration, and positive-end expiratory pressure delivered by the ventilator while being suctioned. In turn, this reduces the occurrence of suction-induced hypoxemia.

Another advantage of this system is a reduced risk of infection, even when the same catheter is used many times. Because the catheter remains in a protective sleeve, gloves are not required.

To perform the procedure, gather a closed suction control valve, a T-piece to connect the artificial airway to the ventilator breathing circuit, and a catheter sleeve that encloses the catheter and has connections at each end for the control valve and T-piece. Then follow these steps:
• Remove the closed suction system from its wrapping. Attach the control valve to the connecting tubing.
• Depress the thumb suction control valve and keep it depressed while setting the suction pressure to the desired level.
• Connect the T-piece to the ventilator breathing circuit, making sure that the irrigation port is closed; then connect the T-piece to the patient's endotracheal or tracheostomy tube, as shown at upper right.

• With one hand keeping the T-piece parallel to the patient's chin, use the thumb and index finger of the other hand to advance the catheter through the tube and into the patient's tracheobronchial tree, as shown below. It may be necessary to gently retract the catheter sleeve as you advance the catheter.

• While continuing to hold the T-piece and control valve, apply intermittent suction and withdraw the catheter until it reaches its fully extended length in the sleeve. Repeat the procedure as necessary.
• To instill normal saline solution into the airway, advance the catheter approximately 6″ (15 cm) into the tube and inject the solution into the irrigation port. Suction as needed.
• After suctioning is complete, flush the catheter by maintaining suction while slowly introducing normal saline or sterile water into the irrigation port.
• Place the thumb control valve in the off position.
• Dispose of and replace the suction equipment and supplies according to hospital policy. Change the closed suction system every 24 hours to minimize the risk of infection.

Tracheal suctioning at home

If a patient can't mobilize secretions effectively by coughing, he may have to perform tracheal suctioning at home using either clean or aseptic technique. Most patients use clean technique; they perform thorough hand washing and may don a clean glove. However, a patient with poor hand-washing technique, recurrent respiratory infections, recent surgery, or a compromised immune system may need to use aseptic technique.

Clean technique

Because the cost of disposable catheters can be prohibitive, many patients reuse disposable catheters, but the practice remains controversial. If the catheter has thick secretions adhering to it, the patient may clean it with Control III, a quaternary compound.

An alternative to disposable catheters is to use nondisposable, red rubber catheters. Consult institutional policy regarding the care and cleaning of suction catheters in the home setting. Some protocols recommend soaking such catheters in soapy water, then placing them in boiling water for 10 minutes; or soaking them in 70% alcohol for 3 to 5 minutes, then rinsing in normal saline solution.

Supplies needed

Obviously, the supplies needed will vary with the technique used. If the patient will be using clean technique he'll need suction catheter kits (or clean gloves, suction catheters, and a basin), and distilled water. If he'll be using sterile technique, the suction catheters and gloves will need to be sterile, as will the basin and the water (or normal saline).

The type of suction machine necessary will depend upon the patient's needs. You'll need to evaluate the amount of suction the machine provides, how easy it is to clean, the volume of the collection bottles, how much it costs, and whether the machine has an overflow safety device to prevent secretions from entering the compressor. You'll also need to determine whether the patient needs a machine that operates on batteries and, if so, how long the batteries will last, and if and how they can be recharged.

Nursing goals

Before discharge, the patient and his family should demonstrate the suctioning procedure. They also need to recognize the indications for suctioning, the signs and symptoms of infection, the importance of adequate hydration, and when to use adjunct therapy, such as aerosol therapy, chest physiotherapy, oxygen therapy, or a hand-held resuscitation bag. At discharge, arrange for a home health care provider and a durable medical equipment vendor to follow up with the patient.

---

blood; and a "red currant jelly" appearance indicates *Klebsiella* infection. When sputum contains blood, note whether it is streaked or well mixed. Also indicate how often blood appeared.

If the patient's heart rate and rhythm are being monitored, observe for arrhythmias. Should they occur, stop suctioning and ventilate the patient.

After suctioning

• After the procedure, hyperoxygenate the patient being maintained on a ventilator with the hand-held resuscitation bag or by using the ventilator's sigh mode, as described earlier.
• Readjust the FIO_2 and, for ventilated patients, the tidal volume, to the ordered settings.
• After suctioning the lower airway, assess the patient's need for upper airway suctioning. If the cuff of the endotracheal or tracheostomy tube is inflated, suction the upper airway before deflating the cuff with a syringe. (See "Oronasopharyngeal suction" in this chapter for more information.) Always change the catheter and sterile glove before resuctioning the lower airway *to avoid introducing microorganisms into the lower airway.*
• Discard the gloves and the catheter in the waterproof trash bag. Clear the connecting tubing by aspirating the remaining saline solution or water. Discard and replace suction equipment and supplies according to hospital policy. Wash your hands.
• Auscultate lungs bilaterally and take vital signs, if indicated, *to assess the procedure's effectiveness.*

Special considerations

Raising the patient's nose into the sniffing position helps align the larynx and pharynx and may facilitate passing the catheter during nasotracheal suctioning. If the patient's condition permits, have an assistant extend the patient's head and neck above his shoulders. The patient's lower jaw may need to be moved up and forward. If the patient is responsive, ask him to stick out his tongue *so he will not be able to swallow the catheter during insertion.*

During suctioning, the catheter typically is advanced as far as the mainstem bronchi. However, because of tracheobronchial anatomy, the catheter tends to enter the right mainstem bronchi instead of the left. Using an angled catheter (such as a Coude or Bronchitrac L) may help you guide the catheter into the left mainstem bronchus. Rotating the patient's head to the right seems to have a limited effect.

Studies show that instillation of normal saline solution into the trachea before suctioning may stimulate the patient's cough but does not liquefy the patient's secretions. Keeping the patient adequately hydrated and using bronchial hygiene techniques seems to have a greater effect on mobilizing secretions.

In addition to the closed tracheal method, oxygen insufflation offers a new approach to suctioning. Oxygen insufflation suctioning uses a double lumen catheter that allows oxygen insufflation during the suctioning procedure.

Do not allow the collection container on the suction machine to become more than ¾ full *to keep from damaging the machine.*

Home care
See *Tracheal suctioning at home.*

Complications
Because oxygen is removed along with secretions, the patient may experience hypoxemia and dyspnea. Anxiety may alter respiratory patterns. Cardiac arrhythmias can result from hypoxia and stimulation of the vagus nerve in the tracheobronchial tree. Tracheal or bronchial trauma can result from traumatic or prolonged suctioning.

Patients with compromised cardiovascular or pulmonary status are at risk for hypoxemia, arrhythmias, hypertension, or hypotension. Patients with a history of nasopharyngeal bleeding, who are taking anticoagulants, who have a recent tracheostomy, or who have a blood dyscrasia incur an increased risk of bleeding as a result of suctioning. Use caution when suctioning patients who have increased intracranial pressure because it may increase pressure further.

If the patient experiences laryngospasm or bronchospasm (rare complications) during suctioning, disconnect the suction catheter from the connecting tubing and allow the catheter to act as an airway. Discuss with the patient's doctor the use of bronchodilators or lidocaine to reduce the risk of this complication.

Documentation
Record the date and time of the procedure, the technique used, and the reason for suctioning; amount, color, consistency, and odor (if any) of the secretions; any com-

plications and the nursing action taken; and pertinent data regarding the patient's subjective response to the procedure.

OTHER TREATMENTS
Oxygen administration

A patient will need oxygen therapy when hypoxemia results from a respiratory or cardiac emergency or an increase in metabolic function.

In a *respiratory emergency,* oxygen administration enables the patient to reduce his ventilatory effort. When conditions such as atelectasis or adult respiratory distress syndrome impair diffusion, or when lung volumes are decreased from alveolar hypoventilation, this procedure boosts alveolar oxygen levels.

In a *cardiac emergency,* oxygen therapy helps meet the increased myocardial work load as the heart tries to compensate for hypoxemia. Oxygen administration is particularly important for a patient whose myocardium is already compromised — perhaps from a myocardial infarction or cardiac arrhythmia.

When *metabolic demand* is high — in cases of massive trauma, burns, or high fever, for instance — oxygen administration supplies the body with enough oxygen to meet its cellular needs. This procedure also increases oxygenation in the patient with a reduced blood oxygen-carrying capacity, perhaps from carbon monoxide poisoning or sickle cell crisis.

The adequacy of oxygen therapy is determined by arterial blood gas (ABG) analysis, oximetry, and clinical examinations. The patient's condition and age will help determine the method of administration.

Equipment
The equipment needed depends on the type of delivery system ordered (see *Guide to oxygen delivery systems,* pages 352 to 355) and includes selections from the following list: oxygen source (wall unit, cylinder, liquid tank, or concentrator) ■ flowmeter ■ adapter, if using a wall unit, or a pressure-reduction gauge, if using a cylinder ■ sterile humidity bottle and adapters ■ sterile distilled water ■ OXYGEN PRECAUTION sign ■ appropriate oxygen delivery system (a nasal cannula, simple mask, partial rebreather mask, or nonrebreather mask for low-flow and variable oxygen concentrations; a venturi mask, aerosol mask, tracheostomy collar, T tube, tent, or oxyhood for high-flow and specific oxygen concentrations) ■ small-diameter and large-diameter connection tubing ■

(Text continues on page 355.)

Guide to oxygen delivery systems

Patients may receive oxygen through one of several administration systems. Each has its own benefits, drawbacks, and indications for use. Advantages and disadvantages of each system are compared below and on the following pages.

Nasal cannula
Oxygen is delivered through plastic cannulas in the patient's nostrils.

Advantages: safe and simple; comfortable and easily tolerated; nasal prongs can be shaped to fit any face; effective for low oxygen concentrations; allows movement, eating, and talking; inexpensive and disposable.

Disadvantages: can't deliver concentrations higher than 40%; can't be used in complete nasal obstruction; may cause headaches or dry mucous membranes if flow rate exceeds 6 liters/minute; can dislodge easily.

Administration guidelines: Ensure patency of the patient's nostrils with a flashlight. If patent, hook the cannula tubing behind the patient's ears and under the chin. Slide the adjuster upward under the chin to secure the tubing. If using an elastic strap to secure the cannula, position it over the ears and around the back of the head. Avoid applying too tightly, which can result in excess pressure on facial structures and cannula occlusion as well. With a nasal cannula, oral breathers achieve the same oxygen delivery as nasal breathers.

Simple mask
Oxygen flows through an entry port at the bottom of the mask and exits through large holes on the sides of the mask.

Adjustable strap

Tubing

Advantages: can deliver concentrations of 40% to 60%.

Disadvantages: hot and confining; may irritate patient's skin; tight seal that may cause discomfort is required for higher oxygen concentration; interferes with talking and eating; impractical for long-term therapy because of imprecision.

Administration guidelines: Select the mask size that offers the best fit. Place the mask over the patient's nose, mouth, and chin, and mold the flexible metal edge to the bridge of the nose. Adjust the elastic band around the head to hold the mask firmly but comfortably over the cheeks, chin, and bridge of the nose. For elderly or cachectic patients with sunken cheeks, tape gauze pads to the mask over the cheek area to try to create an airtight seal. Without this seal, room air dilutes the oxygen, preventing delivery of the prescribed concentration. A minimum of 5 liters/minute is required in all masks to flush expired carbon dioxide from the mask so the patient doesn't rebreathe it.

Guide to oxygen delivery systems *(continued)*

Partial rebreather mask

The patient inspires oxygen from a reservoir bag along with atmospheric air and oxygen from the mask. The first third of exhaled tidal volume enters the bag; the rest exits the mask. Because air entering the reservoir bag comes from the trachea and bronchi, where no gas exchange occurs, the patient rebreathes the oxygenated air he just exhaled.

Exhalation port
Oxygen tubing
Reservoir bag

Advantages: effectively delivers concentrations of 40% to 60%; openings in mask allow patient to inhale room air if oxygen source fails.

Disadvantages: tight seal required for accurate oxygen concentration may cause discomfort; interferes with eating and talking; hot and confining; may irritate skin; bag may twist or kink; impractical for long-term therapy.

Administration guidelines: Follow procedures listed for the simple mask. If the reservoir bag collapses more than slightly during inspiration, raise the flow rate until you see only a slight deflation. Marked or complete deflation indicates insufficient oxygen flow; carbon dioxide will accumulate in the mask and bag. Keep the reservoir bag from twisting or kinking. Ensure free expansion by making sure it lies outside the patient's gown and bedcovers.

Nonrebreather mask

On inhalation, a one-way valve opens, directing oxygen from a reservoir bag into the mask. On exhalation, gas exits the mask through the one-way valve and enters the atmosphere. The patient only breathes air from the bag.

One-way flaps
Oxygen tubing
Reservoir bag

Advantages: delivers the highest possible oxygen concentration (60% to 90%) short of intubation and mechanical ventilation; effective for short-term therapy; doesn't dry mucous membranes; can be converted to a partial rebreather mask, if necessary, by removing the one-way flap.

Disadvantages: requires a tight seal, which may be difficult to maintain and may cause discomfort; may irritate the patient's skin; impractical for long-term therapy.

Administration guidelines: Follow procedures listed for the simple mask. Make sure the mask fits very snugly. Make sure the one-way valves or flaps are secure and functioning. Because the mask excludes room air, valve malfunction can cause carbon dioxide buildup and suffocate an unconscious patient. If the reservoir bag collapses more than slightly during inspiration, raise the flow rate until you see only a slight deflation. Marked or complete deflation indicates an insufficient flow rate. Keep the reservoir bag from twisting or kinking. Ensure free expansion by making sure it lies outside the patient's gown and bedcovers.

(continued)

Guide to oxygen delivery systems *(continued)*

CPAP mask

This system allows the spontaneously breathing patient to receive continuous positive airway pressure (CPAP) with or without an artificial airway.

Head strap
Inlet valve
Oxygen tubing
Position-independent PEEP valve
Adjustable inflation valve

Advantages: noninvasively improves arterial oxygenation by increasing functional residual capacity; allows the patient to avoid intubation; allows the patient to talk and cough without interrupting positive pressure.

Disadvantages: requires a tight fit, which may cause discomfort; heightened risk of aspiration if the patient vomits; increased risk of pneumothorax, diminished cardiac output, and gastric distention; contraindicated in patients with chronic obstructive pulmonary disease, bullous lung disease, low cardiac output, or tension pneumothorax.

Administration guidelines: Place one strap behind the patient's head and the other strap over his head to ensure a snug fit. Attach one latex strap to the connector prong on one side of the mask. Then, use one hand to position the mask on the patient's face while using the other hand to connect the strap to the other side of the mask. After the mask is applied, assess the patient's respiratory, circulatory, and GI function every hour. Watch for signs of pneumothorax, decreased cardiac output, a drop in blood pressure, and gastric distention.

Transtracheal oxygen

The patient receives oxygen through a catheter inserted into the base of his neck in a simple outpatient procedure.

Thyroid cartilage
Cricoid cartilage

Advantages: supplies oxygen to the lungs throughout the respiratory cycle; provides continuous oxygen without hindering mobility; doesn't interfere with eating or talking; doesn't dry mucous membranes; catheter can easily be concealed by a shirt or scarf.

Disadvantages: not suitable for use in patients at risk for bleeding or those with severe bronchospasm, uncompensated respiratory acidosis, pleural herniation into the base of the neck, or high corticosteroid dosages.

Administration guidelines: After insertion, obtain a chest X-ray to confirm placement. Monitor the patient for bleeding, respiratory distress, pneumothorax, pain, coughing, or hoarseness. Don't use the catheter for about 1 week following insertion to decrease the risk of subcutaneous emphysema.

Guide to oxygen delivery systems *(continued)*

Venturi mask
The mask is connected to a Venturi device that mixes a specific volume of air and oxygen.

- Elastic head strap
- Vent holes
- Wide-bore tubing

Advantages: delivers highly accurate oxygen concentration despite patient's respiratory pattern because the same amount of air is always entrained; dilute jets can be changed or dial turned to change oxygen concentration; doesn't dry mucous membranes; humidity or aerosol can be added.

Disadvantages: confining and may irritate skin; oxygen concentration may be altered if mask fits loosely, tubing kinks, oxygen intake ports become blocked, flow is insufficient, or patient is hyperpneic; interferes with eating and talking; condensate may collect and drip on the patient if humidification is used.

Administration guidelines: Make sure that the oxygen flow rate is set at the amount specified on each mask and that the Venturi valve is set for the desired fraction of inspired oxygen.

Aerosols
A face mask, hood, tent, or tracheostomy tube or collar is connected to wide-bore tubing that receives aerosolized oxygen from a jet nebulizer. The jet nebulizer, which is attached near the oxygen source, adjusts air entrainment in a manner similar to the Venturi device.

- Tracheostomy collar

Advantages: administers high humidity; gas can be heated (when delivered through artificial airway) or cooled (when delivered through a tent).

Disadvantages: condensate collected in the tracheostomy collar or T tube may drain into the tracheostomy; the weight of the T tube can put stress on the tracheostomy tube.

Administration guidelines: Guidelines vary with the type of nebulizer used, including the ultrasonic, large volume, small volume, and in-line. When using a high-output nebulizer, watch for signs of overhydration, pulmonary edema, crackles, and electrolyte imbalance.

---

flashlight (for nasal cannula) ▪ water-soluble lubricant ▪ gauze pads and tape (for oxygen masks) ▪ jet adapter for Venturi mask (if adding humidity) ▪ optional: oxygen analyzer.

Preparation of equipment
Although a respiratory therapist typically is responsible for setting up, maintaining, and managing the equipment, you need a working knowledge of the oxygen system being used.

Check the oxygen outlet port *to verify flow.* Pinch the tubing near the prongs *to ensure that an audible alarm will sound if the oxygen flow stops.*

Implementation
- Assess the patient's condition. In an emergency, verify that he has an open airway before administering oxygen.
- Explain the procedure to the patient and let him know why he needs oxygen *to ensure his cooperation.*
- Check the patient's room *to make sure it's safe for oxygen administration.* Whenever possible, replace electrical de-

Types of home oxygen therapy

Home oxygen therapy can be administered using an oxygen tank, an oxygen concentrator, or liquid oxygen.

Oxygen tank
Commonly used for patients who need oxygen on a standby basis or who need a ventilator at home, the oxygen tank has several disadvantages, including its cumbersome design and the need for frequent refills. Because oxygen is stored under high pressure, the oxygen tank also poses a potential hazard.

Oxygen concentrator
The oxygen concentrator extracts oxygen molecules from room air. It can be used for low oxygen flow (less than 4 liters/minute) and doesn't need to be refilled with oxygen. However, because the oxygen concentrator runs on electricity, it won't function during a power failure.

Liquid oxygen
This option is used commonly by patients who are oxygen-dependent but still mobile. The system includes a large liquid reservoir for home use. When the patient wants to leave the house, he fills a portable unit worn over the shoulder; this supplies oxygen for up to several hours, depending on the liter flow.

---

vices with nonelectric ones and post a NO SMOKING sign in the patient's room. If the patient is a child and is in an oxygen tent, remove all toys that may produce a spark. *Oxygen supports combustion and the smallest spark can cause a fire.*

• Place an OXYGEN PRECAUTION sign over the patient's bed and on the door to his room.

• Assist in placing the oxygen delivery device on the patient. Make sure it fits properly and is stable.

• Monitor the patient's response to oxygen therapy. Check his ABG values during initial adjustments of oxygen flow. Once the patient is stabilized, pulse oximetry may be used instead. Check the patient frequently for signs of hypoxia, such as decreased level of consciousness, increased heart rate, arrhythmias, restlessness, perspiration, dyspnea, use of accessory muscles, yawning or flared nostrils, cyanosis, and cool, clammy skin.

• Observe the patient's skin integrity *to prevent skin breakdown on pressure points from the oxygen delivery device.* Wipe moisture or perspiration from the patient's face and from the mask as needed.

• If the patient will be receiving oxygen at a concentration above 60% for more than 24 hours, watch carefully for signs of oxygen toxicity. Remind the patient frequently to cough and deep breathe *to prevent atelectasis.* Also, *to prevent the development of serious lung damage,* measure ABG values repeatedly *to determine whether high oxygen concentrations are still necessary.*

Special considerations
Never administer oxygen at more than 2 liters/minute by nasal cannula to a patient with chronic lung disease unless you have a specific order to do so. *This is because some patients with chronic lung disease have become dependent on a state of hypercapnia and hypoxia to stimulate their respirations; therefore, supplemental oxygen could cause them to stop breathing.* However, long-term oxygen therapy of 12 to 17 hours daily may help patients with chronic lung disease to sleep better, survive longer, and experience a reduced incidence of pulmonary hypertension.

When monitoring a patient's response to a change in oxygen flow, check the pulse oximetry monitor or measure ABG values 20 to 30 minutes after adjusting the flow. In the interim, monitor the patient closely for any adverse response to the change in oxygen flow.

Home care
Before discharging a patient who will receive home oxygen therapy, make sure you know the types of oxygen therapy, the kinds of services that are available to him, and the service schedules offered by local home suppliers. Together with the doctor and the patient, choose the device best-suited to the patient. (See *Types of home oxygen therapy.*)

If the patient will be receiving transtracheal oxygen therapy, teach him how to properly clean and care for the catheter. (See *Transtracheal catheter care.*) Tell the patient to keep the skin surrounding the insertion site clean and dry to prevent infection.

No matter which device the patient uses, you'll need to evaluate his and his family's ability and motivation to administer oxygen therapy at home. Make sure they understand the reason the patient is receiving oxygen and the safety issues for administering oxygen. Teach them how to properly use and clean the equipment and supplies.

Transtracheal catheter care

Teach the patient with a transtracheal catheter how to care for the catheter as well as the skin surrounding the catheter. If the patient has a Heimlich Micro-Trach, tell him to clean around the catheter twice a day using a soapy cotton-tipped applicator and water. He also needs to irrigate the catheter while it's in place, two to three times a day, using normal saline solution. Tell him that this serves to loosen secretions and stimulate coughing. Instruct the patient to change the catheter once a month.

SCOOP catheter

If the patient has a SCOOP catheter, tell him to clean it two to three times a day to keep it free of mucus. Tell him that, before he begins cleaning, he should put on a nasal cannula, disconnect the oxygen tubing from the catheter, and then connect it to the cannula. Instruct the patient to irrigate the catheter by instilling 1½ ml of normal saline solution into the catheter, as shown in the illustration below. Forewarn him that this may make him cough.

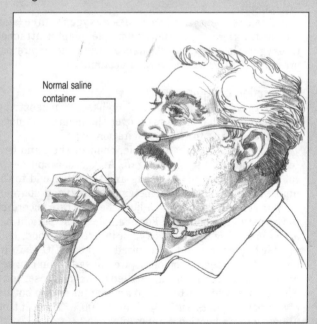

Normal saline container —

Next, tell him to insert a cleaning rod (which he's cleaned beforehand) through the catheter as far as possible and then to pull it back.

Cleaning rod —

After he has removed and reinserted the rod three times, tell him to remove the rod, instill 1½ ml of normal saline solution into the catheter, and then reconnect the oxygen tubing to the catheter. As a final step, instruct him to clean the rod with antimicrobial soap and to store it in a dry place.

In addition to cleaning the catheter while it remains in place, the patient with a SCOOP 1 catheter needs to remove the catheter at least once weekly—the patient with a SCOOP 2 catheter at least once daily—for a more thorough cleaning. (The SCOOP 2 catheter has extra side holes to facilitate oxygen distribution.) After the catheter is removed, tell the patient to use antimicrobial soap, a cleaning rod, and lukewarm tap water to clean the catheter.

Reminders

Remind the patient never to remove or insert a SCOOP catheter while oxygen is flowing through it. Rather, he should put on a nasal cannula, disconnect the catheter from the oxygen source, and then remove the catheter. Next, he should insert a second SCOOP catheter, coated with water-soluble lubricant. Once the second catheter is secured, he can resume oxygen delivery through the catheter.

If your patient will be discharged with oxygen for the first time, make sure his health insurance covers home oxygen. If it doesn't, find out what criteria he must meet to obtain coverage. Without a third-party payer, the patient may not be able to afford home oxygen therapy.

How to apply a hand-held resuscitation bag and mask

Place the mask over the patient's face so that the apex of the triangle covers the bridge of his nose and the base lies between his lower lip and chin.

Make sure that the patient's mouth remains open underneath the mask. Attach the bag to the mask and to the tubing leading to the oxygen source.

Or, if the patient has a tracheostomy or endotracheal tube in place, remove the mask from the bag and attach the hand-held resuscitation bag directly to the tube.

Documentation
Record the date and time of oxygen administration; the type of delivery device; the oxygen flow rate; the patient's vital signs, skin color, respiratory effort, and lung sounds; subjective patient response before and after initiation of therapy; and any patient or family teaching.

Manual ventilation

A hand-held resuscitation bag is an inflatable device that can be attached to a face mask or directly to an endotracheal or tracheostomy tube to allow manual delivery of oxygen or room air to the lungs of a patient who can't breathe by himself. Usually used in an emergency, manual ventilation also can be performed while the patient is disconnected temporarily from a mechanical ventilator, such as during a tubing change, during transport, or before suctioning. In such instances, use of the hand-held resuscitation bag maintains ventilation. Oxygen administration with a resuscitation bag can help improve a compromised cardiorespiratory system.

Equipment
Hand-held resuscitation bag ▪ mask ▪ oxygen source (wall unit or tank) ▪ oxygen tubing ▪ nipple adapter attached to oxygen flowmeter ▪ optional: positive end-expiratory pressure (PEEP) valve, oxygen accumulator.

Preparation of equipment
Unless the patient is intubated or has a tracheostomy, select a mask that fits snugly over the mouth and nose. Attach the mask to the resuscitation bag.

If oxygen is readily available, connect the hand-held resuscitation bag to the oxygen. Attach one end of the tubing to the bottom of the bag and the other end to the nipple adapter on the flowmeter of the oxygen source.

Turn on the oxygen and adjust the flow rate according to the patient's condition. For example, if the patient has a low partial pressure of oxygen in arterial blood, he'll need a higher fraction of inspired oxygen (FIO_2). To increase the concentration of inspired oxygen, you can add an oxygen accumulator (also called an oxygen reservoir). This device, which attaches to an adapter on the bottom of the bag, permits an FIO_2 of up to 100%. Then, if time allows, set up suction equipment.

Implementation
● Before using the hand-held resuscitation bag, check the patient's upper airway for foreign objects. If present, remove them *because this alone may restore spontaneous*

respirations in some instances. Also, foreign matter or secretions can obstruct the airway and impede resuscitation efforts. Suction the patient *to remove any secretions that may obstruct the airway.* If necessary, insert an oropharyngeal or nasopharyngeal airway *to maintain airway patency.* If the patient has a tracheostomy or endotracheal tube in place, suction the tube.

• If appropriate, remove the bed's headboard and stand at the head of the bed *to help keep the patient's neck extended and to free space at the side of the bed for other activities, such as cardiopulmonary resuscitation.*

• Tilt the patient's head backward, if not contraindicated, and pull his jaw forward *to move the tongue away from the base of the pharynx and prevent obstruction of the airway.* (See *How to apply a hand-held resuscitation bag and mask.*)

• Keeping your nondominant hand on the patient's mask, exert downward pressure *to seal the mask against his face.* For the adult patient, use your dominant hand to compress the bag every 5 seconds *to deliver about 1 liter of air.* For a child, deliver 15 breaths/minute, or one compression of the bag every 4 seconds; for the infant, 20 breaths/minute, or one compression every 3 seconds. Infants and children should receive 250 to 500 cc of air with each bag compression.

• Deliver breaths with the patient's own inspiratory effort, if any is present. Don't attempt to deliver a breath as the patient exhales.

• Observe the patient's chest *to ensure that it rises and falls with each compression.* If ventilation fails to occur, check the fit of the mask and the patency of the patient's airway; if necessary, reposition the patient's head and ensure patency with an oral airway.

Special considerations

Avoid neck hyperextension if the patient has a possible cervical injury; instead, use the jaw-thrust technique to open the airway. If you need both hands to keep the patient's mask in place and maintain hyperextension, use the lower part of your arm to compress the bag against your side.

Observe for vomiting through the clear part of the mask. If vomiting occurs, stop the procedure immediately, lift the mask, wipe and suction vomitus, and resume resuscitation.

Underventilation commonly occurs because the hand-held resuscitation bag is difficult to keep positioned tightly on the patient's face while ensuring an open airway. What's more, the volume of air delivered to the patient varies with the type of bag used and the hand size of the person compressing the bag. An adult with a small or medium-sized hand may not consistently deliver 1 liter of air. For these reasons, have someone assist with the procedure, if possible. (See *Using a PEEP valve.*)

Using a PEEP valve

Add positive end-expiratory pressure (PEEP) to manual ventilation by attaching a PEEP valve to the resuscitation bag. This may improve oxygenation if the patient hasn't responded to increased fraction of inspired oxygen levels. Always use a PEEP valve to manually ventilate a patient who has been receiving PEEP on the ventilator.

Complications

Aspiration of vomitus can result in pneumonia, and gastric distention may result from air forced into the patient's stomach.

Documentation

In an emergency, record the date and time of the procedure; manual ventilation efforts; any complications and the nursing action taken; and the patient's response to treatment, according to your hospital's protocol for respiratory arrest.

In a nonemergency, record the date and time of the procedure, the reason and duration the patient was disconnected from mechanical ventilation and received manual ventilation, any complications and the nursing action taken, and the patient's tolerance for the procedure.

 Humidifiers

Humidifiers, which deliver a maximum amount of water vapor without producing particulate water, are used to prevent drying and irritation of the upper airway in conditions where the upper airway is inflamed, such as croup, or when secretions are particularly thick and tenacious.

Some humidifiers heat the water vapor, which raises the moisture-carrying capacity of gas and thus increases the amount of humidity delivered to the patient. Room humidifiers add humidity to an entire room, while humidifiers added to gas lines humidify only the air being delivered to the patient. (See *Comparing humidifiers.*)

Equipment
Humidifier ■ bottled distilled water, or tap water if the unit has a demineralizing capability ■ container for waste water ■ bleach ■ white vinegar.

Preparation of equipment
For a bedside humidifier: Open the reservoir and add sterile distilled water to the fill line; then close the reservoir. Keep all room windows and doors closed tightly to maintain adequate humidification. Then plug the unit into the electrical outlet.

For a heated vaporizer: Remove the top and fill the reservoir to the fill line with tap water. Replace the top securely. Then place the vaporizer about 4 feet from the patient, directing the steam toward but not directly onto the patient. Place the unit in a spot where it can't be overturned *to avoid hot water burns.* This is especially important if children will be in the room.

Plug the unit into an electrical outlet. Steam should soon rise from the unit into the air. Close all windows and doors to maintain adequate humidification.

For a diffusion head humidifier: Unscrew the humidifier reservoir and add sterile distilled water to the appropriate level. (If using a disposable unit, screw the cap with the extension onto the top of the unit.) Then screw the reservoir back onto the humidifier and attach the flowmeter to the oxygen source.

Screw the humidifier onto the flowmeter until the seal is tight. Then set the flowmeter at a rate of 2 liters/minute and check for gentle bubbling.

Next, check the positive-pressure release valve by occluding the end valve on the humidifier. The pressure should back up into the humidifier, signaled by a high-pitched whistle. If this doesn't occur, tighten all connections and try again.

For a cascade bubble diffusion humidifier: Unscrew the cascade reservoir and add sterile distilled water to the fill line. Screw the top back onto the reservoir. Then plug in the heater unit, and set the temperature between 95° F (35° C) and 100.4° F (38° C).

Implementation
• Check to be sure that the humidifier or vaporizer has been prepared properly.

For a bedside humidifier
• Direct the humidifier unit's nozzle away from the patient's face (but toward the patient) for effective treatment. Check for a fine mist emission from the nozzle, which indicates proper operation.
• Check the unit every 4 hours for proper operation, and the water level every 8 hours. When refilling, unplug the unit, discard any old water, wipe with a disinfectant, rinse the reservoir container, and refill with sterile distilled water as necessary.
• Keep the unit cleaned and refilled with sterile water *to reduce the risk of bacterial growth.* Replace the unit every 7 days and send used units for proper decontamination.

For a heated vaporizer
• Check the unit every 4 hours for proper functioning.
• If steam production seems insufficient, unplug the unit, discard the water and refill with half distilled water and half tap water, or clean the unit well.
• Check the water level in the unit every 8 hours. To refill, unplug the unit, discard any old water, wipe with a disinfectant, rinse the reservoir container, and refill with tap water as necessary.

For a diffusion head humidifier
• Attach the oxygen delivery device to the humidifier and then to the patient. Then adjust the flowmeter to the appropriate oxygen flow rate.
• Check the reservoir every 4 hours. If the water level drops too low, empty the remaining water, rinse the jar, and refill it with sterile water. (As the reservoir water level decreases, the evaporation of water in the gas decreases, reducing humidification of the delivered gas.)
• Change the humidification system regularly *to prevent bacterial growth and invasion.*
• Periodically assess the patient's sputum; *if too thick, it can hinder mobilization and expectoration.* If this occurs, the patient requires a device that can provide higher humidity.

For a cascade bubble diffusion humidifier
• Assess the temperature of the inspired gas near the patient's airway every 2 hours when used in critical care and every 4 hours when used in general patient care. If the cascade becomes too hot, drain the water and replace it. *Overheated water vapor can cause respiratory tract burns.*
• Check the reservoir's water level every 2 to 4 hours, and fill as necessary. *If the water level falls below the*

Comparing humidifiers

TYPE	DESCRIPTION AND USES	ADVANTAGES AND DISADVANTAGES
Bedside	• Spinning disc splashes water against baffle, creating small drops and increasing evaporation; motor disperses mist to directly humidify room air	**Advantages** • May be used with all oxygen masks and nasal cannulas • Easy to operate • Inexpensive **Disadvantages** • Produces humidity inefficiently • Can't be used for patient with bypassed upper airway • May harbor bacteria and molds
Heated vaporizer	• Provides direct humidification to room air by heating the water in the reservoir	**Advantages** • May be used with all oxygen masks and nasal cannulas • Easy to operate • Inexpensive **Disadvantages** • Can't guarantee the amount of humidity delivered • Risk of burn injury if the machine is knocked over
Diffusion head	• In-line humidifier most commonly used with low-flow oxygen delivery systems; gas flows through porous diffuser in reservoir to increase gas-liquid interface; provides humidification to patients using a nasal cannula or oxygen mask (except the Venturi mask)	**Advantages** • Easy to use • Inexpensive **Disadvantages** • Provides only 20% to 30% humidity at body temperature • Can't be used for a patient with bypassed upper airway
Cascade bubble diffusion	• Gas is forced through plastic grid in reservoir of warmed water to create fine bubbles; commonly used in patients receiving mechanical ventilation or continuous positive airway pressure therapy	**Advantages** • Delivers 100% humidity at body temperature • The most effective of all evaporative humidifiers **Disadvantages** • If correct water level isn't maintained, mucosa can become irritated

minimum water level mark, humidification will decrease to that of room air.
• Be alert for condensation buildup in the tubing, which can result from the very high humidification produced by the cascade.
• Check the tubing frequently and empty the condensate as necessary *so it cannot drain into the patient's respiratory tract, encourage growth of microorganisms, or obstruct dependent sections of tubing.* To do so, disconnect the tubing, drain the condensate into a container, and dispose of it properly. Never drain the condensate into the humidification system.

• Change the cascade regularly according to your hospital's policy.

Special considerations
Because it creates a humidity level comparable to that of ambient air, the diffusion head humidifier is only used for oxygen flow rates greater than 4 liters/minute.

Because the bedside humidifier doesn't deliver a precise amount of humidification, assess the patient regularly *to determine the effectiveness of therapy.* Ask him if he has noticed any improvement and evaluate his sputum.

Like the bedside humidifier, the heated vaporizer doesn't deliver a precise amount of humidification, so assess the patient regularly by asking if he's feeling better and by examining his sputum.

Keep in mind that a humidifier, if not kept clean, can cause or aggravate respiratory problems, especially for people allergic to molds. Refer to your hospital's policy for changing and disposing of humidification equipment.

Home care
Make sure the patient and his family understand the reason for using a humidifier and that they know how to use the equipment. Give the patient specific, written guidelines concerning all aspects of home care.

Instruct a patient using a bedside humidifier at home to fill it with plain tap water and to periodically use sterile distilled water *to prevent mineral buildup*. Also advise him to run white vinegar through the unit *to help clean it, prevent bacterial buildup, and dissolve deposits.*

Tell the patient to rinse a heated vaporizer unit with bleach and water every 5 days. Also run white vinegar through it *to help clean it, prevent bacterial buildup and dissolve any deposits.*

Complications
Cascade humidifiers can cause aspiration of tubal condensation and, if the air is heated, can cause pulmonary burns. Humidifiers, if contaminated, can cause infection.

Documentation
Record the date and time when humidification began and was discontinued; the type of humidifier; the flow rate (of a gas system); thermometer readings (if heated); any complications and the nursing action taken; and the patient's reaction to humidification.

Nebulizer therapy

An established component of respiratory care, nebulizer therapy aids bronchial hygiene by restoring and maintaining mucous blanket continuity; hydrating dried, retained secretions; promoting expectoration of secretions; humidifying inspired oxygen; and delivering medications. The therapy may be administered through nebulizers that have a large or small volume, are ultrasonic, or are placed inside ventilator tubing.

Ultrasonic nebulizers are electrically driven and use high-frequency vibrations to break up surface water into particles. The resultant dense mist can penetrate the smaller airways and is useful for hydrating secretions

and inducing a cough. Large-volume nebulizers are used to provide humidity for an artificial airway, such as a tracheostomy, and small-volume nebulizers are used to deliver medications, such as bronchodilators. In-line nebulizers are used to deliver medications to patients who are being mechanically ventilated. In this instance, the nebulizer is placed in the inspiratory side of the ventilatory circuit, as close to the endotracheal tube as possible.

Many questions still exist regarding aerosol therapy, including what type of fluid to use, the types of medications that can be delivered, and the effectiveness of therapy. (See *Comparing nebulizers.*)

Equipment
For an ultrasonic nebulizer: ultrasonic gas-delivery device ∎ large-bore oxygen tubing ∎ nebulizer couplet compartment.

For a large-volume nebulizer (such as Venturi jet): pressurized gas source ∎ flowmeter ∎ large-bore oxygen tubing ∎ nebulizer bottle ∎ sterile distilled water ∎ heater (if ordered) ∎ in-line thermometer (if using heater).

For a small-volume nebulizer (such as a mini-nebulizer): pressurized gas source ∎ flowmeter ∎ oxygen tubing ∎ nebulizer cup ∎ mouthpiece or mask ∎ normal saline solution ∎ prescribed medication.

For an in-line nebulizer: pressurized gas source ∎ flowmeter ∎ nebulizer cup ∎ normal saline solution ∎ prescribed medication.

Preparation of equipment
For an ultrasonic nebulizer: Fill the couplet compartment on the nebulizer to the level indicated.

For a large-volume nebulizer: Fill the water chamber to the indicated level with sterile distilled water. Avoid using saline solution *to prevent corrosion*. Add a heating device, if ordered, and place a thermometer in-line between the outlet port and the patient, as close to the patient as possible, *to monitor the actual temperature of the inhaled gas and to avoid burning the patient*. If the unit will supply oxygen, analyze the flow at the patient's end of the tubing *to ensure delivery of the prescribed oxygen percentage*.

For a small-volume nebulizer: Draw up the prescribed medication, inject it into the nebulizer cup, and add the prescribed amount of saline solution or water. Attach the mouthpiece, mask, or other gas-delivery device.

For an in-line nebulizer: Draw up the medication and diluent, remove the nebulizer cup, quickly inject the medication, and then replace the cup. If using an intermittent positive-pressure breathing machine, attach the mouthpiece and mask to the machine.

Comparing nebulizers

TYPE	DESCRIPTION AND USES	ADVANTAGES AND DISADVANTAGES
Ultrasonic	• Uses high-frequency sound waves to create an aerosol mist	**Advantages** • Provides 100% humidity • About 20% of its particles reach the lower airways • Loosens secretions **Disadvantages** • May precipitate bronchospasms in the asthmatic patient • Infants have increased risk of overhydration
Large volume (Venturi jet)	• Supplies cool or heated moisture to a patient whose upper airway has been bypassed by endotracheal intubation or a tracheostomy, or who has recently been extubated	**Advantages** • Provides 100% humidity with cool or heated devices • Provides oxygen and aerosol therapy • Can be used for long-term therapy **Disadvantages** • Nondisposable units increase risk of bacterial growth • Condensate can collect in large-bore tubing • If correct water level isn't maintained in reservoir, mucosal irritation may result from breathing hot, dry air • Infants have increased risk of overhydration from mist
Small volume (mini-nebulizer, Maxi-mist)	• Hand-held device, used to deliver aerosolized medication	**Advantages** • Conforms to patient's physiology, allowing him to inhale and exhale on his own • Can cause less air trapping than medication administered by intermittent positive-pressure breathing • May be used with compressed air, oxygen, or compressor pump • Compact and disposable **Disadvantages** • Procedure takes a long time if patient needs nurse's assistance • Medication distributed unevenly if patient doesn't breathe properly

Implementation

• Explain the procedure to the patient and wash your hands.

• Take the patient's vital signs and auscultate his lung fields *to establish a baseline*. If possible, place the patient in a sitting or high Fowler's position to encourage full lung expansion and promote aerosol dispersion. Encourage the patient to take slow, even breaths during the treatment.

Ultrasonic nebulizer

• Before beginning, administer an inhaled bronchodilator (metered dose inhaler or small-volume nebulizer) *to prevent bronchospasm.*

• Turn on the machine and check the outflow port *to ensure proper misting.*

• Check the patient frequently during the procedure *to observe for adverse reactions.* Watch for labored respirations *because ultrasonic nebulizer therapy may hydrate retained secretions and obstruct airways.* Take the patient's vital signs and auscultate his lung fields.

• Encourage the patient to cough and expectorate, or suction as needed.

Large-volume nebulizer

• Attach the delivery device to the patient.
• Encourage the patient to cough and expectorate, or suction as needed.
• Check the water level in the nebulizer at frequent intervals and refill or replace as indicated. When refilling a reusable container, discard the old water *to prevent infection from bacterial or fungal growth,* and refill the container to the indicator line with sterile distilled water.
• Change the nebulizer unit and tubing according to hospital policy *to prevent bacterial contamination.*
• If the nebulizer is heated, tell the patient to report any warmth, discomfort, or hot tubing *because these may indicate a heater malfunction.* Use the in-line thermometer to monitor the temperature of the gas the patient is inhaling. If you turn off the flow for more than 5 minutes, unplug the heater *to avoid overheating the water and burning the patient when the aerosol is resumed.*

Small-volume nebulizer

• After attaching the flowmeter to the gas source, attach the nebulizer to the flowmeter and then adjust the flow to at least 10 liters/minute *to ensure adequate functioning* but not more than 14 liters/minute to prevent excess venting.
• Check the outflow port *to ensure adequate misting.*
• Remain with the patient during the treatment, which lasts 15 to 20 minutes, and take his vital signs *to detect any adverse reaction to the medication.*
• Encourage the patient to cough and expectorate, or suction as necessary.
• Change the nebulizer cup and tubing according to hospital policy *to prevent bacterial contamination.*

In-line nebulizer

• Turn on the machine and check the outflow port *to ensure proper misting.*
• Remain with the patient during the treatment, which lasts 15 to 20 minutes, and take his vital signs *to detect any adverse reaction to the medication.*
• Encourage the patient to cough and suction excess secretions as necessary.
• Auscultate the patient's lungs *to evaluate the effectiveness of therapy.*

Special considerations

When using high-output nebulizers, such as an ultrasonic nebulizer, in pediatric patients or in patients with a delicate fluid balance, be alert for signs of overhydration (exhibited by unexplained weight gain occurring over several days after the beginning of therapy), pulmonary edema, crackles, and electrolyte imbalance.

Also, if oxygen is being delivered concomitantly, the fraction of inspired oxygen (FIO_2) may be diluted if the flow is not adequate. Therefore, if the mist disappears when the patient inhales, increase the gas flow.

Complications

Nebulized particulates can irritate the mucosa in some patients and cause bronchospasm and dyspnea. Other complications include airway burns (when heating elements are used), infection from contaminated equipment (although rare), and adverse reactions from medications.

Documentation

Record the date, time, and duration of therapy; type and amount of medication; FIO_2, or oxygen flow, if administered; baseline and subsequent vital signs and breath sounds; and patient's response to treatment.

 # Chest physiotherapy

This procedure includes postural drainage, chest percussion and vibration, and coughing and deep breathing exercises. Together, these techniques mobilize and eliminate secretions, reexpand lung tissue, and promote efficient use of respiratory muscles. Of critical importance to the bedridden patient, chest physiotherapy (PT) helps prevent or treat atelectasis and may also help prevent pneumonia — respiratory complications that can seriously impede recovery.

Postural drainage performed in conjunction with percussion and vibration encourages peripheral pulmonary secretions to empty by gravity into the major bronchi or trachea, and is accomplished by sequential repositioning of the patient. Usually, secretions drain best with the patient positioned so the bronchi are perpendicular to the floor. Lower and middle lobe bronchi usually empty best with the patient in the head-down position; upper lobe bronchi, in the head-up position.

Percussing the chest with cupped hands mechanically dislodges thick, tenacious secretions from the bronchial walls. Vibration can be used with percussion or as an alternative to it in a patient who is frail, in pain, or recovering from thoracic surgery or trauma.

Candidates for chest PT include patients who expectorate large amounts of sputum, such as those with bronchiectasis and cystic fibrosis. The procedure has not been proven effective in treating patients with status asthmaticus, lobar pneumonia, or acute exacerbations of chronic bronchitis when the patient has scant secretions and is being mechanically ventilated. Chest PT has little value for treating patients with stable, chronic bronchitis.

Contraindications may include active pulmonary bleeding with hemoptysis and the immediate posthemorrhage stage, fractured ribs or an unstable chest wall, lung contusions, pulmonary tuberculosis, untreated pneumothorax, acute asthma or bronchospasm, lung abscess or tumor, bony metastasis, head injury, and recent myocardial infarction.

Equipment
Stethoscope ▪ pillows ▪ tilt or postural drainage table (if available) or adjustable hospital bed ▪ emesis basin ▪ facial tissues ▪ suction equipment, as needed ▪ equipment for oral care ▪ trash bag ▪ optional: sterile specimen container, mechanical ventilator, supplemental oxygen.

Preparation of equipment
Gather the equipment at the patient's bedside. Set up suction equipment, if needed, and test its function.

Implementation
• Explain the procedure to the patient, provide privacy, and wash your hands.
• Auscultate the patient's lungs *to determine baseline respiratory status.*
• Position the patient as ordered. In generalized disease, drainage usually begins with the lower lobes, continues with the middle lobes, and ends with the upper lobes. In localized disease, drainage begins with the affected lobes and then proceeds to the other lobes *to avoid spreading the disease to uninvolved areas.* (See *Positioning patients for postural drainage,* pages 366 and 367.)
• Instruct the patient to remain in each position for 10 to 15 minutes. During this time, perform percussion and vibration, as ordered. (See *Performing percussion and vibration.*)
• After postural drainage, percussion, or vibration, instruct the patient to cough *to remove loosened secretions.* First, tell him to inhale deeply through his nose and then exhale in three short huffs. Then have him inhale deeply again and cough through a slightly open mouth. Three consecutive coughs are highly effective. An effective cough sounds deep, low, and hollow; an ineffective one, high-pitched. Have the patient perform exercises for about 1 minute and then rest for 2 minutes. Gradually progress to a 10-minute exercise period four times daily.
• Provide oral hygiene *because secretions may taste foul or have a stale odor.*
• Auscultate the patient's lungs *to evaluate the effectiveness of therapy.*

Performing percussion and vibration

To perform percussion, instruct the patient to breathe slowly and deeply, using the diaphragm, *to promote relaxation.* Hold your hands in a cupped shape, with fingers flexed and thumbs pressed tightly against your index fingers. Percuss each segment for 1 to 2 minutes by alternating your hands against the patient in a rhythmic manner. Listen for a hollow sound on percussion *to verify correct performance of the technique.*

To perform vibration, ask the patient to inhale deeply and then exhale slowly through pursed lips. During exhalation, firmly press your fingers and the palms of your hands against the chest wall. Tense the muscles of your arms and shoulders in an isometric contraction *to send fine vibrations through the chest wall.* Vibrate during five exhalations over each chest segment.

Positioning patients for postural drainage

The following illustrations show you the various postural drainage positions and the areas of the lungs affected by each.

Lower lobes: Posterior basal segments

Elevate the foot of the bed 30 degrees. Have the patient lie prone with his head lowered. Position pillows under his chest and abdomen. Percuss his lower ribs on both sides of his spine.

Lower lobes: Lateral basal segments

Elevate the foot of the bed 30 degrees. Instruct the patient to lie on his abdomen with his head lowered and his upper leg flexed over a pillow for support. Then have him rotate a quarter turn upward. Percuss his lower ribs on the uppermost portion of his lateral chest wall.

Lower lobes: Anterior basal segments

Elevate the foot of the bed 30 degrees. Instruct the patient to lie on his side with his head lowered. Then place pillows as shown (above, right). Percuss with a slightly cupped hand over his lower ribs just beneath the axilla. If an acutely ill patient has trouble breathing in this position, adjust the bed to an angle he can tolerate. Then begin percussion.

Lower lobes: Superior segments

With the bed flat, have the patient lie on his abdomen. Place two pillows under his hips. Percuss on both sides of his spine at the lower tip of his scapulae.

Right middle lobe: Medial and lateral segments

Elevate the foot of the bed 15 degrees. Have the patient lie on his left side with his head down and his knees flexed. Then have him rotate a quarter turn backward. Place a pillow beneath him. Percuss with your hand moderately cupped over the right nipple. For a woman, cup your hand so that its heel is under the armpit and your fingers extend forward beneath the breast.

Positioning patients for postural drainage *(continued)*

Left upper lobe: Superior and inferior segments, lingular portion

Elevate the foot of the bed 15 degrees. Have the patient lie on his right side with his head down and knees flexed. Then have him rotate a quarter turn backward. Place a pillow behind him, from shoulders to hips. Percuss with your hand moderately cupped over his left nipple. For a woman, cup your hand so that its heel is beneath the armpit and your fingers extend forward beneath the breast.

Anterior view

Upper lobes: Anterior segments

Make sure the bed is flat. Have the patient lie on his back with a pillow folded under his knees. Then have him rotate slightly away from the side being drained. Percuss between his clavicle and nipple.

Anterior view

Upper lobes: Apical segments

Keep the bed flat. Have the patient lean back at a 30-degree angle against you and a pillow. Percuss with a cupped hand between his clavicles and the top of each scapula.

Posterior view

Upper lobes: Posterior segments

Keep the bed flat. Have the patient lean over a pillow at a 30-degree angle. Percuss and clap his upper back on each side.

Posterior view

Special considerations

For optimal effectiveness and safety, modify chest PT according to the patient's condition. For example, initiate or increase the flow of supplemental oxygen, if indicated. Also, suction the patient who has an ineffective cough reflex. If the patient tires quickly during therapy, shorten the sessions *because fatigue leads to shallow respirations and increased hypoxia.*

Maintain adequate hydration in the patient receiving chest PT *to prevent mucus dehydration and promote easier mobilization.* Avoid performing postural drainage immediately before or within 1½ hours after meals *to avoid nausea and aspiration of food or vomitus.*

Because chest percussion can induce bronchospasm, any adjunct treatment (for example, intermittent positive-pressure breathing, aerosol, or nebulizer therapy) should precede chest PT.

Refrain from percussing over the spine, liver, kidneys, or spleen *to avoid injury to the spine or internal organs.* Also avoid performing percussion on bare skin or the female patient's breasts. Percuss over soft clothing (but not over buttons, snaps, or zippers) or place a thin towel over the chest wall. Remember to remove jewelry that might scratch or bruise the patient.

Explain coughing and deep breathing exercises preoperatively, so the patient can practice them when he's pain-free and better able to concentrate. Postoperatively, splint the patient's incision using your hands or, if possible, teach the patient to splint it himself *to minimize pain during coughing.*

Complications

During postural drainage in head-down positions, pressure on the diaphragm by abdominal contents can impair respiratory excursion and lead to hypoxia or postural hypotension. The head-down position also may lead to increased intracranial pressure, which precludes the use of chest PT in a patient with acute neurologic impairment. Vigorous percussion or vibration can cause rib fracture, especially in the patient with osteoporosis. In an emphysematous patient with blebs, coughing could lead to pneumothorax.

Documentation

Record the date and time of chest PT; positions for secretion drainage and length of time each is maintained; chest segments percussed or vibrated; color, amount, odor, and viscosity of secretions produced, and presence of any blood; any complications and nursing actions taken; and the patient's tolerance of treatment.

Chest tube insertion

The pleural space normally contains a thin layer of lubricating fluid that allows the lungs to move without friction during respiration. An excess of fluid (hemothorax or pleural effusion), air (pneumothorax), or both in this space alters intrapleural pressure and causes partial or complete lung collapse.

Chest tube insertion permits the drainage of air or fluid from the pleural space. Usually performed by a doctor with a nurse assisting, this procedure requires sterile technique. The insertion site varies, depending on the patient's condition and the doctor's judgment. For pneumothorax, the second intercostal space provides the usual site because air rises to the top of the intrapleural space. For hemothorax or pleural effusion, the sixth to the eighth intercostal spaces are common sites because fluid settles to the lower levels of the intrapleural space. For removal of air and fluid, a chest tube is inserted into a high and a low site. Following insertion, one or more chest tubes are connected to a thoracic drainage system that removes air, fluid, or both from the pleural space and prevents backflow into that space, thus promoting lung reexpansion. (See "Thoracic drainage," in this chapter.)

Equipment

Two pairs of sterile gloves ■ sterile drape ■ povidone-iodine solution ■ vial of 1% lidocaine ■ 10-ml syringe ■ alcohol sponge ■ 22G 1″ needle ■ 25G 5⁄8″ needle ■ sterile scalpel (usually with #11 blade) ■ sterile forceps ■ two rubber-tipped clamps for each chest tube inserted ■ sterile 4″ × 4″ gauze pads ■ two sterile 4″ × 4″ drain dressings (gauze pads with slit) ■ 3″ or 4″ sturdy, elastic tape ■ 1″ adhesive tape for connections ■ chest tube of appropriate size (#16 to #20 French catheter for air or serous fluid; #28 to #40 French catheter for blood, pus, or thick fluid), with or without a trocar ■ sterile Kelly clamp ■ suture material (usually 2-0 silk with cutting needle) ■ thoracic drainage system ■ sterile drainage tubing, 6′ (1.8 m) long, and connector ■ sterile Y connector (for two chest tubes on the same side) ■ optional: antimicrobial ointment, petroleum gauze.

Preparation of equipment

Check the expiration date on the sterile packages and inspect for tears. In a nonemergency situation, make sure that the patient has signed the appropriate consent form. Then assemble all equipment in the patient's room and set up the thoracic drainage system. Place it next to the patient's bed below the chest level *to facilitate drainage.*

Implementation

• Explain the procedure to the patient, provide privacy, and wash your hands.

• Record baseline vital signs and respiratory assessment.

• Position the patient appropriately. (See *Positioning the patient for chest tube insertion.*)

• Place the chest tube tray on the overbed table. Open it using sterile technique.

• The doctor puts on sterile gloves and prepares the insertion site by cleaning the area with povidone-iodine solution.

• Wipe the rubber stopper of the lidocaine vial with an alcohol pad. Then invert the bottle and hold it for the doctor to withdraw the anesthetic.

• After the doctor anesthetizes the site, he makes a small incision and inserts the chest tube. Then he either immediately connects the chest tube to the thoracic drainage system or momentarily clamps the tube close to the patient's chest until he can connect it to the drainage system. He may then secure the tube to the skin with a suture.

• As the doctor is inserting the chest tube, reassure the patient and assist the doctor as necessary.

• Open the packages containing the 4″ × 4″ drain dressings and gauze pads, and put on sterile gloves. If desired, apply antimicrobial ointment to the insertion site. Then place two 4″ × 4″ drain dressings around the insertion site, one from the top and the other from the bottom. Place several 4″ × 4″ gauze pads on top of the drain dressings. Tape the dressings, covering them completely.

Positioning the patient for chest tube insertion

If the patient has a *pneumothorax,* place him in high Fowler's, semi-Fowler's, or the supine position. The doctor will insert the tube in the anterior chest at the midclavicular line in the second to the third intercostal space.

If the patient has a *hemothorax,* have him lean over the overbed table or straddle a chair with his arms dangling over the back. The doctor will insert the tube in the fourth to sixth intercostal space at the midaxillary line.

For either pneumothorax or hemothorax, the patient may lie on his unaffected side with his arms extended over his head.

If the patient has had a *thoracotomy,* the doctor usually will insert one or two chest tubes during surgery (typically a basilar tube and an apical tube). The patient will be positioned on his unaffected side with his arms elevated.

Semi-Fowler's position

Insertion site for pneumothorax

Leaning forward

Insertion site for hemothorax

Lying on unaffected side

Insertion site for pneumothorax — Insertion site for hemothorax

• Tape the chest tube to the patient's chest distal to the insertion site *to help prevent accidental dislodgment of the tube.*
• Tape the junction of the chest tube and the drainage tube *to prevent their separation.*

• Coil the drainage tubing and secure it to the bed linen with tape and a safety pin, providing enough slack for the patient to move and turn. *These measures prevent the drainage tubing from getting kinked or dropping to the floor, which would impair drainage into the bottle, and they help prevent accidental dislodgment of the chest tube.*

Performing needle thoracentesis

For a patient with life-threatening tension pneumothorax, a needle thoracentesis temporarily relieves pleural pressure until a doctor can insert a chest tube.

How needle thoracentesis works

A needle attached to a flutter valve is inserted into the affected pleural space. (If no flutter valve is available, one can be made from a perforated finger cot or glove and attached with a rubber band.) Trapped air escapes via the flutter valve when the patient exhales, instead of being retained under pressure. The flutter valve also prevents more air from entering the patient's involved lung during inhalation.

How to perform the procedure

If a doctor isn't available, you may need to perform this procedure. Here's how to proceed.

• Clean the skin around the second intercostal space at the midclavicular line with povidone-iodine solution. Use a circular motion, starting at the center and working outward.
• Insert a sterile 16G (or larger) needle over the superior portion of the rib and through the tissue covering the pleural cavity. The vein, artery, and nerve lie behind the rib's inferior border.
• Listen for a hissing sound. This signals the needle's entry into the pleural cavity.
• If you're using a flutter valve, secure it to the needle. The arrow on the valve indicates the direction of airflow.
• Place a sterile glove on the distal end of the valve to collect the drainage.
• Leave the needle in place until a chest tube can be inserted.

• Immediately after the drainage system is connected, instruct the patient to take a deep breath, hold it momentarily, and slowly exhale *to assist drainage of the pleural space and lung reexpansion.*
• After the procedure, a portable chest X-ray is done *to check tube position.*
• Take the patient's vital signs every 15 minutes for 1 hour, then as his condition indicates. Auscultate his lungs at least every 4 hours following the procedure *to assess air exchange in the affected lung.* Diminished or absent breath sounds indicate that the lung hasn't reexpanded.

Special considerations

If the patient's chest tube comes out, immediately cover the site with $4'' \times 4''$ gauze pads and tape them in place. Stay with the patient and monitor his vital signs every 10 minutes. Observe the patient for signs of tension pneumothorax (hypotension, distended neck veins, absent breath sounds, tracheal shift, hypoxemia, weak and rapid pulse, dyspnea, tachypnea, diaphoresis, and chest pain). Instruct another staff member to notify the doctor and gather equipment needed to reinsert the tube. (See also *Performing needle thoracentesis.*)

Place the rubber-tipped clamps at the bedside. If a drainage bottle breaks, a commercial system cracks, or a tube disconnects, clamp the chest tube momentarily as close to the insertion site as possible. *Because no air or liquid can escape from the pleural space while the tube is clamped,* observe the patient closely for signs of tension pneumothorax while the clamp is in place.

A piece of petroleum gauze may be wrapped around the tube at the insertion site *to make an airtight seal.*

The tube may be clamped with large, smooth, rubber-tipped clamps for several hours before removal. *This allows time to observe the patient for signs of respiratory distress, an indication that air or fluid remains trapped in the pleural space.* A chest tube is usually removed within 7 days of insertion *to prevent infection along the tube tract.* (See *Removing a chest tube.*)

Documentation

Record the date and time of chest tube insertion, the insertion site, drainage system used, presence of drainage and bubbling, vital signs and auscultation findings, any complications, and the nursing action taken.

Thoracic drainage

Because negative pressure in the pleural cavity exerts a suction force that keeps the lungs expanded, any chest trauma that upsets this pressure may cause lung collapse. Consequently, one or more chest tubes may be surgically inserted and then connected to a thoracic drainage system. Thoracic drainage uses gravity and possibly suction to restore negative pressure and remove any material that collects in the pleural cavity. An underwater seal in the drainage system allows air and fluid to escape from the pleural cavity, but doesn't allow air to reenter. The system may include one, two, or three bottles to collect drainage, create a water seal, and control suction. Or it may be a self-contained, disposable system that combines the features of a multibottle system in a compact, one-piece unit. Because you're less likely to use a bottle system, the procedure here details use of a disposable system. (See *Comparing closed drainage systems,* page 372.)

Specifically, thoracic drainage may be ordered to remove accumulated air, fluids (blood, pus, chyle, serous fluids, gastric juices), or solids (blood clots) from the pleural cavity; to restore negative pressure in the pleural cavity; or to reexpand a partially or totally collapsed lung.

Equipment

Thoracic drainage system (Pleur-evac, Argyle, Ohio, or Thora-Klex system, which can function as gravity draining systems or be connected to suction to enhance chest drainage) ■ sterile distilled water (usually 1 liter) ■ adhesive tape ■ sterile clear plastic tubing ■ bottle or system rack ■ two rubber-tipped Kelly clamps ■ sterile 50-ml catheter-tip syringe ■ suction source, if ordered.

Preparation of equipment

Check the doctor's order to determine the type of drainage system to be used and specific procedural details. If appropriate, request the drainage system and suction system from the central supply department. Collect the appropriate equipment and take it to the patient's bedside.

Implementation

• Explain the procedure to the patient, and wash your hands.
• Maintain sterile technique throughout the entire procedure, and whenever you make changes in the system or alter any of the connections *to avoid introducing pathogens into the pleural space.*

Removing a chest tube

Once the patient's lung has reexpanded, you may assist the doctor in removing the chest tube. To do so, first obtain the patient's vital signs and perform a respiratory assessment. Then, after explaining the procedure to the patient, you'll administer an analgesic, as ordered, 30 minutes before tube removal. Then follow the steps listed below:
• Place the patient in semi-Fowler's position or on his unaffected side.
• Place a linen-saver pad under the affected side *to protect the linen from drainage and to provide a place to put the chest tube after removal.*
• Put on clean gloves and remove the chest tube dressings, being careful not to dislodge the chest tube. Discard soiled dressings.
• The doctor puts on sterile gloves, holds the chest tube in place with sterile forceps, and cuts the suture anchoring the tube.
• Make sure the chest tube is securely clamped, and then instruct the patient to perform Valsalva's maneuver by exhaling fully and bearing down. *Valsalva's maneuver effectively increases intrathoracic pressure.*
• The doctor holds an airtight dressing, usually petroleum gauze, *so that he can cover the insertion site with it immediately after removing the tube.* After he removes the tube and covers the insertion site, secure the dressing with tape. Be sure to cover the dressing completely with tape *to make it as airtight as possible.*
• Dispose of the chest tube, soiled gloves, and equipment according to hospital policy.
• Take vital signs, as ordered, and assess the depth and quality of the patient's respirations. Assess the patient carefully for signs and symptoms of pneumothorax, subcutaneous emphysema, or infection.

To set up a commercially prepared disposable system
• Open the packaged system and place it on the floor in the rack supplied by the manufacturer *to avoid accidentally knocking it over or dislodging the components.* After the system is prepared, it may be hung from the side of the patient's bed.
• Remove the plastic connector from the short tube that's attached to the water-seal chamber. Using a 50-ml catheter-tip syringe, instill sterile distilled water into the water-seal chamber until it reaches the 2-cm mark, or

Comparing closed drainage systems

One-bottle system

The one-bottle system is the easiest drainage system to use. It drains by gravity, combining drainage collection and the water-seal chamber. This system is not recommended for excessive drainage.

Two-bottle system

The two-bottle system collects drainage in the first bottle and uses the second bottle as the water-seal chamber. This system is not recommended for excessive drainage.

Three-bottle system

In the three-bottle system, the first bottle collects drainage, the second bottle acts as the water-seal chamber, and the third bottle is the suction-control chamber. This system can handle excessive drainage.

Disposable drainage systems

Commercially prepared disposable systems combine drainage collection, water seal, and suction control in one unit, as shown here. These systems ensure patient safety with positive- and negative-pressure relief valves and have a prominent air-leak indicator. Some systems produce no bubbling sound.

the mark specified by the manufacturer. The Ohio and Thora-Klex systems are ready to use but, with the Thora-Klex system, 15-ml of sterile water may be added to help detect air leaks. Replace the plastic connector.

• If suction is ordered, remove the cap (also called the muffler or atmosphere vent cover) on the suction-control chamber *to open the vent.* Next, instill sterile distilled water until it reaches the 20-cm mark or the ordered level, and recap the suction-control chamber.

• Using the long tube, connect the patient's chest tube to the closed drainage collection chamber. Secure the connection with tape.

• Connect the short tube on the drainage system to the suction source and turn on the suction. Gentle bubbling should begin in the suction chamber, *indicating that the correct suction level has been reached.*

To manage closed chest underwater seal drainage

• Repeatedly note the character, consistency, and amount of drainage in the drainage collection chamber.

• Mark the drainage level in the drainage collection chamber by noting the time and date at the drainage level on the chamber every 8 hours (or more often) if there is a large amount of drainage.

• Check the water level in the water-seal chamber every 8 hours. If necessary, carefully add sterile distilled water until the level reaches the 2-cm mark indicated on the water-seal chamber of the commercial system.

• Check for fluctuation in the water-seal chamber as the patient breathes. Normal fluctuations of 2″ to 4″ (about 5 to 10 cm) reflect pressure changes in the pleural space during respiration. To check for fluctuation when a suction system is being used, momentarily disconnect the suction system so the air vent is opened, and observe for fluctuation.

• Check for intermittent bubbling in the water-seal chamber. This occurs normally when the system is removing air from the pleural cavity. If bubbling isn't readily apparent during quiet breathing, have the patient take a deep breath or cough. Absence of bubbling indicates that the pleural space has sealed.

• Check the water level in the suction-control chamber. Detach the chamber or bottle from the suction source; when bubbling ceases, observe the water level. If necessary, add sterile distilled water to bring the level to the −20-cm line, or as ordered.

• Check for gentle bubbling in the suction control chamber *because it indicates that the proper suction level has been reached.* Vigorous bubbling in this chamber increases the rate of water evaporation.

• Periodically check that the air vent in the system is working properly. *Occlusion of the air vent results in a*

buildup of pressure in the system that could cause the patient to develop a tension pneumothorax.

• Coil the system's tubing and secure it to the edge of the bed with a rubber band or tape and a safety pin. Avoid creating dependent loops, kinks, or pressure on the tubing *because they may interfere with chest drainage.* Avoid lifting the drainage system above the patient's chest *because fluid may flow back into the pleural space.*

• Be sure to keep two rubber-tipped clamps at the bedside. These are used to clamp the chest tube if a bottle breaks or the commercially prepared system cracks, or to locate an air leak in the system.

• Encourage the patient to cough frequently and breathe deeply *to help drain the pleural space and expand the lungs.*

• Instruct him to sit upright *for optimal lung expansion* and to splint the insertion site while coughing *to minimize pain.*

• Check the rate and quality of the patient's respirations and auscultate his lungs periodically *to assess air exchange in the affected lung.* Diminished or absent breath sounds may indicate that the lung has not reexpanded.

• Tell the patient to report any breathing difficulty immediately. Notify the doctor immediately if the patient develops cyanosis, rapid or shallow breathing, subcutaneous emphysema, chest pain, or excessive bleeding.

• When clots are visible, you may be able to strip (or milk) the tubing, depending on your hospital's policy. This is a controversial procedure because it creates high negative pressure that could suck viable lung tissue into the drainage ports of the tube, with subsequent ruptured alveoli and pleural air leak. Strip the tubing only when clots are visible. Use an alcohol sponge or lotion as a lubricant on the tube and pinch it between your thumb and index finger about 2″ (5 cm) from the insertion site. Using the other thumb and index finger, compress the tubing as you slide your fingers down the tube or use a mechanical stripper. After stripping, release the thumb and index finger pinching the tube near the insertion site.

• Check the chest tube dressing at least every 8 hours. Palpate the area surrounding the dressing for crepitus or subcutaneous emphysema, which indicates that air is leaking into the subcutaneous tissue surrounding the insertion site. Change the dressing if necessary or according to hospital policy.

• Encourage active or passive range-of-motion (ROM) exercises for the patient's arm or the affected side if he has been splinting the arm. Usually, the thoractomy patient will splint his arm to decrease his discomfort.

• Give ordered pain medication as needed *for comfort and to help with deep breathing, coughing, and ROM exercises.*

• Remind the ambulatory patient to keep the drainage system below chest level and to be careful not to disconnect the tubing *to maintain the water seal.* With a suction system, the patient must stay within range of the length of tubing attached to a wall outlet or portable pump.

Special considerations

Instruct staff and visitors to avoid touching the equipment *to prevent complications from separated connections.*

If excessive continuous bubbling is present in the water-seal chamber, especially if suction is being used, rule out a leak in the drainage system. Try to locate the leak by clamping the tube momentarily at various points along its length. Begin clamping at the tube's proximal end and work down toward the drainage system, paying special attention to the seal around the connections. If any connection is loose, push it back together and tape it securely. *The bubbling will stop when a clamp is placed between the air leak and the water seal.* If you clamp along the tube's entire length and the bubbling doesn't stop, the drainage unit may be cracked and need replacement.

If the commercially prepared drainage collection chamber fills, replace it. To do this, double-clamp the tube close to the insertion site (use two clamps facing in opposite directions), exchange the system, remove the clamps, and retape the bottle connection. Never leave the tubes clamped for more than a minute or two *to prevent a tension pneumothorax, which may occur when clamping stops air and fluid from escaping.*

If the commercially prepared system cracks, clamp the chest tube momentarily with the two rubber-tipped clamps at the bedside (placed there at the time of tube insertion). Place the clamps close to each other near the insertion site; they should face in opposite directions *to provide a more complete seal.* Observe the patient for altered respirations while the tube is clamped. Then replace the damaged equipment. (Prepare the new unit before clamping the tube.)

Instead of clamping the tube, you can submerge the distal end of the tube in a container of normal saline solution *to create a temporary water seal while you replace the bottle.* Check your hospital's policy for the proper procedure.

Complications

Tension pneumothorax may result from excessive accumulation of air, drainage, or both, and eventually may exert pressure on the heart and aorta, causing a precipitous fall in cardiac output.

Documentation

Record the date and time thoracic drainage began, type of system used, amount of suction applied to the pleural cavity, presence or absence of bubbling or fluctuation in the water-seal chamber, initial amount and type of drainage, and the patient's respiratory status.

At the end of each shift, record the frequency of system inspection; how frequently chest tubes were milked or stripped; amount, color, and consistency of drainage; presence or absence of bubbling or fluctuation in the water-seal chamber; the patient's respiratory status; condition of the chest dressings; pain medication, if given; and any complications and the nursing action taken.

Selected references

American Heart Association, Emergency Cardiac Care Committee and Subcommittees. "Guidelines for Cardiopulmonary Resuscitation and Emergency Cardiac Care, I: Introduction," *JAMA* 16(268):2172-83, October 1992.

Campbell, E.J., et al. "Subjective Effects of Humidification of Oxygen for Delivery by Nasal Cannula: A Prospective Study," *Chest* 93(2):289-93, February 1988.

Carroll, P. "Safe Suctioning," *Nursing89* 19(9):48-51, September 1989.

Craven, R., and Hirnle, C. *Fundamentals of Nursing: Human Health and Function.* Philadelphia: J.B. Lippincott Co., 1992.

Diagnostics: A Comprehensive Manual of Laboratory Tests and Diagnostic Procedures, 3rd ed. Springhouse, Pa.: Springhouse Corp., 1994.

Diseases. Springhouse, Pa.: Springhouse Corp., 1993.

Erickson, R.S. "Mastering the Ins and Outs of Chest Drainage," Part 1. *Nursing89* 19(5):36-44, May 1989.

Gift, A.G., et al. "Sensations During Chest Tube Removal," *Heart & Lung* 20(2):131-37, March 1991.

Guyton, A.C. *Textbook of Medical Physiology,* 8th ed. Philadelphia: W.B. Saunders Co., 1991.

Hess, D., et al. "The Effect of Hand Size, Resuscitator Brand, and Use of Two Hands on Volumes Delivered During Adult Bag-Valve Ventilation," *Respiratory Care* 34(9):805-10, September 1989.

Ignatavicius, D., and Bayne, M. *Medical-Surgical Nursing: A Nursing Process Approach.* Philadelphia: W.B. Saunders Co., 1991.

Illustrated Manual of Nursing Practice, 2nd ed. Springhouse, Pa.: Springhouse Corp., 1994.

Jaffe, A., ed. *Textbook of Advanced Cardiac Life Support,* 2nd ed. Dallas: American Heart Association, 1990.

Kacmarek, R.M., et al. *The Essentials of Respiratory Care,* 3rd ed. St. Louis: Mosby, Inc., 1990.

Kersten, L. *Comprehensive Respiratory Nursing: A Decision-Making Approach.* Philadelphia: W.B. Saunders Co., 1989.

Kim, M.J., et al. *Pocket Guide to Nursing Diagnoses.* St. Louis: Mosby, Inc., 1989.

Kozier, B., and Erb, G. *Techniques in Clinical Nursing: A Nursing Process Approach,* 3rd ed. Menlo Park, Calif.: Addison-Wesley Publishing Co., 1989.

Lewis, S., and Collier, I. *Medical-Surgical Nursing: Assessment and Management of Clinical Problems*, 3rd ed. St. Louis: Mosby, Inc., 1992.

Miracle, V., and Allnutt, D. "Using a Manual Resuscitator Correctly," *Nursing90* 20(5):49-51, May 1990.

Nurse's PhotoLibrary: A Looseleaf Update System. Springhouse, Pa.: Springhouse Corp., 1993.

Nursing94 Drug Handbook. Springhouse, Pa.: Springhouse Corp., 1994.

Pasterkamp, H., et al. "Nomenclature Used by Health Care Professionals to Describe Breath Sounds in Asthma," *Chest* 92(2):346-52, August 1987.

Pierce, J.D., et al. "Effects of Two Chest Tube Clearance Protocols on Drainage in Patients after Myocardial Revascularization Surgery," *Heart & Lung* 20(2):125-30, March 1991.

Rapid Assessment. Clinical Skillbuilders Series. Springhouse, Pa.: Springhouse Corp., 1991.

Respiratory Support. Clinical Skillbuilders Series. Springhouse, Pa.: Springhouse Corp., 1991.

Shapiro, B., et al. *Clinical Applications of Respiratory Care.* St. Louis: Mosby, Inc., 1991.

Sparks, S., and Taylor, C. *Nursing Diagnosis Reference Manual,* 2nd ed. Springhouse, Pa.: Springhouse Corp., 1993.

Stevens, S.A., and Becker, K.L. "How to Perform Picture-Perfect Respiratory Assessment," *Nursing88* 18(1):57-63, January 1988.

Swearingen, P., and Keen, J., eds. *Manual of Critical Care,* 2nd ed. St. Louis: Mosby, Inc., 1991.

Teplitz, L. "Update: Are Milking and Stripping Chest Tubes Necessary?" *Focus On Critical Care* 18(6):506-11, December 1991.

Traver, G.A., et al. *Respiratory Care: A Clinical Approach.* Rockville, Md.: Aspen Pubs., Inc., 1991.

CHAPTER 9

NEUROLOGIC CARE

DIANE BROADBENT FRIEDMAN, RN, MSN, CS

Introduction

Effective neurologic care aims to preserve and restore optimal nervous system function. And precise nursing skills, meticulously applied, are indispensable to achieving effective care. More and more, these nursing skills require mastery of sophisticated techniques and equipment.

Neurologic assessment

Appropriate supportive care requires that you assess and document neurologic vital signs. At the same time, you also need to assess other systems for complications of neurologic dysfunction.

Be sure to assess neurologic vital signs—especially the patient's orientation level. Many neurologic patients experience changes in perception—ranging from confusion to psychosis—from neurologic dysfunction. Unaddressed, this disorientation further impairs the patient's ability to participate in his recovery. Recognizing this will help you intervene appropriately.

To record and track assessment findings, use special neurologic assessment forms or flowcharts. In common use at most hospitals, these charts separate and grade components of a neurologic assessment, assisting the nurse and other caregivers to quickly recognize changes in neurologic status and to plan subsequent care.

Respiratory assessment constitutes an important part of an overall neurologic assessment. That's because patients with neurologic damage—especially those with traumatic brain or spinal cord injuries—are at considerable risk for respiratory complications. These injuries may depress the respiratory control center and paralyze the muscles used for breathing. As a result, brain tissue, which is especially sensitive to blood oxygen levels, can quickly be damaged by inadequate oxygenation.

Thorough respiratory care goes hand in hand with neurologic care. Frequent position changes, chest physiotherapy, and tracheal suctioning are typical interventions. Additional techniques for preventing complications and promoting comfort include pain management and therapeutic touch.

Rehabilitation

Neurologic rehabilitation begins on admission and touches all aspects of daily care. Because neurologic impairment can alter every area of function, the patient's identity may disintegrate. Consequent rehabilitation procedures must address the psychosocial and physiologic changes associated with the patient's condition—a task that requires enormous time and patience.

The success of rehabilitation efforts may hinge largely on the patient's ability to adapt to significant—even profound—changes. Keep in mind that various factors influence this adaptation: the patient's age, the deficit itself, and available support systems—to name a few. Another ingredient needed for effective rehabilitation is sensitive and skilled nursing care. Such care can dramatically improve the patient's prospects of positive adaptation and recovery.

MONITORING
Neurologic vital signs

Neurologic vital signs supplement the routine measurement of temperature, pulse rate, and respirations by evaluating the patient's level of consciousness (LOC), pupillary activity, and level of orientation to place, time, date, situation, and person. They provide a simple, indispensable tool for quickly checking the patient's neurologic status.

LOC—the degree of response to stimuli—reflects brain stem function and usually provides the first sign of central nervous system deterioration. Changes in *pupillary activity*—pupil size, shape, equality, and response to light—may signal increased intracranial pressure (ICP). *Level of orientation* evaluates higher cerebral functions and processing abilities.

Evaluating muscle strength and tone, reflexes, and posture also may help identify nervous system damage. Finally, ongoing assessment of routine vital signs helps detect neurologic changes or trends. In particular, respiratory rate and pattern can help locate brain lesions and determine their size.

Equipment

Penlight ■ thermometer ■ sterile cotton ball or cotton-tipped applicator ■ stethoscope ■ sphygmomanometer ■ pupil size chart ■ optional: pencil or pen.

Implementation

● Explain the procedure to the patient, even if he's unresponsive. Then wash your hands and provide privacy.

Using the Glasgow coma scale

The Glasgow coma scale provides a standard reference for assessing or monitoring a patient with suspected or confirmed brain injury. You measure three responses to stimuli—eye opening, motor response, and verbal response—and assign a number to each of the possible responses within these categories. A score of 3 is the lowest and 15 is the highest. A score of 7 or less indicates coma. This scale is commonly used in the emergency department, at the scene of an accident, and for periodic evaluation of the hospitalized patient.

CHARACTERISTIC	RESPONSE	SCORE
Eye opening	• Spontaneous	4
	• To verbal command	3
	• To pain	2
	• No response	1
Best motor response	• Obeys commands	6
	• To painful stimuli	
	Localizes pain; pushes stimulus away	5
	Flexes and withdraws	4
	Abnormal flexion	3
	Extension	2
	No response	1
Best verbal response (Arouse patient with painful stimuli, if necessary)	• Oriented and converses	5
	• Disoriented and converses	4
	• Uses inappropriate words	3
	• Makes incomprehensible sounds	2
	• No response	1
	Total:	3 to 15

Assess LOC and orientation

• Assess the patient's LOC by evaluating his responses. Use standard guidelines, such as the Glasgow coma scale. (See *Using the Glasgow coma scale.*) Begin by measuring the patient's response to verbal, light tactile (touch), or painful (nail bed pressure) stimuli. First, ask the patient his full name. If he responds appropriately, assess his orientation to place, time, date, and situation. Ask the patient where he is and then what day, season, and year it is. (Expect disorientation to affect the sense of date first, then time, place, caregivers, and finally self.) When the patient responds verbally, assess the quality of replies. For example, garbled words indicate difficulty with the motor nerves that govern speech muscles. Rambling responses indicate difficulty with thought processing and organization.

• Assess the patient's ability to understand and follow one-step commands that require a motor response. For example, ask him to open and close his eyes or stick out his tongue. Note whether the patient can maintain his LOC. If you must gently shake the patient to keep him focused on your verbal commands, he may sustain neurologic compromise.

• If the patient doesn't respond to commands, apply a painful stimulus. With moderate pressure, squeeze the nail beds on fingers and toes, and note his response. Check motor responses bilaterally *to rule out monoplegia (paralysis of a single area) and hemiplegia (paralysis of one side of the body).*

Examine pupils and eye movement

• Ask the patient to open his eyes. If he doesn't respond, gently lift his upper eyelids. Inspect each pupil for size and shape, and compare the two for equality. To evaluate pupil size more precisely, use a chart showing the various pupil sizes (in increments of 1 mm, with the normal diameter ranging from 2 to 6 mm). Remember, pupil size varies considerably, and some patients have normally unequal pupils (anisocoria). Also see if the pupils are positioned in, or deviated from, the midline.

• Test the patient's direct light response. First, darken the room. Then hold each eyelid open in turn, keeping the other eye covered. Swing the penlight from the patient's ear toward the midline of the face. Shine the light directly into the eye. Normally, the pupil constricts immediately. When you remove the penlight, the pupil should

dilate immediately. Wait about 20 seconds before testing the other pupil *to allow it to recover from reflex stimulation.*
• Now test consensual light response. Hold both eyelids open, but shine the light into one eye only. Watch for constriction in the other pupil, *which indicates proper nerve function at the optic chiasm.*
• Brighten the room and have the conscious patient open his eyes. Observe the eyelids for ptosis or drooping. Then check extraocular movements. Hold up one finger and ask the patient to follow it with his eyes alone. As you move the finger up, down, laterally, and obliquely, see if the patient's eyes track together to follow your finger (conjugate gaze). Watch for involuntary jerking or oscillating eye movements (nystagmus).
• Check accommodation. Hold up one finger midline to the patient's face and several feet away. Have the patient focus on your finger. Then gradually move your finger toward his nose while he still focuses on your finger. This should cause his eyes to converge and both pupils to constrict equally.
• Test the corneal reflex by rapidly moving the palm of your hand toward the patient's open eyes. *This forces a cushion of air against the corneas, which normally causes an immediate blink reflex.* Repeat for the other eye.
• If the patient is unconscious, test the oculocephalic (doll's eye) reflex. Hold the patient's eyelids open. Then quickly, but gently, turn the patient's head to one side, then the other. If the patient's eyes move in the opposite direction from the side to which you turn the head—eyes move right when the head moves left—the reflex is intact.
◆ *Nursing alert.* Never test the doll's eye reflex if you know or suspect that the patient has a cervical spine injury. ◆

Evaluate motor function
• If the patient is conscious, test his grip strength in both hands at the same time. Extend your hands, ask the patient to squeeze your fingers as hard as he can, and compare the strength of each hand. Grip strength is usually slightly stronger in the dominant hand.
• Test arm strength by having the patient close his eyes and hold his arms straight out in front of him with the palms up. See if either arm drifts downward or pronates, *which indicates muscle weakness.*
• Test leg strength by having the patient raise his legs, one at a time, against gentle downward pressure from your hand. Gently push down on each leg at the midpoint of the thigh *to evaluate muscle strength.*
• If the patient is unconscious, estimate the strength of spontaneous and reflex movements. Apply a painful stimulus to elicit movement. Exert pressure on each fingernail bed with a pencil or pen. If the patient withdraws from this stimulus, compare the strength of each limb.

Identifying warning postures

Decorticate and decerebrate posturing are ominous signs of central nervous system deterioration.

Decorticate (abnormal flexion)
In decorticate posturing, the patient's arms are adducted and flexed, with the wrists and fingers flexed on the chest. The legs may be stiffly extended and internally rotated, with plantar flexion of the feet.

The decorticate posture may indicate a lesion of the frontal lobe, internal capsule, or cerebral peduncles.

Decerebrate (extension)
In decerebrate posturing, the patient's arms are adducted and extended with the wrists pronated and the fingers flexed. One or both of the legs may be stiffly extended, with plantar flexion of the feet.

The decerebrate posture may indicate lesions of the upper brain stem.

◆ *Nursing alert.* If decorticate or decerebrate posturing develops in response to painful stimuli, notify the doctor immediately. (See *Identifying warning postures.*) ◆
• Flex and extend the extremities on both sides *to evaluate muscle tone.*
• Test the plantar reflex in all patients. Stroke the lateral aspect of the sole of the patient's foot with your thumbnail or another moderately sharp object. Normally, this elicits flexion of all toes. Watch for a positive Babinski's sign—

dorsiflexion of the great toe with fanning of the other toes—*which indicates an upper motor neuron lesion.*
• Test for Brudzinski's and Kernig's signs in patients suspected of having meningitis.

Complete the neurologic examination
• Take the patient's temperature, pulse rate, respiration rate, and blood pressure. Especially note his pulse pressure—the difference between systolic pressure and diastolic pressure—*because widening pulse pressure can indicate increasing ICP.*

Special considerations
◆ *Nursing alert.* If the previously stable patient suddenly develops a change in neurologic or routine vital signs, further assess his condition, and notify the doctor immediately. ◆

Documentation
Baseline data require detailed documentation; subsequent notes can be brief unless the patient's condition changes. Record the patient's LOC and orientation, pupillary activity, motor function, and routine vital signs, as hospital policy directs. To save time while keeping complete records, the hospital may let you use abbreviations. Use only commonly understood abbreviations and terms to avoid misinterpretation of the patient's status. Examples include the following:
• A + O × 4—alert and oriented to person, place, time, and date
• PERRLA—pupils equal, round, reactive to light and accommodation
• PERL—pupils equal, reactive to light
• EOM—extraocular movements
    Also describe the patient's behavior—difficult to arouse by gentle shaking, sleepy, unresponsive to painful stimuli.

TREATMENTS
Seizure management

When a patient has a generalized seizure, nursing care aims to protect him from injury and prevent serious complications. Appropriate care also includes observation of seizure characteristics to help determine the area of the brain involved.
    Seizures are classified as partial or generalized. Partial seizures are usually unilateral, involving a localized or focal area of the brain. A *jacksonian* seizure, for ex-

ample, has a focal onset and progresses in stepwise fashion, reflecting the spread of seizure activity in the brain. Generalized seizures involve the entire brain and are known as *absence (petit mal)* and *tonic-clonic (grand mal)* seizures. An absence seizure occurs most often in children and usually begins with a brief change in level of consciousness. A tonic-clonic seizure typically begins with a loud cry. Then the patient falls and loses consciousness. Tonic and clonic movements and autonomic nervous system dysfunction follow. Prolonged seizure activity—known as status epilepticus—requires emergency medical intervention.
    Patients considered at risk for seizures include those with a history of seizures and those with conditions that may predispose them to seizures. These conditions include hypoglycemia, hypoxia, electrolyte imbalances, drug or alcohol withdrawal, and central nervous system trauma. Patients at risk for seizures need precautionary measures to help prevent injury if a seizure occurs. (See *Precautions for generalized seizures.*)

Equipment
Oral airway ▪ suction equipment ▪ equipment for I.V. line insertion ▪ 1 liter of normal saline solution ▪ anticonvulsant, such as diazepam, phenytoin, or phenobarbital, as ordered ▪ emergency resuscitation equipment ▪ 50-ml bolus of dextrose 50% in water, as ordered ▪ 100-mg bolus of thiamine, as ordered ▪ pillows, side rail pads, blankets, or other soft material ▪ optional: endotracheal intubation set.

Implementation
• If you're with a patient when he experiences an aura, help him into bed, raise the side rails, and adjust the bed flat. If he's away from his room, lower him to the floor and place a pillow, blanket, or other soft material under his head *to keep it from hitting the floor.*
• Stay with the patient during the seizure, and be ready to intervene if complications, such as airway obstruction, develop. If necessary, have another staff member obtain the appropriate equipment and notify the doctor.
• If the patient is in the beginning of the tonic phase and if according to hospital protocol, you may insert an oral airway into his mouth *so his tongue doesn't block his airway.* If an oral airway isn't available, don't try to hold his mouth open or place your hands inside *because you may be bitten.* Once the patient's jaw becomes rigid, don't try to force the airway into place *because you may break his teeth or cause other injury.* Some clinicians advocate waiting until the seizure subsides before inserting the airway.
• Move sharp or hard objects out of the patient's way, and loosen his clothing.

Precautions for generalized seizures

By taking appropriate precautions, you can help protect a patient from injury, aspiration, and airway obstruction should he have a seizure. Plan your precautions using information obtained from the patient's history. What kind of seizure has the patient had before? Is he aware of exacerbating factors? Sleep deprivation, missed doses of anticonvulsants, even upper respiratory infections can increase seizure frequency in some persons who have had seizures. Was his previous seizure an acute episode or did it result from a chronic condition?

Gather the equipment

Based on answers provided in the patient's history, you can tailor your precautions to his needs. Start by gathering the appropriate equipment, including a hospital bed with full-length side rails, commercial side rail pads or six bath blankets (four for a crib), adhesive tape, an oral airway, and oral or nasal suction equipment.

Bedside preparations

Now carry out the precautions you think appropriate for the patient. Remember that a patient with preexisting seizures who's being admitted for a change in medication, treatment of an infection, or detoxification may have an increased risk of seizures.

• Explain the reasons for the precautions to the patient.

• *To protect the patient's limbs, head, and feet from injury if he has a seizure while in bed,* cover the side rails, headboard, and footboard with side rail pads or bath blankets. If you use blankets, keep them in place with adhesive tape. Be sure to keep the side rails raised while the patient is in bed *to prevent falls.* Keep the bed in a low position *to minimize any injuries that may occur if the patient climbs over the rails.*

• Place an airway at the patient's bedside, or tape it to the wall above the bed, according to your hospital's protocol. Keep suction equipment nearby *in case you need to establish a patent airway.* Explain to the patient how the airway will be used.

• If the patient has frequent or prolonged seizures, prepare an I.V. heparin lock *to facilitate administration of emergency medications.*

If a seizure begins

• If the patient experiences a typical seizure warning sign, such as an aura, help him into his bed and raise the side rails. Make sure he knows to put on his call light and immediately get into bed if he experiences an aura when you're not nearby.

• If the patient is confused and walking about after a seizure begins, walk with him and guide him back to his bed; don't try to restrain him.

• If the patient becomes cyanotic, have oxygen available at the bedside *to provide maximum saturation as soon as possible.*

• Never attempt to insert an airway once the seizure itself has started.

• *Alert:* Many clinicians disapprove of using airways, reasoning that seizure onset is commonly so rapid that there's no time to insert such a device before the patient's jaws clench shut. Rather than try to pry the jaws apart, these clinicians advocate waiting until after the seizure passes, then opening the jaws and turning the patient on his side. This also avoids upsetting the patient, who may feel traumatized by an artificial airway. Little research has been done to establish the efficacy of one method over another.

• Don't forcibly restrain the patient or restrict his movements during the seizure, *because the force of the patient's tonic-clonic movements against restraints may cause muscle strain or even joint dislocation.*

• Continually assess the patient during the seizure. Observe the earliest symptom, such as head or eye deviation, as well as how the seizure progresses, what form it takes, and how long it lasts. *Your description may help determine the seizure's type and cause.*

• After the tonic-clonic phase, maintain a patent airway by turning the patient on his side and applying suction. *He'll be less likely to aspirate vomitus if he's on his side.*

• If ordered, establish an I.V. line and infuse normal saline solution at a keep-vein-open rate.

• If the seizure lasts longer than 10 minutes, administer an anticonvulsant, as ordered. (See *Administering emergency anticonvulsants,* page 382.)

• For a patient known to be diabetic, administer 50 ml of dextrose 50% in water by I.V. push, as ordered. For a patient known to be an alcoholic, a 100-mg bolus of thiamine may stop the seizure.

• If the seizure is prolonged and the patient becomes hypoxemic, begin resuscitation measures. Rarely, the patient may require endotracheal intubation.

Administering emergency anticonvulsants

A seizure that lasts longer than 10 minutes, or two seizures that occur without the patient's awakening in the interval, signals a condition known as status epilepticus, which requires emergency intervention. After ensuring a patent airway, you'll need to administer an anticonvulsant, such as diazepam or phenytoin, as ordered. If these drugs are ineffective, phenobarbital may be given.

Diazepam

Give an adult 5 to 20 mg of diazepam by slow I.V. push at a rate of 2 to 5 mg/minute, as ordered. You can repeat this dose every 5 to 10 minutes to a maximum dose of 60 mg.

For an elderly or debilitated patient, wait 20 to 30 minutes to repeat the dose. For a child age 5 or older, give 0.5 to 1 mg every 2 to 5 minutes to a total of 10 mg. Repeat this pattern in 2 to 4 hours. For an infant older than 1 month, administer 0.5 mg every 2 to 5 minutes to a total dose of 5 mg. This pattern may be repeated in 2 to 4 hours. Do not give intramuscularly.

Some clinicians prefer to administer lorazepam in children (0.5 mg/kg I.V., repeatable in 15 minutes), because it's less likely to cause respiratory depression than diazepam. However, the manufacturer does not recommend its use for this indication in children under age 18.

Phenytoin

If the doctor orders phenytoin for an adult, administer 150 to 200 mg (or 8 to 18 mg/kg) by direct I.V. injection at a rate of 50 mg/minute. After 30 minutes, you may administer another 100 to 150 mg at the same rate. For a child, give 10 to 15 mg/kg at 0.5 to 1.5 mg/kg/minute. The maximum daily dose is 20 mg/kg. Do not give intramuscularly.

Intravenous diazepam has a rapid onset—less than 1 minute—but its duration of action is only about 30 minutes. Phenytoin's onset is slower (30 minutes to 1 hour) but its duration is 8 to 12 hours. If ordered, both drugs may be given simultaneously—diazepam followed by phenytoin—as long as they're not given in the same syringe.

Phenobarbital

Give an adult 200 to 600 mg by I.V. push. Keep infusion rate below 60 mg/minute. For a child, the usual dose is 15 to 25 mg/kg I.V., given over 10 to 15 minutes.

• If the seizure continues despite medical treatment, you may need to prepare the patient for general anesthesia to stop seizure activity. Electroencephalogram monitoring should be performed in the neurologic intensive care unit *to determine when the seizure activity stops.*

Special considerations

After the seizure, monitor vital signs and mental status every 15 to 30 minutes for 2 hours. If the patient remains obtunded for more than 2 hours, notify the doctor. When the patient does awaken, reorient and reassure him because he may be anxious, afraid, or embarrassed. Ask him about his aura or activities preceding the seizure. The type of aura (auditory, visual, gustatory, olfactory, or somatic) helps pinpoint the site in the brain where the seizure originated.

Because a seizure commonly indicates an underlying disorder, such as meningitis or a metabolic or electrolyte imbalance, a complete diagnostic workup will be ordered if the cause of the seizure isn't evident.

Complications

The patient may experience an injury, respiratory difficulty, and decreased mental capability.

Common injuries include scrapes and bruises suffered when the patient hits objects during the seizure and traumatic injury to the tongue caused by biting. If you suspect a serious injury, such as a fracture or deep laceration, notify the doctor and arrange for appropriate evaluation and treatment.

Changes in respiratory function may include aspiration, airway obstruction, and hypoxemia. After the seizure, complete a full respiratory assessment, notifying the doctor if you suspect a problem.

Expect most patients to experience a postictal period of decreased mental status lasting 30 minutes to 24 hours. Reassure your patient that this does not indicate incipient brain damage.

Documentation

Note that the patient requires seizure precautions; also record all precautions taken. Record the date and time a seizure began, as well as its duration and any precipitating factors. Identify any sensation that may be considered an aura. Describe any involuntary behavior occurring at onset, such as lip smacking, chewing movements, or hand and eye movements. Record any incontinence occurring during the seizure.

Note the patient's response to the seizure, the medications given, any complications resulting from the medications or the seizure, and any interventions performed. Finally, note the patient's postseizure mental status.

 # Pain management

When a patient feels severe pain, he seeks medical help not only because he wants relief but also because he believes the pain signals a serious problem. This perception produces anxiety, which in turn increases the pain. To assess and manage pain properly, the nurse must depend on the patient's subjective description in addition to objective tools.

Several interventions can be used to manage pain. These include analgesics, emotional support, comfort measures, and cognitive techniques to distract the patient. Severe pain usually requires a narcotic analgesic. Invasive measures such as epidural analgesia (see Chapter 5, Drug administration) or patient-controlled analgesia (see Chapter 6, Intravascular therapy) may also be required.

Equipment
Pain assessment tool or scale ■ oral hygiene supplies ■ water ■ nonnarcotic analgesic (such as aspirin or acetaminophen) ■ optional: patient-controlled analgesia (PCA) device; mild narcotic (such as oxycodone or codeine); strong narcotic (such as methadone, levorphanol, morphine, or hydromorphone).

Implementation
• Explain to the patient how pain medications work together with other pain management therapies to provide relief. Also explain that management aims to keep pain at a low level to permit optimal bodily function.
• Assess the patient's pain by asking key questions and noting his response to the pain. For instance, ask him to describe the duration, severity, and source of his pain. Look for physiologic or behavioral clues to the pain's severity. (See *How to assess pain*.)
• Develop nursing diagnoses. Appropriate nursing diagnostic categories include pain, anxiety, activity intolerance, fear, potential for injury, knowledge deficit, powerlessness, and self-care deficit.
• Work with the patient to develop a nursing care plan, using interventions appropriate to the patient's life-style. These may include prescribed medications, emotional

How to assess pain

To assess pain properly, you'll need to consider the patient's description and your observations of the patient's physical and behavioral responses. Start by asking the following series of key questions (bearing in mind that the patient's responses will be shaped by his prior experiences, self-image, and beliefs about his condition):
• Where is the pain located? How long does it last? How often does it occur?
• What does the pain feel like? (Have the patient describe it.)
• What relieves the pain or makes it worse?
• How do you usually get relief from it?

Ask the patient to rank his pain on a scale of 0 to 10, with 0 denoting lack of pain and 10 denoting the worst pain level. This helps the patient verbally evaluate pain therapies.

Observe the patient's behavioral and physiologic responses to pain. Physiologic responses may be sympathetic or parasympathetic.

Behavioral responses
These include altered body position, moaning, sighing, grimacing, withdrawal, crying, restlessness, muscle twitching, and immobility.

Sympathetic responses
These are commonly associated with mild to moderate pain and include pallor, elevated blood pressure, dilated pupils, skeletal muscle tension, dyspnea, tachycardia, and diaphoresis.

Parasympathetic responses
These are commonly associated with severe, deep pain and include pallor, decreased blood pressure, bradycardia, nausea and vomiting, weakness, dizziness, and loss of consciousness.

support, comfort measures, cognitive techniques, and education about pain and its management. Emphasize the importance of maintaining good bowel habits, respiratory function, and mobility *because pain may exacerbate any problems in these areas.*
• Implement your care plan. Because individuals respond to pain differently, you'll find that what works for one person may not work for another.

Give medications
• If the patient is allowed oral intake, begin with a non-narcotic analgesic, such as acetaminophen or aspirin every 4 to 6 hours as ordered.
• Then, if the patient needs more relief than a nonnarcotic analgesic provides, you may administer a mild narcotic (such as oxycodone or codeine) as ordered.
• If the patient needs still more pain relief, you may administer a strong narcotic (such as methadone, levorphanol, morphine, or hydromorphone) as prescribed. Administer oral medications if possible. Check the appropriate drug information for each medication you administer.
• If ordered, teach the patient to use a PCA device. *Such a device can help the patient manage his pain and decrease his anxiety.*

Provide emotional support
• Show your concern by spending time talking with the patient. Because of his pain and his inability to manage it, the patient may be anxious and frustrated. Such feelings worsen his pain.

Perform comfort measures
• Periodically reposition the patient *to reduce muscle spasms and tension and to relieve pressure on bony prominences.* Increasing the angle of the bed can reduce the pull on an abdominal incision, diminishing pain. If appropriate, elevate a limb *to reduce swelling, inflammation, and pain.*
• Give the patient a back massage *to help relax tense muscles.*
• Perform passive range-of-motion exercises *to prevent stiffness and further loss of mobility, relax tense muscles, and provide comfort.*
• Provide oral hygiene. Keep a fresh water glass or cup at the bedside. *Many medications tend to dry the mouth.*
• Wash the patient's face and hands.

Use cognitive therapy
• Help the patient enhance the effect of analgesics by using such techniques as distraction, guided imagery, deep breathing, and relaxation. You can easily use these "mind-over-pain" techniques at the bedside. Choose whichever method the patient feels most comfortable with. If possible, start these techniques when the patient feels little or no pain. If he feels persistent pain, begin with short, simple exercises. Before beginning, dim the lights, remove the patient's restrictive clothing, and eliminate noise from the environment.
• For *distraction,* have the patient recall an interesting or pleasant experience or focus his attention on an enjoyable activity. For instance, have him use music as a distraction by turning on the radio when the pain begins. Have him close his eyes and concentrate on listening, raising or lowering the volume as his pain increases or subsides. Note, however, that distraction is usually effective only against brief pain episodes lasting less than 5 minutes.
• For *guided imagery,* help the patient concentrate on a peaceful, pleasant image. Encourage him to concentrate on the details of the image he has selected by asking about its sight, sound, smell, taste, and touch. The positive emotions evoked by this exercise minimize pain.
• For *deep breathing,* have the patient stare at an object, then slowly inhale and exhale as he counts aloud to maintain a comfortable rate and rhythm. Have him concentrate on the rise and fall of his abdomen. Encourage him to feel more and more weightless with each breath while he concentrates on the rhythm of his breathing or on any restful image.
• For *muscle relaxation,* have the patient focus on a particular muscle group. Then ask him to tense the muscles and note the sensation. After 5 to 7 seconds, tell him to relax the muscles and concentrate on the relaxed state. Have him note the difference between the tense and relaxed states. After he tenses and relaxes one muscle group, have him proceed to another and another until he's covered his entire body.

Special considerations
Evaluate your patient's response to pain management. If he's still in pain, reassess him and alter your care plan as appropriate.

Remind the patient that results of cognitive therapy techniques improve with practice. Help the patient through the initial sessions.

Remember that patients receiving narcotic analgesics are at risk for developing tolerance, dependence, or addiction. The patient with acute pain may have a smaller risk of dependence or addiction than the patient with chronic pain.

If a patient receiving an opioid analgesic experiences abstinence syndrome when the drug is withdrawn abruptly, suspect physical dependence. The signs and symptoms include anxiety, irritability, chills and hot flashes, excessive salivation and tearing, rhinorrhea, sweating, nausea, vomiting, and seizures. These signs and symptoms are likely to begin in 6 to 12 hours and peak in 24 to 72 hours. To reduce the risk of dependence, discontinue a narcotic by decreasing the dose gradually each day. Also, you may switch to an oral narcotic and decrease its dose gradually.

If a patient becomes addicted, his behavior will be characterized by compulsive drug use and a craving for the drug to experience effects other than pain relief. A patient demonstrating such behavior usually has a pre-existing problem that's exacerbated by the narcotic use. Discuss the addicted patient's problem with support personnel, and make appropriate referrals to experts.

During periods of intense pain, the patient's ability to concentrate diminishes. If your patient experiences such pain, help him to select a cognitive technique that's simple to use. Once he selects a particular technique, encourage him to use it consistently.

Complications
The most common adverse effects of analgesics include respiratory depression (the most serious), sedation, constipation, nausea, and vomiting.

Documentation
Document each step of the nursing process. Describe the subjective information you elicited from the patient, using his own words. Note the location, quality, and duration of the pain, as well any precipitating factors.

Record your nursing diagnoses, and include the pain relief method selected. Summarize your actions and the patient's response. If the patient's pain wasn't relieved, note alternate treatments to consider the next time pain occurs. Also record any complications of drug therapy.

Transcutaneous electrical nerve stimulation

Transcutaneous electrical nerve stimulation (TENS) is based on the gate theory of pain, which proposes that painful impulses pass through a "gate" in the brain. TENS is done with a portable, battery-powered device that transmits painless electrical current to peripheral nerves or directly to a painful area over relatively large nerve fibers. This treatment effectively alters the patient's perception of pain by blocking painful stimuli traveling over smaller fibers. Used for patients after surgery and those with chronic pain, a TENS device reduces the need for analgesic drugs and may allow the patient to resume normal activities. (See *Positioning TENS electrodes,* page 386.) Typically, a course of TENS treatments lasts 3 to 5 days. Some conditions, such as phantom limb pain, may require continuous stimulation; other conditions such as a painful arthritic joint require shorter periods (3 to 4 hours).

The TENS device is contraindicated in patients with cardiac pacemakers because it can interfere with pacemaker function. The procedure is also contraindicated for pregnant patients because its effect on the fetus is unknown. It's also contraindicated in patients who are senile. TENS should be used cautiously in all patients with cardiac disorders. TENS electrodes should not be placed on the head or neck of patients with vascular disorders or seizure disorders. Recent studies have raised questions about the efficacy of TENS treatments.

Equipment
Transcutaneous electrical nerve stimulator ▪ alcohol sponges ▪ electrodes ▪ electrode gel ▪ warm water and soap ▪ lead wires ▪ charged battery pack ▪ battery recharger ▪ adhesive patch or nonallergenic tape.

Commercial TENS kits are available. They include the stimulator, lead wires, electrodes, spare battery pack, battery recharger, and sometimes the adhesive patch.

Preparation of equipment
Before beginning the procedure, always test the battery pack to make sure it's fully charged.

Implementation
● Wash your hands. Provide privacy. If the patient has never seen a TENS unit before, show him the device and explain the procedure.

Before TENS treatment
● With an alcohol sponge, thoroughly clean the skin where the electrode will be applied. Then dry the skin.
● Apply electrode gel to the bottom of each electrode.
● Place the ordered number of electrodes on the proper skin area, leaving at least 2″ (5 cm) between them. Then secure them with the adhesive patch or nonallergenic tape. Tape all sides evenly *so the electrodes are firmly attached to the skin.*
● Plug the pin connectors into the electrode sockets. *To protect the cords,* hold the connectors — not the cords themselves — during insertion.
● Turn the channel controls to the "off" position or to the position recommended in the operator's manual.
● Plug the lead wires into the jacks in the control box.
● Turn the amplitude and rate dials slowly, as the manual directs. (The patient should feel a tingling sensation.) Then adjust the controls on this device to the prescribed settings or to settings that are most comfortable. Most patients select stimulation frequencies of 60 to 100 Hertz.
● Attach the TENS control box to part of the patient's clothing, such as a belt, pocket, or bra.
● *To make sure the device is working effectively,* monitor the patient for signs of excessive stimulation, such as muscular twitches, or signs of inadequate stimulation, signaled by the patient's inability to feel any mild tingling sensation.

Positioning TENS electrodes

In transcutaneous electrical nerve stimulation (TENS), electrodes placed around peripheral nerves (or an incisional site) transmit mild electrical pulses to the brain. The current is thought to block pain impulses. The patient can influence the level and frequency of his pain relief by adjusting the controls on the device.

Typically, electrode placement varies even though patients may have similar complaints. Electrodes can be placed in several ways:

• to cover the painful area or surround it, as with muscle tenderness or spasm or painful joints

• to "capture" the painful area between electrodes, as with incisional pain

In peripheral nerve injury, electrodes should be placed proximal to the injury (between the brain and the injury site) to avoid increasing pain. Placing electrodes in a hypersensitive area also increases pain. In an area lacking sensation, electrodes should be placed on adjacent dermatomes.

The illustrations show combinations of electrode placement (black squares) and areas of nerve stimulation (shaded brown) for low back and leg pain.

After TENS treatment

• Turn off the controls and unplug the electrode lead wires from the control box.
• If another treatment will be given soon, leave the electrodes in place; if not, remove them.
• Clean the electrodes with soap and water, and clean the patient's skin with alcohol sponges. (Don't soak the electrodes in alcohol *because it will damage the rubber.*)
• Remove the battery pack from the unit and replace it with a charged battery pack.

• Recharge the used battery pack *so it's always ready for use.*

Special considerations

If you must move the electrodes during the procedure, turn off the controls first. Follow the doctor's orders regarding electrode placement and control settings. *Incorrect placement of the electrodes will result in inappropriate pain control. Setting the controls too high can cause pain; setting them too low will fail to relieve pain.* Never place the electrodes near the patient's eyes or over the nerves that innervate the carotid sinus or laryngeal or pharyngeal muscles *to avoid interference with critical nerve function.*

If TENS is used continuously for postoperative pain, remove the electrodes at least daily *to check for skin irritation, and provide skin care.*

If appropriate, let the patient study the operator's manual. Teach him how to place the electrodes properly and how to take care of the TENS unit.

Documentation

On the patient's medical record and the nursing care plan, record the electrode sites and the control settings. Document the patient's tolerance to treatment. Also evaluate pain control.

Selected references

American Association of Neuroscience Nurses. *Neuroscience Nursing: Phenomena and Practice.* Edited by Mitchell, P.H., et al. Norwalk, Conn.: Appleton & Lange, 1988.

Clevenger, V. "Nursing Management of Lumbar Drains," *Journal of Neuroscience Nursing* 22(4):227-31, August 1990.

Friedman, D. "Taking the Scare Out of Caring for Seizure Patients," *Nursing88* 18(2):52-60, February 1988.

Illustrated Manual of Nursing Practice, 2nd ed. Springhouse, Pa.: Springhouse Corp., 1994.

Inturrisi, C.E. "Management of Cancer Pain: Pharmacology and Principles of Management," *Cancer* 63(11 Supp.):2308-20, June 1, 1989.

Leppik, I.E. "Status Epilepticus: The Next Decade," *Neurology* 40(5 Supp. 2):4-9, May 1990.

McGuire, L. "Administering Analgesics: Which Drugs Are Right for Your Patient?" *Nursing90* 20(4):34-42, April 1990.

Nurse's PhotoLibrary. Springhouse, Pa.: Springhouse Corp., 1993.

Nursing94 Drug Handbook. Springhouse, Pa.: Springhouse Corp., 1994.

Ropper, A.H., and Kennedy, S.F. *Neurological and Neurosurgical Intensive Care,* 2nd ed. Rockville, Md.: Aspen Pubs., Inc., 1988.

CHAPTER 10

GASTROINTESTINAL CARE

DANIELE SHOLLENBERGER, RN, MSN

Ch 10th

Ch 10

gastrointestinal
Care

Introduction

Gastrointestinal (GI) conditions affect just about everyone at one time or another. These conditions, so intimately tied to psychological health and stability, range from simple changes in bowel habits to life-threatening disorders requiring major surgery and radical life-style changes.

Just as GI conditions vary widely, so does patient care. For example, the patient with simple constipation may need minimal nursing intervention consisting of brief teaching about diet and exercise. However, the patient with colorectal cancer may need ongoing nursing care ranging from encouragement and support during the diagnostic workup to meticulous colostomy care during recovery.

Your role in GI procedures

Therapeutic GI procedures vary greatly, reflecting the wide spectrum of systemic abnormalities. They may involve feeding a patient through a tube, teaching a patient how to use a gastrostomy feeding button, or minimizing a patient's anxiety before abdominal surgery or his discomfort after it.

To carry out responsibilities like these successfully, you need to address both the emotional and the physical needs of the patient. Where to place an incision or which type of colostomy to use have important emotional implications for the patient. Your knowledge of anatomy and physiology, as well as a familiarity with surgical procedures, influences your plan of care and ultimately how the patient responds.

For some GI procedures, you'll need to provide considerable emotional support, especially if they prove uncomfortable or embarrassing to the patient. Helping the patient who is undergoing such a procedure maintain his sense of dignity, while at the same time eliciting his cooperation, requires a skillful blend of compassion and judgment.

For many GI procedures, you'll need to work cooperatively with staff, including the pharmacist, doctors, laboratory personnel, diagnostic technicians, dietitians, and others.

NASAL AND ORAL ACCESS
Nasogastric tube insertion and removal

Usually inserted to decompress the stomach, a nasogastric (NG) tube can prevent vomiting after major surgery. Normally, the patient has the tube for 48 to 72 hours after surgery, by which time peristalsis usually resumes. An NG tube may remain in place for shorter or longer periods, however, depending on its use.

The NG tube has other diagnostic and therapeutic applications, especially in assessing and treating upper GI bleeding, collecting gastric contents for analysis, performing gastric lavage, aspirating gastric secretions, and administering medications and nutrients.

Inserting an NG tube requires close observation of the patient and verification of proper placement. Removing the tube requires careful handling to prevent injury or aspiration. The tube must be inserted with extra care in pregnant patients and in those with an increased risk of complications. For example, the doctor will order an NG tube for a patient with aortic aneurysm, myocardial infarction, gastric hemorrhage, or esophageal varices only if he believes that the benefits outweigh the risks of intubation.

Most NG tubes have a radiopaque marker or strip at the distal end so that the tube's position can be verified by X-ray studies. If the position can't be confirmed, the doctor may order fluoroscopy to verify placement.

The most common NG tubes are the Levin tube, which has one lumen, and the Salem sump tube, which has two lumens, one for suction and drainage and a smaller one for ventilation. Air flows through the vent lumen continuously. This protects the delicate gastric mucosa by preventing a vacuum from forming should the tube adhere to the stomach lining. (See *Types of NG tubes,* page 390.) The Moss tube, which has a triple lumen, is usually inserted during surgery.

Equipment

For inserting an NG tube: tube (usually #14, #16, or #18 French for a normal adult) ▪ towel or linen-saver pad ▪ facial tissues ▪ emesis basin ▪ penlight ▪ 1″ or 2″ nonallergenic tape ▪ gloves ▪ water-soluble lubricant ▪ cup or glass of water with straw (if appropriate) ▪ stethoscope ▪ tongue blade ▪ catheter-tip or bulb syringe or irrigation set ▪ safety pin ▪ ordered suction equipment ▪

Types of NG tubes

The doctor will choose the type and diameter of nasogastric (NG) tube that best suits the patient's needs, including lavage, aspiration, enteral therapy, or stomach decompression. Common choices include the Levin, Salem sump, and Moss tubes.

Levin tube

This rubber or plastic tube has a single lumen, a length of 42" to 50" (107 to 127 cm), and holes at the tip and along the side.

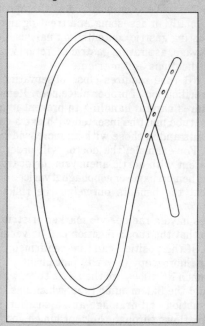

Salem sump tube

This double lumen tube is made of clear plastic and has a blue sump port (pigtail) that allows atmospheric air to enter the patient's stomach. Thus, the tube floats freely and doesn't adhere to or damage gastric mucosa. The larger port of this 48" (122-cm) tube serves as the main suction conduit. The tube has openings at the sides and the tip; markings at 45, 55, 65, and 75 cm; and a radiopaque line to verify placement.

Moss tube

This tube has a radiopaque tip and three lumens. The first, positioned and inflated at the cardia, serves as a balloon inflation port. The second is an esophageal aspiration port. The third is a duodenal feeding port.

optional: metal clamp, ice, warm water, large basin or plastic container, rubber band.

For removing an NG tube: stethoscope ▪ catheter-tip syringe ▪ normal saline solution ▪ towel or linen-saver pad ▪ adhesive remover ▪ optional: clamp.

Preparation of equipment

Inspect the NG tube for defects, such as rough edges or partially closed lumens. Then, check the tube's patency by flushing it with water. *To ease insertion,* increase a stiff tube's flexibility by coiling it around your gloved fingers for a few seconds or by dipping it into warm water. Stiffen a limp tube by briefly chilling it in ice.

Implementation

• Whether you're inserting or removing an NG tube, be sure to provide privacy and wash and glove your hands before inserting the tube.

To insert an NG tube

• Explain the procedure to the patient *to ease anxiety and promote cooperation.* Inform her that she may experience some nasal discomfort, that she may gag, and that her eyes may water. Emphasize that swallowing will ease the tube's advancement.

• Agree on a signal that the patient can use if she wants you to stop briefly during the procedure.

• Gather and prepare all necessary equipment.

• Help the patient into high Fowler's position unless contraindicated.

• Stand at the patient's right side if you're right-handed or at her left side if you're left-handed *to ease insertion.*

• Drape the towel or linen-saver pad over the patient's chest *to protect her gown and bed linens from spills.*

• Have the patient gently blow her nose *to clear her nostrils.*

• Place the facial tissues and emesis basin well within the patient's reach.

• Help the patient face forward with her neck in a neutral position.

• *To determine how long the NG tube must be to reach the stomach,* hold the end of the tube at the tip of the patient's nose. Extend the tube to the patient's earlobe and then down to the xiphoid process.

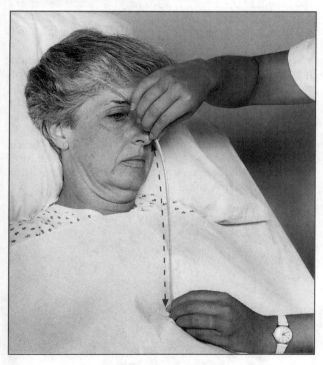

• Mark this distance on the tubing with the tape. (Average measurements for an adult range from 22″ to 26″ [56 to 66 cm].)

• *To determine which nostril will allow easier access,* use a penlight and inspect for a deviated septum or other abnormalities. Ask the patient if she ever had nasal surgery or a nasal injury. Assess airflow in both nostrils by occluding one nostril at a time while the patient breathes through her nose. Choose the nostril with the better airflow.

• Lubricate the first 3″ (7.6 cm) of the tube with a water-soluble gel *to minimize injury to the nasal passages. Using a water-soluble lubricant prevents lipoid pneumonia that may result from aspirating an oil-based lubricant or from accidental slippage of the tube into the trachea.*

• Instruct the patient to hold her head straight and upright.

• Grasp the tube with the end pointing downward, curve it if necessary, and carefully insert it into the more patent nostril.

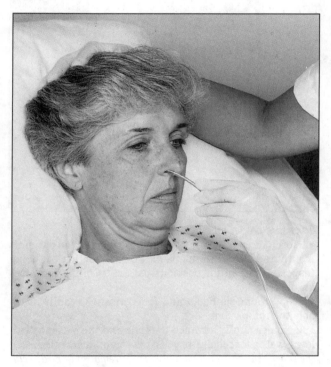

• Aim the tube downward and toward the ear closer to the chosen nostril. Advance it slowly *to avoid pressure on the turbinates and resultant pain and bleeding.*

• When the tube reaches the nasopharynx, you'll feel resistance. Instruct the patient to lower her head slightly *to close the trachea and open the esophagus.* Then, rotate the tube 180 degrees toward the opposite nostril *to redirect it so that the tube won't enter the patient's mouth.*

• Unless contraindicated, offer the patient a cup or glass of water with a straw. Direct her to sip and swallow as you slowly advance the tube (top left, page 392). *This helps the tube pass to the esophagus.* (If you aren't using water, ask the patient to swallow.)

To ensure proper tube placement

• Use a tongue blade and penlight to examine the patient's mouth and throat for signs of a coiled section of tubing (especially in an unconscious patient). Coiling indicates an obstruction.

• Keep an emesis basin and facial tissues readily available for the patient.

• As you carefully advance the tube and the patient swallows, watch for respiratory distress signs, *which may mean the tube is in the bronchus and must be removed immediately.*

• Stop advancing the tube when the tape mark reaches the patient's nostril. *asepto*

• Attach a catheter-tip or bulb syringe to the tube and try to aspirate stomach contents. If you do not obtain stomach contents, position the patient on her left side *to move the contents into the stomach's greater curvature,* and aspirate again (see illustration above at right).

Note: When confirming tube placement, never place the tube's end in a container of water. *If the tube should be mispositioned in the trachea, the patient may aspirate water.* Besides, water without bubbles does not confirm proper placement. *Instead, the tube may be coiled in the trachea or the esophagus.*

• If you still can't aspirate stomach contents, advance the tube 1" to 2" (2.5 to 5 cm). Then inject 10 cc of air into the tube. At the same time, auscultate for air sounds with your stethoscope placed over the epigastric region. *You should hear a whooshing sound if the tube is patent and properly positioned in the stomach.*

• If these tests don't confirm proper tube placement, you'll need X-ray verification.

• Secure the NG tube to the patient's nose with nonallergenic tape (or other designated tube holder). You will need about 4" (10 cm) of 1" tape. Split one end of the tape up the center about 1½" (3.8 cm). Make tabs on the split ends (by folding sticky sides together). Stick the uncut tape end on the patient's nose so that the split in the tape starts about ½" (1.3 cm) to 1½" from the tip of her nose. Crisscross the tabbed ends around the tube. Then apply another piece of tape over the bridge of the nose to secure the tube.

• Alternatively, stabilize the tube with a prepackaged product that secures and cushions it at the nose.

• *To reduce discomfort from the weight of the tube,* tie a slip knot around the tube with a rubber band, and then secure the rubber band to the patient's gown with a safety pin, or wrap another piece of tape around the end of the tube and leave a tab. Then fasten the tape tab to the patient's gown with a safety pin.
• Attach the tube to suction equipment, if ordered, and set the designated suction pressure.

To remove an NG tube
• Explain the procedure to the patient, informing her that it may cause some nasal discomfort and sneezing or gagging.
• Assess bowel function by auscultating for peristalsis or flatus.
• Help the patient into semi-Fowler's position. Then drape a towel or linen-saver pad across her chest *to protect her gown and bed linens from spills.*
• Using a catheter-tip syringe, flush the tube with 10 ml of normal saline solution *to ensure that the tube doesn't contain stomach contents that could irritate tissues during tube removal.*
• Untape the tube from the patient's nose, and then unpin it from her gown.
• Clamp the tube by folding it in your hand.
• Ask the patient to hold her breath *to close the epiglottis.* Then withdraw the tube gently and steadily. (When the distal end of the tube reaches the nasopharynx, you can pull it quickly.)
• When possible, immediately cover and remove the tube *because its sight and odor may nauseate the patient.*

• Assist the patient with thorough mouth care, and clean the tape residue from her nose with adhesive remover.
• For the next 48 hours, monitor the patient for signs of GI dysfunction, including nausea, vomiting, abdominal distention, and food intolerance. GI dysfunction may necessitate reinsertion of the tube.

Special considerations
A helpful device for calculating the correct tube length is Ross-Hanson tape. Place the narrow end of this measuring tape at the tip of the patient's nose. Again, extend the tape to the patient's earlobe and down to the tip of the xiphoid process. Mark this distance on the edge of the tape labeled "nose to ear to xiphoid." The corresponding measurement on the opposite edge of the tape is the proper insertion length.

If the patient has a deviated septum or other nasal condition that prevents nasal insertion, pass the tube orally after removing any dentures, if necessary. Sliding the tube over the tongue, proceed as you would for nasal insertion.

When using the oral route, remember to coil the end of the tube around your hand. *This helps curve and direct the tube downward at the pharynx.*

If your patient lies unconscious, tilt her chin toward her chest *to close the trachea.* Then advance the tube between respirations *to ensure that it doesn't enter the trachea.*

While advancing the tube in an unconscious patient (or in a patient who can't swallow), stroke the patient's neck *to encourage the swallowing reflex and to facilitate passage down the esophagus.*

While advancing the tube, observe for signs that it has entered the trachea, such as choking or breathing difficulties in a conscious patient and cyanosis in an unconscious patient or a patient without a cough reflex. If these signs occur, remove the tube immediately. Allow the patient time to rest; then try to reinsert the tube.

After tube placement, vomiting suggests tubal obstruction or incorrect position. Assess immediately to determine the cause.

Home care
An NG tube may be inserted or removed at home. Indications for insertion include gastric decompression and short-term feeding. A home care nurse or the patient may insert the tube, deliver the feeding, and remove the tube. See *Using an NG tube at home,* page 394.

Complications
Potential complications of prolonged intubation with an NG tube include skin erosion at the nostril, sinusitis, esophagitis, esophagotracheal fistula, gastric ulceration,

lavage
washing out of
cavity

Using an NG tube at home

If your patient will need to have a nasogastric (NG) tube in place at home—for short-term feeding or gastric decompression, for example—find out who will insert the tube. If the patient will have a home care nurse, identify her and, if possible, tell the patient when to expect her.

If the patient or a family member will perform the procedure, you'll need to provide additional instruction and supervision. Use this checklist to assemble your teaching topics:

☐ how and where to obtain equipment needed for home intubation
☐ how to insert the tube
☐ verifying tube placement by aspirating stomach contents
☐ correcting tube misplacement
☐ preparing formula for tube feeding
☐ how to store formula, if appropriate
☐ administering formula through the tube
☐ how to remove and dispose of an NG tube
☐ how to clean and store a reusable NG tube
☐ how to use the NG tube for gastric decompression, if appropriate
☐ how to set up and operate suctioning equipment
☐ troubleshooting suctioning equipment
☐ how to perform mouth care and other hygienic procedures.

and pulmonary and oral infection. Additional complications that may result from suction include electrolyte imbalances and dehydration.

Documentation

Record the type and size of the NG tube and the date, time, and route of insertion. Also note the type and amount of suction, if used, and describe the drainage, including the amount, color, character, consistency, and odor. Note the patient's tolerance of the procedure. When you remove the tube, make sure to record the date and time. Describe the color, consistency, and amount of gastric drainage. Again, note the patient's tolerance of the procedure.

Nasogastric tube care

Providing effective nasogastric (NG) tube care requires meticulous monitoring of the patient and the equipment. Monitoring the patient involves checking drainage from the NG tube and assessing GI function. Monitoring the equipment involves verifying correct tube placement and irrigating the tube to ensure patency and to prevent mucosal damage.

Specific care varies only slightly for the most commonly used NG tubes: the single-lumen Levin tube and the double-lumen Salem sump tube.

Equipment
Irrigant (usually normal saline solution) ■ irrigant container ■ 60-ml catheter-tip syringe ■ bulb syringe ■ suction equipment ■ lemon-glycerin swabs or toothbrush and toothpaste ■ petroleum jelly ■ 1½" or 1" nonallergenic tape ■ water-soluble lubricant ■ gloves ■ stethoscope ■ linen-saver pad ■ optional: emesis basin.

Preparation of equipment
Make sure the suction equipment works properly. (See *Common gastric suction devices*.) When using a Salem sump tube with suction, connect the larger, primary lumen (for drainage and suction) to the suction equipment and select the appropriate setting, as ordered (usually low constant suction). If the doctor doesn't specify the setting, follow the manufacturer's directions. A Levin tube usually calls for intermittent low suction.

Implementation
● Explain the procedure to the patient and provide privacy.
● Wash your hands and put on gloves.

To irrigate the NG tube
● Review the irrigation schedule (usually every 4 hours), if the doctor orders this procedure.
● Inject 10 cc of air and auscultate the epigastric area with a stethoscope and aspirate stomach contents *to check correct positioning in the stomach and to prevent the patient from aspirating the irrigant.*
● Measure the amount of irrigant in the bulb syringe or in the 60-ml catheter-tip syringe (usually 30 ml) *to maintain an accurate intake and output record.*
● When using suction with a Salem sump tube or a Levin tube, unclamp and disconnect the tube from the suction equipment while holding it over a linen-saver pad or an emesis basin *to collect any drainage.*

Patency = open

Common gastric suction devices

A variety of portable or wall-mounted suction devices are available for applying negative pressure to nasogastric (NG) and other drainage tubes. Two common types are shown here.

Portable suction machine
In the portable suction machine, a vacuum created intermittently by an electric pump draws gastric contents up the NG tube and into the collecting bottle.

On-off switch
High-low power switch
Indicator light
Connecting tube
Collecting container

Stationary suction machine
A stationary wall-unit apparatus can provide intermittent or continuous suction. On-off switches and variable power settings let you set and adjust the suction force on either machine.

On-off switch
Suction setting (intermittent to continuous)
Connecting tube
Collecting container

• Slowly instill the irrigant into the NG tube. (When irrigating the Salem sump tube, you may instill small amounts of solution into the vent lumen without interrupting suction; however, you should instill greater amounts into the larger, primary lumen.)

• Gently aspirate the solution with the bulb syringe or 60-ml catheter-tip syringe or connect the tube to the suction equipment, as ordered. *Gentle aspiration prevents excessive pressure on a suture line and on delicate gastric mucosa.*

• Reconnect the tube to suction after completing irrigation.

To instill a solution through the NG tube
• If the doctor orders *instillation,* inject the solution, and do not aspirate it. Note the amount of instilled solution as "intake" on the intake and output record.

• Reattach the tube to suction as ordered.

• After attaching the Salem sump tube's primary lumen to suction, instill 10 to 20 cc of air into the vent lumen *to verify patency.* Listen for a soft hiss in the vent. If you don't hear this sound, suspect a clogged tube; recheck patency by instilling 10 ml of normal saline solution and 10 to 20 cc of air in the vent.

To monitor patient comfort and condition
• Provide mouth care once a shift or as needed. Depending on the patient's condition, use lemon-glycerin swabs to clean his teeth or assist him to brush them with

toothbrush and toothpaste. Coat the patient's lips with petroleum jelly *to prevent dryness from mouth breathing.*

• Change the tape securing the tube as needed or at least daily. Clean the skin, apply fresh tape, and dab water-soluble lubricant on the nostrils as needed.

• Regularly check the tape that secures the tube *because sweat and nasal secretions may loosen the tape.*

• Assess bowel sounds regularly (every 4 to 8 hours) *to verify GI function.*

• Measure the drainage amount and update the intake and output record every 8 hours. Be alert for electrolyte imbalances with excessive gastric output.

• Inspect gastric drainage. Note color, consistency, odor, and amount. Normal gastric secretions have no color or appear yellow-green from bile and have a mucoid consistency. Immediately report any drainage with a coffee-bean color. *This may indicate bleeding.* If you suspect that the drainage contains blood, use a screening test (such as Hematest) for occult blood according to your hospital's protocol.

Special considerations

Irrigate the NG tube with 30 ml of irrigant before and after instilling medication. (See "Instillation of drugs through a nasogastric tube," Chapter 5.) Wait about 30 minutes, or as ordered, after instillation before reconnecting the suction equipment *to allow sufficient time for the medication to be absorbed.*

When no drainage appears, check the suction equipment for proper function. Then, holding the NG tube over a linen-saver pad or an emesis basin, separate the tube and the suction source. Check the suction equipment by placing the suction tubing in an irrigant container. If the apparatus draws the water, check the NG tube for proper function. Be sure to note the amount of water drawn into the suction container on the intake and output record.

A dysfunctional NG tube may be clogged or incorrectly positioned. Attempt to irrigate the tube, reposition the patient, or rotate and reposition the tube. However, if the tube was inserted during surgery, avoid this maneuver *to ensure that the movement doesn't interfere with gastric or esophageal sutures.* Notify the doctor.

If you can ambulate the patient and interrupt suction, disconnect the NG tube from the suction equipment. Clamp the tube *to prevent stomach contents from draining out of the tube.*

If the patient has a Salem sump tube, watch for gastric reflux in the vent lumen when pressure in the stomach exceeds atmospheric pressure. This problem may result from a clogged primary lumen or from a suction system that's set up improperly. Assess the suction equipment for proper functioning. Then, irrigate the NG tube and instill 30 cc of air into the vent tube *to maintain patency.*

Don't attempt to stop reflux by clamping the vent tube. Unless contraindicated, elevate the patient's torso more than 30 degrees, and keep the vent tube above his midline *to prevent a siphoning effect.*

Complications

Epigastric pain and vomiting may result from a clogged or improperly placed tube. Any NG tube — the Levin tube in particular — may move and aggravate esophagitis, ulcers, or esophageal varices, causing hemorrhage. Perforation may result from aggressive intubation. Dehydration and electrolyte imbalances may result from removing body fluids and electrolytes by suctioning. Pain, swelling, and salivary dysfunction may signal parotitis, which occurs in dehydrated, debilitated patients. Intubation can cause nasal skin breakdown and discomfort and increased mucous secretions. Aspiration pneumonia may result from gastric reflux. Vigorous suction may damage the gastric mucosa and cause significant bleeding, possibly interfering with endoscopic assessment and diagnosis.

Documentation

Regularly record tube placement confirmation (usually every 4 to 8 hours). Keep a precise record of fluid intake and output, including the instilled irrigant in fluid input. Track the irrigation schedule and note the actual time of each irrigation. Describe drainage color, consistency, odor, and amount. Also note tape change times and condition of the nares.

Gastric lavage

After poisoning or a drug overdose, especially in patients who have central nervous system depression or an inadequate gag reflex, gastric lavage flushes the stomach and removes ingested substances through a nasogastric (NG) tube. For patients with gastric or esophageal bleeding, lavage with tepid or iced water or normal saline solution may be used to stop bleeding. However, some controversy exists over the effectiveness of iced lavage for this purpose. (See *Is iced lavage effective?*) Typically, this procedure is done in the emergency department or intensive care unit by a doctor, gastroenterologist, or a nurse, although the wide-bore lavage tube is almost always inserted by the gastroenterologist.

Gastric lavage is contraindicated after ingestion of a corrosive substance (such as lye, ammonia, or mineral acids) because the NG tube may perforate the already compromised esophagus.

Correct NG tube placement is essential for patient safety because accidental misplacement (in the lungs, for example) followed by lavage can be fatal. Other complications of gastric lavage include bradyarrhythmias and aspiration of gastric fluids.

Equipment

Lavage setup (two graduated containers for drainage, three pieces of large-lumen rubber tubing, Y connector, and a clamp or hemostat) ■ 2 to 3 liters of normal saline solution or tap water, as ordered ■ I.V. pole ■ basin of ice, if ordered ■ Ewald tube or any large-lumen gastric tube, typically #36 to #40 French (see *Using wide-bore gastric tubes,* page 398) ■ water-soluble lubricant or anesthetic ointment ■ stethoscope ■ ½" nonallergenic tape ■ 50-ml bulb or catheter-tip syringe ■ gloves ■ linen-saver pad or towel ■ Yankauer or tonsil-tip suction device ■ suction apparatus ■ labeled specimen container ■ laboratory request form ■ norepinephrine ■ optional: patient restraints, charcoal tablets.

A prepackaged, syringe-type irrigation kit may be used for lavage. For poisoning or a drug overdose, however, the lavage setup may be more appropriate to use *because it's a faster and more effective means of diluting and removing the harmful substance.*

Preparation of equipment

Set up the lavage equipment. (See *Preparing for gastric lavage,* page 399.)

If iced lavage is ordered, chill the desired irrigant (water or normal saline solution) in a basin of ice.

Lubricate the end of the NG tube with the water-soluble lubricant or anesthetic ointment.

Implementation

• Explain the procedure to the patient, provide privacy, and wash your hands.
• Put on gloves.
• Drape the towel or linen-saver pad over the patient's chest *to protect him from spills.*
• The doctor inserts the NG tube nasally and advances it slowly and gently *because forceful insertion may injure tissues and cause epistaxis.* He then checks the tube's placement by injecting about 30 cc of air into the tube with the bulb syringe and then auscultating the patient's abdomen with a stethoscope. If the tube is in place, he'll hear the sound of air entering the stomach.
• *Because the patient may vomit when the NG tube reaches the posterior pharynx during insertion,* be prepared to suction the airway immediately with either a Yankauer or a tonsil-tip suction device.
• Once the NG tube passes the posterior pharynx, assist the patient into Trendelenburg's position and turn him

---

Is iced lavage effective?

Some experts question the effectiveness of using an iced irrigant for gastric lavage to treat GI bleeding. Here's why.

Iced irrigating solutions stimulate the vagus nerve, which triggers increased hydrochloric acid secretion. In turn, this stimulates gastric motility, which can irritate the bleeding site.

Some clinicians prefer using unchilled normal saline solution (which may prevent rapid electrolyte loss) or even water if the patient must avoid sodium. These clinicians point out that no research exists to support the use of iced irrigant to stop acute GI bleeding.

---

toward his left side in a three-quarter prone posture. *This position minimizes passage of gastric contents into the duodenum and may prevent the patient from aspirating vomitus.*
• After securing the NG tube nasally or orally and making sure the irrigant inflow tube on the lavage setup is clamped, connect the unattached end of this tube to the NG tube. Allow the stomach contents to empty into the drainage container before instilling any irrigant. *This confirms proper tube placement and decreases the risk of overfilling the stomach with irrigant and inducing vomiting.* If you're using a syringe irrigation set, aspirate stomach contents with a 50-ml bulb or catheter-tip syringe before instilling the irrigant.
• Once you confirm proper tube placement, begin gastric lavage by instilling about 250 ml of irrigant *to assess the patient's tolerance and prevent vomiting.* If you're using a syringe, instill about 50 ml of solution at a time until you've instilled between 250 and 500 ml.
• Clamp the inflow tube and unclamp the outflow tube *to allow the irrigant to flow out.* If you're using the syringe irrigation kit, aspirate the irrigant with the syringe and empty it into a calibrated container. Measure the outflow amount to be sure that it at least equals the amount of irrigant you instilled. *This prevents accidental stomach distention and vomiting.* If the drainage amount falls significantly short of the instilled amount, reposition the tube until sufficient solution flows out. Gently massage the abdomen over the stomach to promote outflow.
• Repeat the inflow-outflow cycle until returned fluids appear clear. *This signals that the stomach no longer holds harmful substances or that bleeding has stopped.*

Using wide-bore gastric tubes

If you need to deliver a large volume of fluid rapidly through a gastric tube (when irrigating the stomach of a patient with profuse gastric bleeding or poisoning, for example), a wide-bore gastric tube usually serves best. Typically inserted orally, these tubes remain in place only long enough to complete the lavage and evacuate stomach contents.

Ewald tube
In an emergency, using this single-lumen tube with several openings at the distal end allows you to aspirate large amounts of gastric contents quickly.

Levacuator tube
This tube has two lumens. Use the larger lumen for evacuating gastric contents; the smaller, for instilling an irrigant.

Edlich tube
This single-lumen tube has four openings near the closed distal tip. A funnel or syringe may be connected at the proximal end. Like the Ewald tube, the Edlich tube lets you withdraw large quantities of gastric contents quickly.

● Assess the patient's vital signs, urine output, and level of consciousness (LOC) every 15 minutes. Notify the doctor of any changes.
● If ordered, remove the NG tube.

Special considerations
To control GI bleeding, the doctor may order continuous irrigation of the stomach with an irrigant and a vasoconstrictor, such as norepinephrine. After the stomach absorbs norepinephrine, the portal system delivers the drug directly to the liver, where it's metabolized. *This prevents the drug from circulating systemically and initiating a hypertensive response.* Or the doctor may use an alternate drug-delivery method, directing you to clamp the outflow tube for a prescribed period after instilling the irrigant and the vasoconstrictive medication and before withdrawing it. *This allows the mucosa time to absorb the drug.*

Never leave a patient alone during gastric lavage. Observe continuously for any changes in his LOC, and monitor vital signs frequently *because the natural vagal response to intubation can depress the patient's heart rate.*

If you need to restrain the patient, secure restraints on the same side of the bed or stretcher *so that you can free them quickly without moving to the other side of the bed.* Avoid restraining the patient in a "spread eagle" position, *which would prevent him from turning and leave him at risk for aspirating vomitus.*

Remember also to keep tracheal suctioning equipment nearby and watch closely for airway obstruction caused by vomiting or excess oral secretions. Throughout gastric lavage, you may need to suction the oral cavity frequently *to ensure an open airway and prevent aspiration.* For the same reasons, and if he doesn't exhibit an adequate gag reflex, the patient may require an endotracheal tube before the procedure.

When aspirating the stomach for ingested poisons or drugs, be sure to save the contents in a labeled container to send to the laboratory for analysis. If ordered, after lavage to remove poisons or drugs, mix charcoal tablets with the irrigant (whether it's water or normal saline solution) and administer the mixture through the NG tube. The charcoal will absorb remaining toxic substances. The tube may be clamped temporarily, allowed to drain via gravity, attached to intermittent suction, or removed.

When performing gastric lavage to stop bleeding, keep precise intake and output records *to determine the amount of bleeding.* When the patient has large volumes of fluid instilled and withdrawn, serum electrolyte or arterial blood gas levels (or both) may be measured during or at the end of lavage.

Complications

Vomiting and subsequent aspiration, the most common complication of gastric lavage, occurs more often in a groggy patient. Bradyarrhythmias also may occur. After iced lavage especially, the patient's body temperature may drop, thereby triggering cardiac arrhythmias.

Documentation

Record the date and time of lavage; the size and type of NG tube used; the volume and type of irrigant; and the amount of drained gastric contents. Record this information on the intake and output record sheet, and include your observations, noting, for example, color and consistency of drainage. Also keep precise records of the patient's vital signs and LOC, any drugs instilled through the tube, the time the tube was removed, and how well the patient tolerated the procedure.

 Feeding tube insertion and removal

Inserting a feeding tube nasally or (sometimes) orally into the stomach or duodenum allows a patient who can't or won't eat to receive nourishment. The feeding tube also permits supplemental feedings in a patient who has exceptionally high nutritional requirements—an unconscious patient or one with extensive burns, for example. Typically, the procedure is done by a nurse, as ordered. The preferred feeding tube route is nasal, but the oral route may be used for patients with such conditions as a deviated septum or a head or nose injury.

The doctor may order duodenal feeding when the patient can't tolerate gastric feeding or when he expects gastric feeding to produce aspiration. Absence of bowel sounds or possible intestinal obstruction contraindicates using a feeding tube.

Feeding tubes differ somewhat from standard nasogastric tubes. Made of silicone, rubber, or polyurethane, feeding tubes have small diameters and great flexibility. This reduces oropharyngeal irritation, necrosis from pressure on the tracheoesophageal wall, distal esophageal irritation, and discomfort from swallowing. To facilitate passage, some feeding tubes are weighted with tungsten, and some need a guide wire to keep them from curling in the back of the throat.

These small-bore tubes usually have radiopaque markings and a water-activated coating, which provides a lubricated surface.

EQUIPMENT

 Preparing for gastric lavage

Prepare the lavage setup as follows:
• Connect one of the three pieces of large-lumen tubing to the irrigant container.
• Insert the Y connector stem in the other end of the tubing.
• Connect the remaining two pieces of tubing to the free ends of the Y connector.
• Place the unattached end of one of the tubes into one of the drainage containers. (Later, you'll connect the other piece of tubing to the patient's gastric tube.)
• Clamp the tube leading to the irrigant.
• Suspend the entire setup from the I.V. pole, hanging the irrigant container at the highest level.

Equipment

For insertion: feeding tube (#6 to #18 French, with or without guide) ■ linen-saver pad ■ gloves ■ nonallergenic tape ■ water-soluble lubricant ■ cotton-tipped applicators ■ skin preparation (such as tincture of benzoin) ■ facial tissues ■ penlight ■ small cup of water with straw, or ice chips ■ emesis basin ■ 60-ml syringe ■ stethoscope.

During use: mouthwash or saltwater solution ■ toothbrush.

For removal: linen-saver pad ■ tube clamp ■ bulb syringe.

Preparation of equipment

Have the proper size tube available. Usually, the doctor orders the smallest-bore tube that will allow free passage of the liquid feeding formula. Read the instructions on the tubing package carefully *because tube characteristics vary according to the manufacturer.* (For example, some tubes have marks at the appropriate lengths for gastric, duodenal, and jejunal insertion.)

Examine the tube *to make sure it's free of defects, such as cracks or rough or sharp edges.* Next, run water through the tube. *This checks for patency, activates the coating, and allows for easier removal of the guide.*

Implementation

● Explain the procedure to the patient and show him the tube *so he knows what to expect and can cooperate more fully.*
● Provide privacy and wash your hands. Put on gloves.
● Assist the patient into semi-Fowler's (or high Fowler's) position.
● Place a linen-saver pad across the patient's chest *to protect him from spills.*
● *To determine the tube length needed to reach the stomach,* first extend the distal end of the tube from the tip of the patient's nose to his earlobe. Coil this portion of the tube around your fingers *so the end will remain curved until you insert it.* Then extend the uncoiled portion from the earlobe to the xiphoid process. Use a small piece of nonallergenic tape to mark the total length of these two portions.

To insert the tube nasally

● Using the penlight, assess nasal patency. Inspect nasal passages for a deviated septum, polyps, or other obstructions. As the patient breathes through his nose, occlude one nostril, then the other, *to determine which has the better airflow.* Assess the patient's history of nasal injury or surgery.
● Lubricate the curved tip of the tube (and the feeding tube guide, if appropriate) with a small amount of water-soluble lubricant *to ease insertion and prevent tissue injury.*

● Ask the patient to hold the emesis basin and facial tissues in case he needs them.
● *To advance the tube,* insert the curved, lubricated tip into the more patent nostril and direct it along the nasal passage toward the ear on the same side. When it passes the nasopharyngeal junction, turn the tube 180 degrees *to aim it downward into the esophagus* and advance it. Then, give him a small cup of water with a straw, or ice chips. Direct him to sip the water or suck on the ice and swallow frequently, without clamping his teeth down on the tube. *This will ease the tube's passage.* Advance the tube as he swallows.

To insert the tube orally

● Have the patient lower his chin *to close his trachea,* and ask him to open his mouth.
● Place the tip of the tube at the back of the patient's tongue, give water, and instruct the patient to swallow, as above.

To position the tube

● Keep passing the tube until the tape marking the appropriate length reaches the patient's nostril or lips.
● *To check tube placement,* attach the syringe filled with 10 cc of air to the end of the tube. Gently inject the air into the tube as you auscultate the patient's abdomen with the stethoscope about 3″ (7.6 cm) below the sternum. Listen for a whooshing sound, *which signals that the tube reached its target in the stomach.* If the tube remains coiled in the esophagus, you'll feel resistance when you inject the air, or the patient may belch.
● If you hear the whooshing sound, gently try to aspirate gastric secretions. Successful aspiration confirms correct tube placement. If no gastric secretions return, the tube may be in the esophagus. You'll need to advance the tube or reinsert it before proceeding.
● After confirming proper tube placement, remove the tape marking the tube length.
● Tape the tube to the patient's nose and remove the guide wire. *Note:* In some cases, X-rays may be ordered to verify tube placement.
● *To advance the tube to the duodenum,* especially a tungsten-weighted tube, position the patient on his right side. *This lets gravity assist tube passage through the pylorus.* Move the tube forward 2″ to 3″ (5 to 7.6 cm) hourly until X-ray studies confirm duodenal placement. (An X-ray film must confirm placement before feeding begins *because duodenal feeding can cause nausea and vomiting if accidentally delivered to the stomach.*)
● Apply skin preparation to the patient's cheek before securing the tube with tape. *This helps the tube adhere to the skin and also prevents irritation.*

• Tape the tube securely to the patient's cheek *to avoid excessive pressure on his nostrils.*

To remove the tube
• Protect the patient's chest with a linen-saver pad.
• Flush the tube with air, clamp or pinch it *to prevent fluid aspiration during withdrawal,* and withdraw it gently but quickly.
• Promptly cover and discard the used tube.

Special considerations
Flush the feeding tube every 8 hours with up to 60 ml of normal saline solution or water *to maintain patency.* Retape the tube at least daily and as needed. Alternate taping the tube toward the inner and outer side of the nose *to avoid constant pressure on the same nasal area.* Inspect the skin for redness and breakdown.

Provide nasal hygiene daily using the cotton-tipped applicators and water-soluble lubricant *to remove crusted secretions.* Assist the patient with oral hygiene at least twice daily. Help him brush his teeth, gums, and tongue with mouthwash or a mild saltwater solution.

If the patient can't swallow the feeding tube, use a guide *to aid insertion.*

Precise feeding-tube placement is especially important *because small-bore feeding tubes may slide into the trachea without causing immediate signs or symptoms of respiratory distress, such as coughing, choking, gasping, or cyanosis.* However, the patient will usually cough if the tube enters the larynx. To be sure that the tube clears the larynx, ask the patient to speak. If he can't, the tube is in the larynx. Withdraw the tube at once and reinsert.

When aspirating gastric contents to check tube placement, pull gently on the syringe plunger *because negative pressure may collapse a small-bore feeding tube or traumatize the stomach lining or bowel.* If you meet resistance during aspiration, stop the procedure *because resistance may result simply from the tube lying against the stomach wall.* If the tube coils above the stomach, you'll be unable to aspirate stomach contents. To rectify this, change the patient's position or withdraw the tube a few inches, readvance it, and try to aspirate again. If the tube was inserted with a guide wire, do not use the guide wire to reposition the tube. The doctor may do so, using fluoroscopic guidance.

Home care
If your patient will use a feeding tube at home, make appropriate home care nursing referrals and teach the patient and caregivers how to use and care for a feeding tube. Help them understand how to obtain equipment, to insert and remove the tube, to prepare and store feeding formula, and to troubleshoot tube position and patency.

Complications
Prolonged intubation may lead to skin erosion at the nostril, sinusitis, esophagitis, esophagotracheal fistula, gastric ulceration, and pulmonary and oral infection.

Documentation
For tube insertion, record the date, time, tube type and size, site of insertion, area of placement, and confirmation of proper placement. Also record the name of the person performing the procedure. For tube removal, record the date and time and describe the patient's tolerance of the procedure.

Tube feedings

This procedure involves delivery of a liquid feeding formula directly to the stomach (known as gastric gavage), duodenum, or jejunum. Gastric gavage typically is indicated for a patient who can't eat normally because of dysphagia or oral or esophageal obstruction or injury. Gastric feedings also may be given to an unconscious or intubated patient or to a patient recovering from GI tract surgery who can't ingest food orally.

Duodenal or jejunal feedings decrease the risk of aspiration because the formula bypasses the pylorus. Jejunal feedings result in reduced pancreatic stimulation; thus, the patient may require an elemental diet.

Usually, patients receive gastric feedings on an intermittent schedule. For duodenal or jejunal feedings, however, most patients seem to better tolerate a continuous slow drip.

Liquid nutrient solutions come in various formulas for administration through a nasogastric tube, small-bore feeding tube, gastrostomy or jejunostomy tube, percutaneous endoscopic gastrostomy or jejunostomy tube, or gastrostomy feeding button. (For more information, see "Transabdominal tube feeding and care" later in this chapter. Also see *Managing tube feeding problems,* page 402.) Tube feeding is contraindicated in patients who have no bowel sounds or suspected intestinal obstruction.

Equipment
For gastric feedings: feeding formula ■ graduated container ■ 120 ml of water ■ gavage bag with tubing and flow regulator clamp ■ towel or linen-saver pad ■ 60-ml syringe ■ stethoscope ■ optional: infusion controller and tubing set (for continuous administration), adapter to connect gavage tubing to feeding tube.

For duodenal or jejunal feedings: feeding formula ■ enteral administration set containing a gavage container,

Managing tube feeding problems

COMPLICATION	INTERVENTIONS
Aspiration of gastric secretions	• Discontinue feeding immediately. • Perform tracheal suction of aspirated contents if possible. • Notify the doctor. Prophylactic antibiotics and chest physiotherapy may be ordered. • Check tube placement before feeding to prevent complication.
Tube obstruction	• Flush the tube with warm water or cranberry juice. If necessary, replace the tube. • Flush the tube with 50 ml of water after each feeding to remove excess sticky formula, which could occlude the tube.
Nasal or pharyngeal irritation or necrosis	• Provide frequent oral hygiene using mouthwash or lemon-glycerin swabs. Use petroleum jelly on cracked lips. • Change the tube's position. If necessary, replace the tube.
Vomiting, bloating, diarrhea, or cramps	• Reduce the flow rate. • Administer metoclopramide to increase GI motility. • Warm the formula. • For 30 minutes after feeding, position the patient on his right side with his head elevated to facilitate gastric emptying. • Notify the doctor. He may want to reduce the amount of formula being given during each feeding.
Constipation	• Provide additional fluids if the patient can tolerate them. • Administer a bulk-forming laxative. • Increase fruit, vegetable, or sugar content of the feeding.
Electrolyte imbalance	• Monitor serum electrolyte levels. • Notify the doctor. He may want to adjust the formula content to correct the deficiency.
Hyperglycemia	• Monitor blood glucose levels. • Notify the doctor of elevated levels. • Administer insulin if ordered. • The doctor may adjust the sugar content of the formula.

drip chamber, roller clamp or flow regulator, and tube connector ▪ I.V. pole ▪ 60-ml syringe with adapter tip ▪ water ▪ optional: pump administration set (for an enteral infusion pump), Y connector, antidiarrheal medication (such as paregoric, tincture of opium, or diphenoxylate hydrochloride).

For nasal and oral care: cotton-tipped applicators ▪ water-soluble lubricant ▪ lemon-glycerin swabs ▪ petroleum jelly.

A bulb syringe or large catheter-tip syringe may be substituted for a gavage bag if necessary. The doctor may order an infusion pump *to ensure accurate delivery of prescribed formula.*

Preparation of equipment
Be sure to refrigerate formulas prepared in the dietary department or pharmacy. Refrigerate commercial formulas only after opening them.

Check the date on all formula containers. Discard expired commercial formula. Use powdered formula within 24 hours of mixing. Always shake the container well *to mix the solution thoroughly.*

Allow the formula to warm to room temperature before administration. Never warm it over direct heat *because heat may curdle the formula or change its chemical composition. Also, hot formula may injure the patient.*

Pour 60 ml of water into the graduated container. After closing the flow clamp on the administration set, pour the appropriate amount of formula into the gavage bag. Hang no more than a 4- to 6-hour supply at one time *to prevent bacterial growth.*

Open the flow clamp on the administration set *to remove air from the lines. This keeps air from entering the patient's stomach and causing distention and discomfort.*

Implementation
• Provide privacy and wash your hands.
• Inform the patient that he will receive nourishment through the tube, and explain the procedure to him. If possible, give him a schedule of subsequent feedings.
• If the patient has a nasal or oral tube, cover his chest with a towel or linen-saver pad *to protect him and the bed linens from spills.*
• Assess the patient's abdomen for bowel sounds and distention.

To deliver a gastric feeding
• Elevate the bed to semi-Fowler's or high Fowler's position *to prevent aspiration by gastroesophageal reflux and to promote digestion.*
• Check placement of the feeding tube *to be sure it hasn't slipped out since the last feeding.* Never give a tube feeding until you're sure the tube is properly positioned in the patient's stomach. *Administering a feeding through a misplaced tube can cause formula to enter the patient's lungs.*
• *To check tube patency and position,* remove the cap or plug from the feeding tube, and use the syringe to inject 5 to 10 cc of air through the tube. At the same time, auscultate the patient's stomach with the stethoscope. Listen for a whooshing sound to confirm tube positioning in the stomach. Also aspirate stomach contents to confirm tube patency and placement.
• *To assess gastric emptying,* aspirate and measure residual gastric contents. Reinstill any aspirate obtained.
• Connect the gavage bag tubing to the feeding tube. Depending on the type of tube used, you may need to use an adapter to connect the two.
• If you're using a bulb or catheter-tip syringe, remove the bulb or plunger and attach the syringe to the pinched-off feeding tube *to prevent excess air from entering the patient's stomach, causing distention.* If you're using an infusion controller, thread the tube from the formula container through the controller according to the manufacturer's directions. Purge the tubing of air and attach it to the feeding tube.

• Open the regulator clamp on the gavage bag tubing and adjust the flow rate appropriately. When using a bulb syringe, fill the syringe with formula and release the feeding tube *to allow formula to flow through it.* The height at which you hold the syringe will determine flow rate. When the syringe is three-quarters empty, pour more formula into it.
• To prevent air from entering the tube and the patient's stomach, never allow the syringe to empty completely. If you're using an infusion controller, set the flow rate according to the manufacturer's directions. Always administer a tube feeding slowly—typically 200 to 350 ml over 10 to 15 minutes, depending on the patient's tolerance and the doctor's order—*to prevent sudden stomach distention, which can cause nausea, vomiting, cramps, or diarrhea.*
• After administering the appropriate amount of formula, flush the tubing by adding about 60 ml of water to the gavage bag or bulb syringe. *This maintains the tube's patency by removing excess formula, which could occlude the tube.*
• If you're administering a continuous feeding, flush the feeding tube every 4 hours *to help prevent tube occlusion.* Monitor gastric emptying every 4 hours.
• To discontinue gastric feeding (depending on the equipment you're using), close the regulator clamp on the gavage bag tubing, disconnect the syringe from the feeding tube, or turn off the infusion controller.
• Cover the end of the feeding tube with its plug or cap *to prevent leakage and contamination of the tube.*
• Leave the patient in semi-Fowler's or high Fowler's position for at least 30 minutes.
• Rinse all reusable equipment with warm water. Dry it and store it in a convenient place for the next feeding. Change equipment every 24 hours or according to the hospital's policy.

To deliver a duodenal or jejunal feeding
• Elevate the head of the bed and place the patient in the low Fowler's position.
• Open the enteral administration set and hang the gavage container on the I.V. pole.
• If you're using a nasoduodenal tube, measure its length *to check tube placement.* Remember that you may not get any residual when you aspirate the tube.
• Open the flow clamp and regulate the flow to the desired rate. To regulate the rate using a volumetric infusion pump, follow the manufacturer's directions for setting up the equipment. Most patients receive small amounts initially, with volumes increasing gradually once tolerance is established.
• Flush the tube every 4 hours with water *to maintain patency and provide hydration.* A needle catheter jejunos-

tomy tube may require flushing every 2 hours *to prevent formula buildup inside the tube.* A Y connector may be useful for frequent flushing. Attach the continuous feeding to the main port and use the side port for flushes.

Special considerations
If the feeding solution doesn't initially flow through a bulb syringe, attach the bulb and squeeze it gently to start the flow. Then remove the bulb. Never use the bulb to force the formula through the tube.

If the patient becomes nauseated or vomits, stop the feeding immediately. The patient may vomit if the stomach becomes distended from overfeeding or delayed gastric emptying.

To reduce oropharyngeal discomfort from the tube, allow the patient to brush his teeth or care for his dentures regularly, and encourage frequent gargling. If the patient is unconscious, administer oral care with lemon-glycerin swabs every 4 hours. Use petroleum jelly on dry, cracked lips. (Remember: Dry mucous membranes may indicate dehydration, which requires increased fluid intake.) Clean the patient's nostrils with cotton-tipped applicators, apply lubricant along the mucosa, and assess the skin for signs of breakdown.

During continuous feedings, assess the patient frequently for abdominal distention. Flush the tubing by adding about 50 ml of water to the gavage bag or bulb syringe. *This maintains the tube's patency by removing excess formula, which could occlude the tube.*

If the patient develops diarrhea, administer small, frequent, less concentrated feedings, or administer bolus feedings over a longer time. Also, make sure that the formula isn't cold and that proper storage and sanitation practices have been followed. The loose stools associated with tube feedings make extra perineal and skin care necessary. Giving paregoric, tincture of opium, or diphenoxylate hydrochloride may improve the condition. Changing to a formula with more fiber may eliminate liquid stools.

If the patient becomes constipated, the doctor may increase the fruit, vegetable, or sugar content of the formula. Assess the patient's hydration status *because dehydration may produce constipation.* Increase fluid intake as necessary. If the condition persists, administer an appropriate drug or enema, as ordered.

Drugs can be administered through the feeding tube. Except for enteric-coated drugs or sustained-release medications, crush tablets or open and dilute capsules in water before administering them. Be sure to flush the tubing afterward *to ensure full instillation of medication.* Keep in mind that some drugs may change the osmolarity of the feeding formula and cause diarrhea.

Small-bore feeding tubes may kink, making instillation impossible. If you suspect this problem, try changing the patient's position, or withdraw the tube a few inches and restart. Never use a guide wire to reposition the tube.

Constantly monitor the flow rate of a blended or high-residue formula *to determine if the formula is clogging the tubing as it settles. To prevent such clogging,* squeeze the bag frequently to agitate the solution.

Glycosuria, hyperglycemia, and diuresis can indicate an excessive carbohydrate level, leading to hyperosmotic dehydration, which may be fatal. Collect urine specimens every 4 to 6 hours, and blood specimens, as ordered. Monitor urine and blood glucose levels *to assess glucose tolerance.* (A patient with a serum glucose level of less than 200 mg/100 ml and without glycosuria is considered stable.) Also monitor serum electrolytes, blood urea nitrogen, serum glucose, serum osmolality, and other pertinent findings *to determine the patient's response to therapy and assess his hydration status.*

Check the flow rate hourly to ensure correct infusion. (With an improvised administration set, use a time tape to record the rate *because it's difficult to get precise readings from an irrigation container or enema bag.*)

For duodenal or jejunal feeding, most patients tolerate a continuous drip better than bolus feedings. *Bolus feedings can cause such complications as hyperglycemia, glucosuria, and diarrhea.*

Until the patient acquires a tolerance for the formula, you may need to dilute it to half or three-quarters strength to start, and increase it gradually. Patients under stress or who are receiving steroids may experience a pseudodiabetic state. Assess them frequently to determine the need for insulin.

Home care
Patient education for home tube feeding includes instructions on an infusion control device to maintain accuracy, use of the syringe or bag and tubing, care of the tube and insertion site, and formula-mixing. Formula may be mixed in an electric blender according to package directions. Formula not used within 24 hours must be discarded. If the formula must hang for more than 8 hours, advise the patient to use a gavage or pump administration set with an ice pouch to decrease the incidence of bacterial growth. Tell him to use a new bag daily.

Family members should be instructed in signs and symptoms to report to the doctor or home care nurse, as well as measures to take in an emergency.

Complications
Erosion of esophageal, tracheal, nasal, and oropharyngeal mucosa can result if tubes are left in place for a long

time. If possible, use smaller-lumen tubes *to prevent such irritation. Check hospital policy regarding the frequency of changing feeding tubes to prevent complications.*

Using the gastric route, frequent or large-volume feedings can cause bloating and retention. Dehydration, diarrhea, and vomiting can cause metabolic disturbances. Glycosuria, cramping, and abdominal distention usually indicate intolerance.

Using the duodenal or jejunal route, clogging of the feeding tube is common. The patient may experience metabolic, fluid, and electrolyte abnormalities including hyperglycemia, glycosuria, hyperosmolar dehydration, coma, edema, hypernatremia, and essential fatty acid deficiency.

The patient also may experience dumping syndrome, in which a large amount of hyperosmotic solution in the duodenum causes excessive diffusion of fluid through the semipermeable membrane and results in diarrhea. In a patient with low serum albumin levels, these symptoms may result from low oncotic pressure in the duodenal mucosa.

Documentation

On the intake and output sheet, record the date, volume of formula, and volume of water. In your notes, include abdominal assessment (including tube exit site, if appropriate); amount of residuals; verification of tube placement; amount, type, and time of feeding; and tube patency. Discuss the patient's tolerance to the feeding, including nausea, vomiting, cramping, diarrhea, and distention. Note the result of blood and urine tests, hydration status, and any drugs given through the tube. Include the date and time of administration set changes, oral and nasal hygiene, and results of specimen collections.

Nasoenteric-decompression tube insertion and removal

The nasoenteric-decompression tube is inserted nasally and advanced beyond the stomach into the intestinal tract. It's used to aspirate intestinal contents for analysis and to treat intestinal obstruction. The tube may also help to prevent nausea, vomiting, and abdominal distention after GI surgery. A doctor will usually insert or remove a nasoenteric-decompression tube, but sometimes, a nurse will remove it.

A balloon or rubber bag at one end of the tube holds mercury (or air or water) to stimulate peristalsis and facilitate the tube's passage through the pylorus and into the intestinal tract. (See *Common types of nasoenteric-decompression tubes,* page 406.)

Equipment

Sterile 10-cc syringe ▪ 21G needle ▪ nasoenteric-decompression tube ▪ container of water ▪ 5 to 10 ml of mercury or water, as ordered ▪ suction-decompression equipment ▪ gloves ▪ towel or linen-saver pad ▪ water-soluble lubricant ▪ 4″ × 4″ gauze pad ▪ ½″ nonallergenic tape ▪ bulb syringe or 60-ml catheter-tip syringe ▪ stethoscope ▪ cotton-tipped applicators ▪ rubber band ▪ safety pin ▪ clamp ▪ specimen container ▪ optional: basin of ice or warm water, penlight, waterproof marking pen, glass of water with straw, ice chips, local anesthetic.

Preparation of equipment

Stiffen a flaccid tube by chilling it in a basin of ice *to facilitate insertion.* To make a stiff tube flexible, dip it into warm water.

To check the tube's balloon for leaks, inject 10 cc of air into the balloon with a 10-cc syringe and 21G needle. Immerse the balloon in a container of water and watch for air bubbles. Bubble-free water means a leak-free balloon. Then remove the balloon from the water. Mercury, air, or water are then added to the balloon with a syringe, depending on the type of tube used. Follow the manufacturer's recommendations.

Set up suction-decompression equipment, if ordered, and make sure it works properly.

Implementation

• Explain the procedure to the patient, forewarning him that he may experience some discomfort. Provide privacy and adequate lighting. Wash your hands and put on gloves.

• Position the patient as the doctor specifies. The most common positions to facilitate tube insertion are semi-Fowler's or high Fowler's positions. You may also need to help the patient hold his neck in a hyperextended position.

• Protect the patient's chest with a linen-saver pad or towel.

• Agree with the patient on a signal that can be used to stop the insertion briefly if necessary.

To assist with insertion

• The doctor assesses the patency of the patient's nostrils. To evaluate which nostril has better airflow in a conscious patient, he holds one nostril closed and then the other as the patient breathes. In an unconscious patient, he examines each nostril with a penlight *to check for polyps, a deviated septum, or other obstruction.*

Common types of nasoenteric-decompression tubes

The type of nasoenteric-decompression tube chosen for your patient will depend on the size of the patient and his nostrils, the estimated duration of intubation, and the reason for the procedure. For example, to remove viscous material from the patient's intestinal tract, the doctor may select a tube with a wide bore and a single lumen.

Whichever tube you use, you'll need to provide good mouth care and check the patient's nostrils often for signs of irritation. If you see any signs of irritation, re-tape the tube so it doesn't cause tension. Then, lubricate the nostril. Or check with the doctor to see if the tube can be inserted through the other nostril.

Most tubes are impregnated with a radiopaque mark so that placement can be confirmed easily by X-ray or other imaging technique. The following are among the most commonly used types of nasoenteric-decompression tubes.

Cantor tube

This single-lumen, 10′ (3 m) long tube has a balloon that can hold mercury at its distal tip. The Cantor tube may be used to relieve bowel obstructions and to aspirate intestinal contents.

Harris tube

Measuring only 6′ (1.8 m) long, this single-lumen tube (top right) also ends with a balloon that holds mercury. Used chiefly for treating a bowel obstruction, the Harris tube allows lavage of the intestinal tract—usually with a Y tube attached.

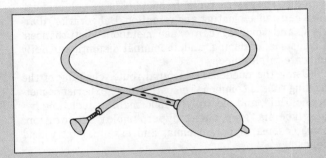

Miller-Abbott tube

This 10′ tube has two lumens: one for inflating the distal balloon with air and one for instilling mercury or water. Also used for bowel obstruction, the tube allows aspiration of intestinal contents.

Dennis tube

This three-lumen sump tube is used to decompress the intestinal tract before or after GI surgery. Each lumen is marked to denote its use: irrigation, drainage, and balloon inflation.

• *To decide how far the tube must be inserted to reach the stomach*, the doctor places the tube's distal end at the tip of the patient's nose and then extends the tube to the earlobe and down to the xiphoid process. He either marks the tube with a waterproof marking pen or holds it at this point.

• The doctor applies water-soluble lubricant to the first few inches of the tube *to reduce friction and tissue trauma and to facilitate insertion.*

• If the balloon already contains mercury or water, the doctor holds it so the fluid runs to the bottom. Then he pinches the balloon closed *to retain the fluid as the insertion begins.*

• Direct the patient to breathe through his mouth or to pant as the balloon enters his nostril. After the balloon begins its descent, the doctor releases his grip on it, *allowing the weight of the fluid to pull the tube into the nasopharynx.* When the tube reaches the nasopharynx, the doctor instructs the patient to lower his chin and to swallow. In some cases, the patient may sip water through a straw *to facilitate swallowing as the tube advances.* After the tube reaches the trachea, however, the patient won't be offered water. *This prevents injury from aspiration.* The doctor continues to advance the tube slowly *to prevent it from curling or kinking in the stomach.*

• *To confirm the tube's passage into the stomach,* the doctor aspirates stomach contents with a bulb syringe.

• When the doctor confirms proper placement of a Miller-Abbott tube, he injects the appropriate amount of mercury (commonly between 2 and 5 ml) into the balloon lumen.

• *To keep the tube out of the patient's eyes and to help avoid undue skin irritation,* fold a 4″ × 4″ gauze pad in half and tape it to the patient's forehead with the fold directed toward the patient's nose. The doctor can slide the tube through this sling, leaving enough slack for the tube to advance.

• Position the patient, as directed, *to help advance the tube.* Commonly, the patient will lie on his right side until the tube clears the pylorus (about 2 hours). The doctor confirms passage by X-ray.

• After the tube clears the pylorus, the doctor may direct you to advance it 2″ to 3″ (5 to 7.6 cm) every hour and to reposition the patient until the premeasured mark reaches the patient's nostril. Gravity and peristalsis will help to advance the tube. (Notify the doctor if you cannot advance the tube.)

• Be sure to keep the remaining premeasured length of tube well lubricated *to ease passage and prevent irritation.*

• Avoid taping the tube while it advances to the premeasured mark, unless the doctor directs you to do so.

• After the tube progresses the necessary distance, the doctor will order an X-ray *to confirm tube positioning.* Once

the tube's in place, secure the external tubing with tape *to prevent further progression.*

• Loop a rubber band around the tube and pin the rubber band to the patient's gown with a safety pin.

• If ordered, attach the tube to intermittent suction.

To remove the tube

• Assist the patient into semi-Fowler's or high Fowler's position. Drape a linen-saver pad or towel across the patient's chest.

• Put on gloves.

• Clamp the tube and disconnect it from the suction. *This prevents the patient from aspirating any gastric contents that leak from the tube during withdrawal.*

• If your patient has a double-lumen Miller-Abbott tube or a triple-lumen Dennis tube, attach a 10-ml syringe to the balloon port and withdraw the mercury. Place the mercury in a specimen container and follow your hospital's protocol for safe disposal. (If you're working with a single-lumen Cantor or Harris tube, you'll withdraw the mercury after you remove the tube.)

• Slowly withdraw between 6″ and 8″ (15.2 and 20.3 cm) of the tube. Wait 10 minutes and withdraw another 6″ to 8″. Wait another 10 minutes. Continue this procedure until the tube reaches the patient's esophagus (with about 18″ [45.7 cm] of the tube remaining inside the patient). At this point, you can gently withdraw the tube completely with the mercury in the balloon.

Special considerations

For a double- or triple-lumen tube, note which lumen accommodates balloon inflation and which accommodates drainage.

An alternate method for removing a single-lumen tube is to withdraw it gently into the pharynx. Ask the patient to open his mouth. Then grasp the tube and mercury balloon and gently pull them outside of the patient's mouth. Remove mercury from the bag with a needle and syringe. Then pull the tube and empty balloon through the patient's nose. Never forcibly remove a tube if you meet resistance. Notify the doctor.

Apply a local anesthetic, if ordered, to the nostril or the back of the throat *to dull sensations and the gag reflex for intubation.* Letting the patient gargle with a liquid anesthetic or hold ice chips in his mouth for a few minutes serves the same purpose.

Mercury can be disposed of only by a licensed hazardous-waste disposal company. Put the container of mercury into a plastic bag, and send it to the appropriate department for disposal.

Complications

Nasoenteric-decompression tubes may cause reflux esophagitis, nasal or oral inflammation, and nasal, laryngeal, or esophageal ulceration.

Documentation

Record the date and time the nasoenteric-decompression tube was inserted and by whom. Note the patient's tolerance of the procedure; the type of tube used; the suction type and amount; and the color, amount, and consistency of drainage. Also note the date, time, and name of the person removing the tube and the patient's tolerance of the removal procedure.

Nasoenteric-decompression tube care

The patient with a nasoenteric-decompression tube needs special care and continuous monitoring to ensure tube patency, to maintain suction and bowel decompression, and to detect such complications as fluid-electrolyte imbalances related to aspiration of intestinal contents. Precise intake and output records form an integral part of the patient's care. Frequent mouth and nose care is also essential to provide comfort and to prevent skin breakdown. Finally, a patient with a nasoenteric-decompression tube will need encouragement and support during insertion and removal of the tube and while the tube is in place.

Equipment

Suction apparatus with intermittent suction capability (stationary or portable unit) ▪ container of water ▪ intake and output record sheets ▪ mouthwash and water mixture ▪ lemon-glycerin swabs ▪ petroleum jelly or water-soluble lubricant ▪ cotton-tipped applicators ▪ safety pin ▪ tape or rubber band ▪ disposable irrigation set ▪ irrigant ▪ labels for tube lumens ▪ optional: throat comfort measures such as gargle, viscous lidocaine, sour hard candy, throat lozenges, ice collar, or chewing gum.

Preparation of equipment

Assemble the suction apparatus and set up the suction unit. If indicated, test the unit by turning it on and placing the end of the suction tubing in a container of water. If the tubing draws in water, the unit works.

Implementation

● Explain to the patient and his family the purpose of the procedure. Answer questions clearly and thoroughly *to ease anxiety and enhance cooperation.*

● After inserting the tube, have the patient lie quietly on his right side for about 2 hours *to promote the tube's passage.* After the tube advances past the pylorus, the patient's activity level may increase, as ordered.

● After the tube advances to the desired position, coil the excess external tubing and secure it to the patient's gown or bed linens with a safety pin attached to tape or a rubber band looped around the tubing. *This may prevent kinks in the tubing, which would interrupt suction.* And once in the desired location, the tube may be taped to the patient's face.

● Maintain slack in the tubing *so the patient can move comfortably and safely in bed.* Show him how far he can move without dislodging the tube.

● After securing the tube, connect it to the tubing on the suction machine *to begin decompression.*

● Check the suction machine at least every 2 hours *to confirm proper functioning and to ensure continued tube patency and bowel decompression.* Excessive negative pressure may draw the mucosa into the tube openings, impair the suction's effectiveness, and injure the mucosa. By using intermittent suction, you may circumvent these problems. To check functioning in an intermittent suction unit, look for drainage in the connecting tube and for drainage dripping into the collecting container. Empty the container every 8 hours and measure the contents.

● After decompression and before extubation, as ordered, provide a clear-to-full liquid diet *to assess bowel function.*

● Record intake and output accurately *to monitor the patient's fluid balance.* If you irrigate the tube, its length may prohibit aspiration of the irrigant, so record the amount of instilled irrigant as "intake." Typically, normal saline solution supersedes water as the preferred irrigant *because water, which is hypotonic, may increase electrolyte loss through osmotic action, especially if you irrigate the tube often.*

● Observe the patient for signs and symptoms of disorders related to suctioning and intubation. These signs and symptoms may suggest dehydration, a fluid-volume deficit, or a fluid-electrolyte imbalance: dry skin and mucous membranes, decreased urine output, lethargy, exhaustion, and fever.

● Watch for signs and symptoms of pneumonia related to the patient's inability to clear his pharynx or cough effectively with a tube in place. Be alert for fever, chest pain, tachypnea or labored breathing, and diminished breath sounds over the affected area.

• Observe drainage characteristics, including amount, color, consistency, odor, and any unusual changes.

• Provide mouth care frequently (at least every 4 hours). *This increases patient comfort and promotes a healthy oral cavity. If the tube remains in place for several days, mouth-breathing will leave the patient's lips, tongue, and other tissues dry and cracked.*

• Encourage the patient to brush his teeth or rinse his mouth with the mouthwash and water mixture.

• Lubricate the patient's lips with either lemon-glycerin swabs or petroleum jelly applied with a cotton-tipped applicator.

• At least every 4 hours, gently clean and lubricate the patient's external nostrils with either petroleum jelly or water-soluble lubricant on a cotton-tipped applicator *to prevent skin breakdown.*

• Watch for peristalsis to resume, signaled by bowel sounds, passage of flatus, decreased abdominal distention, and possibly, a spontaneous bowel movement. *These signs may require tube removal.*

Special considerations

For a Miller-Abbott tube, clamp the lumen leading to the mercury balloon and label DO NOT TOUCH. Label the other lumen SUCTION. *Marking the tube in this way may prevent accidentally instilling irrigant into the wrong lumen and possibly rupturing the mercury balloon.*

If the suction machine works improperly, replace it immediately. If the machine works properly but no drainage accumulates in the collection container, suspect an obstruction in the tube.

As ordered, irrigate the tube with the irrigation set *to clear the obstruction.* (See *Clearing a nasoenteric-decompression tube obstruction.*)

If your patient is ambulatory and his tube connects to a portable suction unit, he may move short distances while connected to the unit. Or, if feasible and ordered, the tube can be disconnected and clamped for a brief time while he moves about.

If the tubing irritates the patient's throat or makes him hoarse, offer relief with mouthwash, gargles, viscous lidocaine, sour hard candy, throat lozenges, an ice collar, or chewing gum, as appropriate.

If the balloon at the end of the tube protrudes from the anus, notify the doctor. Most likely, the tube can be disconnected from suction, the proximal end severed, and the remaining tube removed gradually through the anus either manually or by peristalsis.

Complications

Besides fluid-volume deficit, electrolyte imbalance, and pneumonia, potential complications include mercury poi-

TROUBLESHOOTING

Clearing a nasoenteric-decompression tube obstruction

If your patient's nasoenteric-decompression tube appears to be obstructed, notify the doctor right away. He may order measures, such as these, to restore patency quickly and efficiently.

First, disconnect the tube from the suction source and irrigate with normal saline solution. Use gravity flow to help clear the obstruction unless ordered otherwise.

If irrigation doesn't reestablish patency, the tube may be obstructed by its position against the gastric mucosa. To rectify this, tug slightly on the tube to move it away from the mucosa.

If gentle tugging doesn't restore patency, the tube may be kinked and may need additional manipulation. Before proceeding, though, take these precautions:

• Never reposition or irrigate a nasoenteric-decompression tube (without a doctor's order) in a patient who has had GI surgery.

• Avoid manipulating a tube in a patient who had the tube inserted during surgery. To do so may disturb new sutures.

• Don't try to reposition the tube in a patient who was difficult to intubate (because of an esophageal stricture, for example).

soning (from a ruptured mercury-filled balloon) and intussusception of the bowel (from the weight of the mercury in the balloon).

Documentation

Record the frequency and type of mouth and nose care given. Describe the therapeutic effect, if any. Document in your notes the amount, color, consistency, and odor of the drainage obtained each time you empty the collection container.

Record the amount of drainage on the intake and output sheet. Always write down the amount of any irrigant or other fluid introduced through the tube or taken orally by the patient.

If the suction machine malfunctions, note the length of time it didn't appear to be functioning and the nursing action taken. Document the amount and character of any vomitus. Also note the patient's tolerance of the tube's insertion and removal.

RECTAL ACCESS
Rectal tube insertion and removal

Whether GI hypomotility simply slows the normal release of gas and feces or results in paralytic ileus, inserting a rectal tube may relieve the discomfort of distention and flatus.

Decreased motility may result from various medical or surgical conditions, certain medications (such as atropine sulfate), or even swallowed air.

Conditions that contraindicate using a rectal tube include recent rectal or prostatic surgery, recent myocardial infarction, and diseases of the rectal mucosa.

Equipment
Stethoscope ■ linen-saver pads ■ drape ■ water-soluble lubricant ■ commercial kit or #22 to #32 French rectal tube of soft rubber or plastic ■ container (emesis basin, plastic bag, or water bottle with vent) ■ tape ■ gloves.

Implementation
• Bring all equipment to the patient's bedside, provide privacy, and wash your hands.
• Explain the procedure and encourage the patient to relax.
• Check for abdominal distention. Using the stethoscope, auscultate for bowel sounds.
• Place the linen-saver pads under the patient's buttocks *to absorb any drainage that may leak from the tube.*
• Position the patient in left-lateral Sims' position *to facilitate rectal tube insertion.*
• Put on gloves.
• Drape the patient's exposed buttocks.
• Lubricate the rectal tube tip with water-soluble lubricant *to ease insertion and prevent rectal irritation.*
• Lift the patient's right buttock *to expose the anus.*
• Insert the rectal tube tip into the anus, advancing the tube 2″ to 4″ (5 to 10 cm) into the rectum. Direct the tube toward the umbilicus *along the anatomic course of the large intestine.*
• As you insert the tube, tell the patient to breathe slowly and deeply, or suggest that he bear down as he would for a bowel movement *to relax the anal sphincter and ease insertion.*
• Using tape, secure the rectal tube to the buttocks. Then attach the tube to the container *to collect possible leakage.*
• Remove the tube after 15 to 20 minutes. If the patient reports continued discomfort or if gas wasn't expelled, you can repeat the procedure in 2 or 3 hours if ordered.

• Clean the patient, and replace soiled linens and the linen-saver pad. Be sure the patient feels as comfortable as possible. Again, check for abdominal distention and listen for bowel sounds.
• If you will reuse the equipment, clean it and store it in the bedside cabinet; otherwise discard the tube.

Special considerations
Inform the patient about each step and reasssure him throughout the procedure *to encourage cooperation and promote relaxation.*

Fastening a plastic bag (like a balloon) to the external end of the tube lets you observe gas expulsion. Leaving a rectal tube in place indefinitely does little to promote peristalsis, can reduce sphincter responsiveness, and may lead to permanent sphincter damage or pressure necrosis of the mucosa.

Repeat insertion periodically *to stimulate GI activity.* If the tube fails to relieve distention, notify the doctor.

Documentation
Record the date and time that you insert the tube. Jot down the amount, color, and consistency of any evacuated matter. Describe the patient's abdomen — hard, distended, soft, or drumlike on percussion. Note bowel sounds before and after insertion.

TRANSABDOMINAL ACCESS
Transabdominal tube feeding and care

To access the stomach, duodenum, or jejunum, the doctor may place a tube through the patient's abdominal wall. This may be done surgically or percutaneously.

Gastrostomy or jejunostomy tubes are usually placed during intra-abdominal surgery. The tube may be used for feeding during the immediate postoperative period or it may provide long-term enteral access, depending on what type of surgery the patient had. Typically, the doctor will suture the tube in place to prevent gastric contents from leaking.

In contrast, a percutaneous endoscopic gastrostomy (PEG) or jejunostomy (PEJ) tube can be inserted endoscopically without the need for laparotomy or general anesthesia. Typically, the insertion is done in the endoscopy suite or at the patient's bedside. A PEG or PEJ tube may be used for nutrition, drainage, and decompression. Contraindications to endoscopic placement include obstruction (such as an esophageal stricture or duodenal blockage), previous gastric surgery, morbid obesity, and ascites. These conditions would necessitate surgical placement.

With either type of tube placement, feedings may begin after about 24 hours (or when peristalsis resumes).

After a time, the tube may need replacement, and the doctor may recommend a similar tube, such as a Foley or a mushroom catheter, or a gastrostomy button — a skin-level feeding tube. (See "Gastrostomy feeding button care" in this chapter.)

Nursing care includes providing skin care at the tube site, maintaining the feeding tube, administering feeding, monitoring the patient's response to feeding, adjusting the feeding schedule, and preparing the patient for self-care after discharge.

Equipment

For feeding: feeding formula ■ large-bulb or catheter-tip syringe ■ 120 ml of water ■ 4″ × 4″ gauze pads ■ soap ■ skin protectant ■ antibacterial ointment ■ nonallergenic tape ■ gravity-drip administration bags ■ mouthwash, toothpaste, or mild salt solution ■ gloves ■ optional: enteral infusion pump.

For decompression: suction apparatus with tubing and straight drainage collection set.

Preparation of equipment

Always check the expiration date on commercially prepared feeding formulas. If the formula has been prepared by the dietitian or pharmacist, check the preparation time and date. Discard any opened formula or solution that's more than 1 day old.

Commercially prepared administration sets and enteral pumps allow continuous formula administration. Place the desired amount of formula into the gavage container and purge air from the tubing. To avoid formula contamination, hang only a 4- to 6-hour supply of formula at a time.

Implementation

• Provide privacy and wash your hands.
• Explain the procedure to the patient. Tell him, for example, that feedings usually start at a slow rate and increase as tolerated. After he tolerates continuous feedings, he may progress to intermittent feedings to prepare him for home management, as ordered.
• Assess for bowel sounds before feeding, and monitor for abdominal distention.
• Ask the patient to sit, or assist him into the semi-Fowler's position, for the entire feeding. *This helps to prevent esophageal reflux and pulmonary aspiration of the formula.* For an intermittent feeding, have the patient

maintain this position throughout the feeding and for 1 hour after.
• Put on gloves. Before starting the feeding, measure residual gastric contents. Attach the syringe to the feeding tube and aspirate. If the contents measure more than twice the amount infused, hold the feeding and recheck in 1 hour. Then, if residual contents remain too high, notify the doctor. Chances are the formula isn't being absorbed properly.
• With PEJ or jejunostomy tube feedings, keep in mind that residual contents will be minimal.
• Allow 30 ml of water to flow into the feeding tube *to establish patency.*
• Be sure to administer formula at room temperature. *Cold formula may cause cramping.*

Intermittent feedings

• Allow gravity to help the formula flow over 30 to 45 minutes. *Faster infusions may cause bloating, cramps, or diarrhea.*
• Begin intermittent feeding with a low volume (200 ml) daily. According to the patient's tolerance, increase the volume per feeding, as needed, *to reach the desired calorie intake.*
• When the feeding finishes, flush the feeding tube with 30 to 60 ml of water. *This maintains patency and provides hydration.*
• Cap the tube *to prevent leakage.*
• Rinse the feeding administration set thoroughly with hot water *to avoid contaminating subsequent feedings.* Allow the tube to dry between feedings.

Continuous feedings

• Measure residual gastric contents every 4 hours.
• To administer the feeding with a pump, set up the equipment according to the manufacturer's guidelines, and fill the feeding bag. To administer the feeding by gravity, fill the container with formula and purge air from the tubing.
• Monitor the gravity drip rate or pump infusion rate frequently *to ensure accurate delivery of formula.*
• Flush the feeding tube with 30 to 60 ml of water every 4 hours *to maintain patency and to provide hydration.*
• Monitor intake and output *to anticipate and detect fluid or electrolyte imbalances.*

Decompression

• To decompress the stomach, connect the PEG port to the suction device with tubing or straight gravity drainage tubing. Jejunostomy feeding may be given simultaneously via the PEJ port of the dual-lumen tube.

Caring for the PEG or PEJ site

The exit site of a percutaneous endoscopic gastrostomy (PEG) or percutaneous endoscopic jejunostomy (PEJ) tube requires routine observation and care. Follow these care guidelines:
• Change the dressing daily while the tube is in place.
• After removing the dressing, carefully slide the tube's outer bumper away from the skin about ½″ (1 cm).

Outer bumper Inner bumper
Abdominal wall Stomach wall

• Examine the skin around the tube. Look for redness and other signs of infection or erosion.
• Gently depress the skin surrounding the tube and inspect for drainage (see illustration at right). Initially after implantation, expect minimal wound drainage. This should subside in about 1 week.
• Inspect the tube for wear and tear. (A tube that wears out will need replacement.)

• Clean the site with the prescribed cleaning solution. Then apply povidone-iodine ointment over the exit site, according to your hospital's guidelines.
• Rotate the outer bumper 90 degrees *(to prevent repeating the same tension on the same skin area)*, and slide the outer bumper back over the exit site.
• If leakage appears at the PEG site, or if the patient risks dislodging the tube, apply a sterile gauze dressing over the site. Do not put sterile gauze underneath the outer bumper. Loosening the anchor in this way allows the feeding tube free play, which could lead to wound abscess.
• Write the date and time of the dressing change on the tape.

Tube exit site care
• Provide daily skin care.
• Gently remove the dressing by hand. Never cut away the dressing over the catheter because *you may inadvertently cut the tube or the sutures holding the tube in place.*
• At least daily and as needed, clean the skin around the tube's exit site using a 4″ × 4″ gauze pad soaked in the prescribed cleaning solution. When healed, wash the skin around the exit site daily with soap. Rinse the area with water and pat dry. Apply skin protectant, if necessary, and antibacterial ointment to the catheter at the exit site *to prevent or treat skin maceration.*
• Anchor a gastrostomy or jejunostomy tube to the skin with nonallergenic tape *to prevent peristaltic migration of the tube.* This also prevents tension on the suture anchoring the tube in place.

• Coil the tube, if necessary, and tape it to the abdomen *to prevent pulling and contamination of the tube.* PEG and PEJ tubes have toggle-bolt-like internal and external bumpers that make tape anchors unnecessary. (See *Caring for the PEG or PEJ site.*)

Special considerations
If the patient vomits, stop the feeding immediately and assess his condition. Also stop the feeding if he complains of nausea, feeling too full, or regurgitation. Flush the feeding tube and attempt to restart the feeding again in 1 hour (measure residual gastric contents first). You may have to decrease the volume or rate of feedings. If dumping syndrome develops, which includes nausea, vomiting, cramps, pallor, and diarrhea, the feedings may have been given too quickly.

Teaching the patient about syringe feeding

If the patient plans to feed himself by syringe when he returns home, you'll need to teach him how to do this before he's discharged. Here are some points to emphasize.

Initial instructions

First, show the patient how to clamp the feeding tube, remove the syringe's bulb or plunger, and place the tip of the syringe into the feeding tube. Then, instill between 30 and 60 ml of water into the feeding tube to be sure it stays open and patent.

Next, tell him to pour the feeding solution into the syringe and begin the feeding (see illustration at top right). As the solution flows into the stomach, show him how to tilt the syringe to allow air bubbles to escape. Describe the discomfort that air bubbles may cause.

Tips for free flow

When about one-fourth of the feeding solution remains, direct the patient to refill the syringe. Caution him to avoid letting the syringe empty completely. Doing so may result in abdominal cramping and gas.

Demonstrate how to increase and decrease the solution's flow rate by raising or lowering the syringe. Explain also that he may need to dilute a thick solution to promote free flow.

Finishing the procedure

Inform the patient that the feeding should take at least 15 minutes. If it takes less time, dumping syndrome may result.

Show the patient the steps needed to finish the feeding, including how to flush the tube with water, clamp the tube, and clean the equipment for later use. Naturally, if he's using disposable gear, urge him to discard it properly. Review how to store unused feeding solution if appropriate.

Provide oral hygiene frequently. Brush all surfaces of the teeth, gums, and tongue at least twice daily using mouthwash, toothpaste, or mild salt solution.

You can administer most tablets and pills through the tube by crushing them and diluting as necessary. (The exception: enteric-coated or sustained-released drugs, which lose their effectiveness when crushed.) Medications should be in liquid form for administration.

Control diarrhea resulting from dumping syndrome by using continuous pump or gravity-drip infusions, diluting the feeding formula, or adding antidiarrheal medications.

Home care

Instruct the patient and family members or other caregivers in all aspects of enteral feedings, including tube maintenance and site care. Specify signs and symptoms to report to the doctor, define emergency situations, and review actions to take.

When the tube needs replacement, advise the patient that the doctor may insert a replacement gastrostomy button or a latex, indwelling, or mushroom catheter after removing the initial feeding tube. The procedure may be done in the doctor's office or the hospital endoscopy suite.

As the patient's tolerance to tube feeding improves, he may wish to try syringe feedings rather than intermittent feedings. If appropriate, teach him how to feed himself by this method. (See *Teaching the patient about syringe feeding*, page 413.)

Complications

Common complications include GI or other systemic problems, mechanical malfunction, and metabolic disturbances. Cramping, nausea, vomiting, bloating, and diarrhea may result from medication; a rapid infusion rate; formula contamination, osmolarity, or inappropriate temperature; fat malabsorption; or intestinal atrophy from malnutrition. Constipation may result from inadequate hydration or insufficient exercise. Vitamin and mineral deficiencies, glucose tolerance, and fluid and electrolyte imbalances may follow bouts of diarrhea or constipation.

Systemic problems may result from pulmonary aspiration, infection at the tube exit site, or contaminated formula. Proper positioning during feeding, verification of tube placement, meticulous skin care, and aseptic formula preparation help to prevent these complications.

Typical mechanical problems include tube dislodgment, obstruction, or impairment. For example, a PEG or PEJ tube may migrate if the external bumper loosens. Occlusion may result from incompletely crushed and liquefied medication particles or inadequate tube flushing. Further, the tube may rupture or crack from age, drying, or frequent manipulation.

Documentation

On the intake and output record, record the date, time, and amount of each feeding and the fluid volume instilled. Maintain total volumes for nutrients and water separately to allow calculation of nutrient intake. In your notes, document the type of formula, the infusion method and rate, the patient's tolerance of the procedure and formula, and the amount of residual gastric contents. Also record complications and abdominal assessment findings. Note patient-teaching topics covered.

Gastrostomy feeding button care

The gastrostomy feeding button serves as an alternative feeding device for an ambulatory patient receiving long-term enteral feedings. Approved by the Food and Drug Administration for 6-month implantation, the feeding button can replace the gastrostomy tube if necessary.

The button has a mushroom dome at one end and two wing tabs and a flexible safety plug at the other. When inserted into an established stoma, the button lies almost flush with the skin; only the safety plug's top is visible.

The button usually can be inserted into a stoma in less than 15 minutes. Besides its cosmetic appeal, the device is easily maintained, reduces skin irritation and breakdown, and has a smaller risk of dislodgment and migration than an ordinary feeding tube. A one-way, antireflux valve mounted just inside the mushroom dome prevents accidental leakage of gastric contents. The device usually requires replacement after 3 to 4 months, most often because the antireflux valve wears out.

Equipment

Gastrostomy feeding button of the correct size (all three sizes, if the correct one isn't known) ■ obturator ■ water-soluble lubricant ■ gloves ■ feeding accessories, including adapter, feeding catheter, food syringe or bag, and formula ■ catheter clamp ■ cleaning equipment, including water, a syringe, cotton-tipped applicator, pipe cleaner, and mild soap or povidone-iodine solution ■ optional: pump to provide continuous infusion over several hours.

Implementation

● Explain the insertion and feeding procedures to the patient. Tell him the doctor will perform the initial insertion.

● Wash your hands and put on gloves. (See *How to reinsert a gastrostomy feeding button.*)

● Attach the adapter and feeding catheter to the syringe or feeding bag. Clamp the catheter and fill the syringe

How to reinsert a gastrostomy feeding button

If your patient's gastrostomy feeding button pops out (with coughing for instance), either you or he will need to reinsert the device. Here are some steps to follow.

Prepare the equipment
Collect the feeding button, an obturator, and water-soluble lubricant. If the button will be reinserted, wash it with soap and water and rinse it thoroughly.

Safety plug

Mushroom dome
Antireflux valve

Insert the button
• Check the depth of the patient's stoma *to make sure you have a feeding button of the correct size.* Then, clean around the stoma.
• Lubricate the obturator with a water-soluble lubricant, and distend the button several times *to ensure patency of the antireflux valve within the button.*
• Lubricate the mushroom dome and the stoma. Gently push the button through the stoma into the stomach.

Obturator
Abdominal wall

• Remove the obturator by gently rotating it as you withdraw it, *to keep the antireflux valve from adhering to it.* If the valve sticks nonetheless, gently push the obturator back into the button until the valve closes.
• After removing the obturator, check the valve to make sure it's closed. Then close the flexible safety plug, which should be relatively flush with the skin surface.

• If you need to administer a feeding right away, open the safety plug and attach the feeding adapter and feeding tube. Deliver the feeding as ordered.

Feeding catheter

Feeding adapter

Safety plug

or bag and catheter with formula. Refill the syringe before it's empty. *These steps prevent air from entering the stomach and distending the abdomen.*

• Open the safety plug and attach the adapter and feeding catheter to the button. Elevate the syringe or feeding bag above stomach level, and gravity-feed the formula for 15 to 30 minutes, varying the height as needed *to alter the flow rate.* Use a pump for continuous infusion or for feedings lasting several hours.

• After feeding, flush the button with 10 ml of water and clean the inside of the feeding catheter with a cotton-tipped applicator and water *to preserve patency and to dislodge formula or food particles,* and lower the syringe or bag below stomach level *to allow burping.* Remove the adapter and feeding catheter. The antireflux valve should prevent gastric reflux. Then snap the safety plug in place *to keep the lumen clean and prevent leakage if the antireflux valve fails.* If the patient feels nauseated or vomits after feeding, vent the button with the adapter and feeding catheter *to control emesis.*

• Wash the catheter and syringe or feeding bag in warm soapy water and rinse thoroughly. Clean the catheter and adapter with a pipe cleaner. Rinse well before using for the next feeding. Soak the equipment once a week according to manufacturer's recommendations.

Special considerations
If the button pops out while feeding, reinsert it, estimate the formula already delivered, and resume feeding.

Once daily, clean the peristomal skin with mild soap and water or povidone-iodine, and let the skin air-dry for 20 minutes, *to avoid skin irritation.* Also clean the site whenever spillage from the feeding bag occurs.

Home care
Before discharge, be sure the patient can insert and care for the gastrostomy feeding button. If necessary, teach him or a family member how to reinsert the button by first practicing on a model. Offer written instructions and answer his questions on obtaining replacement supplies.

Documentation
Record feeding time and duration, amount and type of feeding formula used, and patient tolerance. Maintain intake and output records, as necessary. Note the appearance of the stoma and surrounding skin.

Colostomy and ileostomy care

A patient with an ascending or transverse colostomy or an ileostomy may wear an external pouch to collect emerging fecal matter, which will be watery or pasty. Besides collecting waste matter, the pouch helps to control odor and to protect the stoma and peristomal skin. Most disposable pouching systems can be used from 2 to 7 days. Some models last even longer—up to 14 days.

Any pouching system needs immediate changing if a leak develops. And every pouch needs emptying when it's one-third to one-half full. The patient with an ileostomy may need to empty his pouch four or five times daily.

Naturally, the best time to change the pouching system is when the bowel is least active, usually between 2 and 4 hours after meals. After a few months, most patients can predict the best changing time.

Pouching-system selection should consider which system provides the best adhesive seal and skin protection for the individual patient. The type of pouch selected depends on the stoma's location and structure, availability of supplies, wear time, consistency of effluent, personal preference, and finances.

Equipment
Pouching system ■ stoma measuring guide ■ stoma paste (if drainage is watery to pasty or stoma secretes excess mucus) ■ plastic bag ■ water ■ washcloth and towel ■ closure clamp ■ toilet or bedpan ■ water or pouch cleaning solution ■ gloves ■ facial tissues ■ optional: ostomy belt, paper tape, mild nonmoisturizing soap, skin shaving equipment, liquid skin sealant, pouch deodorant.

Pouching systems may be drainable or closed-bottomed, disposable or reusable, adhesive-backed, and one-piece or two-piece. (See *Comparing ostomy pouching systems.*)

Implementation
Begin the following procedures by providing privacy and emotional support.

To fit the pouch and skin barrier
• For a pouch with an attached skin barrier, measure the stoma with the stoma measuring guide. Select the opening size that matches the stoma.

• For an adhesive-backed pouch with a separate skin barrier, measure the stoma with the measuring guide and select the opening that matches the stoma. Trace the selected size opening onto the paper back of the skin barrier's adhesive side. Cut out the opening. (If the pouch

Comparing ostomy pouching systems

Manufactured in many shapes and sizes, ostomy pouches are fashioned for comfort, safety, and easy application. For example, a disposable closed-end pouch may meet the needs of a patient who irrigates, who wants added security, or who wants to discard the pouch after each bowel movement. Another patient may prefer a reusable, drainable pouch. Some commonly available pouches are described below.

Disposable pouches

The patient who must empty his pouch often (because of diarrhea or a new colostomy or ileostomy) may prefer a one-piece, drainable, disposable pouch with a closure clamp attached to a skin barrier (below, left).

These transparent or opaque, odor-proof, plastic pouches come with attached adhesive or karaya seals. Some pouches have microporous adhesive or belt tabs. The bottom opening allows for easy draining. This pouch may be used permanently or temporarily, until stoma size stabilizes.

Also disposable and also made of transparent or opaque odor-proof plastic, a one-piece disposable closed-end pouch (above, right) may come in a kit with adhesive seal, belt tabs, skin barrier, or carbon filter for gas release. A patient with a regular bowel elimination pattern may choose this style for additional security and confidence.

A two-piece disposable drainable pouch with separate skin barrier, shown below, permits frequent changes and also minimizes skin breakdown. Also made of transparent or opaque odor-proof plastic, this style comes with belt tabs and usually snaps to the skin barrier with a flange mechanism.

Reusable pouches

Typically manufactured from sturdy, opaque, nonallergenic plastic, the reusable pouch comes with a separate custom-made faceplate and O-ring, as shown below. Some pouches have a pressure valve for releasing gas. The device has a 1- to 2-month life span, depending on how frequently the patient empties the pouch.

Reusable equipment may benefit a patient who needs a firm faceplate or who wishes to minimize cost. However, many reusable ostomy pouches aren't odor-proof.

Applying a skin barrier and pouch

Fitting a skin barrier and ostomy pouch properly can be done in a few steps. Shown below is a two-piece pouching system with flanges, which is in common use.

Measure the stoma using a measuring guide.

Trace the appropriate circle carefully on the back of the skin barrier.

Cut the circular opening in the skin barrier. Bevel the edges to keep them from irritating the patient.

Remove the backing from the skin barrier and moisten it or apply barrier paste, as needed, along the edge of the circular opening.

Center the skin barrier over the stoma, adhesive side down, and gently press it to the skin.

Gently press the pouch opening onto the ring until it snaps into place.

has precut openings, which can be handy for a round stoma, select an opening that's ⅛" larger than the stoma. If the pouch comes without an opening, cut the hole ⅛" wider than the measured tracing.) The cut-to-fit system works best for an irregularly shaped stoma.

• For a two-piece pouching system with flanges, see *Applying a skin barrier and pouch*.

• Avoid fitting the pouch too tightly *because the stoma has no pain receptors. A constrictive opening could injure the stoma or skin tissue without the patient feeling warning discomfort*. Also avoid cutting the opening too big *because this may expose the skin to fecal matter and moisture*.

• The patient with a descending or sigmoid colostomy who has formed stool and whose ostomy doesn't secrete much mucus may choose to wear only a pouch. In this case, make sure that the pouch opening closely matches the stoma size.

• Between 6 weeks and 1 year after surgery, the stoma will shrink to its permanent size. Then pattern-making preparations will be unnecessary unless the patient gains weight, has additional surgery, or injures the stoma.

To apply or change the pouch

• Collect all equipment.

• Wash your hands and provide privacy.

• Explain the procedure to the patient. As you perform each step, explain what you are doing and why *because the patient will eventually perform the procedure himself*.

• Put on gloves.

• Remove and discard the old pouch. Wipe the stoma and peristomal skin gently with a facial tissue.

• Carefully wash and dry the peristomal skin. Inspect the peristomal skin and stoma. Shave surrounding hair, if necessary, *to promote a better seal and avoid skin irritation from hair pulling against the adhesive*.

• If applying a separate skin barrier, peel off the paper backing of the prepared skin barrier, center the barrier over the stoma, and press gently to ensure adhesion.

• You may want to outline the stoma or the back of the skin barrier (depending on the product) with a thin ring of stoma paste *to provide extra skin protection*. (Skip this step if the patient has a sigmoid or descending colostomy, formed stool, and little mucus.)

• Remove the paper backing from the adhesive side of the pouching system and center the pouch opening over the stoma. Press gently to secure.

• For a pouching system with flanges, align the lip of the pouch flange with the bottom edge of the skin barrier flange. Gently press around the circumference of the pouch flange, beginning at the bottom, until the pouch securely adheres to the barrier flange. (The pouch will click into its secured position.) Holding the barrier

against the skin, gently pull on the pouch *to confirm the seal between flanges*.

• Encourage the patient to stay quietly in position for about 5 minutes *to improve adherence. The patient's body warmth also helps to improve adherence and soften a rigid skin barrier*.

• Attach an ostomy belt to further secure the pouch, if desired. (Some pouches have belt loops, and others have plastic adapters for belts.)

• Leave a bit of air in the pouch *to allow drainage to fall to the bottom*.

• Apply the closure clamp, if necessary.

• If desired, apply paper tape in a picture-frame fashion to the pouch edges *for additional security*.

To empty the pouch

• Tilt the bottom of the pouch upward and remove the closure clamp.

• Turn up a cuff on the lower end of the pouch and allow it to drain into the toilet or bedpan.

• Wipe the bottom of the pouch and reapply the closure clamp.

• If desired, the bottom portion of the pouch can be rinsed with cool tap water. Do not aim water up near the top of the pouch *because this may loosen the seal on the skin*.

• A two-piece flanged system can also be emptied by unsnapping the pouch. Let the drainage flow into the toilet.

• Release flatus through the gas release valve if the pouch has one. Otherwise, release flatus by tilting the pouch bottom upward, releasing the clamp, and expelling the flatus. To release flatus from a flanged system, loosen the seal between the flanges. (Some pouches have gas release valves.)

• Never make a pinhole in a pouch to release gas. *This destroys the odor-proof seal.*

Special considerations

After performing and explaining the procedure to the patient, encourage the patient's increasing involvement in self-care.

Use adhesive solvents and removers only after patch-testing the patient's skin because *some products may irritate the skin or produce hypersensitivity reactions*. Consider using a liquid skin sealant, if available, *to give skin tissue additional protection from drainage and adhesive irritants*.

Remove the pouching system if the patient reports burning or itching beneath it or purulent drainage around the stoma. Notify the doctor or therapist of any skin irritation, breakdown, rash, or unusual appearance of the stoma or peristomal area.

Use commercial pouch deodorants, if desired. However, most pouches are odor-free, and odor should only be evident when you empty the pouch or if it leaks. Before discharge, suggest that the patient avoid odor-causing foods such as fish, eggs, onions, and garlic.

If the patient wears a reusable pouching system, suggest that he obtain two or more systems *so he can wear one while the other dries after cleaning with soap and water or a commercially prepared cleaning solution.*

Complications
Failing to fit the pouch properly over the stoma or improper use of a belt can injure the stoma. Be alert for a possible allergic reaction to adhesives and other ostomy products.

Documentation
Record the date and time of the pouching system change; note the character of drainage, including color, amount, type, and consistency. Also describe the appearance of the stoma and the peristomal skin. Document patient teaching. Describe the teaching content. Record the patient's response to self-care, and evaluate his learning progress.

Colostomy irrigation

This procedure can serve two purposes: it allows a patient with a descending or sigmoid colostomy to regulate bowel function, and it's used to clean the large bowel before and after tests, surgery, or other procedures.

Colostomy irrigation may begin as soon as bowel function resumes after surgery. However, most clinicians recommend waiting until bowel movements are more predictable. Initially, the nurse or the patient irrigates the colostomy at the same time every day, recording the amount of output and any spillage between irrigations. Between 4 and 6 weeks may pass before colostomy irrigation establishes a predictable elimination pattern.

Equipment
Colostomy irrigation set (contains an irrigation drain or sleeve, an ostomy belt [if needed] to secure the drain or sleeve, water-soluble lubricant, drainage pouch clamp, and irrigation bag with clamp, tubing, and cone tip) ■ 1,000 ml (about 30 oz or 1 quart) of tap water irrigant warmed to about 100° F (37.8° C) ■ normal saline solution (for cleansing enemas) ■ I.V. pole or wall hook ■ washcloth and towel ■ water ■ ostomy pouching system ■ linen-saver pad ■ gloves ■ optional: bedpan or chair, mild non-moisturizing soap, rubber band or clip, small dressing or bandage, stoma cap.

Preparation of equipment
Depending on the patient's condition, colostomy irrigation may be performed in bed using a bedpan or in the bathroom using the chair and the toilet.

Set up the irrigation bag with tubing and cone tip. If irrigation will take place with the patient in bed, place the bedpan beside the bed and elevate the head of the bed between 45 and 90 degrees, if allowed. If irrigation will take place in the bathroom, have the patient sit on the toilet or on a chair facing the toilet, whichever he finds more comfortable.

Fill the irrigation bag with warmed tap water (or normal saline solution, if the irrigation is for bowel cleansing). Hang the bag on the I.V. pole or wall hook. The bottom of the bag should be at the patient's shoulder level *to prevent the fluid from entering the bowel too quickly.* Most irrigation sets also have a clamp that regulates the flow rate.

Prime the tubing with irrigant *to prevent air from entering the colon and possibly causing cramps and gas pains.*

Implementation
● Explain every step of the procedure to the patient *for teaching purposes, especially since the patient will most likely be irrigating the colostomy himself.*
● Provide privacy and wash your hands.
● If the patient's in bed, place a linen-saver pad under him *to protect the sheets from soiling.*
● Put on gloves.
● Remove the ostomy pouch if the patient uses one.
● Place the irrigation sleeve over the stoma. If the sleeve doesn't have an adhesive backing, secure the sleeve with an ostomy belt. If the patient has a two-piece pouching system with flanges, snap off the pouch and save it. Snap on the irrigation sleeve.
● Place the open-ended bottom of the irrigation sleeve in the bedpan or toilet *to promote drainage by gravity.* If necessary, cut the sleeve so that it meets the water level inside the bedpan or toilet. *Effluent may splash from a short sleeve. From a long sleeve, it may not drain.*
● Lubricate your gloved small finger with water-soluble lubricant and insert the finger into the stoma. If you're teaching the patient, have him do this *to determine the bowel angle at which to insert the cone safely.* Expect the stoma to tighten when the finger enters the bowel and then to relax in a few seconds.
● Lubricate the cone with water-soluble lubricant *to prevent it from irritating the mucosa.*

• Insert the cone into the top opening of the irrigation sleeve and then into the stoma. Angle the cone to match the bowel angle. Insert it gently but snugly.

• Unclamp the irrigation tubing and allow the water to flow slowly. If you don't have a clamp to control the irrigant's flow rate, pinch the tubing *to control the flow.* The water should enter the colon over 10 to 15 minutes. (If the patient reports cramping, slow or stop the flow, keep the cone in place, and have the patient take a few deep breaths until the cramping stops.) Cramping during irrigation may result from a bowel that's ready to empty, water that's too cold, a rapid flow rate, or air in the tubing.

• Have the patient remain stationary for 15 or 20 minutes *so the initial effluent can drain.*

• If the patient's ambulatory, he can stay in the bathroom until all effluent empties, or he can clamp the bottom of the drainage sleeve with a rubber band or clip and return to bed. Explain that *ambulation and activity stimulate elimination.* Suggest that the nonambulatory patient lean forward or massage his abdomen *to stimulate elimination.*

• Wait about 45 minutes for the bowel to finish eliminating the irrigant and effluent. Then remove the irrigation sleeve.

• If the irrigation was intended to clean the bowel, repeat the procedure with warmed normal saline solution until the return solution appears clear.

• Using a washcloth, mild soap, and water, gently clean the area around the stoma. Rinse and dry the area thoroughly with a clean towel.

• Inspect the skin and stoma for changes in appearance. Usually dark pink to red, stoma color may change with the patient's status. Notify the doctor of marked stoma color changes because *a pale hue may result from anemia, and substantial darkening suggests a change in blood flow to the stoma.*

• Apply a clean pouch. Or if the patient has a regular bowel elimination pattern, he may prefer a small dressing, bandage, or commercial stoma cap.

• Discard a disposable irrigation sleeve. Rinse a reusable irrigation sleeve and hang it to dry along with the irrigation bag, tubing, and cone.

Special considerations

Irrigating a colostomy to establish a regular bowel elimination pattern doesn't work for all patients. If the bowel continues to move between irrigations, try decreasing the volume of irrigant. *Increasing the irrigant will not help because it serves only to stimulate peristalsis.* Keep a record of results. Also consider irrigating every other day.

Irrigation may help to regulate bowel function in patients with a descending or sigmoid colostomy *because this is the bowel's stool storage area.* However, a patient

with an ascending or transverse colostomy won't benefit from irrigation. Also, a patient with descending or sigmoid colostomy who is missing part of the ascending or transverse colon may not be able to irrigate successfully because his ostomy may function like an ascending or transverse colostomy.

If diarrhea develops, discontinue irrigations until stools form again. Keep in mind that irrigation alone won't achieve regularity for the patient. He must also observe a complementary diet and exercise regimen.

If the patient has a strictured stoma that prohibits cone insertion, remove the cone from the irrigation tubing and replace it with a soft silicone catheter. Angle the catheter gently 2″ to 4″ (5 to 10 cm) into the bowel to instill the irrigant. Don't force the catheter into the stoma, and don't insert it further than the recommended length *because you may perforate the bowel.*

Complications

Bowel perforation may result if a catheter is incorrectly inserted into the stoma. Fluid and electrolyte imbalances may result from using too much irrigant.

Documentation

Record the date and time of irrigation and the type and amount of irrigant. Note the stoma's color and the character of drainage, including the drainage color, consistency, and amount. Record any patient teaching. Describe teaching content and patient response to self-care instruction. Evaluate the patient's learning progress.

 Continent ileostomy care

An alternative to conventional ileostomy, a continent or pouch ileostomy (also called a Koch ileostomy or an ileal pouch) features an internal reservoir fashioned from the terminal ileum. This procedure may be used for a patient who requires proctocolectomy for chronic ulcerative colitis or multiple polyposis. Other patients may have a traditional ileostomy converted to a pouch ileostomy. This procedure is contraindicated in Crohn's disease or gross obesity. Patients who need emergency surgery and those who cannot care for the pouch are also unlikely to have this procedure.

The length of preoperative hospitalization varies with the patient's condition. Nursing responsibilities include providing bowel preparation, antibiotic therapy, and emotional support. After surgery, nursing responsibilities include ensuring patency of the drainage catheter, assessing GI function, caring for the stoma and peristomal

Understanding pouch construction

Depending on the patient and related factors during intestinal surgery, the doctor may construct a pouch to collect fecal matter internally. To make such a pouch, the doctor loops about 12″ (30.5 cm) of ileum and sutures the inner sides together.

He opens the loop with a U-shaped cut and seams the inside to create a smooth lining. Then he fashions a nipple or valve between what is becoming the pouch and what will be the stoma.

He folds the open ileum over, sews the pouch closed, and fixes the pouch to the abdominal wall.

Because the pouch holds fecal matter in reserve, the patient benefits from not having to change and empty ostomy equipment. Instead, he empties and irrigates the pouch as needed by inserting a catheter though the stoma and into the pouch.

Initially after surgery, the nurse performs this procedure until the patient can do it himself.

Irrigating catheter

Stoma

Ileal pouch

Bladder

Intestine

the suture line heals, the patient learns how to drain the pouch himself.

Equipment
Leg drainage bag ■ bedside drainage bag ■ normal saline solution ■ 50-ml catheter-tip syringe ■ extra continent ileostomy catheter ■ 20-ml syringe with adapter ■ 4″ × 4″ × 1″ foam dressing and Montgomery straps ■ precut drain dressing ■ gloves ■ water-soluble lubricant ■ graduated container ■ skin sealant ■ optional: commercial catheter securing device.

Implementation
Nursing interventions for the patient having a continent ileostomy range from standard preoperative and postoperative care to pouch care and patient teaching.

Preoperative care
• Reinforce and, if necessary, supplement the doctor's explanation of a continent ileostomy and its implications for the patient. (See *Understanding pouch construction.*)
• Assess patient and family attitudes related to the operation and to the forthcoming change in the patient's body image.
• Provide encouragement and support.

Postoperative care
• When the patient returns to his room, attach the drainage catheter emerging from the ileostomy to continuous gravity drainage.
• A leg drainage bag may be attached to the patient's thigh during ambulation.
• Irrigate the catheter with 30 ml of normal saline solution, as ordered and as necessary, *to prevent catheter obstruction and to allow fluid return by gravity.* During the early postoperative period, keep the pouch empty *to allow the suture lines to heal and to prevent rapid pouch expansion.* At first, drainage will be serosanguineous.
• Monitor fluid intake and output.
• Check the catheter frequently once the patient begins eating solid food *to ensure that mucus or undigested food particles don't block it.*
• If the patient complains of abdominal cramps, distention, and nausea — symptoms of bowel obstruction — the catheter may be clogged. Gently irrigate with 20 to 30 ml of water or normal saline solution until the catheter drains freely. Then move the catheter slightly or rotate it gently *to help clear the obstruction.* Finally, try milking the catheter. If these measures fail, notify the doctor.
• Check the stoma frequently for color, edema, and bleeding. Normally pink to red, a stoma that turns dark red or blue-red may have a compromised blood supply.

skin, managing pain resulting from surgery, and if necessary, perineal skin care.

Usually, daily patient teaching on pouch intubation and drainage begins soon after surgery. Continuous drainage is maintained for about 2 to 6 weeks to allow the suture lines to heal. During this period, a drainage catheter is attached to low intermittent suction. After

• To care for the stoma and peristomal skin, put on gloves. Remove the dressing, gently clean the peristomal area with water, and pat dry. Use a skin sealant around the stoma *to prevent skin irritation.*

• One way to apply a stoma dressing is to slip a precut drain dressing around the catheter to cover the stoma. Cut a hole slightly larger than the lumen of the catheter in the center of a 4" × 4" × 1" piece of foam. Disconnect the catheter from the drainage bag and insert the distal end of the catheter through the hole in the foam. Slide the foam pad onto the dressing. Secure the foam in place with Montgomery straps. Secure the catheter by wrapping the strap ties around it or by using a commercial catheter securing device. Then reconnect the catheter to the drainage bag. (The drainage catheter will be removed by the surgeon when he determines that the suture line has healed.)

• Assess the peristomal skin for irritation from moisture.

• *To reduce discomfort from gas pains,* encourage ambulation. Also recommend that the patient avoid swallowing air (*to minimize gas pains*) by chewing food well, limiting conversation while eating, and not drinking from a straw.

Draining the pouch

• Provide privacy, carefully explain the procedure to the patient, and wash your hands.

• Put on gloves.

• Have the patient with a pouch conversion sit on the toilet *to help him feel more at ease during the procedure.*

• Remove the stoma dressing.

• Encourage the patient to relax his abdominal muscles *to allow the catheter to slide easily into the pouch.*

• Lubricate the tip of the drainage catheter tip with the water-soluble lubricant and insert it in the stoma. Gently push the catheter downward. (The direction of insertion may vary depending on the patient.)

• When the catheter reaches the nipple valve of the internal pouch or reservoir (after about 2" or 2½" [5 or 6.4 cm]), you'll feel resistance. Instruct the patient to take a deep breath as you exert gentle pressure on the catheter to insert it through the valve. If this fails, have the patient lie supine and rest for a few minutes. Then, with the patient still supine, try to insert the catheter again.

• Gently advance the catheter to the suture marking made by the surgeon.

• Let the pouch drain completely. This usually takes 5 to 10 minutes. With thick drainage or a clogged catheter, the process may take 30 minutes.

• If the tube clogs, irrigate using the 50-ml catheter-tip syringe with 30 ml of water or normal saline solution. Also, rotate and milk the tube. If these measures fail, then remove, rinse, and reinsert the catheter.

• Remove the catheter after completing drainage.

• Measure output, subtracting the amount of irrigant used.

• Rinse the catheter thoroughly with warm water.

• Clean the peristomal area and apply a fresh stoma dressing.

Predischarge teaching

• Be sure the patient can properly intubate and drain the pouch himself.

• Provide the patient with the appropriate equipment. If the postoperative drainage catheter is still in place, teach the patient how to care for it properly.

• Be sure the patient has a pouch-draining schedule, and give him appropriate pamphlets or video instructions on pouch care.

• Make sure he feels comfortable calling the doctor, nurse, or appropriate other caregivers with questions or problems.

• Tell the patient where to obtain supplies.

• Refer the patient to a local ostomy group.

• Provide dietary counseling.

Special considerations

Never aspirate fluid from the catheter *because the resulting negative pressure may damage inflamed tissue.*

The first few times you intubate the pouch, the patient may be tense, making insertion difficult. Encourage relaxation. To shorten drainage time, have the patient cough, press gently on his abdomen over the pouch, or suddenly tighten his abdominal muscles and then relax them.

Keep an accurate record of intake and output *to ensure fluid and electrolyte balance.* The average daily output should be 1,000 ml. Report inadequate or excessive output (more than 1,400 ml daily).

Complications

Common postoperative complications include obstruction, fistula, pouch perforation, nipple valve dysfunction, abscesses, and bacterial overgrowth in the pouch.

Documentation

Record the date, time, and all aspects of preoperative and postoperative care including condition of the stoma and peristomal skin, diet, medications, intubations, patient teaching, and discharge planning.

 T-tube care

The T tube may be placed in the common bile duct after cholecystectomy. This tube facilitates biliary drainage during healing. The surgeon inserts the short end (the crossbar) of the T tube in the common bile duct and draws the long end through the incision. The tube then connects to a closed gravity drainage system. (See *Understanding T-tube placement*.) Postoperatively, the tube remains in place between 7 and 14 days.

Equipment

Graduated collection container ▪ small plastic bag ▪ sterile gloves and clean gloves ▪ clamp ▪ sterile 4″ × 4″ gauze pads ▪ transparent dressings ▪ rubber band ▪ normal saline solution ▪ sterile cleaning solution ▪ two sterile basins ▪ povidone-iodine sponges ▪ sterile precut drain dressings ▪ nonallergenic paper tape ▪ skin protectant, such as petroleum jelly, zinc oxide, or aluminum-based gel ▪ optional: Montgomery straps.

Preparation of equipment

Assemble equipment at the bedside. Open all sterile equipment. Place one sterile 4″ × 4″ gauze pad in each sterile basin. Using sterile technique, pour 50 ml of cleaning solution into one basin and 50 ml of normal saline into the other basin. Tape a small plastic bag on the table to use for refuse.

Implementation
• Provide privacy and explain the procedure to the patient. Wash your hands thoroughly.

To empty drainage
• Put on clean gloves.
• Place the graduated collection container under the outlet valve of the drainage bag. Without contaminating the clamp, valve, or outlet valve, empty the bag's contents completely into the container and reseal the outlet valve. Carefully measure and record the character, color, and amount of drainage. Discard gloves.

To re-dress the T tube
• Wash your hands thoroughly *to prevent bacterial contamination of the incision*. Put on clean gloves.
• Without dislodging the T tube, remove old dressings, and dispose of them in the small plastic bag. Remove the clean gloves.
• Wash your hands again and put on sterile gloves. From this point on, follow strict aseptic technique *to prevent bacterial contamination of the incision*.
• Inspect the incision and tube site for signs of infection. Assess for wound dehiscence or evisceration.

Understanding T-tube placement

The T tube is placed in the common bile duct, anchored to the abdominal wall, and connected to a closed drainage system.

Incision

Common bile duct

T tube

Duodenum

Bile drainage bag

- Use the prescribed sterile solution to clean and remove dried matter or drainage from around the tube. Start at the tube site and gently wipe outward in a continuous motion *to prevent recontamination of the incision.*
- Use normal saline solution to rinse off the prescribed cleaning solution. Dry the area with a sterile 4″ × 4″ gauze pad and discard all used materials.
- Using a circular motion, wipe the incision site with a povidone-iodine sponge. Allow the area to dry thoroughly.
- Lightly apply a skin protectant, such as petroleum jelly, *to protect the skin from injury caused by draining bile.*
- Apply a sterile precut drain dressing on each side of the T tube *to absorb drainage.*
- Apply a sterile 4″ × 4″ gauze pad or transparent dressing over the T tube and the drain dressings. Be careful not to put the dressing over the open end of the T tube *because it connects to the closed drainage system.*
- Secure the dressings with the nonallergenic paper tape or Montgomery straps if necessary.

To clamp the T tube

- As ordered, occlude the tube lightly with a clamp or wrap a rubber band around the end. *Clamping the tube 1 hour before and after meals diverts bile back to the duodenum to aid digestion.*
- *To ensure patient comfort and safety,* check bile drainage amounts regularly. Be alert for such signs of obstructed bile flow as chills, fever, tachycardia, nausea, right-upper-quadrant fullness and pain, jaundice, dark foamy urine, and clay-colored stools. Report them immediately. (See *Managing T-tube obstruction.*)

Special considerations

Normal daily bile drainage ranges from 500 to 1,000 ml of viscous, green-brown liquid. The T tube usually drains 300 to 500 ml of blood-tinged bile in the first 24 hours after surgery. Report drainage that exceeds 500 ml in the first 24 hours after surgery. This amount typically declines to 200 ml or less after 4 days. Monitor fluid, electrolyte, and acid-base status carefully.

To prevent excessive bile loss (over 500 ml in first 24 hours) or backflow contamination, secure the T-tube drainage system at abdominal level. Bile will flow into the bag only when biliary pressure increases. As ordered, return excessive bile drainage (between 1,000 and 1,500 ml daily) to the patient mixed with chilled fruit juice or, if possible, through a nasogastric tube.

Provide meticulous skin care and frequent dressing changes. Observe for bile leakage, which may indicate obstruction. Assess tube patency and site condition hourly for the first 8 hours and then every 4 hours until the doctor removes the tube. Protect the skin edges and avoid excessive taping *to prevent shearing the skin.*

TROUBLESHOOTING

Managing T-tube obstruction

If your patient's T tube blocks after cholecystectomy, notify the doctor and take these steps while you wait for him to arrive.
- Unclamp the T tube (if it was clamped before and after a meal) and connect the tube to a closed gravity-drainage system.
- Inspect the tube carefully to detect any kinks or obstructions.
- Prepare the patient for possible T-tube irrigation or direct X-ray of the common bile duct (cholangiography). Briefly describe these measures to reduce the patient's apprehension and promote cooperation.
- Provide encouragement and support.

Monitor all urine and stools for color changes. Assess for icteric skin and sclera, *which may signal jaundice.*

Loose bowels occur commonly in the first few weeks after surgery. Teach the patient about reportable signs of T-tube and biliary obstruction.

Complications

Obstructed bile flow, skin excoriation or breakdown, tube dislodgment, drainage reflux, and infection are the most common complications related to a biliary T tube.

Documentation

Record the date and time of each dressing change. Note the appearance of the wound and surrounding skin. Write down the color, character, and volume of bile collected. Also record the color of skin and mucous membranes around the T tube. Record any complaints of nausea or pain. Keep a precise record of temperature trends, the patient's coloring, and the amount and frequency of urination and bowel movements.

Selected references

Camp, D., and Otten, N. "How to Insert and Remove Nasogastric Tubes," *Nursing90* 20(9):59-64, September 1990.

Rombeau, J., et al. *Atlas of Nutritional Support Techniques.* Boston: Little, Brown & Co., 1989.

RENAL AND UROLOGIC CARE

MARY BETH MODIC, RN, MSN

fluid
electrolytes
acid-base balance
elimination
&w

Based on the results of continued patient assessment, you can make valid clinical decisions and establish priorities that will contribute to a positive outcome. Your ability to assess a situation, analyze it critically, and establish priorities probably has the greatest impact on the success of the nursing process.

Introduction

Because the renal and urologic systems produce, transport, collect, and excrete urine, their dysfunction will impair fluid, electrolyte, and acid-base balance and the elimination of waste. To restore or facilitate effective function of these systems, treatment of renal and urologic disorders usually involves temporary or permanent insertion of a urinary, peritoneal, or vascular catheter or tube. Catheterization also allows monitoring of renal and urologic systems and aids diagnosis of dysfunction.

Helping the patient cope

One goal in caring for a patient with a renal or urologic disorder is helping him accept an invasive procedure or adjust to a new body image. Begin to meet this goal by assessing the amount and kind of information he needs and can absorb about the procedure. Then present or reinforce this information and tell him what to expect.

For example, before insertion of an indwelling catheter, tell the patient that he'll feel pressure during insertion, that the catheter will cause a sense of fullness or the urge to void, that he must avoid dislodging the catheter, and that the collection bag must be at lower-than-bladder level.

In a patient with a severe and chronic disorder, treatment usually requires permanent changes, such as urinary diversion, which may seriously affect his body image. To manage such a patient effectively, you must help him cope with any distressing changes by helping him recognize the health benefits of the treatment. For example, a stoma may be initially unappealing, but you can help the patient see that living with the stoma is easier than living with the disease or symptoms that caused him to seek treatment in the first place.

Managing the procedure

Performing procedures skillfully is only one aspect of successfully managing renal and urologic disorders. You must also understand the purpose of each step of the procedure, the physiologic and scientific principles that support the procedure, and the associated indications, contraindications, and clinical ramifications.

Additionally, you must accurately assess the patient's status, plan the appropriate approach to the procedure, implement the procedure, and evaluate its overall effect on the patient.

URINARY CATHETERS
Insertion of an indwelling catheter

Also known as a Foley or retention catheter, an indwelling catheter remains in the bladder to provide continuous urine drainage. A balloon inflated at the catheter's distal end prevents it from slipping out of the bladder after insertion. Indwelling catheters are used most often to relieve bladder distention caused by urine retention and to allow continuous urine drainage when the urinary meatus is swollen from childbirth, surgery, or local trauma. Other indications for an indwelling catheter include urinary tract obstruction (by a tumor or enlarged prostate), urine retention or infection from neurogenic bladder paralysis caused by spinal cord injury or disease, and any illness in which the patient's urine output must be monitored closely.

An indwelling catheter is inserted using sterile technique and only when absolutely necessary. Insertion should be performed with extreme care to prevent injury and infection.

Equipment

Sterile indwelling catheter (latex or silicone #10 to #22 French [average adult sizes are #16 to #18 French]) ▪ syringe filled with 5 to 8 ml of normal saline solution ▪ washcloth ▪ towel ▪ soap and water ▪ two linen-saver pads ▪ sterile gloves ▪ sterile drape ▪ sterile fenestrated drape ▪ sterile cotton-tipped applicators (or cotton balls and plastic forceps) ▪ povidone-iodine or other antiseptic cleaning agent ▪ urine receptacle ▪ sterile water-soluble lubricant ▪ sterile drainage collection bag ▪ intake and output sheet ▪ adhesive tape ▪ optional: urine-specimen container and laboratory request form, leg band with Velcro closure, gooseneck lamp.

Prepackaged sterile disposable kits are available and usually contain all the necessary equipment. The syringes in these kits are prefilled with normal saline solution.

Preparation of equipment

Check the order on the patient's chart *to determine if a catheter size or type has been specified.* Then wash your hands, select the appropriate equipment, and assemble it at the patient's bedside.

Implementation

• Explain the procedure to the patient and provide privacy. Check his chart and ask when he voided last. Percuss and palpate the bladder *to establish baseline data.* Ask if he feels the urge to void.

• *So that you can see the urinary meatus clearly in poor lighting,* place a gooseneck lamp next to the patient's bed.

• Place the female patient in the supine position, with her knees flexed and separated and her feet flat on the bed, about 2′ (61 cm) apart. If she finds this position uncomfortable, have her flex one knee and keep the other leg flat on the bed. You may need an assistant to help the patient stay in position or to direct the light. Place the male patient in the supine position with his legs extended and flat on the bed. Ask the patient to hold the position *to give you a clear view of the urinary meatus and to prevent contamination of the sterile field.*

• Use the washcloth to clean the patient's genital area and perineum thoroughly with soap and water. Dry the area with the towel. Then, wash your hands.

• Place the linen-saver pads on the bed between the patient's legs and under the hips. *To create the sterile field,* open the prepackaged kit or equipment tray and place it between the female patient's legs or next to the male patient's hip. If the sterile gloves are the first item on the top of the tray, put them on. Place the sterile drape under the patient's hips. Then drape the patient's lower abdomen with the sterile fenestrated drape so that only the genital area remains exposed. Take care not to contaminate your gloves.

• Open the rest of the kit or tray. Put on the sterile gloves if you haven't already done so.

• Tear open the packet of povidone-iodine or other antiseptic cleaning agent, and use it to saturate the sterile cotton balls or applicators. Be careful not to spill the solution on the equipment.

• Open the packet of water-soluble lubricant and apply it to the catheter tip; attach the drainage bag to the other end of the catheter. (If you're using a commercial kit, the drainage bag may be attached.) Make sure all tubing ends remain sterile, and be sure the clamp at the emptying port of the drainage bag is closed *to prevent urine leakage from the bag.* Some drainage systems have an airlock chamber *to prevent bacteria from traveling to the bladder from urine in the drainage bag.*

• Before inserting the catheter, inflate the balloon with normal saline solution *to inspect it for leaks.* To do this, attach the saline-filled syringe to the luer-lock, then push the plunger and check for seepage as the balloon expands. Aspirate the saline *to deflate the balloon.* Also inspect the

catheter for resiliency. *Rough, cracked catheters can injure the urethral mucosa during insertion, which can predispose the patient to infection.*

• For the female patient, separate the labia majora and labia minora as widely as possible with the thumb, middle, and index fingers of your nondominant hand *so you have a full view of the urinary meatus.* Keep the labia well separated throughout the procedure, *so they don't obscure the urinary meatus or contaminate the area once it's cleaned.*

• With your dominant hand, use a sterile, cotton-tipped applicator (or pick up a sterile cotton ball with the plastic forceps) and wipe one side of the urinary meatus with a single downward motion. Wipe the other side with another sterile applicator or cotton ball in the same way. Then wipe directly over the meatus with still another sterile applicator or cotton ball. Take care not to contaminate your sterile glove.

• For the male patient, hold the penis with your nondominant hand. If he's uncircumcised, retract the foreskin. Then gently lift and stretch the penis to a 60-degree to 90-degree angle. Hold the penis in this way throughout the procedure *to straighten the urethra and maintain a sterile field.*

• Use your dominant hand to clean the glans with a sterile cotton-tipped applicator or a sterile cotton ball held in forceps. Clean in a circular motion, starting at the urinary meatus and working outward.
• Repeat the procedure using another sterile applicator or cotton ball and taking care not to contaminate your sterile glove.
• Pick up the catheter with your dominant hand and prepare to insert the lubricated tip into the urinary meatus. *To facilitate insertion by relaxing the sphincter,* ask the patient (male or female) to cough as you insert the catheter. Tell the patient to breathe deeply and slowly *to further relax the sphincter and prevent spasms.* Hold the catheter close to its tip *to ease insertion and control its direction.*

♦ *Nursing alert.* Never force a catheter during insertion. Maneuver it gently as the patient bears down or coughs. If you still meet resistance, stop the procedure and notify the doctor. Strictures, sphincter spasms, misplacement in the vagina (in females), or an enlarged prostate (in males) may cause resistance. ♦
• For the female patient, advance the catheter about 2" to 3" (5 to 7.6 cm) — while continuing to hold the labia apart — until urine begins to flow (top right).

• For the male patient, advance the catheter about 6" to 8" (15.2 to 20.3 cm) until urine begins to flow. If the foreskin was retracted, be sure to replace it *to prevent compromised circulation and painful swelling.*

• When urine stops flowing, attach the saline-filled syringe to the luer-lock.
• Push the plunger and inflate the balloon *to keep the catheter in place in the bladder* (see top left illustration, page 430).

♦ *Nursing alert.* Never inflate a balloon without first establishing urine flow, *which assures you that the catheter is in the bladder, not in the urethral channel.* ♦

• Hang the collection bag below bladder level *to prevent urine reflux into the bladder, which can cause infection, and to facilitate gravity drainage of the bladder.* Make sure the tubing doesn't get tangled in the bed's side rails.

• Tape the catheter to the female patient's thigh *to prevent possible tension on the urogenital trigone.*

• Tape the catheter to the male patient's thigh or lower abdomen *to prevent pressure on the urethra at the penoscrotal junction, which can lead to formation of urethrocutaneous fistulas* (see illustration at top right).

• Also tape the catheter, as stated, to prevent traction on the bladder and alteration in the normal direction of urine flow in males.

• As an alternative, secure the catheter to the patient's thigh using a leg band with a Velcro closure. *This decreases skin irritation, especially in patients with long-term indwelling catheters.*

• Dispose of all used supplies properly.

Special considerations

Several types of catheters are available with balloons of various sizes. Each type has its own method of inflation and closure. For example, in one type of catheter, sterile solution or air is injected through the inflation lumen; then the end of the injection port is folded over itself and fastened with a clamp or rubber band.

Note: Injecting a catheter with air makes identifying leaks difficult and doesn't guarantee deflation of the balloon for removal.

A similar catheter is inflated by penetrating a seal in the end of the inflation lumen with a needle or the tip of the solution-filled syringe. Another type of balloon catheter self-inflates when a prepositioned clamp is loosened. The balloon size determines the amount of solution needed for inflation, and the exact amount is usually printed on the distal extension of the catheter used for inflating the balloon.

If necessary, ask the female patient to lie on her side with her knees drawn up to her chest during the catheterization procedure. *This position may be especially helpful for elderly or disabled patients, such as those with severe contractures* (see illustration on page 431).

If the doctor orders a urine specimen for laboratory analysis, obtain it from the urine receptacle with a specimen collection container at the time of catheterization, and send it to the laboratory with the appropriate laboratory request form. Connect the drainage bag when urine stops flowing.

Inspect the catheter and tubing periodically while they're in place *to detect compression or kinking that could obstruct urine flow.* Explain the basic principles of gravity drainage *so that the patient realizes the importance of keeping the drainage tubing and collection bag lower than his bladder at all times.* If necessary, provide the patient with detailed instructions for performing clean intermittent self-catheterization.

For monitoring purposes, empty the collection bag at least every 8 hours. Excessive fluid volume may require more frequent emptying *to prevent traction on the catheter,* which would cause the patient discomfort, and *to prevent injury to the urethra and bladder wall.* Some hospitals encourage changing catheters at regular intervals, such as every 30 days, if the patient will have long-term continuous drainage.

♦ *Nursing alert.* Observe the patient carefully for adverse reactions, such as hypovolemic shock, caused by removing excessive volumes of residual urine. Check the hospital's policy beforehand to determine the maximum amount of urine that may be drained at one time (some hospitals limit the amount to 700 to 1,000 ml). Whether or not to limit the amount of urine drained is currently controversial. Clamp the catheter at the first sign of an adverse reaction, and notify the doctor. ♦

Home care
If the patient will be discharged with a long-term indwelling catheter, teach him and his family all aspects of daily catheter maintenance, including care of the skin and urinary meatus, signs and symptoms of urinary tract infection or obstruction, how to irrigate the catheter (if appropriate), and the importance of adequate fluid intake to maintain patency. Explain that a home care nurse should visit every 4 to 6 weeks, or more often if needed, to change the catheter.

Complications
Urinary tract infection can result from the introduction of bacteria into the bladder. Improper insertion can cause traumatic injury to the urethral and bladder mucosa. Bladder atony or spasms can result from rapid decompression of a severely distended bladder.

Documentation
Record the date, time, and size and type of indwelling catheter used. Also describe the amount, color, and other characteristics of urine emptied from the bladder. Your hospital may require only the intake and output sheet for fluid-balance data. If large volumes of urine have been emptied, describe the patient's tolerance for the procedure. Note whether a urine specimen was sent for laboratory analysis.

 ## Care of an indwelling catheter

Intended to prevent infection and other complications by keeping the catheter insertion site clean, routine catheter care typically is performed daily after the patient's morning bath and immediately after perineal care. (Bedtime catheter care may have to be performed before perineal care.)

Because some studies suggest that catheter care increases the risk of infection and other complications rather than lowers it, many hospitals don't recommend daily catheter care. Thus, individual hospital policy dictates whether or not a patient receives such care. Regardless of the catheter care policy, the equipment and the patient's genitalia require inspection twice daily.

Equipment
For catheter care: povidone-iodine (or other antiseptic cleaning agent) ■ sterile gloves ■ basin ■ eight sterile 4″ × 4″ gauze pads ■ sterile absorbent cotton balls or cotton-tipped applicators ■ leg bag ■ collection bag ■ adhesive tape ■ waste receptacle ■ optional: safety pin, rubber band, gooseneck lamp or flashlight, adhesive remover, antibiotic ointment, specimen container.

For perineal cleaning: washcloth ■ additional basin ■ soap and water.

Commercially prepared catheter care kits containing all necessary supplies are available.

Preparation of equipment

Wash your hands and bring all equipment to the patient's bedside. Open the gauze pads, place several in the first basin, and pour some povidone-iodine or other cleaning agent over them.

Some hospitals specify that, after wiping the urinary meatus with cleaning solution, you should wipe it off with wet, sterile gauze pads *to prevent possible irritation from the cleaning solution.* If this is your hospital's policy, pour water into the second basin, and moisten three more gauze pads.

Implementation

• Explain the procedure and its purpose to the patient.
• Provide privacy and make sure that the lighting is adequate *so you can see the perineum and catheter tubing clearly.* Place a gooseneck lamp at the bedside if needed.
• Inspect the catheter for any problems, and check the urine drainage for mucus, blood clots, sediment, and turbidity. Then pinch the catheter between two fingers *to determine if the lumen contains any material.* If you notice any of these conditions (or if hospital policy requires it), obtain a urine specimen (about 6 oz or 17.4 ml), and notify the doctor.
• Inspect the outside of the catheter where it enters the urinary meatus *for encrusted material and suppurative drainage.* Also inspect the tissue around the meatus for irritation or swelling.
• Remove any adhesive tape securing the catheter to the patient's thigh or abdomen. Inspect the area for signs of adhesive burns—redness, tenderness, or blisters.
• Put on the sterile gloves. Then use a saturated, sterile gauze pad or cotton-tipped applicator to clean the outside of the catheter and the tissue around the meatus. *To avoid contaminating the urinary tract,* always clean by wiping away from—never toward—the urinary meatus. Use a dry gauze pad to remove encrusted material.
♦ *Nursing alert.* Don't pull on the catheter while you're cleaning it. *This can injure the urethra and the bladder wall. It can also expose a section of the catheter that was inside the urethra, so that when you release the catheter, the newly contaminated section will reenter the urethra, introducing potentially infectious organisms.* ♦
• Remove your gloves and tear a piece of adhesive tape from the roll.
• *To prevent skin hypersensitivity or irritation,* retape the catheter to the other thigh or opposite side of the abdomen.

♦ *Nursing alert.* Provide enough slack before securing the catheter to prevent tension on the tubing *to avoid injuring the urethral lumen or bladder wall.* ♦
• Most drainage bags have a plastic clamp on the tubing to attach them to the sheet. If this isn't available, wrap a rubber band around the drainage tubing, insert the safety pin through a loop of the rubber band, and pin the tubing to the sheet below bladder level. Then attach the collection bag, below bladder level, to the bed frame.
• If necessary, clean residue from the previous tape site with adhesive remover. Then dispose of all used supplies in a waste receptacle.

Special considerations

Your hospital may require the use of specific cleaning agents for catheter care, so check the policy manual before beginning this procedure. A doctor's order will also be needed to apply antibiotic ointments to the urinary meatus after cleaning.

Avoid raising the drainage bag above bladder level. *This prevents reflux of urine, which may contain bacteria. To avoid damaging the urethral lumen or bladder wall,* always disconnect the drainage bag and tubing from the bed linen and bed frame before helping the patient out of bed.

When possible, attach a leg bag *to allow the patient greater mobility.* If the patient will be discharged with an indwelling catheter, teach him how to use a leg bag. (See *Teaching about leg bags.*)

Encourage patients with unrestricted fluid intake to increase intake to at least 3,000 ml per day. *This helps flush the urinary system and reduces sediment formation. To prevent urinary sediment and calculi from obstructing the drainage tube,* some patients are placed on an acid-ash diet to acidify the urine. Cranberry juice, for example, may help to promote urinary acidity.

Home care 2x daily

Instruct patients discharged with indwelling catheters to wash the urinary meatus and perineal area with soap and water twice daily and the anal area after each bowel movement.

Complications

Sediment buildup, such as casts or mucus plugs, can occur anywhere in a catheterization system, especially in bedridden and dehydrated patients. *To prevent sediment buildup,* keep the patient well hydrated if he's not on fluid restriction. Change the indwelling catheter as ordered or when malfunction, obstruction, or contamination occurs.

Teaching about leg bags

A urine drainage bag attached to the leg provides the catheterized patient with greater mobility. Because the bag is hidden under clothing, it may also help him feel more comfortable about catheterization. Leg bags are usually worn during the day and are replaced at night with a standard collection device.

If your patient will be discharged with an indwelling catheter, teach him how to attach and remove a leg bag. To demonstrate, you'll need a bag with a short drainage tube, two straps, an alcohol sponge, adhesive tape, and a screw clamp or hemostat.

Attaching the leg bag

• Provide privacy and explain the procedure. Describe the advantages of a leg bag, but caution the patient that a leg bag is smaller than a standard collection device and may have to be emptied more frequently.
• Remove the protective covering from the tip of the drainage tube. Then show the patient how to clean the tip with an alcohol sponge, wiping away from the opening to avoid contaminating the tube. Show him how to attach the tube to the catheter.
• Place the drainage bag on the patient's calf or thigh. Have him fasten the straps securely, and show him how to tape the catheter to his leg. Emphasize that he must leave slack in the catheter to minimize pressure on the bladder, urethra, and other structures. Explain that undue pressure or tension can cause tissue breakdown.
• Also tell him not to fasten the straps too tightly to avoid interfering with his circulation.

Avoiding complications

• Although most leg bags have a valve in the drainage tube that prevents urine reflux into the bladder, urge the

patient to keep the drainage bag lower than his bladder at all times because urine in the bag is a perfect growth medium for bacteria. Caution him also not to go to bed or take long naps while wearing the drainage bag.
• To prevent a full leg bag from damaging the bladder wall and urethra, encourage the patient to empty the bag when it's only half full. He should also inspect the catheter and drainage tube periodically for compression or kinking, which could obstruct urine flow and result in bladder distention.
• Tell the patient to wash the leg bag with soap and water or a bacteriostatic solution before each use.

Acute renal failure may result from a catheter obstructed by sediment. Be alert for sharply reduced urine flow from the catheter. Assess for bladder discomfort or distention.

Urinary tract infection is caused by endogenous or exogenous bacteria introduced into the urethra. This can occur during catheter insertion or from intraluminal or extraluminal migration of bacteria up the catheter. Signs and symptoms vary but may include cloudy urine, hematuria, fever, malaise, tenderness over the bladder, and flank pain.

Documentation

Record the care you performed, any necessary modifications in technique, any patient complaints or comments, and the condition of the perineum and urinary meatus. Note the character of the urine in the drainage bag, any sediment buildup, and whether a specimen was sent for laboratory analysis. Also record fluid intake and output. An hourly record is usually necessary for critically ill patients and those with renal insufficiency who are hemodynamically unstable.

strict aseptic technique (handwritten)

Catheter irrigation

30cc (handwritten)

To avoid introducing microorganisms into the bladder, the nurse irrigates an indwelling catheter only to remove an obstruction, such as a blood clot that develops after bladder, kidney, or prostate surgery.

Equipment

Ordered irrigating solution (such as normal saline solution) ▪ sterile graduated receptacle or emesis basin ▪ sterile bulb syringe or 50-ml catheter-tip syringe ▪ two alcohol sponges ▪ sterile gloves ▪ linen-saver pad ▪ intake-output sheet ▪ optional: basin of warm water.

Commercially packaged sterile irrigating kits are available and usually include irrigating solution, a graduated receptacle, and a bulb or 50-ml catheter-tip syringe. If the volume of irrigating solution instilled must be measured, use a graduated syringe instead of a noncalibrated bulb syringe.

Preparation of equipment

Check the expiration date on the irrigating solution. *To prevent vesical spasms during instillation of solution,* warm it to room temperature. If necessary, place the container in a basin of warm water. Never heat the solution on a burner or in a microwave oven. *Hot irrigating solution can injure the patient's bladder.*

Implementation

(handwritten: 21.00)

• Wash your hands, and assemble the equipment at the bedside. Explain the procedure to the patient, and provide privacy.
• Place the linen-saver pad under the patient's buttocks *to protect the bed linens.*
• Create a sterile field at the patient's bedside by opening the sterile equipment tray or commercial kit. Using aseptic technique, clean the lip of the solution bottle by pouring a small amount of solution into a sink or waste receptacle. Then pour the prescribed amount of solution into the graduated receptacle or emesis basin.
• Place the tip of the syringe into the solution. Squeeze the bulb or pull back the plunger (depending on the type of syringe), and fill the syringe with the appropriate amount of solution (usually 30 ml).
• Open the alcohol sponges; then put on the sterile gloves. Clean the juncture of the catheter and drainage tube with an alcohol sponge *to remove as many bacterial contaminants as possible.*
• Disconnect the catheter and drainage tube by twisting them in opposite directions and carefully pulling them apart without creating tension on the catheter. Do not

let go of the catheter—hold it in your nondominant hand. Then place the end of the drainage tube on the sterile field, making sure not to contaminate the tube.
• Twist the bulb syringe or catheter-tip syringe onto the catheter's distal end.
• Squeeze the bulb or slowly push the plunger of the syringe *to instill the irrigating solution through the catheter.* If necessary, refill the syringe and repeat this step until you've instilled the prescribed amount of irrigating solution.
• Remove the syringe and direct the return flow from the catheter into a graduated receptacle or emesis basin. Don't let the catheter end touch the drainage in the receptacle or become contaminated in any other way.
• Wipe the end of the drainage tube and catheter with the remaining alcohol sponge.
• Wait a few seconds until the alcohol evaporates; then reattach the drainage tubing to the catheter.
• Dispose of all used supplies properly.

Special considerations

Catheter irrigation requires strict aseptic technique to prevent bacteria from entering the bladder. The ends of the catheter and drainage tube and the tip of the syringe must be kept sterile throughout this procedure.

If you encounter any resistance during instillation of the irrigating solution, do not try to force the solution into the bladder. Instead, stop the procedure and notify the doctor. If an indwelling catheter becomes totally obstructed, obtain an order to remove it and replace it with a new one *to prevent bladder distention, acute renal failure, urinary stasis, and subsequent infection.*

The doctor may order a continuous irrigation system. *This decreases the risk of infection by eliminating the need to disconnect the catheter and drainage tube repeatedly.* (See "Continuous bladder irrigation.")

Encourage catheterized patients not on restricted fluid intake to increase intake to 3,000 ml per day *to help flush the urinary system and reduce sediment formation. To keep the patient's urine acidic and help prevent calculus formation,* tell the patient to eat foods containing ascorbic acid, including citrus fruits and juices, cranberry juice, and dark green and deep yellow vegetables.

Documentation

Coca (handwritten)

Note the amount, color, and consistency of return urine flow, and document the patient's tolerance for the procedure. Also note any resistance during instillation of the solution. If the return flow volume is less than the amount of solution instilled, note this on the intake and output balance sheets and in your notes.

Continuous bladder irrigation

Continuous bladder irrigation can help prevent urinary tract obstruction by flushing out small blood clots that form after prostate or bladder surgery. It may also be used to treat an irritated, inflamed, or infected bladder lining.

This procedure requires placement of a triple-lumen catheter. One lumen controls balloon inflation, one allows irrigant inflow, and one allows irrigant outflow. The continuous flow of irrigating solution through the bladder also creates a mild tamponade that may help prevent venous hemorrhage. (See *Setup for continuous bladder irrigation.*) Although the patient typically receives the catheter while he's in the operating room after prostate or bladder surgery, he may have it inserted at bedside if he's not a surgical patient.

Equipment
One 4,000-ml container or two 2,000-ml containers of irrigating solution (usually normal saline solution) or the prescribed amount of medicated solution ■ Y-type tubing made specifically for bladder irrigation ■ alcohol or povidone-iodine sponge.

Normal saline solution is usually prescribed for bladder irrigation after prostate or bladder surgery. Large volumes of irrigating solution are usually required during the first 24 to 48 hours after surgery. *This explains the use of Y-type tubing, which allows immediate irrigation with reserve solution.*

EQUIPMENT

Setup for continuous bladder irrigation

In continuous bladder irrigation, a triple-lumen catheter allows irrigating solution to flow into the bladder through one lumen and flow out through another, as shown in the inset. The third lumen is used to inflate the balloon that holds the catheter in place.

Preparation of equipment

Before starting continuous bladder irrigation, double-check the irrigating solution against the doctor's order. If the solution contains an antibiotic, check the patient's chart *to make sure he's not allergic to the drug.*

Implementation

• Wash your hands. Assemble all equipment at the patient's bedside. Explain the procedure and provide privacy.
• Insert the spike of the Y-type tubing into the container of irrigating solution. (If you have a two-container system, insert one spike into each container.)
• Squeeze the drip chamber on the spike of the tubing.
• Open the flow clamp and flush the tubing *to remove air, which could cause bladder distention.* Then close the clamp.
• To begin, hang the irrigating solution on the I.V. pole.
• Clean the opening to the inflow lumen of the catheter with the alcohol or povidone-iodine sponge.
• Insert the distal end of the Y-type tubing securely into the inflow lumen (third port) of the catheter.
• Make sure the catheter's outflow lumen is securely attached to the drainage bag tubing.
• Open the flow clamp under the container of irrigating solution, and set the drip rate, as ordered.
• *To prevent air from entering the system,* don't allow the primary container to empty completely before replacing it.
• If you have a two-container system, simultaneously close the flow clamp under the nearly empty container and open the flow clamp under the reserve container. *This prevents reflux of irrigating solution from the reserve container into the nearly empty one.* Hang a new reserve container on the I.V. pole and insert the tubing, maintaining asepsis.
• Empty the drainage bag about every 4 hours, or as often as needed. Use sterile technique *to avoid the risk of contamination.*

Special considerations

Check the inflow and outflow lines periodically for kinks *to make sure the solution is running freely.* If the solution flows rapidly, check the lines frequently.

Measure the outflow volume accurately. It should equal or, allowing for urine production, slightly exceed inflow volume. If inflow volume exceeds outflow volume postoperatively, suspect bladder rupture at the suture lines, or renal damage, and notify the doctor immediately.

Also assess outflow for changes in appearance and for blood clots, especially if irrigation is being performed postoperatively to control bleeding. If drainage is bright red, irrigating solution should usually be infused rapidly *with the clamp wide open* until drainage clears. Notify the

doctor immediately if you suspect hemorrhage. If drainage is clear, the solution is usually given at a rate of 40 to 60 drops/minute. The doctor typically specifies the rate for antibiotic solutions.

Complications

Interruptions in a continuous irrigation system can predispose the patient to infection. Obstruction in the catheter's outflow lumen can cause bladder distention.

Documentation

Each time you finish a container of solution, record the date, time, and amount of fluid given on the intake and output record. Also record the time and the amount of fluid each time you empty the drainage bag. Note the appearance of the drainage and any complaints the patient has.

Removal of an indwelling catheter

An indwelling catheter should be removed when bladder decompression is no longer necessary, when the patient can resume voiding, or when the catheter is obstructed. Depending on how long the patient was catheterized, the doctor may order bladder retraining before catheter removal.

Equipment

Absorbent cotton ■ gloves ■ alcohol sponge ■ 10-ml syringe with a luer-lock ■ bedpan ■ optional: clamp for bladder retraining.

Preparation of equipment *Bladder training*

If the doctor orders bladder retraining, follow these steps: Clamp the catheter for 2 hours; then release it for 5 minutes *to empty the bladder.* Repeat the procedure. *This gradual filling and emptying helps restore the bladder's muscle tone.*

Implementation

• Wash your hands. Assemble the equipment at the patient's bedside. Explain the procedure to the patient, and tell him that he may feel slight discomfort. Tell him that you'll check him periodically during the first 8 to 24 hours after catheter removal *to make sure he resumes voiding.* Provide adequate privacy.
• Put on gloves. Attach the syringe to the luer-lock mechanism on the catheter.
• Pull back on the plunger of the syringe. *This deflates the balloon by aspirating the fluid injected at the time of*

catheter insertion. The amount of fluid injected is usually indicated on the tip of the catheter's balloon lumen—it should also be noted on the Kardex and the patient's chart.

• Grasp the catheter with the absorbent cotton and gently pull it from the urethra. Before doing so, offer the patient a bedpan *because catheter removal typically creates a desire to void*.
• Measure and record the amount of urine in the collection bag before discarding it.

Special considerations
Encourage fluid intake *to stimulate urine production, dilute the urine, and help decrease the patient's discomfort when he begins voiding*.

Within 24 hours, the patient should be voiding normally (300 to 400 ml at a time), depending on fluid intake. If he's voiding small amounts (30 to 100 ml every 30 minutes to 1 hour), he's not emptying his bladder completely. Report this to the doctor. He may order a post-voiding catheterization *to remove residual urine*.

After catheter removal, assess the patient for incontinence (or dribbling), urgency, persistent dysuria or bladder spasms, fever, chills, or palpable bladder distention. Report any such findings to the doctor.

Complications
Major complications in removing an indwelling catheter are failure of the balloon to deflate and rupture of the balloon. If the balloon ruptures, cystoscopy is usually performed to ensure removal of any balloon fragments.

Documentation
For bladder retraining, record the date and time the catheter was clamped, the time it was released, and the volume and appearance of the urine. For catheter removal, record the date and time the catheter was removed and the patient's tolerance for the procedure. Record when and how much the patient voided after catheter removal and any problems associated with voiding.

SURGICAL URINARY DIVERSION
Care of nephrostomy and cystostomy tubes

Two urinary diversion techniques—nephrostomy and cystostomy—ensure adequate drainage from the kidneys or bladder and help prevent urinary tract infection or kidney failure. (See *Urinary diversion techniques*, page 438.)

A nephrostomy tube drains urine directly from a kidney when a disorder inhibits the normal flow of urine. The tube is usually placed percutaneously, though sometimes it is surgically inserted through the renal cortex and medulla into the renal pelvis from a lateral incision in the flank. The usual indication is obstructive disease, such as calculi in the ureter or ureteropelvic junction, or an obstructing tumor. Draining urine with a nephrostomy tube also allows kidney tissue damaged by obstructive disease to heal.

A cystostomy tube drains urine from the bladder, diverting it from the urethra. This type of tube is used after certain gynecologic procedures, bladder surgery, prostatectomy, and for severe urethral strictures or traumatic injury. Inserted about 2″ (5 cm) above the symphysis pubis, a cystostomy tube may be used alone or with an indwelling urethral catheter.

Equipment
For dressing changes: 4″ × 4″ gauze pads ■ povidone-iodine solution or povidone-iodine sponges ■ sterile cup or emesis basin ■ paper bag ■ linen-saver pad ■ clean gloves (for dressing removal) ■ sterile gloves (for new dressing) ■ forceps ■ precut 4″ × 4″ drain dressings or transparent semipermeable dressings ■ adhesive tape (preferably hypoallergenic).

For nephrostomy-tube irrigation: 3-ml syringe ■ alcohol sponge or povidone-iodine sponge ■ normal saline solution ■ optional: hemostat.

Commercially prepared sterile dressing kits and povidone-iodine sponges may be available.

Preparation of equipment
Wash your hands and assemble all equipment at the patient's bedside. Open several packages of gauze pads, place them in the sterile cup or emesis basin, and pour the povidone-iodine solution over them. Or open several packages of povidone-iodine sponges. If you're using a commercially packaged dressing kit, open it using aseptic technique. Fill the cup with antiseptic solution.

Open the paper bag and place it away from the other equipment *to avoid contaminating the sterile field*.

Implementation
• Wash your hands, provide privacy, and explain the procedure to the patient.

To change a dressing
• Help the patient to lie on his back (for a cystostomy tube) or the side opposite the tube (for a nephrostomy

Urinary diversion techniques

Nephrostomy and cystostomy can be used to create permanent diversion, to relieve obstruction from an inoperable tumor, or to provide an outlet for urine after cystectomy. Temporary diversion can relieve obstruction from a calculus or ureteral edema. In *cystostomy*, a catheter is inserted percutaneously through the suprapubic area into the bladder. In *nephrostomy*, a catheter is inserted percutaneously through the flank into the renal pelvis.

Cystostomy

Nephrostomy

tube) *so you can see the tube clearly and change the dressing more easily.*
• Place the linen-saver pad under the patient *to absorb excess drainage and keep him dry.*
• Put on the clean gloves. Carefully remove the tape around the tube, and then remove the wet or soiled dressing. Discard the tape and dressing in the paper bag. Remove the gloves and discard them in the bag.
• Put on the sterile gloves. Pick up a saturated pad or dip a dry one into the cup of antiseptic solution.
• To clean the wound, wipe only once with each pad or sponge, moving from the insertion site outward. Discard the used pad or sponge in the paper bag. Don't touch the bag *to avoid contaminating your gloves.*
• Pick up a sterile 4″ × 4″ drain dressing and place it around the tube. If necessary, overlap two drain dressings *to provide maximum absorption.* Or, depending on your hospital's policy, apply a transparent semipermeable dressing over the site and tubing *to allow observation of the site without removing the dressing.*
• Use hypoallergenic tape *to secure the dressing.* Then tape the tube to the patient's lateral abdomen *to prevent tension on the tube.* (See *Taping a nephrostomy tube.*)
• Dispose of all equipment appropriately. Clean the patient as necessary.

To irrigate a nephrostomy tube
• Fill the 3-ml syringe with the normal saline solution.
• Clean the junction of the nephrostomy tube and drainage tube with the alcohol sponge or povidone-iodine sponge, and disconnect the tubes.
• Insert the syringe into the nephrostomy tube opening, and instill 2 to 3 ml of saline solution into the tube.
• Slowly aspirate the solution back into the syringe. *To avoid damaging the renal pelvis tissue,* never pull back forcefully on the plunger.
• If the solution doesn't return, remove the syringe from the tube and reattach it to the drainage tubing *to allow the solution to drain by gravity.*
• Dispose of all equipment appropriately.

Special considerations
Change dressings once a day or more often if needed.
♦ *Nursing alert.* Never irrigate a nephrostomy tube with more than 5 ml of solution *because the capacity of the renal pelvis is usually between 4 and 8 ml.* (Remember: The purpose of irrigation is to keep the tube patent, not to lavage the renal pelvis.) ♦

When necessary, irrigate a cystostomy tube as you would an indwelling catheter. Be sure to perform the irrigation gently *to avoid damaging any suture lines.*

Check a nephrostomy tube frequently for kinks or obstructions. Kinks are likely to occur if the patient lies on the insertion site. Suspect an obstruction when the amount of urine in the drainage bag decreases or the amount of urine around the insertion site increases. Pres-

Taping a nephrostomy tube

To tape a nephrostomy tube directly to the skin, cut a wide piece of hypoallergenic adhesive tape twice lengthwise to its midpoint.

Apply the uncut end of the tape to the skin so that the midpoint meets the tube. Wrap the middle strip around the tube in spiral fashion. Tape the other two strips to the patient's skin on both sides of the tube.

For greater security, repeat this step with a second piece of tape, applying it in the reverse direction. You may also apply two more strips of tape perpendicular to and over the first two pieces.

In any case, always apply another strip of tape lower down on the tube in the direction of the drainage tube to further anchor the tube. Don't put tension on any sutures that prevent tube dislocation.

sure created by urine backing up in the tube can damage nephrons. Gently curve a cystostomy tube *to prevent kinks*.

If a blood clot or mucus plug obstructs a nephrostomy or cystostomy tube, try milking the tube *to restore its patency*. With your nondominant hand, hold the tube securely above the obstruction *to avoid pulling the tube out of the incision*. Then place the flat side of a closed hemostat under the tube, just above the obstruction, pinch the tube against the hemostat, and slide both your finger and the hemostat toward you, away from the patient.

Typically, cystostomy tubes for postoperative urologic patients should be checked hourly for 24 hours *to ensure adequate drainage and tube patency*. To check tube patency,

note the amount of urine in the drainage bag and check the patient's bladder for distention.

Home care

Tell the home care patient that he must clean the insertion site with soap and water, check for skin breakdown, and change the dressing daily; then show him how to take these steps. Also teach him how to change the leg bag or drainage bag. He can use a leg bag during the day and a larger drainage bag at night.

Stress the importance of reporting to the doctor signs of infection (red skin or white, yellow, or green drainage at the insertion site) or tube displacement (drainage that smells like urine).

Whether he uses a drainage bag or larger container, explain that he must wash the device daily with a 1:3 vinegar and water solution, rinse it with plain water, and dry it on a clothes hanger or over the towel rack. *This prevents crystalline buildup.*

Complications
The patient has an increased risk of infection because nephrostomy and cystostomy tubes provide a direct opening to the kidneys and bladder.

Documentation
Describe the color and amount of drainage from the nephrostomy or cystostomy tube, and record any color changes as they occur.

Similarly, if the patient has more than one tube, describe the drainage (color, amount, and character) from each tube separately. If irrigation is necessary, record the amount and type of irrigant used and whether or not you obtained a complete return.

Care of a urinary diversion stoma

Urinary diversions provide an alternative route for urine flow when a disorder, such as an invasive bladder tumor, impedes normal drainage. A permanent urinary diversion is indicated in any condition that requires a total cystectomy. In conditions requiring temporary urinary drainage or diversion, a suprapubic or urethral catheter is usually inserted to divert the flow of urine temporarily. The catheter remains in place until the incision heals.

Urinary diversions may also be indicated for patients with neurogenic bladder, congenital anomaly, traumatic injury to the lower urinary tract, or severe chronic urinary tract infection.

Three types of permanent urinary diversions can be created: ureterostomy, ileal conduit, and continent urinary diversion. (See *Types of permanent urinary diversion.*) Most require the patient to wear a urine-collection appliance and to care for the stoma created during surgery.

Equipment
Soap and warm water ■ waste receptacle (such as an impervious or wax-coated bag) ■ linen-saver pad ■ nonallergenic paper tape ■ povidone-iodine sponges ■ urine collection container ■ rubber catheter (usually #14 or #16 French) ■ ruler ■ scissors ■ urine-collection appliance (with or without antireflux valve) ■ graduated cylinder ■ cottonless gauze pads (some rolled, some flat) ■ washcloth ■ skin barrier in liquid, paste, wafer, or sheet form ■ appliance belt ■ stoma covering (nonadherent gauze pad or panty liner) ■ two pairs of gloves ■ optional: adhesive solvent, irrigating syringe, tampon, hair dryer, electric razor, regular gauze pads, vinegar, deodorant tablets.

Commercially packaged stoma care kits are available.

In place of soap and water, you can use adhesive remover pads, if available, or cotton gauze saturated with adhesive solvent.

Some appliances come with a semipermeable skin barrier (impermeable to liquid but permeable to vapor and oxygen, which is essential for maintaining skin integrity). Wafer-type barriers may offer more protection against irritation than adhesive appliances. For example, a carbon-zinc barrier is economical and easy to apply. Its puttylike consistency allows it to be rolled between the palms to form a "washer" that can encircle the base of the stoma. This barrier can withstand enzymes, acids, and other damaging discharge material. All semipermeable barriers are easily removed along with the adhesive, causing less damage to the skin.

Preparation of equipment
Assemble all the equipment on the patient's overbed table. Tape the waste receptacle to the table for ready access. Provide privacy for the patient, and wash your hands. Measure the diameter of the stoma with a ruler. Cut the opening of the appliance with the scissors—it shouldn't be more than 1/16″ to 1/8″ larger than the diameter of the stoma. Moisten the faceplate of the appliance with a small amount of solvent or water *to prepare it for adhesion.* Performing these preliminary steps at the bedside *allows you to demonstrate the procedure and show the patient that it's not difficult, which will help him relax.*

Implementation
● Wash your hands again. Explain the procedure to the patient as you go along, and offer constant reinforcement and reassurance *to counteract negative reactions that may be elicited by stoma care.*
● Place the bed in a low Fowler's position so the patient's abdomen is flat. *This position eliminates skin folds that could cause the appliance to slip or irritate the skin and allows the patient to observe or participate.*
● Put on the gloves and place the linen-saver pad under the patient's side, near the stoma. Open the drain valve of the appliance being replaced *to empty the urine into the graduated cylinder.* Then, *to remove the appliance,* apply soap and water or adhesive solvent as you gently push the skin back from the pouch. If the appliance is disposable, discard it into the waste receptacle. If it's reus-

Types of permanent urinary diversion

The types of permanent urinary diversion with stomas include ureterostomy, ileal conduit, and continent urinary diversion.

Ureterostomy

A stoma or stomas are formed when ureters are diverted to the abdominal wall or flank. There are five different types of ureterostomy:

• *Flank loop ureterostomy:* Ureters loop as they are brought to the skin surface, forming a stoma.

• *Double-barrel ureterostomy:* Both ureters are brought to the skin surface to form side-by-side stomas.

• *Transureteroureterostomy:* One ureter is anastomosed to the other, which is then brought to the skin surface to form a stoma.

• *Bilateral ureterostomy:* Both ureters are brought to the skin surface to form stomas.

• *Unilateral ureterostomy:* One ureter is brought to the skin surface to form a stoma.

Ileal conduit

A segment of the ileum is excised, and the two ends of the ileum that result from excision of the segment are sutured closed. Then the ureters are dissected from the bladder and anastomosed to the ileal segment. One end of the ileal segment is closed with sutures; the opposite end is brought through the abdominal wall, thereby forming a stoma.

Continent urinary diversion

A tube is formed from part of the bladder wall. One end of the tube is brought to the skin to form the stoma. At the internal end of this tube, a nipple valve is created from the bladder wall so urine won't drain out unless a catheter is inserted through the stoma into the bladder pouch. The urethral neck is sutured closed.

Flank loop ureterostomy

Double-barrel ureterostomy

Transureteroureterostomy

Bilateral ureterostomy

Unilateral ureterostomy

Ileal conduit

Continent urinary diversion

Wicking urine from a stoma

Use a piece of rolled, cottonless gauze or a tampon to wick urine from a stoma. Working by capillary action, wicking absorbs urine while you prepare the patient's skin to hold a urine-collection appliance.

able, clean it with soap and lukewarm water and let it air-dry.

♦ *Nursing alert. To avoid irritating the patient's stoma,* avoid touching it with adhesive solvent. If adhesive remains on the skin, gently rub it off with a dry gauze pad. Discard used gauze pads in the waste receptacle. ♦

• *To prevent a constant flow of urine onto the skin while you're changing the appliance,* wick the urine with an absorbent, lint-free material. (See *Wicking urine from a stoma.*)

• Use water to carefully wash off any crystal deposits that may have formed around the stoma. If urine has stagnated and has a strong odor, use soap to wash it off. Be sure to rinse thoroughly *to remove any oily residue that could cause the appliance to slip.*

• Follow hospital skin care protocol to treat any minor skin problems.

• Dry the peristomal area thoroughly with a gauze pad *because moisture will keep the appliance from sticking.* Use a hair dryer if you wish. Remove any hair from the area with scissors or an electric razor *to prevent hair follicles*

from becoming irritated when the pouch is removed, which can cause folliculitis.

• Inspect the stoma *to see if it's healing properly and to detect complications.* Check the color and the appearance of the suture line, and examine any moisture or effluent. Inspect the peristomal skin for redness, irritation, and intactness.

• Apply the skin barrier. If you apply a wafer or sheet, cut it to fit over the stoma. Remove any protective backing and set the barrier aside with the adhesive side up. If you apply a liquid barrier (such as Skin-Prep), saturate a gauze pad with it and coat the peristomal skin. Move in concentric circles outward from the stoma until you've covered an area 2″ (5 cm) larger than the wafer. Let the skin dry for several minutes — it should feel tacky. Gently press the wafer around the stoma, sticky side down, smoothing from the stoma outward.

• If you're using a barrier paste, open the tube, squeeze out a small amount, and then discard it. Then squeeze a ribbon of paste directly onto the peristomal skin about ½″ (1.3 cm) from the stoma, making a complete circle. Make several more concentric circles outward. Dip your fingers into lukewarm water, and smooth the paste until the skin is completely covered from the edge of the stoma to 3″ to 4″ (7.6 to 10.2 cm) outward. The paste should be ¼″ to ½″ (0.6 to 1.3 cm) thick. Then discard the gloves, wash your hands, and put on new gloves.

• Remove the material used for wicking urine, and place it in the waste receptacle.

• Now place the appliance over the stoma, leaving only a small amount (⅜″ to ¾″ [1 to 2 cm]) of skin exposed.

• Secure the faceplate of the appliance to the skin with paper tape, if recommended. To do this, place a piece of tape lengthwise on each edge of the faceplate so that the tape overlaps onto the skin.

• Apply the appliance belt. Be sure that it's on a level with the stoma. *Applied above or below the stoma, the belt can break the bag's seal, or it can rub or injure the stoma.* The belt should be loose enough for you to insert two fingers between the skin and the belt. *If the belt is too tight, it can irritate the skin or cause internal damage.*

• Dispose of the used materials appropriately.

Special considerations

The patient's attitude toward his urinary diversion stoma plays a big part in determining how well he'll adjust to it. *To encourage a positive attitude,* help him get used to the idea of caring for his stoma and the appliance as though they are natural extensions of himself. When teaching him to perform the procedure, give him written instructions and provide positive reinforcement after he completes each step. Suggest that he perform the procedure in the morning when urine flows most slowly.

Caring for the patient with a continent urinary diversion

In this procedure, an alternative to the traditional ileal conduit, a pouch created from the ascending colon and the terminal ileum serves as a new bladder, which empties through a stoma. To drain urine continuously, several drains are inserted into this reconstructed bladder and left in place for 3 to 6 weeks until the new stoma heals. The patient will be discharged from the hospital with the drains in place. He will return to have them removed and to learn how to catheterize his stoma.

During first hospitalization
• Immediately after surgery, monitor intake and output from each drain. Be alert for decreased output, which may indicate that urine flow is obstructed.
• Watch for common postoperative complications, such as infection or bleeding. Also watch for signs of urinary leakage, which include increased abdominal pain, decreased urine output from the drains, increased abdominal distention, and urine appearing around the drains or midline incision.
• Irrigate the drains as ordered.
• Clean the area around the drains daily—first with povidone-iodine solution and then with sterile water. Apply a dry sterile dressing to the area. Use precut 4″ × 4″ drain dressings around the drain *to absorb leakage.*
• *To increase the patient's mobility and comfort,* connect the drains to a leg bag.

During second hospitalization
• After the patient's drains are removed, teach the patient how to catheterize the stoma. Begin by gathering the following equipment on a clean towel: rubber catheter (usually #14 or #16 French), water-soluble lubricant, washcloth, stoma covering (nonadherent gauze pad or panty liner), nonallergenic adhesive tape, and an irrigating syringe (optional).
• Apply water-soluble lubricant to the catheter tip *to facilitate insertion.*

• Remove and discard the stoma cover. Using the washcloth, clean the stoma and the area around it, starting at the stoma and working outward in a circular motion.
• Hold the urine-collection container under the catheter; then slowly insert the catheter into the stoma. Urine should begin to flow into the container. If it doesn't, gently rotate the catheter or redirect its angle. If the catheter drains slowly, it may be plugged with mucus. Irrigate with sterile saline solution or sterile water *to clear it.* When the flow stops, pinch the catheter closed and remove it.
• Dry the skin if necessary. Apply a sterile gauze pad over the stoma *to keep it clean,* and secure the pad with tape. Alternatively, secure a panty liner to the patient's underwear.

Home care
• Teach the patient how to care for the drains and their insertion sites during the 3 to 6 weeks he'll be at home before their removal, and teach him how to attach them to a leg bag. Also teach him to recognize the signs of infection and obstruction.
• After the drains are removed, teach the patient how to empty the pouch, and direct him to do so on a schedule. Initially, he should catheterize the stoma and empty the pouch every 2 to 3 hours. Later, he should catheterize every 4 hours while awake and also irrigate the pouch each morning and evening. Instruct him to empty the pouch whenever he feels a sensation of fullness.
• Tell the patient that catheters are reusable, but only after they are cleaned. He should clean the catheter thoroughly with warm, soapy water, rinse it thoroughly, and hang it to dry over a clean towel. He should store cleaned and dried catheters in plastic bags. Tell him he can reuse catheters for up to 1 month before discarding them. However, he should immediately discard any catheter that becomes discolored or cracked.

Help the patient choose between disposable and reusable appliances by telling him the advantages and disadvantages of each. Emphasize the importance of correct placement and of a well-fitted appliance *to prevent seepage of urine onto the skin.* When positioned correctly, most appliances remain in place for at least 3 days and for as long as 5 days if no leakage occurs. After 5 days, the appliance should be changed. With the improved adhesives and pouches available, belts aren't always necessary.

Because urine flows constantly, it accumulates quickly, becoming even heavier than stools. *To prevent the weight of the urine from loosening the seal around the stoma and separating the appliance from the skin,* tell the patient to empty the appliance through the drain valve when it is one-third to one-half full.

Instruct the patient to connect his appliance to a urine-collection container before he goes to sleep. *The continuous flow of urine into the container during the night prevents the urine from accumulating and stagnating in the appliance.*

Teach the patient sanitary and dietary measures that can protect the peristomal skin and control the odor that commonly results from alkaline urine, infection, or poor hygiene. Reusable appliances should be washed with soap and lukewarm water, then air-dried thoroughly *to prevent brittleness.* Soaking the appliance in vinegar and water or placing deodorant tablets in it can further dissipate stubborn odors. An acid-ash diet that includes ascorbic acid and cranberry juice may raise urinary acidity, thereby reducing bacterial action and fermentation (the underlying causes of odor). Generous fluid intake also helps to reduce odors by diluting the urine.

If the patient has a continent urinary diversion, be sure you know how to meet his special needs. (See *Caring for the patient with a continent urinary diversion,* page 443.)

Tell the patient about ostomy clubs and the American Cancer Society. Members of these organizations routinely visit hospitals to explain ostomy care and the types of appliances available and to help patients learn to function normally with a stoma.

Home care
The patient or a family member can learn to care for a urinary diversion stoma at home. However, the patient's emotional adjustment to the stoma must be given special consideration before he can be expected to maintain it properly. Arrange for a visiting nurse or an enterostomal therapist to assist the patient at home.

Complications
Because intestinal mucosa is delicate, an ill-fitting appliance can cause bleeding. This is especially likely with an ileal conduit, the most common urinary diversion stoma, *because a segment of the intestine forms the conduit.*

Peristomal skin may become reddened or excoriated from too-frequent changing or improper placement of the appliance, poor skin care, or allergic reaction to the appliance or adhesive. Constant leakage around the appliance can result from improper placement of the appliance or from poor skin turgor.

Documentation
Record the appearance and color of the stoma and whether it's inverted, flush with the skin, or protruding. If it protrudes, note by how much it protrudes above the skin. (The normal range is ½″ to ¾″ [1.3 to 2 cm].) Record the appearance and condition of the peristomal skin, noting any redness or irritation or complaints by the patient of itching or burning.

Document the patient's adjustment to the stoma, and note his participation in stoma care and application of the appliance.

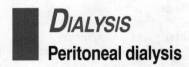

DIALYSIS
Peritoneal dialysis

In patients with acute or chronic renal failure, peritoneal dialysis performs the kidneys' function of removing impurities from the blood. Dialysate—the solution instilled into the peritoneal cavity by a catheter—draws waste products, excess fluid, and electrolytes from the blood across the semipermeable peritoneal membrane. (See *Principles of peritoneal dialysis*.) After a prescribed period, the dialysate is drained from the peritoneal cavity, removing impurities with it. The dialysis procedure is then repeated, using a new dialysate each time, until waste removal is complete and fluid, electrolyte, and acid-base balance have been restored.

The catheter is inserted in the operating room or at the patient's bedside with a nurse assisting. With special preparation, the nurse may perform dialysis, either manually or using an automatic or semiautomatic cycle machine. (Or, in some cases, she may assist the patient with continuous ambulatory peritoneal dialysis.)

Equipment
For catheter placement and dialysis: prescribed dialysate (in 1- or 2-liter bottles or bags, as ordered) ■ warmer, heating pad, or water bath ■ at least three face masks ■ medication, such as heparin, if ordered ■ dialysis administration set with drainage bag ■ two pairs of sterile gloves ■ I.V. pole ■ fenestrated sterile drape ■ vial of 1% or 2% lidocaine ■ povidone-iodine pads ■ 3-ml syringe with 25G 1″ needle ■ scalpel (with #11 blade) ■ ordered type of multi-eyed, nylon, peritoneal catheter (see *Comparing peritoneal dialysis catheters,* page 446) ■ peritoneal stylet ■ sutures or nonallergenic tape ■ povidone-iodine solution (for doctor to prepare abdomen) ■ precut drain dressings ■ protective cap for catheter ■ small, sterile plastic clamp ■ 4″×4″ gauze pads ■ optional: 10-ml syringe with 22G 1½″ needle, protein or potassium supplement, specimen container, label, laboratory request form.

For dressing changes: one pair of sterile gloves ■ ten sterile cotton-tipped applicators or sterile 2″×2″ gauze pads ■ povidone-iodine ointment ■ two precut drain dress-

Principles of peritoneal dialysis

Peritoneal dialysis works by a combination of diffusion and osmosis.

Diffusion

In this process, particles move through a semipermeable membrane from an area of high concentration to an area of low concentration.

In peritoneal dialysis, the water-based dialysate being infused contains glucose, sodium chloride, calcium, magnesium, acetate or lactate, and no waste products. Therefore, the waste products and excess electrolytes in the blood cross through the semipermeable peritoneal membrane into the dialysate. Removing the waste-filled dialysate and replacing it with fresh solution keeps the waste concentration low and encourages further diffusion. Potassium may be added occasionally to maintain serum levels of this element. However, because failing kidneys can't excrete potassium, levels must be monitored closely and adjusted as needed.

Osmosis

In this process, fluids move through a semipermeable membrane from an area of low-solute concentration to an area of high-solute concentration. In peritoneal dialysis, osmosis removes excess water from the patient's blood. Dextrose in the dialysate encourages fluid movement by giving the dialysate a higher solute-particle concentration than the blood.

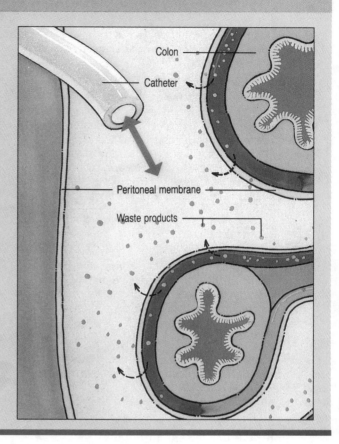

ings ■ adhesive tape ■ povidone-iodine solution or normal saline solution ■ two sterile 4″ × 4″ gauze pads.

All equipment must be sterile. Commercially packaged dialysis kits or trays are available and contain all the equipment needed for catheter placement and dressing changes.

Preparation of equipment

Bring all equipment to the patient's bedside. Make sure the dialysate is at body temperature. *This decreases patient discomfort during the procedure and reduces vasoconstriction of the peritoneal capillaries. Dilated capillaries enhance blood flow to the peritoneal membrane surface, increasing waste clearance into the peritoneal cavity.* To warm the solution, place the container in a warmer or wrap it in a heating pad set at 105° F (40.6° C) for 30 to 60 minutes. You can also place the container in a water bath at 98.6° to 100.4° F (37° to 38° C) for 30 to 60 minutes.

Implementation

• Explain the procedure to the patient. Weigh him and record his vital signs *to establish baseline levels.*

For catheter placement and dialysis

• Have the patient try to urinate. *This reduces the risk of bladder perforation during insertion of the peritoneal catheter and also reduces patient discomfort.* If he can't urinate, and if you suspect that his bladder isn't empty, obtain an order for straight catheterization *to empty his bladder.*
• Place the patient in the supine position, and have him put on one of the sterile face masks.
• Wash your hands.
• Inspect the warmed dialysate, which should appear clear and colorless.
• Put on a sterile face mask. Prepare to add any prescribed medication to the dialysate, using strict aseptic technique *to avoid contaminating the solution.* Commonly,

Comparing peritoneal dialysis catheters

The first step in any type of peritoneal dialysis is insertion of a catheter to allow instillation of dialyzing solution. The surgeon may insert one of three different catheters described below.

Tenckhoff catheter

To implant a Tenckhoff catheter, the surgeon inserts the first 6¾″ (17 cm) of the catheter into the patient's abdomen. The next 2¾″ (7-cm) segment, which may have a Dacron cuff at one or both ends, is imbedded subcutaneously. Within a few days after insertion, the patient's tissues grow around the cuffs, forming a tight barrier against bacterial infiltration. The remaining 3⅞″ (10 cm) of the catheter extends outside of the abdomen and is equipped with a metal adapter at the tip that connects to dialyzer tubing.

Flanged-collar catheter

To insert this kind of catheter, the surgeon positions its flanged collar just below the dermis so that the device extends through the abdominal wall. He keeps the distal end of the cuff from extending into the peritoneum, where it could cause adhesions.

Column-disk peritoneal catheter

To insert a column-disk peritoneal catheter (CDPC), the surgeon rolls up the flexible disk section of the implant, inserts it into the peritoneal cavity, and retracts it against the abdominal wall. The implant's first cuff rests just outside the peritoneal membrane, while its second cuff rests just beneath the skin. Because the CDPC doesn't float freely in the peritoneal cavity, it keeps inflowing dialyzing solution from being directed at the sensitive organs—which increases patient comfort during dialysis.

---

heparin is added *to prevent accumulation of fibrin in the catheter.*
• Prepare the dialysis administration set. (See *Setup for peritoneal dialysis.*)
• Close the clamps on all lines. Place the drainage bag below the patient *to facilitate gravity drainage,* and connect the drainage line to it. Connect the dialysate infusion lines to the bottles or bags of dialysate. Hang the bottles or bags on the I.V. pole at the patient's bedside. *To prime the tubing,* open the infusion lines and allow the solution to flow until all lines are primed. Then close all clamps.
• At this point, the doctor puts on a mask and a pair of sterile gloves. He cleans the patient's abdomen with povidone-iodine solution and drapes it with a sterile drape.

• Wipe the stopper of the lidocaine vial with povidone-iodine and allow it to dry. Invert the vial and hand it to the doctor so he can withdraw the lidocaine, using the 3-ml syringe with the 25G 1″ needle.

• The doctor anesthetizes a small area of the patient's abdomen below the umbilicus. He then makes a small incision with the scalpel, inserts the catheter into the peritoneal cavity — using the stylet to guide the catheter — and sutures or tapes the catheter in place.

• Connect the catheter to the administration set, using strict aseptic technique *to prevent contamination of the catheter and the solution, which could cause peritonitis.*

• Open the drain dressing and the 4″ × 4″ gauze pad packages. Put on the other pair of sterile gloves. Apply the precut drain dressings around the catheter. Cover them with the gauze pads and tape them securely.

• Unclamp the lines to the patient. Rapidly instill 500 ml of dialysate into the peritoneal cavity *to test the catheter's patency.*

• Clamp the lines to the patient. Immediately unclamp the lines to the drainage bag *to allow fluid to drain into the bag.* Outflow should be brisk.

• Having established the catheter's patency, clamp the lines to the drainage bag and unclamp the lines to the patient *to infuse the prescribed volume of solution over a period of 5 to 10 minutes.* As soon as the dialysate container empties, clamp the lines to the patient immediately *to prevent air from entering the tubing.*

• Allow the solution to dwell in the peritoneal cavity for the prescribed time (10 minutes to 4 hours). *This lets excess fluid, electrolytes, and accumulated wastes move from the blood through the peritoneal membrane and into the dialysate.*

• Warm the solution for the next infusion.

• At the end of the prescribed dwell time, unclamp the line to the drainage bag and allow the solution to drain from the peritoneal cavity into the drainage bag.

• Repeat the infusion-dwell-drain cycle immediately after outflow until the prescribed number of fluid exchanges have been completed.

• If the doctor or hospital policy requires a dialysate specimen, you'll usually collect one after every 10 infusion-dwell-drain cycles (*always* during the drain phase), after every 24-hour period, or as ordered. To do this, attach the 10-ml syringe to the 22G 1½″ needle and insert it into the injection port on the drainage line, using strict aseptic technique, and aspirate the drainage sample. Transfer the sample to the specimen container, label it appropriately, and send it to the laboratory with a laboratory request form.

• After completing the prescribed number of exchanges, clamp the catheter, and put on sterile gloves. Disconnect the administration set from the peritoneal catheter. Place

Setup for peritoneal dialysis

the sterile protective cap over the catheter's distal end. (Or the doctor may remove the catheter and place a Deane's prosthesis in its place *to maintain the patency of the tract and to simplify reinsertion of the catheter for the next dialysis treatment.*)

• Dispose of all used equipment appropriately.

Dressing changes

• Explain the procedure to the patient and wash your hands.

• If necessary, carefully remove the old dressings *to avoid putting tension on the catheter and accidentally dislodging it and to avoid introducing bacteria into the tract through movement of the catheter.*

• Put on the sterile gloves.

• Saturate the sterile applicators or the 2″ × 2″ gauze pads with povidone-iodine, and clean the skin around the catheter, moving in concentric circles from the catheter site outward. Remove any crusted material carefully.
• Inspect the catheter site for drainage and the tissue around the site for redness and swelling.
• Apply povidone-iodine ointment to the catheter site with a sterile gauze pad.
• Place two precut drain dressings around the catheter site. Tape the 4″ × 4″ gauze pads over them to secure the dressing.

Special considerations

During and after dialysis, monitor the patient and his response to treatment. Peritoneal dialysis is usually contraindicated in patients who have had extensive abdominal or bowel surgery or extensive abdominal trauma.

Monitor the patient's vital signs every 10 to 15 minutes for the first 1 to 2 hours of exchanges, then every 2 to 4 hours, or more frequently if necessary. Notify the doctor of any abrupt changes in the patient's condition.

To reduce the risk of peritonitis, use strict aseptic technique during catheter insertion, dialysis, and dressing changes. Masks should be worn by all personnel in the room whenever the dialysis system is opened or entered. Change the dressing at least every 24 hours or whenever it becomes wet or soiled. Frequent dressing changes will also help prevent skin excoriation from any leakage.

To prevent respiratory distress, position the patient for maximal lung expansion. Promote lung expansion through turning and deep-breathing exercises.
◆ *Nursing alert.* If the patient suffers severe respiratory distress during the dwell phase of dialysis, drain the peritoneal cavity and notify the doctor. Monitor any patient on peritoneal dialysis who's being weaned from a ventilator. ◆

To prevent protein depletion, the doctor may order a high-protein diet or a protein supplement. He will also monitor serum albumin levels.

Dialysate is available in three concentrations — 4.25% dextrose, 2.5% dextrose, and 1.5% dextrose. The 4.25% solution usually removes the largest amount of fluid from the blood because its glucose concentration is highest. If your patient receives this concentrated solution, monitor him carefully *to prevent excess fluid loss.* Also, some of the glucose in the 4.25% solution may enter the patient's bloodstream, causing hyperglycemia severe enough to require an insulin injection or an insulin addition to the dialysate.

Patients with low serum potassium levels may require the addition of potassium to the dialysate solution *to prevent further losses.*

Monitor fluid volume balance, blood pressure, and pulse *to help prevent fluid imbalance.* Assess fluid balance at the end of each infusion-dwell-drain cycle. Fluid balance is positive if less than the amount infused was recovered; it's negative if more than the amount infused was recovered. Notify the doctor if the patient retains 500 ml or more of fluid for three consecutive cycles or if he loses at least 1 liter of fluid for three consecutive cycles.

Weigh the patient daily *to help you determine how much fluid is being removed during dialysis treatment.* Note the time and any variations in the weighing technique next to his weight on his chart.

If inflow and outflow are slow or absent, check the tubing for kinks. You can also try raising the I.V. pole or repositioning the patient *to increase the inflow rate.* Repositioning the patient or applying manual pressure to the lateral aspects of the patient's abdomen may also help increase drainage. If these maneuvers fail, notify the doctor. Improper positioning of the catheter or an accumulation of fibrin may obstruct the catheter.

Always examine outflow fluid (effluent) for color and clarity. Normally it's clear or pale yellow, but pink-tinged effluent may appear during the first three or four cycles. If the effluent remains pink-tinged, or if it's grossly bloody, suspect bleeding into the peritoneal cavity and notify the doctor. Also notify the doctor if the outflow contains feces, which suggests bowel perforation, or if it's cloudy, which suggests peritonitis. Obtain a sample for culture and Gram stain. Send the sample in a labeled specimen container to the laboratory with a laboratory request form.

Patient discomfort at the start of the procedure is normal. If the patient experiences pain during the procedure, determine when it occurs, its quality and duration, and whether it radiates to other body parts. Then notify the doctor. Pain during infusion usually results from a dialysate that's too cool or acidic. Pain may also result from rapid inflow; slowing the inflow rate may reduce the pain. Severe, diffuse pain with rebound tenderness and cloudy effluent may indicate peritoneal infection. Pain that radiates to the shoulder often results from air accumulation under the diaphragm. Severe, persistent perineal or rectal pain can result from improper catheter placement.

The patient undergoing peritoneal dialysis will require a great deal of assistance in his daily care. *To minimize his discomfort,* perform daily care during a drain phase in the cycle, when the patient's abdomen is less distended.

Complications

Peritonitis, the most common complication, usually follows contamination of the dialysate, but it may develop if solution leaks from the catheter exit site and flows back into the catheter tract.

Protein depletion may result from the diffusion of protein in the blood into the dialysate solution through the peritoneal membrane. As much as ½ oz (15 g) of protein may be lost daily — more in patients with peritonitis.

Respiratory distress may result when dialysate in the peritoneal cavity increases pressure on the diaphragm, which decreases lung expansion.

Constipation is a major cause of inflow-outflow problems; therefore, *to ensure regular bowel movements,* give a laxative or stool softener, as needed.

Excessive fluid loss from the use of 4.25% solution may cause hypovolemia, hypotension, and shock. Excessive fluid retention may lead to blood volume expansion, hypertension, peripheral edema, and even pulmonary edema and congestive heart failure.

Other possible complications include electrolyte imbalance and hyperglycemia, which can be identified by frequent blood tests.

Documentation

Record the amount of dialysate infused and drained, any medications added to the solution, and the color and character of effluent. Also record the patient's daily weight and fluid balance.

Use a peritoneal dialysis flowchart to compute total fluid balance after each exchange. Note the patient's vital signs and tolerance of the treatment and other pertinent observations.

Selected references

Heneghan, G., et al. "The Indiana Pouch: A Continent Urinary Diversion," *Journal of Enterostomal Therapy* 17(6):231-36, November-December 1990.

Illustrated Manual of Nursing Practice, 2nd ed. Springhouse, Pa.: Springhouse Corp., 1994.

Norris, M. "Action Stat! Dialysis Disequilibrium Syndrome," *Nursing89* 19(4):33, April 1989.

Rowland, R.G. "Continent Urinary Reservoirs," *Surgical Clinics of North America* 68(5):891-907, October 1988.

Snyder, T.E. "An Exercise Program for Dialysis Patients," *AJN* 89(3):362-64, March 1989.

Ulrich, B.T., ed. *Nephrology Nursing: Concepts and Strategies.* Norwalk, Conn.: Appleton & Lange, 1988.

ORTHOPEDIC CARE

DORI TAYLOR, RN, PhD, CNA

Introduction

Orthopedics began as a specialty for the prevention and treatment of children's musculoskeletal deformities. However, this branch of medicine has expanded dramatically to include the prevention, treatment, and care of musculoskeletal conditions affecting patients of all ages.

The American Nurses' Association defines orthopedic nursing as the diagnosis and treatment of human responses to actual and potential health problems related to musculoskeletal function. More specifically, orthopedic nursing focuses on promoting wellness and self-care and on preventing further injury and illness in patients with degenerative, traumatic, inflammatory, neuromuscular, congenital, metabolic, and oncologic disorders.

Traditionally, orthopedic nurses have needed to operate special mechanical and traction equipment. Today, such nurses need to understand principles of internal and external fixation, prosthetics, orthotics, immobilization, and implantation.

Despite the evolution of complex surgical procedures and mechanical devices that characterize modern orthopedic care, some things remain the same. A patient hospitalized for any orthopedic procedure—whether it's cast application, traction, or arthroplasty—is vulnerable to similar complications, such as:
• joint stiffness and skin breakdown from impaired physical mobility
• fractures from mishandling of osteoporotic extremities
• neurovascular compromise from pressure on major blood vessels and nerves caused by immobilization devices or compartmental edema
• infection of surgical wounds or skeletal pin tracts
• prolonged healing time from failure to observe sound principles of immobilization.

In addition, the patient's level of understanding and effectiveness of coping skills must be assessed.

Consistent care

Without exception, orthopedic complications can be prevented or minimized by appropriate and consistent assessment, monitoring, and therapy. For example, it's essential to assess the orthopedic patient's neurovascular status at regular intervals; otherwise, the signs and symptoms of neurovascular compromise may go undetected until irreversible damage occurs. Consistent or-

thopedic care remains the surest way to promote rapid healing and successful rehabilitation.

Ready for an emergency

Orthopedic nursing care is characterized by the high incidence of emergency procedures that you're likely to perform. The first step—always—in administering emergency care at the scene of an accident is immediate assessment for a life-threatening condition. Do not move the patient unless danger is imminent, because this might worsen the injury and increase pain. If the patient must be moved, assess him for possible spinal injury so that appropriate transfer techniques can be used. After determining that no life-threatening injury exists, conduct an initial head-to-toe assessment, comparing bilaterally where applicable.

Always evaluate neurovascular status. (Check the five P's: pain, pallor, pulse, paresthesia, and paralysis.) Assess the injury thoroughly, and use strict aseptic technique when caring for all open wounds to prevent infection. If you suspect bone injury, apply a splint to reduce injury and immobilize the bone.

In nonemergencies, performing orthopedic procedures correctly can ease pain, prevent further injury, and encourage proper healing.

SUPPORT PROCEDURES
Triangular sling

Made from a triangular piece of muslin, canvas, or cotton, a sling supports and immobilizes an injured arm, wrist, or hand, and thereby facilitates healing. It may be applied to restrict movement of a fracture or dislocation or to support a muscle sprain. A sling can also support the weight of a splint or help secure dressings.

Equipment

Triangular bandage or commercial sling ■ gauze (for padding) ■ safety pins (tape for children under age 7).

Implementation

• Explain the procedure to the patient and wash your hands.
• If the patient is a child, fold the bandage in half *to make a smaller triangle.* Then follow the steps shown in *Making a sling,* page 452.
• If you anticipate prolonged use of a sling, pad the area under the knot with gauze *to prevent skin irritation.* Place

Making a sling

Place the apex of a triangular bandage behind the patient's elbow on the injured side. Hold one end of the bandage so it extends up toward the patient's neck on the uninjured side and let the other end hang straight down. The bandage's long side should parallel the midline of the patient's body (upper left).

Loop the top corner of the bandage over the shoulder on the uninjured side and around the back of the patient's neck. Then bring the lower end of the bandage over the flexed forearm and up to the shoulder on the injured side (upper right).

Adjust the bandage so that the forearm and upper arm form an angle of slightly less than 90 degrees *to increase venous return from the hand and forearm* and *to facilitate drainage from swelling.* Then tie the two bandage ends at the side of the patient's neck, rather than at the back, *to prevent neck flexion and avoid irritation and pressure over a cervical vertebra* (lower left).

Carefully secure the sling with a safety pin above and behind the elbow. See the illustration (lower right). (For a child under age 7, use tape instead of a pin *to avoid the chance of an injury.*)

the sling outside the shirt collar *to reduce direct pressure on the neck and shoulder.*

• If the arm requires complete immobilization, apply a swathe after placing the arm in a sling. (See *Applying a swathe.*) At regular intervals, check to be sure that the sling stays in proper position. Also assess patient comfort and circulation to the fingers.

Special considerations
Before the patient leaves the hospital, provide an extra triangular bandage. Teach him and a family member or friend how to change the sling. If appropriate, instruct him to change the sling regularly *because a soiled sling can cause irritation and infection.* Also, teach him how to check periodically for axillary skin breakdown.

Documentation
In the patient's chart, record the date, time, and location of sling application, and describe the patient's tolerance of the procedure. Also document circulation to the fingers, noting color and temperature.

 ## Clavicle strap

Also called a figure-eight strap, a clavicle strap reduces and immobilizes fractures of the clavicle. It does this by elevating, extending, and supporting the shoulders in position for healing, known as the *position of attention.* A commercially available figure-eight strap or a 4″ elastic bandage may serve as a clavicle strap. This strap is contraindicated for an uncooperative patient.

Equipment
Powder or cornstarch ▪ figure-eight clavicle strap or 4″ elastic bandage ▪ safety pins, if necessary ▪ tape ▪ cotton batting or padding ▪ marking pen ▪ analgesics, as ordered.

Implementation
• Explain the procedure to the patient and provide privacy.
• Help the patient take off his shirt.
• Assess neurovascular integrity by palpating skin temperature; noting the color of the hand and fingers; palpating the radial, ulnar, and brachial pulses bilaterally; and then comparing the affected with the unaffected side. Also, ask the patient about any numbness or tingling distal to the injury, and assess his motor function. Determine the patient's degree of comfort and administer analgesics, as ordered.

Applying a swathe

To further immobilize an arm after applying a sling, wrap a folded triangular bandage or wide elastic bandage around the patient's upper torso and the upper arm on the injured side. Don't cover the patient's uninjured arm. Make the swathe just tight enough to secure the injured arm to the body. Tie or pin the ends of the bandage just in front of the axilla on the uninjured side.

• Demonstrate how to assume the position of attention. Instruct the patient to sit upright and assume the position of attention gradually *to minimize pain.*
• Gently apply powder or cornstarch, as appropriate, to the axillae and shoulder area *to reduce friction from the clavicle strap.* You can use cornstarch if the patient is allergic to powder.

Types of clavicle straps

Clavicle straps provide support to the shoulder to help heal a fractured clavicle. These straps are available ready-made. They can also be made from a bandage.

Commercially made clavicle straps have a short back panel and long straps that extend around the patient's shoulders and axillae. They have Velcro pads or buckles on the ends for easy fastening.

When making a clavicle strap with a wide elastic bandage, start in the middle of the patient's back. After wrapping the bandage around the shoulders, fasten the ends with safety pins.

To apply a figure-eight strap
• Place the apex of the triangle between the scapulae and drape the straps over the shoulders. Bring the strap with the Velcro or buckle end under one axilla and through the loop; then pull the other strap under the other axilla and through the loop. (See *Types of clavicle straps*.)
• Gently adjust the straps so they support the shoulders in the position of attention.
• Bring the straps back under the axillae toward the anterior chest, making sure they maintain the position of attention.

To apply a 4″ elastic bandage
• Roll both ends of the elastic bandage toward the middle, leaving between 12″ and 18″ (30.5 to 45.7 cm) unrolled.
• Place the unrolled portion diagonally across the patient's back, from right shoulder to left axilla.
• Bring the lower end of the bandage under the left axilla and back over the left shoulder; loop the upper end over the right shoulder and under the axilla.
• Pull the two ends together at the center of the back *so the bandage supports the position of attention.*

To complete a figure-eight strap or elastic bandage
• Secure the ends using safety pins, Velcro pads, or a buckle, depending on the equipment. Make sure a buckle or any sharp edges face away from the skin. Tape the secured ends to the underlying strap or bandage.
• Place cotton batting or padding under the straps, as well as under the buckle or pins, *to avoid skin irritation.*
• Use a pen to mark the strap at the site of the loop of the figure-eight strap, or the site where the elastic bandage crosses on the patient's back. *If the strap loosens, this mark helps you tighten it to the original position.*
• Assess neurovascular integrity, *which may be impaired by a strap that's too tight.* If neurovascular integrity is compromised when the strap is correctly applied, notify the doctor. *He may want to change the treatment.*

Special considerations
If possible, perform the procedure with the patient standing. However, this may not be feasible, because the pain from the fracture can cause syncope.

An adult with a clavicle strap made from an elastic bandage may require a triangular sling *to help support the weight of the arm, enhance immobilization, and reduce pain.* (See "Triangular sling.") For a small child or a confused adult, a well-molded plaster jacket is needed to ensure immobilization. *Inadequate immobilization can cause improper healing.*

Instruct the patient not to remove the clavicle strap. Explain that, with help, he can maintain proper hygiene by lifting segments of the strap to remove the cotton and by washing and powdering the skin daily. Explain that fresh cotton should be applied after cleaning.

For a hospitalized patient, monitor the position of the strap by checking the pen markings every 8 hours. Also assess neurovascular integrity. Teach the outpatient how to assess his own neurovascular integrity and to recognize symptoms to report promptly to the doctor.

Documentation

In the appropriate section of the emergency department sheet or in your notes, record the date and time of strap application, type of clavicle strap, use of powder and padding, bilateral neurovascular integrity before and after the procedure, and instructions to the patient.

Cervical collar

A cervical collar may be used for an acute injury (such as strained cervical muscles) or a chronic condition (such as arthritis or cervical metastasis). Or it may augment such splinting devices as a spine board to prevent potential cervical spine fracture or spinal cord damage.

Designed to hold the neck straight with the chin slightly elevated and tucked in, the collar immobilizes the cervical spine, decreases muscle spasms, and relieves some pain; it also prevents further injury and promotes healing. As symptoms of an acute injury subside, the patient may gradually discontinue wearing the collar, alternating periods of wear with increasing periods of removal, until he no longer needs the collar.

Equipment

Cervical collar, in the appropriate size. (See *Types of cervical collars*.)

Implementation

• Check the patient's neurovascular status before application.
• Instruct the patient to position his head slowly to face directly forward.
• Place the cervical collar in front of the patient's neck *to ensure that the size is correct.*
• Fit the collar snugly around the neck and attach the Velcro fasteners or buckles at the back of the neck.
• Check the patient's airway and his neurovascular status *to ensure that the collar isn't too tight.*

EQUIPMENT

Types of cervical collars

Cervical collars are used to support an injured or weakened cervical spine and to maintain alignment during healing.

Made of rigid plastic, the molded cervical collar holds the patient's neck firmly, keeping it straight, with the chin slightly elevated and tucked in.

The soft cervical collar, made of spongy foam, provides gentler support and reminds the patient to avoid cervical spine motion.

Special considerations

For a sprain or a potential cervical spine fracture, make sure the collar isn't too high in front *because this may hyperextend the neck.* In a neck sprain, such hyperextension may cause ligaments to heal in a shortened position. In a potential cervical spine fracture, hyperextension may cause serious neurologic damage.

Home care

Teach the patient how to apply the collar and how to do a neurovascular check. Name symptoms to report to the doctor. If indicated, advise sleeping without a pillow.

Documentation

Note the type and size of the cervical collar and the time and date of application in your notes. Record the results of neurovascular checks. Document patient comfort, the collar's snugness, and all patient instruction.

Splints

By immobilizing the site of an injury, a splint alleviates pain and allows the injury to heal in proper alignment. It also minimizes possible complications, such as excessive bleeding into tissues, restricted blood flow caused by bone pressing against vessels, and possible paralysis from an unstable spinal cord injury. In cases of multiple serious injuries, a splint or spine board allows caretakers to move the patient without risking further damage to bones, muscles, nerves, blood vessels, and skin.

A splint can be applied to immobilize a simple or compound fracture, a dislocation, or a subluxation. (See *Types of splints.*) During an emergency, any injury even suspected of being a fracture, dislocation, or subluxation should be splinted. No contraindications exist for rigid splints; traction splints are contraindicated for upper extremity injuries and open fractures.

Equipment

Rigid splint, Velcro support splint, spine board, or traction splint ▪ bindings ▪ padding ▪ sandbags or rolled towels or clothing ▪ optional: roller gauze, cloth strips, sterile or clean compress, ice bag.

Several commercial splints are available. In an emergency, any long, sturdy object, such as a tree limb, mop handle, or broom — even a magazine or newspaper — can be used to make a rigid splint for an extremity; a door can be used as a spine board.

Velcro straps, 2″ roller gauze, or 2″ cloth strips can be used as bindings. When improvising, avoid using twine or rope, if possible, *because they can restrict circulation.*

An inflatable semirigid splint, called an air splint, sometimes can be used to secure an injured extremity. (See *Using an air splint,* page 458.)

Implementation

● Obtain a complete history of the injury, if possible, and begin a thorough head-to-toe assessment, inspecting for obvious deformities, swelling or bleeding.
● Ask the patient if he can move the injured area (typically an extremity). Compare it bilaterally with the uninjured extremity, where applicable. Gently palpate the injured area; inspect for swelling, obvious deformities, bleeding, discoloration, and evidence of fracture or dislocation.
● Remove or cut away clothing from the injury site, if necessary. Check neurovascular integrity distal to the site. Explain the procedure to the patient to allay his fears.
● If an obvious bone misalignment causes the patient acute distress or severe neurovascular problems, align the extremity in its normal anatomic position, if possible. Stop doing this, however, if the action causes further neurovascular deterioration. Don't attempt to straighten a dislocation *because movement may damage displaced vessels and nerves.* Also, don't attempt reduction of a contaminated bone end *because this may cause additional laceration of soft tissues, vessels, and nerves, and also may cause gross contamination of deep tissues.*
● Choose a splint that will immobilize the joints above and below the fracture; pad the splint as necessary *to prevent excessive pressure over bony prominences.*

To apply a rigid splint

● Support the injured extremity and apply firm, gentle traction.
● Have an assistant place the splint under, beside, or on top of the extremity, as ordered.
● Tell the assistant to apply the bindings *to secure the splint.* Make sure they don't obstruct circulation.

To apply a spine board

● Pad the spine board (or door) carefully, especially the areas that will support the lumbar region and knees, *to prevent uneven pressure and discomfort.*
● If the patient is lying on his back, place one hand on each side of his head and apply gentle traction to the head and neck, keeping the head aligned with the body. Have one assistant logroll the patient onto his side while another slides the spine board under the patient. Then instruct the assistants to roll the patient onto the board while you maintain traction and alignment.

Types of splints

Three kinds of splints are commonly used to help provide support for injured or weakened limbs, or to help correct deformities.

A *rigid splint* can be used to immobilize a fracture or dislocation in an extremity, as shown. Ideally, two people should apply a rigid splint to an extremity.

A *traction splint* immobilizes a fracture and exerts a longitudinal pull that reduces muscle spasms, pain, and arterial and neural damage. Used primarily for femoral fractures, a traction splint may also be applied for a fractured hip or tibia. Two trained people should apply a traction splint.

A *spine board,* applied for a suspected spinal fracture, is a rigid splint that supports the injured person's entire body. Three people should apply a spine board.

• If the patient is prone, logroll him onto the board so he ends up in a supine position.

• *To maintain body alignment,* use strips of cloth to secure the patient on the spine board; *to keep head and neck aligned,* place sandbags or rolled towels or clothing on both sides of his head.

To apply a traction splint

• Place the splint beside the injured leg. (Never use a traction splint on an arm *because the major axillary plexus of nerves and blood vessels can't tolerate countertraction.*) Adjust the splint to the correct length, and then open and adjust the Velcro straps.

Using an air splint

In an emergency, an air splint can be applied to immobilize a fracture or control bleeding, especially from a forearm or lower leg. This compact, comfortable splint is made of double-walled plastic and provides gentle, diffuse pressure over an injured area. The appropriate splint is wrapped around the affected extremity, secured with Velcro or other strips, then inflated. The fit should be snug enough to immobilize the extremity without impairing circulation.

An air splint may actually control bleeding better than a local pressure bandage. The device's clear plastic construction simplifies inspection of the affected site for bleeding, pallor, or cyanosis. An air splint also allows the patient to be moved without further damage to the injured limb.

• Have an assistant keep the leg motionless while you pad the ankle and foot and fasten the ankle hitch around them. (You may leave the shoe on.)
• Tell the assistant to lift and support the leg at the injury site, as you apply firm, gentle traction.
• While you maintain traction, instruct the assistant to slide the splint under the leg, pad the groin *to avoid excessive pressure on external genitalia,* and gently apply the ischial strap.
• Have the assistant connect the loops of the ankle hitch to the end of the splint.
• Adjust the splint to apply enough traction *to secure the leg comfortably in the corrected position.*
• After applying traction, fasten the Velcro support splints *to secure the leg closely to the splint.*
♦ *Nursing alert.* Don't use a traction splint for a severely angulated femur or knee fracture. ♦

Special considerations
At the scene of an accident, always examine the patient completely for other injuries. Avoid unnecessary movement or manipulation *that may cause additional pain or injury.*

Always consider the possibility of cervical injury in an unconscious patient. If possible, apply the splint before repositioning the patient.

If the patient requires a rigid splint but one isn't available, use another body part as a splint. To splint a leg in this manner, pad its inner aspect and secure it to the other leg with roller gauze or cloth strips.

After applying any type of splint, monitor vital signs frequently *because bleeding in fractured bones and surrounding tissues may cause shock.* Also monitor the neurovascular status of the fractured limb by assessing skin color and checking for numbness in the fingers or toes. *Numbness or paralysis distal to the injury indicates pressure on nerves.* (See *Assessing neurovascular status.*)

Transport the patient as soon as possible to a medical facility. Apply ice to the injury. Regardless of the apparent extent of the patient's injury, don't allow him to eat or drink anything until the doctor evaluates him.

Indications for removal of a splint include evidence of improper application or vascular impairment. Apply gentle traction, and remove the splint carefully under a doctor's direct supervision.

Complications
Multiple transfers and repeated manipulation of a fracture may result in fat embolism, indicated by shortness of breath, agitation, and irrational behavior. This complication usually occurs within 24 to 72 hours of injury or manipulation.

Documentation
Record the circumstances and cause of the injury. Document the patient's complaints, noting whether symptoms are localized. Also record neurovascular status before and after applying the splint. Note the type of wound and the amount and type of drainage, if any. Document the time of splint application. If the bone end should slip into surrounding tissue or if transportation causes any change in the degree of dislocation, be sure to note it.

Casts

A cast is a hard mold that encases a body part, usually an extremity, to provide immobilization without discomfort. It can be used to treat injuries (including fractures), correct orthopedic conditions (such as deformities), or promote healing after general or plastic surgery, amputation, or nerve and vascular repair. (See *Types of cylindrical casts,* page 460.)

Casts may be constructed of plaster, fiberglass, or synthetic materials. Plaster—a commonly used material—is inexpensive, nontoxic, nonflammable, easy to mold, and rarely causes allergic reactions or skin irritation. However, fiberglass is lighter, stronger, and more resilient than plaster. Because fiberglass dries rapidly, it is more difficult to mold, but it can bear body weight immediately, if necessary.

Typically, a doctor applies a cast and a nurse prepares the patient and the equipment and assists during the procedure. With special preparation, a nurse may apply or change a standard cast, but an orthopedist must reduce and set the fracture.

Contraindications for casting may include skin diseases, peripheral vascular disease, diabetes mellitus, open or draining wounds, and susceptibility to skin irritations. However, these aren't strict contraindications; the doctor must weigh the potential risks and benefits for each patient.

Equipment
Tubular stockinette ■ casting material ■ plaster rolls ■ plaster splints (if necessary) ■ bucket of water ■ sink equipped with plaster trap ■ linen-saver pad ■ sheet wadding ■ sponge or felt padding (if necessary) ■ cast scissors, cast saw, and cast spreader (if necessary) ■ pillows or bath blankets ■ optional: rubber gloves, cast stand, moleskin or adhesive tape.

Gather the tubular stockinette, cast material, and plaster splints in the appropriate sizes. Tubular stockinettes range from 2″ to 12″ (5 to 30.5 cm) wide; plaster rolls, from 2″ to 6″ (5 to 15.2 cm) wide; and plaster splints, from 3″ to 6″ (7.6 to 15.2 cm) wide. Wear rubber gloves, especially if applying a fiberglass cast.

Preparation of equipment
Gently squeeze the packaged casting material *to make sure the envelopes don't have any air leaks.* Humid air penetrating such leaks can cause plaster to become stale, which could make it set too quickly, form lumps, fail to bond with lower layers, or set as a soft, friable mass. (Baking a stale plaster roll at a medium temperature for 1 hour can make it usable again.)

Follow the manufacturer's directions for water temperature when preparing plaster. Usually, room temperature or slightly warmer water is best *because it allows the cast to set in about 7 minutes without excessive exothermia.* (Cold water retards the rate of setting and may be used to facilitate difficult molding; warm water speeds the rate of setting and raises skin temperature under the cast.) Place all equipment within the doctor's reach.

Assessing neurovascular status
When assessing an injured extremity, always include the following steps and compare your findings bilaterally:
• Inspect the color of fingers or toes.
• To detect edema, note the size of the digits.
• Simultaneously touch the digits of the affected and unaffected extremities and compare temperature.
• Check capillary refill by pressing on the distal tip of one digit until it's white. Then release the pressure and note how soon the normal color returns. It should return quickly in both the affected and the unaffected extremities.
• Check sensation by touching the fingers or toes and asking the patient how they feel. Note reports of any numbness or tingling.
• To check proprioception, tell the patient to close his eyes; then move one digit and ask him which position it's in.
• To test movement, tell the patient to wiggle his toes or move his fingers.
• Palpate the distal pulses to assess vascular patency.
Record your findings for the affected and the unaffected extremities, using standard terminology to avoid ambiguity. Warmth, free movement, rapid capillary refill, and normal color, sensation, and proprioception indicate sound neurovascular status.

Implementation
• *To allay the patient's fears,* explain the procedure. If plaster is being used, make sure he understands that heat will build under the cast because of a chemical reaction between the water and plaster. Also begin explaining some aspects of proper cast care *to prepare him for patient teaching and to assess his knowledge level.*
• Cover the appropriate parts of the patient's bedding and gown with a linen-saver pad.
• If the cast is applied to the wrist or arm, remove rings that may interfere with circulation in the fingers.
• Assess the condition of the skin in the affected area, noting any redness, contusions, or open wounds. *This will make it easier to evaluate any complaints the patient may have after the cast is applied.*
• If the patient has severe contusions or open wounds, prepare him for a local anesthetic if the doctor will administer one.

Types of cylindrical casts

Made of plaster, fiberglass, or synthetic material, casts may be applied almost anywhere on the body to support a single finger or the entire body. Common casts are shown here.

Hanging arm cast

Shoulder spica

Support bar

Short arm cast

One-and-one-half hip spica

Support bar

Long leg cast

Short leg cast

Single hip spica

• *To establish baseline measurements,* assess neurovascular status. Palpate the distal pulses; assess the color, temperature, and capillary refill of the appropriate fingers or toes; and check neurologic function, including sensation and motion in the affected and unaffected extremities.

• Help the doctor position the limb, as ordered. (Commonly, the limb is immobilized in the neutral position.)

• Support the limb in the prescribed position while the doctor applies the tubular stockinette and sheet wadding. The stockinette, if used, should extend beyond the ends of the cast *to pad the edges.* (If the patient has an open wound or a severe contusion, the doctor may not use the stockinette.) He then wraps the limb in sheet wadding, starting at the distal end, and applies extra wadding to the distal and proximal ends of the cast area, as well as any points of prominence. As he applies the sheet wadding, check for wrinkles.

• If needed, assist the doctor to place an extra layer of sponge or felt padding over the area where the cast scissors will be used.

• Prepare the various cast materials as ordered.

To prepare plaster casting

• Place a roll of plaster casting on its end in the bucket of water. Make sure to immerse it completely. When air bubbles stop rising from the roll, remove it, gently squeeze out the excess water, and hand the casting material to the doctor, who will begin applying it to the extremity. As he applies the first roll, prepare a second roll in the same manner. (Stay at least one roll ahead of the doctor during the procedure.)

• After the doctor applies each roll, he'll smooth it to remove wrinkles, spread the plaster into the cloth webbing, and empty air pockets. If he's using plaster splints, he'll apply them in the middle layers of the cast. Before wrapping the last roll, he'll pull the ends of the tubular stockinette over the cast edges *to create padded ends, prevent cast crumbling, and reduce skin irritation.* He will then use the final roll to keep the ends of the stockinette in place.

To prepare cotton and polyester casting

• Open these casting materials one roll at a time *because cotton and polyester casting must be applied within 3 minutes—before humidity in the air hardens the tape.*

• Immerse the roll in cold water, and squeeze it four times *to ensure uniform wetness.*

• Remove the dripping wet material from the bucket. Tell the patient that it will be applied immediately. Forewarn him that the material will feel warm, giving off heat as it sets.

To prepare fiberglass casting

• If you're using water-activated fiberglass, immerse the tape rolls in tepid water for 10 to 15 minutes *to initiate the chemical reaction that causes the cast to harden.* Open one roll at a time. Avoid squeezing out excess water before application.

• If you're using light-cured fiberglass, you can unroll the material more slowly. This casting remains soft and malleable until it's exposed to ultraviolet light, which sets it.

To complete casting

• As necessary, "petal" the cast's edges *to reduce roughness and to cushion pressure points.* (See *How to petal a cast.*)

• Use a cast stand or the palm of your hand to support the cast in the therapeutic position until it becomes firm to the touch (usually 6 to 8 minutes).

• *To check circulation in the casted limb,* palpate the distal pulse and assess the color, temperature, and capillary refill of the fingers or toes. Determine neurologic status by asking the patient if he's experiencing paresthesia in the extremity or decreased motion of the extremity's

How to petal a cast

Rough cast edges can be cushioned by petaling them with adhesive tape or moleskin. To do this, first cut several 4″ × 2″ (10.2 × 5 cm) strips. Round off one end of each strip to keep it from curling. Then, making sure the rounded end of the strip is on the outside of the cast, tuck the straight end just inside the cast edge.

Smooth the moleskin with your finger until you're sure it's secured inside and out. Repeat the procedure, overlapping the moleskin pieces until you've gone all the way around the cast edge.

uncovered joints. Assess the unaffected extremity in the same manner and compare findings.

• Elevate the limb above heart level with pillows or bath blankets, as ordered, *to facilitate venous return and reduce*

Removing a plaster cast

Typically, a cast is removed when a fracture heals or requires further manipulation. Less common indications include cast damage, a pressure ulcer under the cast, excessive drainage or bleeding, and a constrictive cast.

Explain the procedure to the patient. Tell him he'll feel some heat and vibration as the cast is split with the cast saw. If the patient is a child, tell him the saw is very noisy but will not cut the skin beneath. Warn the patient that when the padding is cut, he'll see discolored skin and signs of poor muscle tone. Reassure him that you'll stay with him. The pictures show how a plaster cast is removed.

First, the doctor cuts one side of the cast, then the other. As he does so, closely monitor the patient's anxiety level.

Next, the doctor opens the cast pieces with a spreader.

Finally, using cast scissors, the doctor cuts through the cast padding.

When the cast is removed, give skin care to remove accumulated dead skin and to begin restoring the extremity's normal appearance.

---

edema. To prevent molding, make sure pressure is evenly distributed under the cast.
• The doctor will then send the patient for X-rays *to ensure proper positioning.*
• Instruct the patient to notify the doctor of any pain, foul odor, drainage, or burning sensation under the cast. (After the cast hardens, the doctor may cut a window in it to inspect the painful or burning area.)
• Pour water from the plaster bucket into a sink containing a plaster trap. Don't use a regular sink *because plaster will block the plumbing.*

Special considerations
A fiberglass cast dries immediately after application. A plaster extremity cast dries in approximately 24 to 48 hours; a plaster spica or body cast, in 48 to 72 hours. During this drying period, the cast must be properly positioned to prevent a surface depression that could cause pressure areas or dependent edema. Neurovascular status must be assessed, drainage monitored, and the condition of the cast checked periodically.

After the cast dries completely, it looks white and shiny and no longer feels damp or soft. Care consists of monitoring for changes in the drainage pattern, preventing skin breakdown near the cast, and averting the complications of immobility.

Patient teaching must begin immediately after the cast is applied and should continue until the patient or a family member can care for the cast.

Never use the bed or a table to support the cast as it sets *because molding can result, causing pressure necrosis of underlying tissue.* Also, don't use rubber- or plastic-covered pillows before the cast hardens *because they can trap heat under the cast.*

If a cast is applied after surgery or traumatic injury, remember that the most accurate way to assess for bleeding is to monitor vital signs. A visible blood spot on the cast can be misleading: One drop of blood can produce a circle 3″ (7.6 cm) in diameter.

The doctor usually removes the cast at the appropriate time, with a nurse assisting. (See *Removing a plaster cast.*) Tell the patient that when the cast is removed, his casted limb will appear thinner and flabbier than the uncasted limb. What's more, his skin will appear yellowish or gray from the accumulated dead skin and oils from the glands near the skin surface. Reassure the patient that with exercise and good skin care, his limb will return to normal.

Home care
Before the patient goes home, teach him how to care for his cast. Tell him to keep the casted limb elevated above heart level to minimize swelling. Raise a casted leg by having the patient lie supine with his leg on top of pillows. Prop a casted arm so that the hand and elbow are higher than the shoulder.

Instruct the patient to call the doctor if he can't move his fingers or toes, if he has numbness or tingling in the affected limb, or if he has symptoms of infection such as a fever, unusual pain, or a foul odor from the cast.

Instruct the patient to maintain muscle strength by continuing any recommended exercises.

If the cast needs repair (if it loosens and slips) or if the patient has any questions about cast care, advise him to notify his doctor.

Warn the patient not to get the cast wet. Moisture will weaken or destroy it.

Urge the patient not to insert anything (such as a back scratcher or powder) into the cast to relieve itching. Foreign matter can damage the skin and cause an infection. Tell him, though, that he can use alcohol on the skin at the cast edges.

Warn the patient not to chip, crush, cut, or otherwise break any area of the cast and not to bear weight on the cast unless instructed to do so by the doctor.

If the patient must use crutches, instruct him to remove throw rugs from the floor and to rearrange furniture to reduce the risk of tripping and falling.

If the patient has a cast on his dominant arm, he may need help with bathing, toileting, eating, and dressing.

Complications
Complications of improper cast application include compartment syndrome, palsy, paresthesia, ischemia, ischemic myositis, pressure necrosis and, eventually, misalignment or nonunion of fractured bones.

Documentation
Record the date and time of cast application and skin condition of the extremity before the cast was applied. Note any contusions, redness, or open wounds; results of neurovascular checks, before and after application, for the affected and unaffected extremities; location of any special devices, such as felt pads or plaster splints; and any patient teaching.

TRACTION AND FIXATION
Mechanical traction

Mechanical traction exerts a pulling force on a part of the body — usually the spine, pelvis, or long bones of the arms and legs. It can be used to reduce fractures, treat dislocations, correct or prevent deformities, improve or correct contractures, or decrease muscle spasms. Depending on the injury or condition, an orthopedist may order either skin or skeletal traction.

Applied directly to the skin and thus indirectly to the bone, skin traction is ordered when a light, temporary, or noncontinuous pulling force is required. Contraindications for skin traction include a severe injury with open wounds, an allergy to tape or other skin traction equipment, circulatory disturbances, dermatitis, and varicose veins.

In skeletal traction, an orthopedist inserts a pin or wire through the bone and attaches the traction equipment to the pin or wire to exert a direct, constant, longitudinal pulling force. Indications for skeletal traction include fractures of the tibia, femur, and humerus. Infections such as osteomyelitis contraindicate skeletal traction.

Nursing responsibilities for this procedure include setting up the traction frame. (See *Traction frames,* page 464.) The design of the patient's bed usually dictates whether to use a claw clamp or I.V.-post-type frame.

Traction frames

You may encounter three types of traction frames, as described below.

Claw-type basic frame
With this frame, claw attachments secure the uprights to the footboard and headboard.

I.V.-type basic frame
With this frame, I.V. posts, placed in I.V. holders, support the horizontal bars across the foot and head of the bed. These horizontal bars then support the two uprights.

I.V.-type Balkan frame
This frame features I.V. posts and horizontal bars (secured in the same manner as those for the I.V.-type basic frame) that support four uprights.

(However, the claw-type Balkan frame is rarely used.) Setup of the specific traction can be done by a nurse with special skills, an orthopedic technician, or by the doctor. Instructions for setting up these traction units usually accompany the equipment. (See *Comparing traction types*). After the patient is placed in the specific type of traction ordered by the orthopedist, the nurse is responsible for preventing complications from immobility; for routinely inspecting the equipment; for adding traction weights, as ordered; and, in patients with skeletal traction, for monitoring the pin insertion sites for signs of infection.

Equipment
For a claw-type basic frame: 102″ (259-cm) plain bar ▪ two 66″ (168-cm) swivel-clamp bars ▪ two upper-panel clamps ▪ two lower-panel clamps.

    For an I.V.-type basic frame: 102″ plain bar ▪ 27″ (68.6-cm) double-clamp bar ▪ 48″ (122-cm) swivel-clamp bar ▪ two 36″ (91.4-cm) plain bars ▪ four 4″ (10-cm) I.V. posts with clamps ▪ cross clamp.

    For an I.V.-type Balkan frame: two 102″ plain bars ▪ two 48″ swivel-clamp bars ▪ five 36″ plain bars ▪ two 27″ double-clamp bars ▪ four 4″ I.V. posts with clamps ▪ eight cross clamps.

    For all frame types: trapeze with clamp ▪ wall bumper or roller.

    For skeletal traction care: sterile cotton-tipped applicators ▪ prescribed antiseptic solution ▪ sterile gauze pads ▪ povidone-iodine solution ▪ optional: antimicrobial ointment.

Preparation of equipment
Arrange with central supply or the appropriate department to have the traction equipment transported to the patient's room on a traction cart. If appropriate, gather the equipment for pin-site care at the patient's bedside. Pin-site care protocols may vary with each hospital or doctor.

Implementation
• Explain the purpose of traction to the patient. Emphasize the importance of maintaining proper body alignment after the traction equipment is set up.

To set up a claw-type basic frame
• Attach one lower-panel and one upper-panel clamp to each 66″ swivel-clamp bar.
• Fasten one bar to the footboard and one to the headboard by turning the clamp knobs clockwise until they are tight and then pulling back on the upper clamp's rubberized bar until it is tight.
• Secure the 102″ horizontal plain bar atop the two vertical bars, making sure the clamp knobs point up.

Comparing traction types

Traction therapy restricts movement of a patient's affected limb or body part and may confine the patient to bed rest for an extended period. The limb is immobilized by pulling with equal force on each end of the injured area—an equal mix of traction and countertraction. Weights provide the pulling force. Countertraction is produced by using other weights or by positioning the patient's body weight against the traction pull.

Skin traction
This procedure immobilizes a body part intermittently over an extended period through direct application of a pulling force on the patient's skin. The force may be applied using adhesive or nonadhesive traction tape or other skin traction devices, such as a boot, belt, or halter.

Adhesive attachment allows more continuous traction, whereas nonadhesive attachment allows easier removal for daily skin care.

Skeletal traction
This procedure immobilizes a body part for prolonged periods by attaching weighted equipment directly to the patient's bones. This may be accomplished with pins, screws, wires, or tongs.

• Using the appropriate clamp, attach the trapeze to the horizontal bar about 2' (0.6 m) from the head of the bed.

To set up an I.V.-type basic frame
• Attach one 4" I.V. post with clamp to each end of both 36" horizontal plain bars.
• Secure an I.V. post in each I.V. holder at the bed corners. Using a cross clamp, fasten the 48" vertical swivel-clamp bar to the middle of the horizontal plain bar at the foot of the bed.
• Fasten the 27" vertical double-clamp bar to the middle of the horizontal plain bar at the head of the bed.
• Attach the 102" horizontal plain bar to the tops of the two vertical bars, making sure the clamp knobs point up.
• Using the appropriate clamp, attach the trapeze to the horizontal bar about 2' from the head of the bed.

To set up an I.V.-type Balkan frame
• Attach one 4" I.V. post with clamp to each end of two 36" horizontal plain bars.
• Secure an I.V. post in each I.V. holder at the bed corners.
• Attach a 48" vertical swivel-clamp bar, using a cross clamp, to each I.V. post clamp on the horizontal plain bar at the foot of the bed.
• Fasten one 36" horizontal plain bar across the midpoints of the two 48" swivel-clamp bars, using two cross clamps.
• Attach a 27" vertical double-clamp bar to each I.V. post clamp on the horizontal bar at the head of the bed.
• Using two cross clamps, fasten a 36" horizontal plain bar across the midpoints of two 27" double-clamp bars.
• Clamp a 102" horizontal plain bar onto the vertical bars on each side of the bed, making sure the clamp knobs point up.
• Use two cross clamps to attach a 36" horizontal plain bar across the two overhead bars, about 2' from the head of the bed.
• Attach the trapeze to this 36" horizontal bar.

After setting up any frame
• Attach a wall bumper or roller to the vertical bar or bars at the head of the bed. *This protects the walls from damage caused by the bed or equipment.*

Caring for the traction patient
• Show the patient how much movement he's allowed and instruct him not to readjust the equipment. Also tell him to report any pain or pressure from the traction equipment.
• At least once a shift, make sure that the traction equipment connections are tight and that no parts touch the bedding, the patient, or other inappropriate portions of the apparatus. Check for impingements, such as ropes rubbing on the footboard or getting caught between pulleys. *Friction and impingement reduce the effectiveness of traction.*
• Inspect the traction equipment *to ensure the correct alignment.*
• Inspect the ropes for fraying, *which can eventually cause a rope to break.*
• Make sure the ropes are positioned properly in the pulley track. *An improperly positioned rope changes the degree of traction.*
• *To prevent tampering and aid stability and security,* make sure that all rope ends are taped above the knot.
• Inspect the equipment regularly to make sure that the traction weights hang freely. *Weights that touch the floor, bed, or each other reduce the amount of traction.*
• About every 2 hours, check the patient for proper body alignment and reposition the patient as necessary. *Misalignment causes ineffective traction and may keep the fracture from healing properly.*
• *To prevent complications from immobility,* assess neurovascular integrity routinely. The patient's condition, the hospital routine, and the doctor's orders determine the frequency of neurovascular assessments.
• Provide skin care, encourage coughing and deep breathing exercises, and assist with ordered range-of-motion exercises for unaffected extremities. Typically, an order for elastic support stockings is written. Check elimination patterns and provide laxatives, as ordered.
• For the patient with skeletal traction, make sure that the protruding pin or wire ends are covered with cork *to prevent them from tearing the bedding or injuring the patient and staff.*
• Check the pin site and surrounding skin regularly for signs of infection.
• If ordered, clean the pin site and surrounding skin. Pin-site care varies, but you'll usually follow guidelines like these: Use sterile technique; avoid digging at pin sites with the cotton-tipped applicator; if ordered, clean the pin site and surrounding skin with a cotton-tipped applicator dipped in ordered antiseptic; if ordered, apply antimicrobial ointment to the pin sites; apply a loose sterile dressing, or dress with sterile gauze pads soaked in povidone-iodine solution. Perform pin-site care as often as necessary, depending on the amount of drainage.

Special considerations
When using skin traction, apply ordered weights slowly and carefully *to avoid jerking the affected extremity. To avoid injury in case the ropes break,* arrange the weights so they don't hang over the patient.

Complications
Immobility during traction may result in pressure ulcers; muscle atrophy, weakness, or contractures; and osteo-

porosis. Immobility can also cause GI disturbances, such as constipation; urinary problems, including stasis and calculi; respiratory problems, such as stasis of secretions and hypostatic pneumonia; and circulatory disturbances, including stasis and thrombophlebitis. Prolonged immobility, especially after traumatic injury, may promote depression or other emotional disturbances. Skeletal traction may cause osteomyelitis originating at the pin or wire sites.

Documentation

In the patient record, document the amount of traction weight used daily, noting the application of additional weights and the patient's tolerance. Document equipment inspections and patient care, including routine checks of neurovascular integrity, skin condition, respiratory status, and elimination patterns. If applicable, note the condition of the pin site and any care given.

External fixation

In external fixation, a doctor inserts metal pins through skin and muscle layers into the broken bones and fixes them to an adjustable external frame that maintains their proper alignment. (See *Types of external fixation devices.*) This procedure is used most commonly to treat open, unstable fractures with extensive soft tissue damage, comminuted closed fractures, and septic, nonunion fractures and to facilitate surgical immobilization of a joint. Specialized types of external fixators may be used to lengthen leg bones or immobilize the cervical spine.

An advantage of external fixation over other immobilization techniques is that it stabilizes the fracture while allowing full visualization and access to open wounds. It also facilitates early ambulation, thus reducing the risk of complications from immobilization.

Equipment

Sterile cotton-tipped applicators ▪ prescribed antiseptic cleaning solution ▪ sterile gauze pads ▪ povidone-iodine solution ▪ optional: antimicrobial ointment.

Equipment varies with the type of fixator used, and the type and location of the fracture. Typically, sets of pins, stabilizing rods, and clips are available from manufacturers. Do not reuse pins.

Preparation of equipment

Make sure that the external fixation set includes all the equipment it's supposed to include. Also make sure that

Types of external fixation devices

The illustrations below show how some common external fixation devices work. The doctor's selection of a device will depend on the severity of the patient's fracture and on the type of bone alignment needed.

Universal day frame

This device is used to manage tibial fractures. The frame allows the doctor to readjust the position of bony fragments by angulation and rotation. The compression-distraction device allows compression and distraction of bony fragments.

Portsmouth external fixation bar

This device is used to manage complicated tibial fractures. The locking nut adjustment on the mobile carriage only allows bone compression, so the doctor must accurately reduce bony fragments before applying the device.

the equipment has been sterilized according to hospital procedure.

Implementation

● Explain the procedure to the patient *to reduce his anxiety.* Emphasize that he'll feel little pain once the fixation device is in place. Assure the patient that his feelings of anxiety are normal and that he will be able to adjust to the apparatus.

● Tell the patient that he will be able to move about with the apparatus in place, which may help him resume normal activities more quickly.

● After the fixation device is in place, perform neurovascular checks every 2 to 4 hours for 24 hours, then every 4 to 8 hours, as appropriate, *to assess for possible neurologic damage.* Assess color, motion, sensation, digital movement, edema, capillary refill, and pulses of the affected extremity. Compare with the unaffected side.

● Apply an ice bag to the surgical site, as ordered, *to reduce swelling, relieve pain, and lessen bleeding.*

● Administer analgesics or narcotics, as ordered, before exercising or mobilizing the affected extremity *to promote comfort.*

● Monitor the patient for pain not relieved by analgesics or narcotics, or for burning, tingling, or numbness, *which may indicate nerve damage or circulatory impairment.*

● Elevate the affected extremity, if appropriate, *to minimize edema.*

● Perform pin-site care, as ordered, *to prevent infection.* Pin-site care varies, but you'll usually follow guidelines like these: Use sterile technique; avoid digging at pin sites with the cotton-tipped applicator; if ordered, clean the pin site and surrounding skin with a cotton-tipped applicator dipped in ordered antiseptic solution; if ordered, apply antimicrobial ointment to pin sites; apply a loose sterile dressing, or dress with sterile gauze pads soaked in povidone-iodine solution. Perform pin-site care as often as necessary, depending on the amount of drainage.

● Also check for redness, tenting of the skin, prolonged or purulent drainage from the pin site, swelling, elevated body or pin-site temperature, and any bowing or bending of pins, which may stress the skin.

Special considerations

Before discharge, teach the patient and family members how to give pin-site care. Although this is a sterile procedure in the hospital, the patient can use clean technique at home. Teach the patient to recognize warning signs of pin-site infection. Tell him to keep the affected limb elevated when sitting or lying down.

Complications

Complications of external fixation include loosening of pins and loss of fracture stabilization, infection of the pin tract or wound, skin breakdown, nerve damage, and muscle impingement.

Documentation

Record the patient's reaction to the apparatus. Assess and document the condition of the pin sites and skin. Also document the patient's reaction to ambulation and understanding of teaching instructions.

 Internal fixation

In this procedure, also known as surgical reduction or open reduction-internal fixation, the doctor implants fixation devices—using no external framework—to stabilize the fracture. Internal fixation devices include nails, screws, pins, wires, and rods, all of which may be used in combination with metal plates. These devices remain in the body indefinitely unless the patient experiences adverse reactions after the healing process is complete. (See *Reviewing internal fixation devices.*)

Typically, internal fixation is used to treat fractures of the face and jaw, spine, bones of the arms and legs, and fractures involving a joint (most commonly, the hip). Internal fixation permits earlier mobilization and can shorten hospitalization, particularly in elderly patients with hip fractures.

Equipment

Ice bag ▪ pain medication (analgesic or narcotic) ▪ incentive spirometer or intermittent positive-pressure breathing (IPPB) device ▪ elastic stockings.

Patients with leg fractures may also need the following: overhead frame with trapeze ▪ pressure-relief mattress ▪ crutches or walker ▪ pillow (hip fractures may require abductor pillows).

Preparation of equipment

Equipment is collected and prepared in the operating room.

Implementation

● Explain the procedure to the patient *to allay his fears.* Tell him what to expect during postoperative assessment and monitoring; teach him how to use an IPPB device or incentive spirometer; and prepare him for proposed exercise and progressive ambulation regimens, if necessary. Instruct him to tell the doctor if he feels pain.

Reviewing internal fixation devices

Choice of a specific internal fixation device depends on the location, type, and configuration of the fracture. In trochanteric or subtrochanteric fractures, for instance, the surgeon may use a hip pin or nail, with or without a screw plate. A pin or plate with extra nails stabilizes the fracture by impacting the bone ends at the fracture site.

In an uncomplicated fracture of the femoral shaft, the surgeon may use an intramedullary rod, as shown at the top of the next column. This device permits early ambulation with partial weight bearing.

Another choice for fixation of a long-bone fracture is a screw plate, shown here on the tibia.

In an arm fracture, the surgeon may fix the involved bones with a plate, rod, or nail. Most radial and ulnar fractures may be fixed with plates, whereas humeral fractures are commonly fixed with rods.

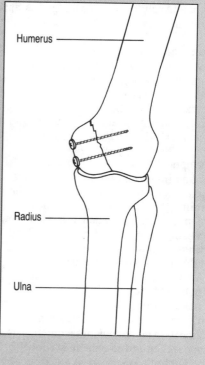

• After the procedure, monitor the patient's vital signs every 2 to 4 hours for 24 hours, then every 4 to 8 hours, according to hospital protocols. *Changes in vital signs may indicate hemorrhage or infection.*
• Monitor fluid intake and output every 4 to 8 hours.
• Perform neurovascular checks every 2 to 4 hours for 24 hours, then every 4 to 8 hours as appropriate. Assess color, motion, sensation, digital movement, edema, capillary refill, and pulses of the affected area. Compare findings with the unaffected side.
• Apply an ice bag to the operative site, as ordered, *to reduce swelling, relieve pain, and lessen bleeding.*

• Administer analgesics or narcotics, as ordered, before exercising or mobilizing the affected area *to promote comfort.*
• Monitor the patient for pain unrelieved by analgesics or narcotics, or for burning, tingling, or numbness, *which may indicate infection or impaired circulation.*
• Elevate the affected limb on a pillow, if appropriate, *to minimize edema.*
• Check surgical dressings for excessive drainage or bleeding. Also check the incision site for signs of infection, such as erythema, drainage, edema, and unusual pain.

• Assist and encourage the patient to perform range-of-motion and other muscle strengthening exercises, as ordered, *to promote circulation, improve muscle tone, and maintain joint function.*

• Teach the patient to perform progressive ambulation and mobilization using an overhead frame with trapeze, or crutches or a walker, as appropriate.

Special considerations

To avoid the complications of immobility after surgery, have the patient use an incentive spirometer or IPPB device. Apply elastic stockings, as appropriate. The patient may also require a pressure-relief mattress.

Home care

Before discharge, instruct the patient and family members about caring for the incisional site, recognizing signs and symptoms of wound infection, administering pain medication, practicing an exercise regimen (if any), and using assistive ambulation devices (such as crutches or a walker), if appropriate.

Complications

Wound infection and, more critically, infection involving metal fixation devices may require reopening the incision, draining the suture line and, possibly, removing the fixation device. Any such infection would require wound dressings and antibiotic therapy. Other complications may include malunion, nonunion, fat or pulmonary embolism, and neurovascular impairment.

Documentation

In the patient record, document perioperative findings on cardiovascular, respiratory, and neurovascular status. Name pain management techniques used. Describe wound appearance and alignment of the affected bone. Document the patient's response to teaching about appropriate exercise, care of the infection site, use of assistive devices (if appropriate), and symptoms that should be reported to the doctor.

OTHER ORTHOPEDIC PROCEDURES
Stump and prosthesis care

Patient care immediately after limb amputation includes monitoring drainage from the stump, positioning the affected limb, assisting with exercises prescribed by a phys-

ical therapist, and wrapping and conditioning the stump. Postoperative care of the stump will vary slightly, depending on the amputation site (arm or leg) and the type of dressing applied to the stump (elastic bandage or plaster cast).

After the stump heals, it requires only routine daily care, such as proper hygiene and continued muscle-strengthening exercises. The prosthesis — once the patient begins to use it — also requires daily care. Typically, a plastic prosthesis, the most common type, must be cleaned and lubricated and checked for proper fit. As the patient recovers from the physical and psychological trauma of amputation, he will need to learn correct procedures for routine daily care of the stump and the prosthesis.

Equipment

For postoperative stump care: pressure dressing ■ tourniquet ■ ABD pad ■ suction equipment, if ordered ■ overhead trapeze ■ 1″ adhesive tape, bandage clips or safety pins ■ sandbags or trochanter roll (for a leg) ■ elastic stump shrinker or 4″ elastic bandage ■ optional: tourniquet (as last resort to control bleeding).

For stump and prosthesis care: mild soap or alcohol sponges ■ stump socks or athletic tube socks ■ two washcloths ■ two towels ■ appropriate lubricating oil.

Implementation

• Perform routine postoperative care — frequently assessing respiratory status and level of consciousness, monitoring vital signs and I.V. infusions, checking tube patency, and providing for the patient's comfort and safety.

Monitor stump drainage

• *Because gravity causes fluid to accumulate at the stump,* frequently check the amount of blood and drainage on the dressing. Notify the doctor if accumulations of drainage or blood increase rapidly. If excessive bleeding occurs, notify the doctor immediately and apply a pressure dressing or compress the appropriate pressure points. If this doesn't control bleeding, use a tourniquet only as a last resort. Keep a tourniquet available, if needed.

• Tape the ABD pad over the moist part of the dressing, as necessary. *This provides a dry area to help prevent bacterial infection.*

• Monitor the suction drainage equipment and note the amount and type of drainage.

Position the extremity

• *To prevent contractures,* position an arm with the elbow extended and the shoulder abducted.

• *To correctly position a leg*, elevate the foot of the bed slightly and place sandbags or a trochanter roll against the hip *to prevent external rotation.*

♦ **Nursing alert.** Don't place a pillow under the thigh to flex the hip *because this can cause hip flexion contracture.* For the same reason, tell the patient to avoid prolonged sitting. ♦

• After a below-the-knee amputation, maintain knee extension *to prevent hamstring muscle contractures.*

• After any leg amputation, place the patient on a firm surface in the prone position for at least 4 hours a day, with his legs close together and without pillows under his stomach, hips, knees, or stump, unless this position is contraindicated. *This position helps prevent hip flexion, contractures, and abduction; it also stretches the flexor muscles.*

Assist with prescribed exercises

• After arm amputation, encourage the patient to exercise the remaining arm *to prevent muscle contractures.* Help the patient perform isometric and range-of-motion (ROM) exercises for both shoulders, as prescribed by the physical therapist, *because use of the prosthesis requires both shoulders.*

• After leg amputation, stand behind the patient and, if necessary, support him with your hands at his waist during balancing exercises.

• Instruct the patient to exercise the affected and unaffected limbs *to maintain muscle tone and increase muscle strength.* The patient with a leg amputation may perform push-ups, as ordered (in the sitting position, arms at his sides), or pull-ups on the overhead trapeze *to strengthen his arms, shoulders, and back in preparation for using crutches.*

Wrap and condition the stump

• If the patient doesn't have a rigid cast, apply an elastic stump shrinker *to prevent edema and shape the limb in preparation for the prosthesis.* Wrap the stump so that it narrows toward the distal end. *This helps to ensure comfort when the patient wears the prosthesis.*

• Instead of using an elastic stump shrinker, you can wrap the stump in a 4" elastic bandage. To do this, stretch the bandage to about two-thirds its maximum length as you wrap it diagonally around the stump, with the greatest pressure distally. (Depending on the size of the leg, you may need to use two 4" bandages.) Secure the bandage with clips, safety pins, or adhesive tape. Make sure the bandage covers all portions of the stump smoothly *because wrinkles or exposed areas encourage skin breakdown.* (See *Wrapping a stump*, page 472.)

• If the patient experiences throbbing after the stump is wrapped, remove the bandage immediately and reapply it less tightly. *Throbbing indicates impaired circulation.*

• Check the bandage regularly. Rewrap it when it begins to bunch up at the end (usually about every 12 hours for a moderately active patient) or every 24 hours.

• After removing the bandage to rewrap it, massage the stump gently, always pushing toward the suture line rather than away from it. *This stimulates circulation and prevents scar tissue from adhering to the bone.*

• When healing begins, instruct the patient to push the stump against a pillow. Then have him progress gradually to pushing against harder surfaces, such as a padded chair, then a hard chair. *These conditioning exercises will help the patient adjust to experiencing pressure and sensation in the stump.*

Care for the healed stump

• Bathe the stump, but never shave it *because a rash or irritation may result.* If possible, bathe the stump at the end of the day *because the warm water may cause swelling, making reapplication of the prosthesis difficult.*

• Rub the stump with alcohol daily *to toughen the skin, reducing the risk of skin breakdown.* (Avoid using powders or lotions *because they can soften or irritate the skin.) Because alcohol may cause severe irritation in some patients,* instruct the patient to watch for and report this sign.

• Inspect the stump for redness, swelling, irritation, and calluses. Report any of these to the doctor. Tell the patient to avoid putting weight on the stump. (The skin should be firm but not taut over the bony end of the limb.)

• Continue muscle-strengthening exercises *so the patient can build the strength he'll need to control the prosthesis.*

• Change the patient's stump socks as necessary *to avoid exposing the skin to excessive perspiration, which can be irritating.* Wash the socks in warm water and gentle nondetergent soap; lay them flat on a towel to dry. *Machine washing or drying may shrink the socks.*

Care for the plastic prosthesis

• Wipe the plastic socket of the prosthesis with a damp cloth and mild soap or alcohol *to prevent bacterial accumulation.*

• Wipe the insert (if the prosthesis has one) with a dry cloth.

• Dry the prosthesis thoroughly; if possible, allow it to dry overnight.

• Maintain and lubricate the prosthesis, as instructed by the manufacturer.

• Check for malfunctions and adjust or repair the prosthesis as necessary *to prevent further damage.*

• Check the condition of the shoe on a foot prosthesis frequently and change it as necessary.

Wrapping a stump

Proper stump care helps protect the limb, reduces swelling, and prepares the limb for a prosthesis. As you perform the procedure, teach it to the patient. Start by obtaining two 4″ elastic bandages. Center the end of the first 4″ bandage at the top of the patient's thigh. Unroll the bandage downward over the stump and to the back of the leg, as shown here.

Make three figure-eight turns to adequately cover the ends of the stump. As you wrap, be sure to include the roll of flesh in the groin area. Use enough pressure to ensure that the stump narrows toward the end so that it fits comfortably into the prosthesis.

Use the second 4″ bandage to anchor the first bandage around the waist. For a below-the-knee amputation, use the knee to anchor the bandage in place. Secure the bandage with clips, safety pins, or adhesive tape. Check the stump bandage regularly, and rewrap it if it bunches at the end.

Apply the prosthesis

• Apply a stump sock. Keep the seams away from bony prominences.
• If the prosthesis has an insert, remove it from the socket, place it over the stump, and insert the stump into the prosthesis.
• If it has no insert, merely slide the prosthesis over the stump. Secure the prosthesis onto the stump according to the manufacturer's directions.

Special considerations

If a patient arrives at the hospital with a traumatic amputation, the amputated part may be saved for possible reimplantation. (See *Caring for an amputated body part.*)

Teach the patient how to care for his stump and prosthesis properly. Make sure he knows the signs and symptoms that indicate problems in the stump. Explain that a 10-lb (4.5-kg) change in body weight will alter his stump size and require a new prosthesis socket *to ensure a correct fit.*

Exercise of the remaining muscles in an amputated limb must begin the day after surgery. A physical therapist will direct these exercises. For example, arm exercises progress from isometrics to assisted ROM to active ROM. Leg exercises include rising from a chair, balancing on one leg, and ROM exercises of the knees and hips.

For a below-the-knee amputation, you may substitute an athletic tube sock for a stump sock by cutting off the elastic band. If the patient has a rigid plaster of paris dressing, perform normal cast care. Check the cast frequently to make sure it doesn't slip off. If it does, apply an elastic bandage immediately and notify the doctor *because edema will develop rapidly.*

Home care

Emphasize to the patient that proper care of his stump can speed healing. Tell the patient to inspect his stump carefully every day, using a mirror. Instruct him to call the doctor if the incision appears to be opening, looks red or swollen, feels warm, is painful to touch, or is

Caring for an amputated body part

After traumatic amputation, a surgeon may be able to reimplant the severed body part through microsurgery. The chance of successful reimplantation is much greater if the amputated part has received proper care.

If a patient arrives at the hospital with a severed body part, first make sure that bleeding at the amputation site has been controlled. Then follow these guidelines for preserving the body part.
• Put on sterile gloves. Place several sterile gauze pads and an appropriate amount of sterile roller gauze in a sterile basin, and pour sterile normal saline or sterile lactated Ringer's solution over them. *Never* use any other solution, and don't try to scrub or debride the part.
• Holding the body part in one gloved hand, carefully pat it dry with sterile gauze. Place saline-soaked gauze pads over the stump; then wrap the whole body part with saline-soaked roller gauze. Wrap the gauze with a sterile towel, if available. Then put this package in a watertight container or bag and seal it.
• Fill another plastic bag with ice and place the part, still in its watertight container, inside. Seal the outer bag. (Always protect the part from direct contact with ice—and *never* use dry ice—*to prevent irreversible tissue damage, which would make the part unsuitable for reimplantation.*) Keep this bag ice-cold until the doctor's ready to do the reimplantation surgery.

Amputated part
(wrapped in sterile gauze)

Outer container

Ice

• Label the bag with the patient's name, identification number, identification of the amputated part, the hospital identification number, and the date and time when cooling began.

Note: The body part must be wrapped and cooled quickly. Irreversible tissue damage occurs after only 6 hours at ambient temperature. However, hypothermic management seldom preserves tissues for more than 24 hours.

---

seeping drainage. Instruct him to continue proper daily stump care.

Tell the patient to massage the stump *toward the suture line* to mobilize the scar and prevent its adherence to bone. Advise him to avoid exposing the skin around the stump to excessive perspiration, which can be irritating. Tell him to change his elastic bandages or stump socks during the day to avoid this.

Tell the patient that he may experience twitching, spasms, or phantom limb pain as his stump muscles adjust to amputation. Advise him that he can decrease these symptoms with heat, massage, or gentle pressure. If his stump is sensitive to touch, tell him to rub it with a dry washcloth for 4 minutes three times a day.

Stress the importance of performing prescribed exercises to help minimize complications, maintain muscle strength and tone, prevent contractures, and promote independence. Also stress the importance of positioning to prevent contractures and edema.

Complications

The most common postoperative complications include hemorrhage, stump infection, contractures, and a swollen or flabby stump. Complications that may develop at any time after an amputation include skin breakdown or irritation from lack of ventilation; friction from an irritant in the prosthesis; a sebaceous cyst or boil from tight socks; psychological problems, such as denial, depression, or withdrawal; and phantom limb pain caused by stimulation of nerves that once carried sensations from the distal part of the extremity.

Documentation

Record the date, time, and specific procedures of all postoperative care, including amount and type of drainage, condition of the dressing, need for dressing reinforcement, and appearance of the suture line and surrounding tissue. Also note any signs of skin irritation or infection, any complications and the nursing action taken, the patient's tolerance for exercises, and his psychological reaction to the amputation.

Looking at total hip replacement

To form a totally artificial hip (here, the McKee-Farrar total hip replacement), the surgeon cements a femoral head prosthesis in place to articulate with a studded cup, which he then cements into the deepened acetabulum. He may avoid using cement by implanting a prosthesis with a porous coating that promotes bony ingrowth.

During routine daily care, document the date, time, type of care given, and condition of the skin and suture line, noting any signs of irritation, such as redness or tenderness. Also note the patient's progress in caring for the stump or prosthesis.

Arthroplasty care

Care of the patient after arthroplasty — surgical replacement of all or part of a joint — helps restore mobility and normal use of the affected extremity; it also helps prevent such complications as infection, phlebitis, and respiratory problems. Arthroplasty care includes maintaining alignment of the affected joint, assisting with exercises, and providing routine postoperative care. An equally important nursing responsibility is teaching home care and exercises that may continue for several years, depending on the type of arthroplasty performed and the patient's condition.

The two most common arthroplastic procedures are cup arthroplasty and total joint replacement. In *cup arthroplasty*, the surgeon inserts a movable cup between the hip joint surfaces. The prosthesis has a porous coating that promotes bone regrowth. This procedure is usually indicated for a young patient who has rheumatoid arthritis, degenerative joint disease from traumatic injury, or an acetabulum fracture.

Total joint replacement (usually of the hip or knee) is commonly performed on patients over age 50. Total hip replacement may be used to treat osteoarthritis and severe crippling rheumatoid arthritis; total knee replacement is commonly used to treat severe pain, joint contractures, and deterioration of joint surfaces, conditions that prohibit full extension or flexion. (See *Looking at total hip replacement.*)

Nursing care after these operations — as well as care after less common surgical procedures (such as shoulder, elbow, wrist, ankle, or finger joint replacement) — requires similar skills.

Equipment

Balkan frame with trapeze ▪ comfort device (such as foam mattress, static air mattress overlay, low-air-loss bed, or sheepskin) ▪ bed sheets ▪ ordered traction apparatus (for example, for Buck's extension) ▪ incentive spirometer or intermittent positive-pressure breathing (IPPB) machine ▪ continuous passive motion (CPM) machine ▪ elastic stocking ▪ sterile dressings ▪ hypoallergenic tape ▪ ice bag ▪ skin lotion ▪ warm water ▪ crutches or walker ▪ pain medications ▪ closed-wound drainage system ▪ I.V. antibiotics ▪ pillow ▪ optional: abduction splint.

Traction is not usually applied after cup arthroplasty or total hip replacement. Instead, the patient may be given CPM treatments, which permit passive joint flexion.

After total knee replacement, a knee immobilizer may be applied in the operating room, or the leg may be placed in CPM.

Preparation of equipment

After the patient goes to the operating room, construct a Balkan frame with a trapeze on his bed frame. *This will allow him some mobility after the operation.* Then make the bed, using a comfort device and clean sheets. If the doctor orders postoperative traction, have the bed taken to the operating room. *This enables immediate placement of the patient on his hospital bed after surgery and eliminates the need for an additional move from his recovery room bed.*

Implementation

● Check vital signs every 30 minutes until they stabilize, then every 2 to 4 hours and routinely thereafter, according to hospital protocol. Report any changes in vital signs *because they may indicate infection and hemorrhage.*

• Encourage the patient to perform deep-breathing and coughing exercises. Assist with incentive spirometry or IPPB treatments, as ordered, *to prevent respiratory complications.*

• Assess neurovascular status every 2 hours for the first 48 hours and then every 4 hours *for signs of complications.* Specifically, check the affected leg for color, temperature, toe movement, sensation, edema, capillary filling, and pedal pulse. Also investigate any complaints of pain, burning, numbness, or tingling.

• Apply the elastic stocking to the unaffected leg, as ordered, *to promote venous return and prevent phlebitis and pulmonary emboli.* Once every 8 hours, remove the stocking, inspect the leg for pressure ulcers, and reapply it.

• Administer pain medications, as ordered.

• For at least 48 hours after surgery, administer I.V. antibiotics, as ordered, *to minimize the risk of wound infection.* Also observe the site for symptoms of phlebitis, such as warmth, swelling, tenderness, redness, and positive Homans' sign.

• Administer anticoagulant therapy, as ordered, *to minimize the risk of thrombophlebitis and embolus formation.* Observe for bleeding.

• Check dressings for excessive bleeding. Circle any drainage on the dressing and mark it with your initials, the date, and the time. As appropriate, apply more sterile dressings, using hypoallergenic tape. Report any excessive bleeding to the doctor.

• Observe the closed-wound drainage system for discharge color. *Proper drainage prevents hematoma. Purulent discharge and fever may indicate infection.* Empty and measure drainage, as ordered, using aseptic technique *to prevent infection.* (For more information, see "Closed-wound drain management," Chapter 4.)

• Monitor fluid intake and output daily, making sure to include wound drainage in the output measurement.

• Apply an ice bag, as ordered, to the affected site for the first 48 hours *to reduce swelling, relieve pain, and control bleeding.*

• Every 2 hours, turn the patient no more than 45 degrees toward each side and keep him in this position as long as he's comfortable. *These position changes enhance comfort, prevent pressure ulcers, and help prevent respiratory complications.*

• Help the patient use the trapeze to lift himself every 2 hours. Then provide skin care for his back and buttocks, using warm water and lotion, as indicated.

• Instruct the patient to perform muscle-strengthening exercises for affected and unaffected extremities, as ordered, *to help maintain muscle strength and range of motion and to help prevent phlebitis.*

• Before ambulation exercises, administer a mild analgesic, as ordered, *because movement is very painful.* Encourage the patient during the exercises.

• Assist the patient with progressive ambulation, using adjustable crutches or a walker when needed for support.

After cup arthroplasty

• Maintain balanced suspension and, if appropriate, Buck's extension traction *to support the leg, reduce muscle spasms, maintain abduction, and increase patient comfort.*

• Keep the affected leg in abduction and in the neutral position *to stabilize the hip and keep the cup and femur head in the acetabulum.* Place a pillow between the patient's legs *to maintain hip abduction.*

• On the day after surgery, teach the patient about CPM exercises, as ordered, *to maintain muscle strength and prepare him for eventual ambulation.* Exercises include quadriceps setting, ankle rotation, and plantar flexion and dorsiflexion of the feet.

After total hip replacement

• If ordered, maintain balanced suspension *to increase patient comfort, reduce muscle spasms, and maintain hip abduction.* Place a pillow or abduction splint between the patient's legs *to help maintain hip abduction.*

• If the patient desires, elevate the head of the bed 45 degrees for comfort. (Some doctors permit 60-degree elevation.) Keep the bed elevated no more than 30 minutes at a time *to prevent excessive hip flexion.*

◆ *Nursing alert.* Don't let the hip flex more than 90 degrees *because the prosthesis may dislocate.* ◆

• Keep the patient in the supine position, with the affected hip in full extension, for 1 hour three times a day and at night. *This will help prevent hip flexion contracture.*

• On the day after surgery, have the patient begin plantar flexion and dorsiflexion exercises of the foot on the affected leg. When ordered, instruct him to begin quadriceps exercises. Progressive ambulation protocols vary. Most patients are permitted to dangle their feet on the first day after surgery and to begin transfer and progressive ambulation with assistive devices on the second day.

After total knee replacement

• Keep the knee immobilized in full extension immediately after surgery. Many hospitals start CPM in the recovery room.

• Elevate the affected leg, as ordered, *to reduce swelling.*

• Instruct the patient to begin quadriceps exercises and straight leg-raising, when ordered (usually on the second postoperative day). Encourage flexion-extension exercises, when ordered (usually after the first dressing change).

• If the doctor orders use of the CPM machine, he will adjust the machine daily *to gradually increase the degree of flexion of the affected leg.* Typically, patients can dangle their feet on the first day after surgery and begin ambulation with partial weight-bearing as tolerated (cemented knee) or toe-touch ambulation only (uncemented knee) by the second day. The patient may need to wear a knee immobilizer for support when walking; otherwise, he should be in CPM for most of the day and night or during waking hours only. Check your hospital's protocol.

Special considerations

Before surgery, explain the procedure to the patient. Emphasize that frequent assessment — including the monitoring of vital signs, neurovascular integrity, and wound drainage — is normal after the operation.

Inform the patient that he'll receive I.V. antibiotics for about 2 days. Also be sure he understands that he'll receive medication around the clock for pain control. Explain the need for immobilizing the affected leg and exercising the unaffected one.

Before discharge, instruct the patient regarding home care and exercises.

Complications

Immobility after arthroplasty may result in such complications as shock, pulmonary embolism, pneumonia, phlebitis, paralytic ileus, urine retention, and bowel impaction. A deep wound or infection at the prosthesis site is a serious complication that may force removal of the prosthesis. Dislocation of a total hip prosthesis may occur after violent hip flexion or adduction or during internal rotation. Signs of dislocation include inability to rotate the hip or bear weight, shortening of the leg, and increased pain.

Fat embolism, a potentially fatal complication resulting from release of fat molecules in response to increased intermedullary canal pressure from the prosthesis, may develop within 72 hours after surgery. Watch for such signs and symptoms as apprehension, diaphoresis, fever, dyspnea, pulmonary effusion, tachycardia, cyanosis, seizures, decreased level of consciousness, and a petechial rash on the chest and shoulders.

Documentation

Record the patient's neurovascular status, maintenance of traction (for cup arthroplasty and hip replacement), or knee immobilization (for knee replacement). Note also the condition of the dressings and the drainage system and the application of ice bags. Describe the patient's position (especially the position of the affected leg), skin care and condition, respiratory care and condition, and the use of elastic stockings. Document all exercises performed and their effect; also record ambulatory efforts, the type of support used, and the amount of traction weight.

On the appropriate flowchart, record vital signs and fluid intake and output. Note the turning and skin care schedule and the current exercise and ambulation program. Also include the doctor's orders for the amount of traction weight and the degree of flexion permitted; update these orders as necessary. Record discharge instructions and how well the patient seems to understand them.

Selected references

Adams, J.C., and Hamblen, D.L. *Outline of Orthopaedics,* 11th ed. New York: Churchill Livingstone, 1990.

Arandottir, G. *Neurobehavioral Assessment in Adult CNS Dysfunction.* St. Louis: C.V. Mosby Co., 1989.

Barangan, J.D. "Factors That Influence Recovery from Hip Fracture During Hospitalization," *Orthopaedic Nursing* 9(5):19-30, September-October 1990.

Basmajian, J. *Therapeutic Exercise,* 5th ed. Baltimore: Williams & Wilkins Co., 1989.

Baum, C., et al. *Human Performance Deficits: Occupational Therapy Assessment and Intervention.* Thorofare, N.J.: Charles B. Slack, Inc., 1989.

Crenshaw, A.H., ed. *Campbell's Operative Orthopaedics,* 8th ed. St. Louis: Mosby-Year Book, Inc., 1991.

Davis, C.M. *Patient-Practitioner Interaction: An Experiential Manual for Developing the Art of Health Care.* Thorofare, N.J.: Charles B. Slack, Inc., 1989.

Dubrovskis, V., and Wells, D. "Hip Fracture in the Elderly: Program Planning Puts These Patients on Their Feet Again," *Canadian Nurse* 84(5):20-22, May 1988.

Errico, T.J., et al., eds. *Spinal Trauma.* Philadelphia: J.B. Lippincott Co., 1991.

Hansell, M.J. "Fractures and the Healing Process," *Orthopaedic Nursing* 7(1):43-50, January-February 1988.

Illustrated Manual of Nursing Practice, 2nd ed. Springhouse, Pa.: Springhouse Corp., 1994.

"Internal Fixation for Open Fractures," *Patient Care* 21(14):25, September 15, 1988.

Medhat, A., et al. "Factors That Influence the Level of Activities in Persons with Lower Extremity Amputation," *Rehabilitation Nursing* 15(1):13-18, January-February 1990.

Moncor, C., and Williams, H.J. "Cervical Spine Management in Patients with Rheumatoid Arthritis," *Physical Therapy* 68(4): 509-15, April 1988.

Morton, P.G. *Health Assessment in Nursing,* 2nd ed. Springhouse, Pa.: Springhouse Corp., 1993.

Pastorino, C., et al. "Scope of Orthopaedic Nursing Practice," *Orthopaedic Nursing* 9(6):11-13, November-December 1990.

Patient Teaching Loose-leaf Library. Springhouse, Pa.: Springhouse Corp., 1990.

Rockwood, C.A., and Green, D.P., eds. *Fractures in Adults,* 3rd ed. Philadelphia: J.B. Lippincott Co., 1990.

Rockwood, C.A., and Matsen, F.A., eds. *The Shoulder.* Philadelphia: W.B. Saunders Co., 1990.

Sherk, H.H., ed. *Lasers in Orthopaedics.* Philadelphia: J.B. Lippincott Co., 1990.

Weinstein, J.N., and Wiesel, S.W., eds. *The Lumbar Spine.* Philadelphia: W.B. Saunders Co., 1990.

Zaslav, K., et al. "General Principles of Management of Fractures and Dislocations," in *Principles of Orthopaedic Practice,* vol. 1. Edited by Dee, R., et al. New York: McGraw-Hill Book Co., 1988.

EYE, EAR, AND NOSE CARE

REBECCA McCASKEY, RN, BA, MEd

Introduction

Because the eyes transmit about 70% of the sensory information reaching the brain, visual impairment can severely limit a patient's ability to function independently and to perceive and react to his surroundings. Similarly, untreated hearing loss can drastically impair communication and social interaction. Inner-ear disorders may disrupt equilibrium and the ability to move freely. And nasal disorders can interfere with respiration, reduce vitality, and cause marked discomfort.

When caring for a patient with a sensory loss, remember that he's actually experiencing multiple impairments. That's because sensory impairment brings about perceptual impairment. The combined loss significantly alters a person's daily activities and threatens his security and self-image.

Because eye, ear, and nose disorders are as common as they are troublesome, you're likely to perform the procedures presented in this chapter whether you practice in a hospital, clinic, extended-care facility, or other setting. You may be called on to assist with or perform eye, ear, or nose procedures in situations ranging from emergencies to routine checkups. These procedures call for the utmost care and precision to prevent infection and injury and to preserve function.

Overcome perceptual barriers

Performing procedures that diagnose, treat, or even briefly cause sensory impairment requires you to give clear, simple instructions and explanations. You'll also need to give ample reassurance to a patient who's certain to feel apprehensive about his ability to care for himself and function independently. In an emergency, effective communication becomes even more important because you'll be dealing with a patient suddenly disoriented by sensory and perceptual impairments.

Provide patient teaching

You can make an important contribution to the patient's understanding of eye, ear, and nasal disorders. As you implement various procedures, inform your patient about preventive care measures. Help him to recognize signs and symptoms of sensory disorders. Urge him to schedule regular examinations to detect problems early. And remind him to use safety equipment at work and, as appropriate, at home.

EYE CARE
Hot and cold eye compresses

Whether applied hot or cold, eye compresses are soothing and therapeutic. Hot compresses may be used to relieve discomfort. Because heat increases circulation (which enhances absorption and decreases inflammation), hot compresses may promote drainage of superficial infections. On the other hand, cold compresses can reduce swelling or bleeding and relieve itching. Because cold numbs sensory fibers, cold compresses may be ordered to ease periorbital discomfort between prescribed doses of pain medication. Typically, a hot or cold compress should be applied for 20-minute periods, four to six times a day. Ocular infection calls for the use of aseptic technique.

Equipment

For hot compresses: gloves ■ prescribed solution, usually sterile water or normal saline solution ■ sterile bowl ■ sterile 4″ × 4″ gauze pads ■ towel.

For cold compresses: small plastic bag (such as a sandwich bag) or glove ■ ice chips ■ ½″ (1.3 cm) nonallergenic tape ■ towel ■ sterile 4″ × 4″ gauze pads ■ sterile water, normal saline solution, or prescribed ophthalmic irrigant ■ gloves.

Preparation of equipment

For hot compresses: Place a capped bottle of sterile water or normal saline solution in a bowl of hot water or under a stream of hot, tap water. Allow the solution to become warm, not hot (no higher than 120° F [49° C]). Pour the warm water or saline solution into a sterile bowl, filling the bowl about halfway. Place some sterile gauze pads in the bowl.

For cold compresses: Place ice chips in a plastic bag (or a glove if necessary) to make an ice pack. Keep the ice pack small *to avoid excessive pressure on the eye.* Remove excess air from the bag or glove and knot the open end. Cut a piece of nonallergenic tape *to secure the ice pack.* Place all equipment on the bedside stand near the patient.

Implementation

● Explain the procedure to the patient, make him comfortable, and provide privacy.
● When applying hot compresses, have the patient sit, if possible. When applying cold compresses, have the patient lie supine. Support his head with a pillow, and turn

his head slightly to the unaffected side. *This position will help to hold the compress in place.*

• If the patient has an eye patch, remove it.

• Drape a towel around the patient's shoulders *to catch any spills.* Wash your hands and put on gloves.

To apply hot compresses

• Take two 4″×4″ gauze pads from the basin. Squeeze out the excess solution.

• Instruct the patient to close his eyes. Gently apply the pads—one on top of the other—to the affected eye. (If the patient complains that the compress feels too hot, remove it immediately.)

• Change the compress every few minutes, as necessary, for the prescribed length of time. After removing each compress, check the skin for signs that the compress solution is too hot.

To apply cold compresses

• Moisten the middle of one of the sterile 4″×4″ gauze pads with the sterile water, normal saline solution, or ophthalmic irrigating solution. *This helps to conduct the cold from the ice pack.* Keep the edges dry *so that they can absorb excess moisture.*

• Tell the patient to close his eyes; then place the moist gauze pad over the affected eye.

• Place the ice pack on top of the gauze pad and tape it in place. If he complains of pain, remove the ice pack. Some patients may have an adverse reaction to cold.

• After 15 to 20 minutes, remove the tape, ice pack, and gauze pad and discard them.

To conclude the procedure

• Use the remaining sterile 4″×4″ gauze pads to clean and dry the patient's face.

• If ordered, apply ophthalmic ointment.

• If ordered, apply an eye patch. (See *Applying an eye patch.*)

Special considerations

When applying hot compresses, change the prescribed solution as frequently as necessary *to maintain a constant temperature.*

If ordered to apply moist, cold compresses directly to the patient's eyelid, fill a bowl with ice and water and soak 4″×4″ gauze pads in it. Place a compress directly on the lid; change compresses every 2 to 3 minutes.

Home care

When teaching a patient to apply warm compresses at home, explain that he can substitute a clean bowl and washcloth for the sterile equipment.

If both eyes are infected, emphasize using separate equipment for each eye (two bowls of prescribed solution and individual compresses). Inform the patient that this will keep him from passing infection back and forth between eyes. Also direct him to wash his hands thoroughly after treating each eye.

Documentation

Record the time and duration of the procedure. Describe the eye's appearance before and after treatment. Name any ointments (and amounts) or dressings applied to the eye. Also note the patient's tolerance of the procedure.

 Eye irrigation

Used mainly to flush secretions, chemicals, and foreign bodies from the eye, eye irrigation also provides a way to administer medications for corneal and conjunctival disorders. In an emergency, tap water may serve as an irrigant.

The amount of solution needed to irrigate an eye depends on the contaminant. Secretions require a moderate volume; major chemical burns require a copious amount. Usually, an I.V. bottle or bag of normal saline solution (with I.V. tubing attached) supplies enough solution for continuous irrigation of a chemical burn. (See *Three devices for eye irrigation,* page 482.)

Equipment

Gloves ▪ towels ▪ eyelid retractor ▪ cotton balls or facial tissues ▪ optional: litmus paper, proparacaine hydrochloride topical anesthetic.

For moderate-volume irrigation: prescribed sterile ophthalmic irrigant ▪ cotton-tipped applicators.

For copious irrigation: one or more 1,000-ml bottles or bags of normal saline solution ▪ standard I.V. infusion set without needle.

Commercially prepared bottles of sterile ophthalmic irrigant are available. All solutions should be at body temperature: 98.6° F (37° C).

Preparation of equipment

Read the label on the sterile ophthalmic irrigant. Double-check its sterility, strength, and expiration date.

For moderate-volume irrigation: Remove the cap from the irrigant container and place the container within easy reach. (Be sure to keep the tip of the container sterile.)

For copious irrigation: Use sterile technique to set up the I.V. tubing and the bag or bottle of normal saline

Applying an eye patch

With a doctor's order, you may apply an eye patch for various reasons: to protect the eye after injury or surgery, to prevent accidental damage to an anesthetized eye, to promote healing, to absorb secretions, or to prevent the patient from touching or rubbing his eye.

A thicker patch, called a pressure patch, may be used to help corneal abrasions heal, compress postoperative edema, or control hemorrhage from traumatic injury. Application requires an ophthalmologist's prescription and supervision.

To apply a patch, choose a gauze pad of appropriate size for the patient's face, place it gently over the closed eye.

For increased protection of an injured eye, you should place a plastic or metal shield (as shown below) on top of the gauze pads and apply tape over the shield.

Secure the patch with two or three strips of tape. Extend the tape from midforehead across the eye to below the earlobe. A pressure patch, which is markedly thicker than a single-thickness gauze patch, exerts extra tension against the closed eye. After placing the initial gauze pad, you'll need to build it up with additional gauze pieces (as shown above, at right). Tape it firmly so that the patch exerts even pressure against the closed eye.

Occasionally, you may use a head dressing to secure a pressure patch. The dressing applies additional pressure or, in burn patients, holds the patch in place without tape.

---

solution. Hang the container on an I.V. pole, fill the I.V. tubing with the solution, and adjust the drip regulator valve *to ensure an adequate but not forceful flow.* Place all other equipment within easy reach.

Implementation

• Wash your hands, put on gloves, and explain the procedure to the patient. If the patient has a chemical burn, ease his anxiety by explaining that irrigation prevents further damage.

• Assist the patient in lying supine. Turn his head slightly toward the affected side *to prevent solution flowing over his nose and into the other eye.*
• Place a towel under the patient's head, and let him hold another towel against his affected side *to catch excess solution.*
• Using the thumb and index finger of your nondominant hand, separate the patient's eyelids.

Three devices for eye irrigation

Depending on the type and extent of injury, the patient's eye may need to be irrigated using different devices.

Squeeze bottle

For moderate-volume irrigation—to remove eye secretions, for example—apply sterile ophthalmic irrigant to the eye directly from the squeeze bottle container. Direct the stream at the inner canthus and position the patient so the stream washes across the cornea and exits at the outer canthus.

I.V. tube

For copious irrigation—to treat chemical burns, for example—set up an I.V. bag and tubing without a needle. Use the procedure described for moderate irrigation to flush the eye for at least 15 minutes.

Morgan lens

Connected to irrigation tubing, a Morgan lens permits continuous lavage and also delivers medication to the eye. Use an adapter to connect the lens to the I.V. tubing and the solution container. Begin the irrigation at the prescribed flow rate. To insert the device, ask the patient to look down as you insert the lens under the upper eyelid. Then have her look up as you retract and release the lower eyelid over the lens.

• If ordered, instill proparacaine hydrochloride eyedrops *as a comfort measure.* Use them only once *because repeated use retards healing.*

• *To irrigate the conjunctival cul-de-sac,* continue holding the eyelids apart with your thumb and index finger.

• *To irrigate the upper eyelid (the superior fornix)* use an eyelid retractor. Steady the hand holding the retractor by resting it on the patient's forehead. *The retractor prevents the eyelid from closing involuntarily when solution touches the cornea and conjunctiva.*

Moderate irrigation

• Holding the bottle of sterile ophthalmic irrigant about 1″ (2.5 cm) from the eye, direct a constant, gentle stream at the inner canthus *so that the solution flows across the cornea to the outer canthus.*

• Evert the lower eyelid and then the upper eyelid *to inspect for retained foreign particles.*

• Remove any foreign particles by gently touching the the conjunctiva with sterile, wet, cotton-tipped applicators. Do not touch the cornea.

• Resume irrigating the eye until it's clean of all visible foreign particles.

Copious irrigation

• Hold the control valve on the I.V. tubing about 1″ above the eye, and direct a constant, gentle stream of normal saline solution at the inner canthus *so that the solution flows across the cornea to the outer canthus.*

• Ask the patient to rotate his eye periodically while you continue the irrigation. This action may dislodge foreign particles.

• Evert the lower and then the upper eyelid to inspect for retained foreign particles. (This inspection is especially important when the patient has caustic lime in his eye.)

Aftercare

• After eye irrigation, gently dry the eyelids with cotton balls or facial tissues, wiping from the inner to the outer canthus. Use a new cotton ball or tissue for each wipe. *This reduces the patient's need to rub his eye.*

• Remove and discard your gloves.

• When indicated, arrange for follow-up care.

• Wash your hands *to avoid burning from residual chemical contaminants.*

Special considerations

When irrigating both eyes, have the patient tilt his head toward the side being irrigated to avoid cross-contamination.

For chemical burns, irrigate each eye for at least 15 minutes with normal saline solution *to dilute and wash out the harsh chemical.* If the patient can't identify the specific chemical, use litmus paper *to determine if the chemical is acidic or alkaline, or to be sure that the eye has been irrigated adequately.* (After irrigating any chemical, note the time, date, and chemical for your own reference *in case you develop contact dermatitis.*)

Documentation

Note the duration of irrigation, the type and amount of solution, and characteristics of the drainage. Record your assessment of the patient's eye before and after irrigation. Also note his response to the procedure.

EAR CARE
Ear irrigation

Irrigating the ear involves washing the external auditory canal with a stream of solution to clean the canal of discharges, to soften and remove impacted cerumen, or to dislodge a foreign body. Sometimes, irrigation aims to relieve localized inflammation and discomfort. The procedure must be performed carefully to avoid causing the patient discomfort or vertigo, to prevent maceration of tissue that lines the canal, and to avoid increasing the risk of otitis externa. Because irrigation may contaminate the middle ear if the tympanic membrane is ruptured, an otoscopic examination always precedes ear irrigation.

This procedure is contraindicated when a vegetable foreign body (such as a pea, a bean, or a corn kernel) obstructs the auditory canal. These foreign bodies are *hygroscopic* — that is, they attract and absorb moisture. In contact with an irrigant or other solution, they swell, causing intense pain and complicating removal of the object by irrigation. The procedure is contraindicated also if the patient has a cold, fever, ear infection, or an injured or ruptured tympanic membrane.

Equipment

Ear irrigation syringe (rubber bulb) ▪ otoscope ▪ prescribed irrigant ▪ large basin ▪ linen-saver pad and bath towel ▪ emesis basin ▪ cotton balls or cotton-tipped applicators ▪ 4″ × 4″ gauze pad ▪ optional: adjustable light (such as a gooseneck lamp), container for irrigant, tubing, clamp, and catheter with ear tip.

Wear gloves if you expect contact with infected matter.

How to irrigate the ear canal

Follow these guidelines for irrigating the ear canal.
• Gently pull the auricle up and back *to straighten the ear canal.* (For a child, pull the ear down and back.)
• Have the patient hold an emesis basin beneath the ear to catch returning irrigant. Position the tip of the irrigating syringe at the meatus of the auditory canal. Be sure not to occlude the meatus *because you'll impede backflow and increase pressure in the canal.*

• Point the tip of the syringe upward and toward the posterior ear canal. *This angle prevents damage to the tympanic membrane and also guards against pushing debris farther into the canal.*

• Direct a steady stream of irrigant against the side of the ear canal and inspect the return fluid for cloudiness, cerumen, blood, or foreign matter.

Preparation of equipment
Select the appropriate syringe, and obtain the prescribed irrigant. Put the container of irrigant into the large basin filled with hot water *to warm the solution to body temperature:* 98.6° F (37° C). Avoid extreme temperature changes *because they can affect inner ear fluids, causing nausea and dizziness.*

Test the temperature of the solution by sprinkling a few drops on your inner wrist. Inspect equipment (syringe or catheter tips) for breaks or cracks; inspect all metal tips for roughness.

Implementation
• Explain the procedure to the patient, provide privacy, wash your hands, and put on gloves (if necessary).
• If you haven't already done so, use the otoscope to inspect the auditory canal to be irrigated.
• Help the patient to a sitting position. *To prevent the solution from running down his neck,* tilt his head slightly forward and toward the affected side. If he can't sit, have him lie on his back and tilt his head slightly forward and toward the affected ear.
• Make sure that you have adequate lighting.
• If the patient is sitting, place the linen-saver pad— covered with the bath towel—on his shoulder and upper arm, under the affected ear. If he's lying down, cover his pillow and the area under the affected ear.
• Have the patient hold the emesis basin close to his head under the affected ear.
• *To avoid getting foreign matter into the ear canal,* clean the auricle and the meatus of the auditory canal with a cotton ball or cotton-tipped applicator moistened with normal saline or the prescribed irrigating solution.
• Draw the irrigant into the syringe and expel any air.
• Straighten the auditory canal; then insert the syringe tip and start the flow. (See *How to irrigate the ear canal.*)
• During the irrigation, observe the patient for signs of pain or dizziness. If he reports either, stop the procedure immediately.
• When the syringe is empty, remove it and inspect the return flow. Then, refill the syringe, and continue the irrigation until the return flow is clear. Never use more than 500 ml of irrigant during this procedure.
• Remove the syringe, and inspect the ear canal for cleanliness with the otoscope.
• Dry the patient's auricle and neck.
• Remove the bath towel and linen-saver pad. Help the seated patient lie on his affected side with the 4″ × 4″ gauze pad under his ear *to promote drainage of residual debris and solution.*

Special considerations

Avoid dropping or squirting irrigant on the tympanic membrane. *This may startle the patient and cause discomfort.* If you're using an irrigating catheter instead of a syringe, adjust the flow of solution to a steady, comfortable rate with a flow clamp. Don't raise the container more than 6″ (15.2 cm) above the ear. *If the container is higher, the resulting pressure may damage the tympanic membrane.*

If the doctor directs you to place a cotton pledget in the ear canal *to retain some of the solution,* pack the cotton loosely. Instruct the patient not to remove it.

If irrigation doesn't dislodge impacted cerumen, the doctor may order you to instill several drops of glycerin, carbamide peroxide (Debrox), or a similar preparation two to three times daily for 2 to 3 days, and then to irrigate the ear again.

Complications

Possible complications include vertigo, nausea, skin maceration, otitis externa, and otitis media (if the patient has a perforated or ruptured tympanic membrane). Forceful instillation of irrigant can rupture the tympanic membrane.

Documentation

Record the date and time of irrigation. Note which ear you irrigated. Also note the volume and the solution used, the appearance of the canal before and after irrigation, the appearance of the return flow, the patient's tolerance of the procedure, and any comments he made about his condition, especially related to his hearing acuity.

NOSE CARE
Nasal irrigation

Irrigation of the nasal passages with warm normal saline solution soothes irritated mucous membranes and washes away crusted mucus, secretions, and foreign matter. Left unattended, these deposits may impede sinus drainage and airflow and cause headaches, infections, and unpleasant odors. Routine irrigation reduces the infection risk and increases comfort and ease of breathing. Irrigation may be done with a bulb syringe or an electronic oral irrigating device.

Nasal irrigation benefits patients with chronic nasal conditions — such as sinusitis, rhinitis, Wegener's granulomatosis, and Sjögren's syndrome. In addition, it may help long-term users of some inhalant drugs (such as cocaine or nose drops containing phenylephrine chloride) and those who regularly inhale toxins or allergens — paint fumes, sawdust, pesticides, or coal dust, for example.

Contraindications to nasal irrigation may include recent sinus surgery, advanced destruction of the sinuses, frequent nosebleeds, and foreign bodies in the nasal passages (which could be driven farther into the passages by the irrigant). However, some patients with these conditions may benefit from irrigation.

Equipment

Bulb syringe or an oral irrigating device (such as a Water Pik) ▪ rigid or flexible disposable irrigation tips (for one-patient use) ▪ normal saline solution ▪ plastic sheet ▪ apron or towels ▪ facial tissues ▪ bath basin ▪ gloves.

Preparation of equipment

Warm the normal saline solution to about 105° F (40.5° C). If you're irrigating with a bulb syringe, draw some irrigant into the bulb and then expel it. *This will rinse any residual solution from the previous irrigation and warm the bulb.*

If you're using an oral irrigating device, plug the instrument into an electrical outlet in an area near the patient. Then, run about 1 cup of normal saline solution through the tubing *to rinse residual solution from the lines and warm the tubing.* Next, fill the reservoir of the device with warm normal saline solution.

Implementation

- Wash your hands and put on gloves.
- Explain the procedure to the patient.
- Have the patient sit comfortably near the equipment in a position that allows the bulb or catheter tip to enter his nose and the returning irrigant to flow into the bath basin or sink. (See *Positioning the patient for nasal irrigation,* page 486.)
- Remind him to keep his mouth open and to breathe rhythmically during irrigation. *This causes the soft palate to seal the throat, allowing the irrigant to stream out the opposite nostril and carry discharge with it.*
- Instruct the patient not to speak or swallow during the irrigation *to avoid forcing infectious material into the sinuses or eustachian tubes.*
- *To avoid injuring the nasal mucosa,* remove the irrigating tip from the patient's nostril if he has to sneeze or cough.

To use a bulb syringe

- Fill the bulb syringe with normal saline solution and insert the tip about ½″ (1.3 cm) into the patient's nostril.
- Squeeze the bulb until a gentle stream of warm irrigant washes through the nose. Avoid forceful squeezing, *which*

Positioning the patient for nasal irrigation

Whether you're teaching a patient to perform nasal irrigation with a bulb syringe or an oral irrigating device, the irrigation will progress more easily once the patient learns how to hold her head for safety, comfort, and effectiveness.

Help the patient to sit upright with her head bent forward over the basin or sink and well-flexed on her chest. Her nose and ear should be on the same vertical plane.

Explain that she's less likely to breathe in the irrigant when holding her head in this position. Additionally, this position should keep the irrigant from entering the eustachian tubes, which will now lie above the level of the irrigation stream.

may drive debris from the nasal passages into the sinuses or eustachian tubes and introduce infection. Alternate nostrils until the return irrigant runs clear.
• Inspect returning irrigant. Changes in color, viscosity, or volume may signal an infection and should be reported to the doctor. Also report blood or necrotic material.

To use an oral irrigation device
• Insert the irrigation tip into the nostril about ½″ to 1″ (1.3 to 2.5 cm) and turn on the irrigating device. Begin with a low pressure setting (increasing the pressure as needed) *to obtain a gentle stream of irrigant.* Again, be careful not to drive material from the nose into the sinuses or eustachian tubes. Irrigate both nostrils.
• Inspect returning irrigant. Changes in color, viscosity, or volume may signal an infection and should be reported to the doctor. Also report blood or necrotic material.

To conclude the procedure
• After irrigation, have the patient wait for a few minutes before blowing excess fluid from both nostrils at once. *Gentle blowing through both nostrils prevents fluid or pressure buildup in the sinuses. This action also helps to loosen and expel crusted secretions and mucus.*
• Clean the bulb syringe and irrigating device with disinfectant as recommended. Rinse and dry.

Special considerations
Expect fluid to drain from the patient's nose for a brief time after the irrigation and before he blows his nose.

Be sure to insert the irrigation tip far enough to ensure that the irrigant cleans the nasal membranes before draining out. The amount of normal saline solution used for an irrigation varies depending on the amount of crusted mucus. A typical amount ranges from 500 to 1,000 ml.

Home care
To continue nasal irrigations at home, teach the patient how to prepare normal saline solution. Tell him to fill a clean 1-liter plastic bottle with tap water or distilled water (4 cups + 1 oz = 1 liter), add 1½ tsp of table salt, and shake the solution until the salt dissolves. Teach him how to disinfect used irrigation devices.

Documentation
Write down the time and duration of the procedure and the amount of irrigant used. Describe the appearance of the returned solution. Record your assessment of the patient's comfort level and breathing ease before and after the procedure. Document patient-teaching content.

Nasal packing

In the highly vascular nasal mucosa, even seemingly minor injuries can cause major bleeding and blood loss. When routine therapeutic measures — such as direct pressure, cautery, or vasoconstrictive medications—fail to control epistaxis (nosebleed), the patient's nose may have to be packed to stop anterior bleeding (which runs out of the nose) or posterior bleeding (which runs down the throat). If blood drains into the nasopharyngeal area or the lacrimal ducts, the patient may appear to bleed from the mouth and eyes as well.

Most nasal bleeding originates at a plexus of arterioles and venules in the anteroinferior septum. Only about 1 in 10 nosebleeds occurs in the more vascular posterior nose, which usually bleeds more heavily than the anterior location.

A nurse typically assists a doctor with anterior or posterior nasal packing, depending on the bleeding site. (See *Types of nasal packing,* page 488.) Or she may assist with nasal balloon catheterization, a procedure that applies pressure to a posterior bleeding site. (See *Nasal balloon catheters,* page 489.)

Whichever procedure the patient undergoes, the nurse should provide ongoing encouragement and support to reduce his discomfort and anxiety. In addition, the nurse should perform ongoing assessment to determine the procedure's success and detect possible complications.

Equipment

For anterior and posterior packing: gowns ■ goggles ■ masks ■ sterile gloves ■ prepackaged nasal packing kit, head and neck examination kit, or sterile tray ■ nasal speculum ■ headlamp ■ sterile bayonet forceps ■ suction apparatus (with sterile suction-connecting tubing and sterile nasal aspirator tip) ■ two sterile towels ■ normal saline solution ■ sterile bowl ■ local anesthetic spray or vial of local anesthetic solution (such as lidocaine with epinephrine or a decongestant with a vasoconstrictor, such as phenylephrine) ■ cotton pledgets ■ electrocautery device or silver nitrate pledgets ■ antibiotic ointment ■ 10-ml syringe with a 22G 1½" needle ■ sedative or tranquilizer ■ water-soluble lubricant ■ sterile cotton-tipped applicators ■ nonallergenic tape ■ emesis basin ■ facial tissues ■ mouth care supplies.

For anterior packing: ½" (1.3 cm) petroleum gauze (3' to 4' [0.9- to 1.2-m] strip), nasal tampons, or absorbable nasal pack (Surgicel, Gelfoam, or thrombin) ■ small flexible catheter ■ normal saline solution or antibiotic solution.

For posterior packing: sterile 4" × 4" gauze pads or dental roll ■ sterile 2" × 2" gauze pads ■ long heavy silk sutures ■ two small flexible catheters ■ two single- or double-chamber nasal balloon catheters ■ normal saline solution ■ two hemostats ■ 30-ml syringe.

For emergency bedside use: flashlight ■ scissors ■ hemostat.

Preparation of equipment

Wash your hands. Assemble all equipment at the patient's bedside. Be sure the headlamp works. Plug in the suction apparatus and connect the tubing from the collection bottle to the suction source. Test the suction equipment to be sure it works properly. At the bedside, create a sterile field. (Use the sterile towels or the sterile tray.) Using sterile technique, place all sterile equipment on the sterile field.

If the doctor will inject a local anesthetic rather than spray it, place the 22G 1½" needle attached to the 10-ml syringe on the sterile field. When the doctor readies the syringe, clean the stopper on the anesthetic vial and hold the vial so he can withdraw the anesthetic. *This practice allows the doctor to avoid touching his sterile gloves to the nonsterile vial.*

Open the packages containing sterile suction-connecting tubing and aspirating tip and place them on the sterile field. Fill the sterile bowl with the normal saline solution *so the suction tubing can be flushed as necessary.*

If the patient needs posterior packing and you don't have premade packing, wash your hands, put on sterile gloves, and make a posterior pack by rolling a sterile 2" × 2" gauze pad. The pack should be 1½" (3.75 cm) long and 1" (2.5 cm) in diameter. Trim excess gauze with sterile scissors. Secure the roll with the three 18" (46-cm) lengths of silk suture. Tie a suture at each end and one in the middle of the roll; don't trim the suture ends. Thoroughly lubricate the anterior or posterior packing with antibiotic ointment.

If the patient needs a nasal balloon catheter, test the balloon for leaks by inflating the catheter with normal saline solution. Remove the solution before insertion.

Implementation

● Ensure that all persons caring for the patient wear gowns, gloves, and eye protection during insertion of packing *to prevent possible contamination from splattered blood.*

● Check the patient's vital signs and observe for hypotension with postural changes. *Hypotension suggests significant blood loss.* Also monitor airway patency *because the patient will be at risk for aspirating or vomiting swallowed blood.*

● Explain the procedure to the patient and offer reassurance *to reduce his anxiety and promote cooperation.*

● If ordered, administer a sedative or tranquilizer *to reduce the patient's anxiety and decrease sympathetic stimulation, which can exacerbate a nosebleed.*

● Help the patient sit with his head tilted forward *to minimize blood drainage into the throat and avoid aspiration.*

(Text continues on page 490.)

Types of nasal packing

Depending on its source, your patient's nosebleed may be controlled with anterior or posterior nasal packing.

Anterior nasal packing
The doctor may treat an anterior nosebleed by packing the anterior nasal cavity with a 3′ to 4′ (0.9- to 1.2-m) strip of antibiotic-impregnated petroleum gauze or with a nasal tampon.

A nasal tampon is made of tightly compressed absorbent material with a central breathing tube. The doctor inserts a lubricated tampon along the floor of the nose and, with the patient's head tilted backward, instills 5 to 10 ml of antibiotic or normal saline solution. The tampon expands as a result, stopping the bleeding. It should be moistened periodically, and the central breathing tube should be suctioned regularly.

In a child or a patient with blood dyscrasias, the doctor may fashion an absorbable pack by moistening a gauzelike, regenerated cellulose material with a vasoconstrictor. Applied to a visible bleeding point, this substance will swell to form a clot. Because it's absorbable, the packing doesn't need removal.

Posterior nasal packing
Posterior packing consists of a gauze roll shaped and secured by three sutures (one suture at each end and one in the middle) or a balloon-type catheter. To insert the packing, the doctor advances one or two soft catheters into the patient's nostrils. When the catheter tips appear in the nasopharynx, the doctor grasps them with a Kelly clamp or bayonet forceps and pulls them forward

through the patient's mouth. He secures the two end sutures to the catheter tip and draws the catheter back through the patient's nostrils.

This step brings the packing into place with the end sutures hanging from the patient's nostril. (The middle suture emerges from the patient's mouth to free the packing, when needed.)

The doctor may weight the nose sutures with a clamp. Then he will pull the packing securely into place behind the soft palate and against the posterior end of the septum (nasal choana).

Finally, after he examines the patient's throat (to ensure that the uvula hasn't been forced under the packing), he will insert anterior packing and secure the whole apparatus by tying the posterior pack strings around rolled gauze or a dental roll at the nostrils.

Anterior packing

Rolled gauze

Posterior packing

Nasal balloon catheters

To control posterior epistaxis, the doctor may use a balloon catheter instead of nasal packing. Self-retaining and disposable, the catheter may have a single or a double balloon to apply pressure to bleeding nasal tissues. Less commonly, the doctor may insert a balloon-tipped urinary drainage catheter (a #14 to #16 French with a 30-ml balloon for an adult). If bleeding remains uncontrolled, arterial ligation, cryotherapy, or arterial embolization may be needed.

Once inserted and inflated, the single-balloon catheter shown below compresses the blood vessels while a soft, collapsible external bulb prevents the catheter from dislodging posteriorly.

After placement and inflation with saline solution (not air because it will leak slowly), the posterior portion of the double-balloon device (shown at the top of the next column) secures the catheter in the nasopharynx while the anterior balloon compresses bleeding vessels. This catheter has a central airway for breathing comfort.

Assisting with insertion

To assist with inserting a single- or double-balloon catheter, prepare the patient as you would for nasal packing. Take care to discuss the procedure thoroughly to alleviate the patient's anxiety and promote his cooperation.

Explain that the catheter tip will be lubricated with an antibiotic or water-soluble lubricant to ease passage and to prevent infection.

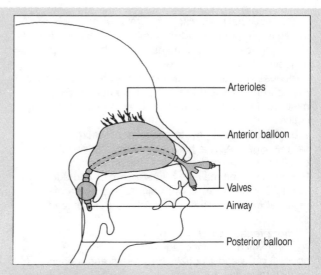

Providing routine care

The tip of the single-balloon catheter will be inserted in the nostrils until it reaches the posterior pharynx. Then, the balloon will be inflated with normal saline solution, pulled gently into the posterior nasopharynx and secured at the nostrils with the collapsible bulb (or with a hemostat). With a double-balloon catheter, the posterior balloon is inflated with normal saline solution; then the anterior balloon is inflated.

Check catheter placement routinely. Assess the nostrils for irritation or erosion. Remove secretions by gently suctioning the airway of a double-balloon catheter or by dabbing away crusted external secretions if the patient has a catheter without an airway.

To prevent damage to nasal tissue, the doctor may order the balloon deflated for 10 minutes every 24 hours. If bleeding recurs or remains uncontrolled, reinflate the balloon and contact the doctor. He may add packing in front of or around the balloon.

Recognizing complications

Complications associated with nasal balloon catheters are similar to those associated with nasal packing. The patient may report difficulty breathing, swallowing, or eating, and the nasal mucosa may sustain damage from pressure. Balloon deflation may dislodge clots and nasal debris into the oropharynx, which could prompt coughing, gagging, or vomiting.

Preventing recurrent nosebleeds

Before your patient's discharge, review the following self-care guidelines to minimize his chances for recurrent nosebleeds at home, on the job, or in school.

• Because nosebleeds can result from dry mucous membranes, suggest that the patient use a cool-mist room vaporizer or humidifier as needed, especially in dry environments.

• Teach the patient how to minimize pressure on nasal passages. Advise him, for instance, to avoid constipation and consequent straining at stool. Recommend maintaining a fiber-rich diet and adequate fluid intake. Also warn him to forgo extreme physical exertion for 24 hours after the nosebleed stops.

• Other precautionary measures include avoiding aspirin (which has anticoagulant properties) for about 5 days and alcoholic beverages and tobacco as well for at least 5 days.

• If the patient develops a nosebleed despite these precautions, tell him to keep his head higher than his heart. He should use a thumb and forefinger to press the soft portion of the nostrils together and against the facial bones. (Recommend against direct pressure if he has a facial injury or nasal fracture.) He should maintain pressure for up to 10 minutes and then apply ice wrapped in a plastic bag or washcloth to his nose (because cold facilitates coagulation).

• Turn on the suction apparatus and attach the connecting tubing *so the doctor can aspirate the nasal cavity to remove clots before locating the bleeding source.*

• To inspect the nasal cavity, the doctor will insert a nasal speculum. He will open the speculum *to dilate the cavity.* If he can see the bleeding site, the doctor calls the episode an "anterior bleed."

For anterior nasal packing

• Help the doctor try to control bleeding by chemical cautery with silver nitrate pledgets, electrocautery, or a vasoconstricting agent such as phenylephrine (topical), lidocaine with epinephrine (injected), or cocaine (topical).

• To enhance the vasoconstrictor's action, apply manual pressure to the nose for about 10 minutes. (See *Preventing recurrent nosebleeds.*)

• If bleeding persists, you may assist with insertion of an absorbable nasal pack directly on the bleeding site. The material will swell, forming an artificial clot.

• If these methods prove unsuccessful, prepare to assist the doctor with insertion of anterior nasal packing. (Even if only one side is bleeding, both sides may require packing to apply sufficient pressure to the bleeding site.)

• While the patient has the anterior pack in place, use the cotton-tipped applicators to apply petroleum jelly to his lips and nostrils *to prevent drying and cracking.*

For posterior nasal packing

• Wash your hands and put on sterile gloves.

• If the doctor identifies the bleeding source in the posterior nasal cavity, lubricate the soft catheters *to ease insertion.*

• Instruct the patient to open his mouth and pant during catheter insertion *to minimize gagging as the doctor advances the catheters into the patient's nostrils.*

• Assist the doctor, as directed, to insert the packing.

• Tape the sutures that protrude from the patient's mouth to his cheek. Leave enough slack to permit comfortable talking, chewing, and swallowing. *The slack also prevents stress on the sutures, which could cut the patient's lips or soft palate or cause the posterior pack to slip into the airway.*

• Help the patient assume a comfortable position. Assess him for airway obstruction or any respiratory changes.

• Monitor his vital signs *to detect hemodynamic changes that may indicate hypovolemia or hypoxemia.*

Special considerations

Test the patient's call bell to be sure he can summon help if needed. Also keep emergency equipment (a flashlight, scissors, and hemostats) at the patient's bedside *to speed packing removal in case the posterior pack slides and obstructs the airway.* To remove a posterior pack quickly, cut the sutures and pull the pack out through the patient's mouth.

Once the packing is in place, compile your assessment data carefully to help detect the underlying cause of nosebleeds. Mechanical factors include a deviated septum, traumatic injury, or a foreign body that produces pressure necrosis. Environmental factors include drying and erosion of the nasal mucosa. Other possible causes are upper respiratory tract infection, anticoagulant therapy, blood dyscrasias, cardiovascular disorders, tumors of the nasal cavity or paranasal sinuses, hepatic disease, chronic nephritis, and familial hemorrhagic telangiectasis.

If significant blood loss occurs or if the underlying cause remains unknown, expect the doctor to order a complete blood count and coagulation profile as soon as possible. Blood transfusion may be necessary. After the procedure, the doctor may order arterial blood gas analysis to detect any pulmonary complications and arterial oxygen saturation monitoring to assess for hypoxemia. If necessary, prepare to administer supplemental oxygen with a face mask, and give antibiotics and decongestants as ordered.

Because a patient with nasal packing must breathe through his mouth, provide thorough mouth care frequently.

The doctor usually removes anterior nasal packs after 2 days. However, absorbable packs may remain in place for 3 to 5 days. Posterior packing typically remains in place for 4 days. Until the pack is removed, the patient should be on modified bed rest. As ordered, administer moderate doses of nonaspirin analgesics and sedatives along with prophylactic antibiotics *to prevent sinusitis or related infections.*

After an anterior pack is removed, instruct the patient to avoid rubbing or picking his nose, inserting any object (such as a handkerchief or tissue) into his nose, and blowing his nose forcefully for 48 hours or as ordered.

Home care
To boost the patient's confidence in his self-care ability, offer applicable home care guidelines. Try to emphasize nosebleed prevention, if possible.

Complications
The pressure of a posterior pack on the soft palate may lead to hypoxemia. Patients with posterior nosebleeds are at special risk for hypoxemia because they commonly aspirate blood and because posterior packing partially obstructs the upper airway. Hypoxemia can be detected with pulse oximetry. Signs and symptoms include tachycardia, confusion, cyanosis, and restlessness.

Airway obstruction may occur if a posterior or anterior nasal pack slips backward. The patient may complain of difficulty swallowing and pain or discomfort. In patients with posterior packs, otitis media may develop because the pack blocks the eustachian tube openings. Other possible complications include hematotympanum and pressure necrosis of nasal structures, especially the septum.

Sedation may cause hypotension or hypertension in a patient with significant blood loss and may also increase the patient's risk of aspiration.

Documentation
Record the type of pack used to ensure its removal at the appropriate time. On the intake and output record, document the estimated blood loss and all fluid administered. Also note the patient's vital signs, his response to sedation or position changes, results of any laboratory tests, and any drugs administered, including topical agents. Record any unusual findings or complications. Document discharge instructions and clinical follow-up plans.

Selected references

Adams, G., et al. *Fundamentals of Otolaryngology,* 6th ed. Philadelphia: W.B. Saunders Co., 1989.

Blakely, B., and Swanson, R. *Otolaryngology for the House Officer.* Baltimore: Williams & Wilkins Co., 1989.

Flynn, J., and Hackel, R. *Technological Foundations in Nursing.* Norwalk, Conn.: Appleton & Lange, 1990.

Herrin, M. *Ophthalmic Examination and Basic Skills.* Thorofare, N.J.: Charles B. Slack, Inc., 1990.

Illustrated Manual of Nursing Practice, 2nd ed. Springhouse, Pa.: Springhouse Corp., 1994.

McConnell, E. "How to Irrigate the Eye," *Nursing91* 21(3):28, March 1991.

Newell, F.W. *Ophthalmology: Principles and Concepts,* 7th ed. St. Louis: Mosby-Year Book, Inc., 1991.

Nursing94 Drug Handbook. Springhouse, Pa.: Springhouse Corp., 1994.

Paparella, M.M., et al. *Otolaryngology: Head & Neck,* vol. 3, 3rd ed. Philadelphia: W.B. Saunders Co., 1991.

Perry, A., and Potter, P. *Clinical Nursing Skills and Techniques,* 2nd ed. St. Louis: C.V. Mosby Co., 1990.

Phipps, W., et al. *Medical-Surgical Nursing: Concepts and Clinical Practice,* 4th ed. St. Louis: Mosby-Year Book, Inc., 1991.

Sands, J. *Clinical Manual of Medical-Surgical Nursing,* 2nd ed. St. Louis: Mosby-Year Book, Inc., 1991.

U.S. Public Health Service. Office of Clinical Center Communications. *Facts About the Nose and Nasal Irrigation.* Washington, D.C.: U.S. Department of Health and Human Services, 1990.

INDEX

i refers to illustration; t refers to table

i refers to illustration; t refers to table

i refers to illustration; t refers to table

i refers to illustration; t refers to table

i refers to illustration; t refers to table

Riverside Hospital

meet at
Cherry Corner
5:30

2 medical